Steward's Manual of Pediatric Anesthesia

Jerrold Lerman • Charles J. Coté

Steward's Manual of Pediatric Anesthesia

Eighth Edition

Springer

Jerrold Lerman, MD, FRCPC, FANZCA
Professor of Anesthesiology
Department of Anesthesiology
Golisano Children's Hospital of Buffalo, Jacobs School of Medicine and Biomedical Sciences
Buffalo, NY, USA

Charles J. Coté, MD, FAAP
Professor of Anaesthesia (Emeritus), Harvard Medical School, Division of Pediatric Anesthesia, the MassGeneral Hospital for Children, Department of Anesthesia
Critical Care, and Pain Medicine
Massachusetts General Hospital
Boston, MA, USA

ISBN 978-3-032-24544-1 ISBN 978-3-032-24545-8 (eBook)
https://doi.org/10.1007/978-3-032-24545-8

This Springer imprint is published by the registered company Springer Nature Switzerland AG
The registered company address is: Gewerbestrasse 11, 6330 Cham, Switzerland

Preface

We dedicate this eighth edition of the *Manual of Pediatric Anesthesia* to David J. Steward MB BS, FRCPC (1934–2023), who founded the Manual in 1979. At that time, he sought to address an unmet need for a concise yet comprehensive pocketbook guide to pediatric anesthesia for the practicing anesthesiologist. The first edition, which he spearheaded along with members of the department of Anesthesia from the Hospital for Sick Children in Toronto, Ontario, became a must-read supplement for anyone practicing pediatric anesthesia. In subsequent editions, David ensured the content continued to be relevant and practical to appeal to the broadest possible audience by including a comprehensive list of syndromes with anesthetic implications, an online version, and finally by recruiting two editors who continue the Manual in his spirit. Although reluctant to eponymously title the Manual in his name, we decided it was fitting to rename the Manual, *Steward's Manual of Pediatric Anesthesia*, after consulting his wife, Dr. Mary Lou Steward. Thus, what you now hold in your hands is the first edition of *Steward's Manual of Pediatric Anesthesia*.

The Manual outlines the important considerations when anesthetizing infants and children, describes management problems, and presents a course of action for treating many of your pediatric patients. Each chapter also directs you to further in-depth reading. For the resident in training, it provides a compact but comprehensive source of current information concerning pediatric anesthesia practice.

Together, the current editors have a combined total of almost a century of clinical experience in providing perioperative care for children of all ages undergoing all types of surgical and medical procedures. In recent years, our practices have shifted from inpatient to ambulatory surgery, while an increasing fraction of children require our services outside the operating room, from radiology suites to oncology floors.

In preparing this edition, we compiled an evidence-based approach and fused this with our own experience to optimize clinical strategies for each scenario. In many instances, we recommend a course of action for a given clinical situation that is based on what has worked well for us in our differing practices. However, we recognize that others may have different ideas, approaches, and constraints on their practices that may require them to adapt to ensure a successful outcome.

More than 45 years have passed since the first edition of this book, and, yes, many practices have changed. Some have occurred because of the expanding scope of pediatric surgery and the relentless introduction of new anesthetic drugs and technologies, research that has opened new vistas and visions of what constitutes optimal pediatric anesthesia care. In 2026, we can practice evidence-based anesthesia care much of the time, although the art of our subspecialty has never diminished.

Still, questions remain unanswered. The current debate regarding the safety of general anesthetics in the neonate versus what constitutes the safe limits of hypotension and oxygen saturation serves to remind us that challenges remain that we must continue to investigate and address if we are to continue to deliver safe care to our youngest patients.

Children remain the most rewarding patients to manage and are our future. There is great satisfaction from caring for these tiny patients, the reticent child, and the many other children whom you will meet in your daily practice. We hope that this handbook will empower you to deliver the best care possible and to achieve the satisfaction from anesthetizing children.

Buffalo, NY, USA Jerrold Lerman
Quincy, MA, USA Charles J. Coté

Contents

Preparation for Anesthesia 1

Psychological Aspects of Anesthesia for Children

Hospitalization, surgery, and/or medical procedures can have profound emotional consequences for infants and children. Some children demonstrate behavioral disturbances that persist long after the event. The severity of these disturbances is determined by several factors, the most important being the child's age.

Infants younger than 6 months of age are not upset by separation from their parents and readily accept a nurse as a substitute parent. Psychologically, this is probably a good age for major surgery, although prolonged separation may impair parent-child bonding.

Older infants and toddlers (6 months to 5 years) are much more upset by parental separation. However, the anxiety over separation for ambulatory surgery is far less intense than for overnight hospital admission. Explanations of procedures to relieve stress in this age group are not particularly effective; unsurprisingly, these children show the most severe behavior regression after surgery and/or hospitalization.

School-age children are usually less upset by separation and more concerned with the surgery and fear of mutilation. They often have the wildest misconceptions of their surgery. In contrast, adolescents fear losing control, becoming emotional as they are anesthetized, and waking up during surgery or not waking up

J. Lerman, C. J. Coté, *Steward's Manual of Pediatric Anesthesia*,
https://doi.org/10.1007/978-3-032-24545-8_1

at the end. It is for these reasons that we should make it very clear that they will remain unconscious throughout the surgery, not feel pain, and wake up after the surgery.

The type and extent of the surgery are also an important source of anxiety. Major surgery, craniofacial surgery, and urologic procedures are especially distressing for children older than 18 months.

Besides the child's age, hospitalization confers emotional consequences. Ambulatory surgery usually has a negligible emotional effect, whereas repeat hospitalizations and surgeries often cause significant psychological disturbances; a previous bad hospital experience is not quickly forgotten. Prolonged versus brief hospitalizations are much more disturbing, although in-room lodging by the parent is comforting and reduces stress.

Children vary in their responses to impending surgical or medical interventions. Some seek information and participate keenly in preparation programs, benefitting psychologically from the preparation and rendering them cooperative, whereas others maintain an air of disinterest; they have an avoidance coping style (the "silent child"). Children in the latter group may not benefit and indeed may be further sensitized by efforts at psychological preparation. They may benefit most from an anxiolytic premedication (see later discussion).

Psychological Preparation

Preoperative psychological preparation is beneficial in most cases, with parents preparing their children for surgery; the extent to which the child benefits depends on the child's age. The basic goal is to explain to the child what will happen at the hospital in simple, understandable, and reassuring terms. Younger children should not be prepared too far in advance—rather, they should be prepared a day or so beforehand. A host of age-appropriate multimedia modalities are effective anxiolytics including hospital tours, coloring books, puppet shows, and/or audiovisual presentations. Older children and adolescents benefit most from advanced preparation, especially if hospitalization is anticipated.

Preoperative Laboratory Tests

Preoperative laboratory tests are unnecessary for most children. A preoperative Hb is unnecessary as mild anemia neither affects the risk of anesthesia nor the choice of anesthesia technique. However, former preterm infants, older children with systemic diseases, those with a history of anemia, and those at risk for significant blood loss should have a preoperative Hb determination. For those at risk for sickle cell disease whose sickle risk is unknown, a Sickledex should be obtained, and if positive, an Hb electrophoresis is recommended. In menarcheal females, urine (or blood) for pregnancy testing has become required in many centers. In children with complex medical issues and those taking medications that may affect their metabolic status, appropriate laboratory investigations should be conducted as indicated.

Preoperative Feeding Orders

Infants and children should be fasted according to published guidelines (see Table 1.1). Prolonged fasting may lead to hypovolemia, hypoglycemia, an unhappy child, and/or metabolic acidosis, particularly in young former preterm infants. Children may safely be given unlimited clear fluids up to 2 h before induction; recent guidelines have reduced the fasting interval after 5 mL/kg of clear fluids to 1 h before induction, although

Table 1.1 Preoperative fasting intervals for elective surgery

	Fasting interval (h)	Comments
Clear fluids	2[a]	Water, ginger ale, and apple juice; particle-free fluids
Breast milk	4	
Formula/cow's milk	6	Also, dry toast and black tea
Solids	8	

[a]Some have adopted a 1-h fast after 5 mL/kg clear fluids

the added benefit of this practice is unclear. Texting parents the night before surgery ensures that most children comply with the fasting guidelines.

N.B.: Chewing gum should be expectorated; if swallowed, the anesthetic should be delayed 8 h.

Children who are scheduled for afternoon surgery may have a light breakfast (dry toast and clear fluids) early in the morning (6 h prior to their scheduled procedure). These rules must be modified in special cases, for example, for diabetics. Children taking GLP-1 drugs may present with food in the stomach after a normal fast. To minimize this risk, a number of recommendations have been proposed including: (i) holding the dose 1 week prior to anesthesia, (ii) not taking their last dose before surgery, (iii) ingesting only clear fluids for 24 h before surgery, and (iv) gastric ultrasound to confirm that the stomach is empty. Children who require emergency surgery, those with gastrointestinal disease, and any others at increased risk for vomiting during induction should receive intravenous (IV) fluids and a rapid sequence induction. When evaluating injured children, the interval between last ingestion and the injury is the best predictor of the likelihood of stomach contents but verification with gastric ultrasound should be considered. It is prudent to consider establishing IV access in those with cyanotic heart disease to reduce the risks of polycythemia and hyperviscosity.

Preoperative Assessment

Although most children are healthy, some have diseases with important anesthetic implications; a careful preoperative assessment is always indicated and a thorough history should be solicited from both parents. A systems review and a thorough review of the child's chart should be completed to identify medical issues that may complicate their anesthetic (Table 1.2). When a significant medical issue has been identified, the current status of the disease and recent consultations should be summarized. Pertinent historical questions for infants include whether they were full-term at birth and if not, the infant's gestational age at birth, peri-

Table 1.2 Review of the medical history—possible implications for anesthesia

Systems	History	Anesthesia implications
Central nervous system	Seizures	Frequency of seizure and medications, date of last seizure, seizure characteristics, for example, staring spells versus tonic-clonic. Phenytoin may cause resistance to non-depolarizing relaxants and fentanyl, produces gingival hyperplasia and bleeding, and hepatic dysfunction. Ketamine and methohexital are relatively contraindicated
	Hydrocephalus	Possible increased intracranial pressure. Prophylactic antibiotics to prevent shunt infection
	Head injury	Possible raised intracranial pressure. Concussion
	Cerebral tumor	Possible raised intracranial pressure, vomiting, and electrolyte changes. Chemotherapeutic agents and possible drug interactions
	Cerebral palsy	Nutritional status and presence of chronic infections. Possible chronic aspiration, contractures, and surgical positioning difficulties. Intelligence may be normal—careful psychological preparation needed
	Down syndrome	Airway (large tongue and subglottic narrowing). Obstructive sleep apnea (OSA). Congenital heart disease (CHD). Evidence of joint hypermobility and possible atlanto-axial instability. May require parental assistance at induction
	Neuromuscular disease	Difficulty positioning. Repeated surgery. Avoid succinylcholine; rhabdomyolysis possible
	Meningomyelocele	Associated hydrocephalus. Possible latex allergy. Renal infections and/or impaired renal function
Cardiovascular system	Heart murmur	Innocent murmur versus significant defect. Need for prophylactic antibiotics. Risk of paradoxical embolism
	Cyanosis Dyspnea Tachypnea Sweating Difficulty feeding	Avoid fluid restriction. Coagulopathy secondary to hyperviscosity. Reduced response to hypoxemia—caution with premedication Evidence of congestive heart failure. History of digoxin and/or diuretic therapy. Assess digoxin and electrolyte values Review previous cardiac surgery. Review EKG, C-Xray, ECHO, and catheterization results; current activity level. History of arrhythmias, cardiac conduction defects, or pacemaker. Cardiology consult
	Hypertension	Renal disease, coarctation of the aorta, endocrine disease

(continued)

Table 1.2 (continued)

Systems	History	Anesthesia implications
Respiratory system	Prematurity	Risk of perioperative apnea, subglottic stenosis. Determine gestational age at birth and postconceptional age. Anemia
	Respiratory distress syndrome	Residual chronic respiratory disease/bronchopulmonary dysplasia (BPD) and impaired gas exchange. Need for diuretics and supplemental oxygen. History of prolonged ventilation and possible subglottic stenosis
	Recent upper respiratory tract infection	Evidence of acute infection. Reactive airways disease. Increased risk of laryngospasm, bronchospasm, and oxygen desaturation
	Bronchiolitis	Reactive airways and evidence of bronchospasm
	Croup	Possible subglottic stenosis. Avoid intubation, use facemask or laryngeal mask airway (LMA) if possible
	Asthma	Frequency of using β-agonist and other medications, admissions to hospital, and history of corticosteroid therapy. Optimize preoperative status. Avoid intubation if possible. Have a device to administer intraoperative bronchodilator, for example, spacer device
	Cystic fibrosis	Current pulmonary status. Presence of an acute infection. Can the pulmonary status be optimized. Consider regional analgesia. Current drug therapy including steroids. Administer inhaled hypertonic saline (7%); humidify inhaled gases. Nutritional and emotional status. Diabetes. Recover in 30–40° upright position to facilitate respirations. Avoid hospital admission if possible
Gastrointestinal system	Gastroesophageal reflux	Evidence of aspiration pneumonia, reactive airways. Full stomach risk, risk of regurgitation, are they taking GLP-1 drugs?, and need for antacid and H_2-blockers
	Vomiting	Hypovolemia and electrolyte status. Full stomach risk. Nutrition
	Diarrhea	Hypovolemia, hypoglycemia, and electrolyte status
	Liver disease	Altered drug metabolism. Decreased requirements for non-depolarizing relaxants

Genitourinary system Endocrine system	Renal failure	Anemia and coagulopathy, electrolyte abnormality especially hyperkalemia, and volume and acid-base status. Are hypertension, pericardial effusion, or congestive heart failure present? Date of last dialysis. History of infection. Impaired drug excretion
	Bladder/genital surgery	Possible latex allergy. Psychological stress
	Diabetes mellitus	Current status and therapy. Perioperative management. Insulin pump settings. Endocrinologist's consult.
Hematopoietic system	Thyroid disease	Current status and medication. Thyromegaly compressing the airway.
	Pituitary disease	Intracranial pressure. Adrenal insufficiency. Thyroid function. Diabetes insipidus
	Adrenal disease	Need for corticosteroid therapy. Volume and electrolyte status
	Anemia	Severity, etiology, and should surgery be delayed. Hemoglobinopathy. Is a preoperative transfusion indicated?
Muscular system	Bruising or bleeding	Is a coagulopathy present. Hematology consult. Preoperative therapy. Differentiate natural bruising from child abuse
	Sickle cell disease	Trait or disease. Hb electrophoresis results. Transfuse to a Hb of 10 g/dL.
	Muscular dystrophy	Risk of hyperkalemia after succinylcholine <10 yr old. Avoid depolarizing relaxants. Limit dose of non-depolarizing muscle relaxants. Avoid inhalation agents to preclude rhabdomyolysis. Assess ventilatory reserve and cardiac function. Consider postoperative ICU admission
Immune system and allergy	latex allergy	Lips swell with latex balloons; reactions to bananas, eggplant, passion fruit, and other fruits/vegetables suggest latex allergy Possible concurrent latex allergy (Chap. 8)

natal medical problems, if they required a breathing tube, and for how long, and any residual cardiorespiratory issues or surgeries that occurred. A history of prematurity indicates a risk for post-anesthesia apnea and the need to admit overnight and monitor. Tracheal intubation at birth should prompt questions about possible subglottic stenosis. The family history should focus on a history of specific risks including sickle cell disease, problems during anesthesia (malignant hyperthermia, pseudocholinesterase deficiency), or family history of neuromuscular diseases (muscular dystrophy). All medications, nutraceuticals, and drug allergies should be documented. Most medications can be taken with a sip of water on the morning of surgery, for example, anti-seizure medications (see Table 1.3). If they are only taken with food, the

Table 1.3 Medications—possible implications for anesthesia

Medications	Anesthesia implications
Non-opioid analgesics	
Acetylsalicylic acid (ASA, aspirin Non-steroidal anti-inflammatory drugs (NSAIDs)	Prolonged bleeding time due to platelet inactivation; check bleeding time if ASA given within 10 days Decreases platelet aggregation and prolongs bleeding time Effect of antihypertensives may be decreased. Ketorolac decreases diuretic effect of furosemide
Antibiotics	
Aminoglycosides	The "mycins" may potentiate neuromuscular blockade. Renal & ototoxicity.
Clindamycin	Bradycardia when given rapidly. May potentiate non-depolarizing muscle relaxants
Erythromycin	May prolong the effect of alfentanil and midazolam. Decreases theophylline clearance rates. Potentiates anticoagulant effect of warfarin
Gentamicin	May prolong the effect of succinylcholine. Potentiates non-depolarizing muscle relaxants
Vancomycin	Potentiates non-depolarizing muscle relaxants. Rapid administration (<1 h) may cause "red man syndrome" with severe cardiovascular collapse

(continued)

Table 1.3 (continued)

Medications	Anesthesia implications
Anticancer agents	All may cause blood dyscrasia, coagulopathy, anorexia, nausea, stomatitis, and reduced resistance to infection
Doxorubicin (Adriamycin)	Cardiotoxic especially if combined with inhalation agents may cause arrhythmias
Daunorubicin (Cerubidine)	Cardiotoxic especially if combined with inhalation agents, likely when cumulative dose exceeds 250 mg/m^2 (or 150 mg/m^2 plus radiation)
Bleomycin	Pulmonary fibrosis—may be exacerbated by excess oxygen; limit inspired oxygen concentration
Busulfan	Inhibits plasma cholinesterase
Cyclophosphamide	Inhibits plasma cholinesterase
Anticonvulsants	
Phenytoin	May cause blood dyscrasia, hypotension, bradycardia, and arrhythmia
Valproic acid	May cause hypotonia. Hepatotoxic
Antihypertensive drugs	Severe hypotension may occur with potent anesthetics, especially if dehydrated
Captopril	Hyperkalemia with potassium-sparing diuretics (spironolactone). Indomethacin reduces antihypertensive effect
Clonidine	Must not be abruptly withdrawn—severe hypertension may result. Interaction with α-blockers—bradycardia, hypotension
Hydralazine (Apresoline)	May cause systemic lupus erythematosus (SLE)-type syndrome. Decreases tachycardia with atropine
Labetalol	Cimetidine may potentiate labetalol's action
Prazosin (Minipress)	May potentiate effects of ketamine. Diuretics potentiate antihypertensive effect
Antiviral agent	
Acyclovir	Nephrotoxic, bone marrow depression
α-blocking drugs	May cause bronchospasm, attenuate the effects of albuterol. Potentiates cardiac depression caused by inhalation agents. May cause bradycardia with anticholinesterase drugs and hypoglycemia

(continued)

Table 1.3 (continued)

Medications	Anesthesia implications
Calcium channel blockers:	Potentiate non-depolarizing relaxant drugs. Severe bradycardia or heart block with α-blocking drugs. Potentiates cardiac depression with potent inhalation agents or with reduced ionized calcium during rapid FFP infusion. May interact with α-blockers to cause severe cardiac depression
Miscellaneous drugs	
Corticosteroids	Chronic therapy may suppress the hypothalamic pituitary axis; give perioperative steroids
Digoxin	May potentiate bupivacaine toxicity
Diuretics	Hypokalemia may be exacerbated by hyperventilation, predisposes to arrhythmias. Electrolyte disturbances
Acetazolamide (Diamox)	Produces hyperchloremic metabolic acidosis
Theophylline	Severe arrhythmias with inhalational agents
Topical ophthalmic drugs	
Echothiophate iodide	Inhibit plasma cholinesterase. Prolonged apnea with succinylcholine
Phenylephrine	May cause tachycardia and hypertension
Timolol (α-blocker)	May exacerbate asthma

medication may be administered after surgery or parenterally. Herbal supplements may have important perioperative implications (see Table 1.4). Elicit details of any "allergic" reactions; many "allergies" are in fact sensitivities. The majority of rashes associated with an oral antibiotic (e.g., amoxicillin) are nonimmunologic reactions. Throughout the preoperative interview, strive to gain the confidence of the child and the parents; always invite questions from both the parents and the child so as to help establish rapport and confidence.

Table 1.4 Some herbal preparations and their anesthesia implications

Herbal preparation	Indication	Anesthesia implications
Echinacea	URTI prophylaxis	Increased sedation with midazolam
		Decreased metabolism of phenobarbital, phenytoin, and rifampin
		Increases liver damage with hepatotoxic agents
		Immunosuppression with long-term use
St John's wort	Anxiety, depression, and sleep problems	Cardiovascular collapse, delayed awakening due to effect on GABA neurotransmitter
		Severe interactions with antidepressants
		Induces CYP3A4 system leading to increased dose requirements of some drugs, for example, midazolam
Gingko	Improves memory and concentration	Increased surgical bleeding. Concurrent use of NSAIDs not recommended
		Decreases effect of anticonvulsants
Garlic	Cardiac health	Increased surgical bleeding
		Augments ASA, warfarin, and heparin
Ginseng	General health	Hypoglycemic effects in diabetics
		Antiplatelet effects and bleeding
		Hypertension, headaches, and vomiting
Aloe	Skin problems	Allergic skin reactions. GI constipation, bleeding, renal damage with oral use

The Anesthesiologist, Child, and Parents

Anesthesiologists should strive to build a relationship with the parents and child based on warmth, friendliness, empathy, and understanding. How we interact with the child in front of the parents and then involve the parents in our anesthetic prescription may be critically important for a successful outcome. Studies indicate that anesthesiologists vary in their ability to relate to children to minimize their angst. An *empathic approach* to the child before and during medical procedures is preferred (e.g., "*This may be a little uncomfortable and I know you are scared, but we are going to do all we can to help and it will soon be over. We don't mind if you cry*"). The alternative *directive approach* ("*Hold still and be big and brave*") is generally frowned upon.

Direct your attention to the child at the outset, even if he or she is developmentally delayed. Parents appreciate that you focus on their child as the patient, all the while knowing that everything you say to their child is also meant for them. Try to maintain eye contact with the child to establish rapport. Talk in simple terms that the child understands. Older children may be frightened, inflating the size of the incision or the extent of the procedure. They must be reassured that the incision will be small and that they will not awaken during surgery no matter what occurs. Children who are old enough to understand and who have not had surgery appreciate knowing that the surgery will only feel as if it lasted as long as a "blink," that we will not allow them to wake up during the surgery, and that they will feel exhausted for a while after the surgery until they get their energy back. It is best to avoid the phrase *"we will put you to sleep"*—as this may conjure up the events, such as a family pet that never returned! It may also cause them to worry that they might wake up from their *"sleep"* when the operation starts or while it is still in progress. Also avoid presenting the child with unpleasant or difficult choices such as, "*Do you want the needle or the mask?*" Tell the child what you intend to do and then try to meet any special requests (e.g., "*I do not want a needle, I want to go to sleep with the mask*" or "*I'd like to hold the mask myself*"). For all children who are anxious and frightened, offer a premedication (see Table 1.5).

Table 1.5 Premedications and routes of delivery

	Midazolam (mg/kg)	Ketamine (mg/kg)	Clonidine (μg/kg)	Dexmedetomidine (μg/kg)
Intravenous	0.05–0.1	1–2		1 (over 10 minutes)
Intramuscular	0.1–0.2	3–10	2–4	1–4
Oral	0.25–0.75	5–10	2–4	2.5–4
Nasal	0.1–0.2	3–5	4	1–4
Rectal	0.75–1.0	6–10		

See Chap. 3 and Appendix C for addition details

A physical examination should include assessing mouth opening, neck mobility, loose teeth, and heart and lung sounds. Many children become upset at being disrobed; avoid uncovering the child more than necessary for the examination. Ensure that the surgeon has identified the surgical site and confirmed the laterality of the surgery.

Parents play an increasingly active role in the perioperative care of their children and many have preconceived notions about their child's anesthetic. To clarify their understanding and diffuse anxiety, the parents should be assured that their child's anesthetic will be designed specifically for their child, and their safety is paramount. After reviewing their child's medical history, a detailed age-appropriate description of how their child will be anesthetized (by a flavored facemask or IV), monitored (including breathing, heart rate, blood pressure, temperature, the amounts of anesthetics, and oxygen levels), and managed/supervised during and after the surgery by the anesthesiology team should be provided. Carefully explain to the child and parents that they will receive medications to prevent pain, nausea, and vomiting before they awaken from anesthesia. After surgery, they may have an eye patch, stomach tube in their nose, or a catheter in their bladder, which will be inserted during surgery without them feeling it. Any questions that the parents pose should be answered in calm yet understandable terms to reduce parental angst. This in turn often reduces the child's anxiety. The interview should make it clear that their child's well-being will be the focus of our attention throughout the surgery.

Anesthetic Risks and Consent

Anesthesiologists should explain the common side effects from anesthesia, including a possible sore throat, possible damage to teeth (especially if loose), pain, nausea, and vomiting, as well as uncommon risks depending on the nature of the surgery and the child's medical condition. Parents will be comforted by knowing that their child will receive pain medications as well as medications to prevent nausea and vomiting before they emerge from anesthesia. We also caution parents that even though their child may be healthy and have no family history of anesthetic problems, there is always a very remote chance that more serious complications could occur and we continuously monitor for them. In the unlikely event that such an unexpected event occurs, their child will be cared for "to the very best of our ability" with all available resources and they will be kept fully informed.

Many parents are aware of concerns with the "safety" of anesthesia in infants and young children in terms of possible neurocognitive harm. We advise parents that the decision to proceed with surgery in young children is a balance of risks of not operating versus the benefits of the surgery and anesthesia. Most surgery in young children is necessary, and delaying it increases the risks of sequelae. In terms of anesthesia, evidence from large prospective studies has not demonstrated adverse neurocognitive outcomes in children after general anesthesia; there is currently no evidence that anesthetics harm cognitive function in infants and children. Instead, we emphasize that these issues are theoretical regarding humans, that if such a problem were a major issue, then likely this would have been noted many years ago, and that it is far more important for us to focus on maintaining vital signs including blood pressure, oxygen levels in tissues, and blunting the stress response (e.g., adequate analgesia) than to be overly concerned with an as yet unproven problem in infants and children.

Parents should feel comfortable asking questions and expressing their concerns about the proposed anesthetic and risks. A discussion of the risks specific to their child and the anesthetic will place them in perspective. Assurance that their child's anesthesia will be designed specifically for their child, his/her safety, and the surgical requirements will put the parents at ease. Also, inform them that medications to treat postoperative pain and prevent vomiting will be administered before their child is discharged. Every parent will be pleased if you communicate the message, *"We will design your child's anesthetic with his/her medical issues and the needs of the surgeon in mind. We will be with your child at all the time during the anesthetic!"* Informed legal consent must be secured before beginning any anesthetic.

Anxiolysis: Distraction and Premedications

Anxiolysis may be effected based on the child and parent's wishes and the degree of anxiety. Several strategies are available based on the child's age, level of understanding, and local services including distraction (involving Child Life practitioners), premedications, and parental presence at induction of anesthesia.

Distraction

Distraction is widely practiced as an anxiolytic in toddlers, although premedication may be required in some to separate from the parents smoothly, increase cooperation during induction, and decrease posthospitalization behavior disturbances. Many distraction strategies reduce children's anxiety as effectively as a premedication, including iPad tablets, hand-held computer games, television and cartoons, video glasses, music, and magic. Child-life specialists introduce the children to the airway equipment (including a facemask) and flavors to apply in the preoperative unit, use play therapy (with a breathing circuit and mask) and other tools to distract the child's attention and reduce the fear of the unknown.

Topical Local Anesthetics

If an IV is preferred by the child for induction or blood needs to be drawn for testing, topical anesthetic may be applied to the IV site in advance. Topical local anesthetic may be applied to numb the skin before attempting venous cannulation although small children may cry nonetheless (See also Chap. 3 and Appendix C). Children may be calmed by telling them, "*We will put a Band-Aid on in a minute*." The intravenous route can then be used for both premedication (e.g., midazolam) and/or induction of anesthesia.

Premedications

Special Considerations

1. Neurosurgical patients who may have increased ICP should not receive any sedative premedication.
2. Children with a suspected difficult airway or OSA should be sedated with great caution due to the possibility of respiratory depression or airway obstruction. Consider using a pulse oximeter while the child breathes room air.
3. Atropine should not be given intramuscularly to children with a fever because it may exacerbate the fever by abolishing sweating. If indicated, it may be given intravenously at the time of induction.
4. Some children undergoing correction of strabismus are assessed by the ophthalmologist immediately before the operation and should not be premedicated with atropine. They may receive atropine after induction to block the oculocardiac reflex.

Sedatives and Tranquilizers

Numerous premedications and routes of delivery are available and their choice tailored to the child's needs.

Midazolam Oral midazolam is the most widely prescribed sedative premedication for children in North America. The oral dose increases with decreasing age, producing anxiolysis within 10–15 min with little effect noted by 60 min. In infants, midazolam may be applied sublingually with a medicine dropper; this technique ensures rapid oral transmucosal absorption. Intranasal (IN) midazolam (0.1–0.2 mg/kg) is effective, particularly in the uncooperative child, although nasal instillation may be unpleasant and, in older children, may cause nasal irritation. Rectal midazolam (0.75–1 mg/kg) has a less predictable onset. Note that IV midazolam has a peak brain effect in 3 to 5 min, so adequate time must be allowed for repeat dosing.

Ketamine Ketamine (6–10 mg/kg) may be given orally but is usually accompanied by oral atropine to avoid excessive secretions. Ketamine may increase postoperative vomiting. The combination of oral midazolam and oral ketamine produces very effective deep sedation, but the child should be carefully monitored.

Clonidine Oral clonidine premedication (2–4 μg/kg) has a slow onset, up to 90 min. It reduces anesthesia requirements, diminishes cardiovascular responses to tracheal intubation, smooths emergence, reduces emergence delirium, and enhances analgesia. Bradycardia and hypotension have been reported.

Dexmedetomidine As an oral premedication, dexmedetomidine has an onset time faster than after clonidine but slower than midazolam. IN dexmedetomidine (1–4 μg/kg) is also effective with an onset time of 60 min; it reduces emergence delirium and decreases postoperative pain.

Parental Presence at Induction

Although many parents express a desire to be present at induction of anesthesia, evidence suggests that parental presence at induction of anesthesia (PPIA) primarily reduces parental anxiety; it has either no effect or less effect than other strategies (e.g., midazolam) to reduce the child's anxiety. PPIA varies widely among institutions; some only permit PPIA under special circumstances, whereas others allow all parents to be present. The entire surgical team must endorse adopting PPIA, and parents must be informed of their role and responsibilities if they attend the induction. This can be accomplished through a presurgical education program to reduce potential parental disruptions at a time when all attention should be focused on the child. If appropriate, calm and supportive parents may accompany their child to the operating room for the induction. If this is not possible, both the child and the parent's anxieties may be reduced if the child is sedated (e.g., oral midazolam, see Table 1.5). Parents of children with disabilities or children with life-threatening disease (e.g., cancer) can often be of great assistance in accompanying their child to the operating room (OR) and through the induction. Having the child sit on their parent's lap while the parent hugs them while holding their arms at the side allows the parents to feel that they are part of the process in a supportive way, as the facemask is gently applied to the child's face.

The overly anxious parent requires special consideration. Excessive anxiety is often of multifactorial origin and may not be entirely related to the child's present surgical condition. Parents should be forewarned of how their child will appear during induction anesthesia, that is, eyes rolling up, movements of the arms and legs, and turning of the head, which are normal and expected responses.

Parents who remain highly anxious despite our best efforts and are present at induction of anesthesia may do more harm than good. Such anxious parents should be counseled and excluded if possible as their presence will augment the child's anxiety. Adequate preoperative sedation of the child may help the parents agree to this course. There is no benefit for PPIA for any child who has not developed fears of strangers due to their young developmental level or for the child in need of a rapid sequence induction. It must be clear that parental presence during induction is a privilege given at the discretion of the anesthesiologist in what he/she deems to be in the best interests of the child and the child's safety.

Heading to the OR

Allow the child to bring a favorite toy or other security object to the OR. If the child is able, let them walk hand in hand rather than be carried or wheeled; children are quite independent and feel more confident walking. The parents are usually satisfied if their child separates from them calmly and/or sedated.

The noise level (extraneous conversations) in the OR should be minimized during induction. Only one person should talk to the child during induction. Soothing music may help. Select the most appropriate induction technique and proceed without delay after applying monitors: a pulse oximeter may be the only monitor that can be applied in a combative child. Talk to the child throughout the induction as "magic laughing gas" (70% nitrous oxide) is administered. Add 8% sevoflurane to complete the induction when the end-tidal nitrous oxide concentration reaches 50%.

Postoperative Care

The parents should be reunited with their child as soon as the child awakens. Pain and vomiting should be addressed before the parents arrive. The parents should be cautioned that if an emergency occurs in the recovery room, they will be escorted back to the parent waiting room until it is appropriate for them to return. A discussion of what the parents can expect after leaving the hospital and the need to give postoperative oral analgesics is also important.

If the child is transferred to the intensive care unit (ICU), the child may face problems similar to those that adults face: pain, lack of sleep, and, later, boredom. In addition, children have their own special concerns, including separation from their parents if in-room accommodations are not available. Special attention should be directed to pain management, regular visitation by the parents, and provision of toys, games, and other distractions (e.g., television and computer games) as the child's condition improves. Parents of children in the ICU benefit by being kept very well informed of their child's condition and progress, and they must also be continuously updated on their treatment plans.

Suggested Reading

Achule A, Gedeno K, Aweke Z. Management of preoperative anxiety with non-pharmacological methods in pediatric patients in resource-limited settings: a literature review. Ann Med Surg. 2025;87:780–90.

Challa C, Geng-Ramos G, Gray L, et al. Anxiety in children: a review on how to address it in the perioperative setting post-pandemic. Pediatr Anesth. 2023;33:422–6.

Chen H, Zhang J, Li S, Zhang H, Wei L. Non-pharmacological interventions for preoperative anxiety in children: a systematic review and network meta-analysis. J Clin Nursing. 2025;34:1493–507.

Yang C-Q, Yu K-H, Huang R-R, et al. Comparison of different sedatives in children before general anaesthesia for selective surgery: a network meta-analysis. J Clin Pharm Ther. 2022;47:1495–505.

Developmental Anatomy and Physiology

2

Central Nervous System

The central nervous system in neonates differs from that in children and adults. At birth, the neonate's brain is about 25% of the size in adults, doubles in size in the first year, and reaches 90% of adult size by 5 years. Furthermore, myelination of nerve fibers takes about 2 years to complete, the cerebral cortex is less developed, and its cellular elements rapidly mature during the first years of life. Reflexes may be elicited in neonates that are not present in older children. Because the EEG in neonates differs markedly from that in older patients, most neuromonitoring is less reliable in neonates. Although anesthesia-induced neurotoxicity has been demonstrated in animal models, neurotoxicity has not been established in human infants, despite numerous attempts to confirm its existence.

Sensitivity to Pain

In the past, many dismissed the notion that neonates and infants appreciated pain, leading to an undertreatment of pain. However, it is now well established that neonates and infants, including those born prematurely, perceive pain and respond to it with a range of responses including tachycardia, hypertension, increased

J. Lerman, C. J. Coté, *Steward's Manual of Pediatric Anesthesia*,
https://doi.org/10.1007/978-3-032-24545-8_2

intracranial pressure, and neuroendocrine responses, which may exceed the responses observed in adults. Infants demonstrate measurable behavioral responses to pain, e.g., crying, grimacing, and restlessness; these responses have been used as a basis for pain scoring systems. Evidence also suggests that infants subjected to painful procedures, e.g., circumcision, without adequate analgesia may have a reduced threshold to pain as older children and adults; this may be the result of conditioning that alters the infant's central nociceptive processing. Control of intraoperative and postoperative pain, by attenuating the stress responses, may improve survival in infants with critical illnesses. It is for these reasons that optimal analgesia or anesthesia is required for all infants and children during and after *any* painful procedure.

Cranium and Intracranial Pressure

The skull in infants is less rigid than in adults. As a result, an increase in the volume of its contents—blood, cerebral spinal fluid (CSF), and brain tissue—can be accommodated to some extent by expansion of the fontanelles and separation of the suture lines. Intracranial pressure in infants may be assessed by palpating the fontanelles. Normal intracranial pressure (ICP) increases with age: in neonates, 1.5–6 mmHg; in young children, 3–7 mmHg; and in older children and adolescents, 10–15 mmHg.

Cerebral Blood Flow and Intraventricular Hemorrhage

Autoregulation of cerebral blood flow (CBF) is impaired in sick neonates. The threshold below which autoregulation of CBF is impaired in these neonates is unknown, but it is well established that inhalation agents may blunt and even abolish the response completely, rendering CBF pressure-passive. Thus a low blood pressure, combined with hyperventilation in sick neonates during inhalational anesthesia, may lead to cerebral ischemia. In preterm infants, the cerebral vessels are also very fragile, especially in the region of the germinal matrix overlying the caudate nucleus. As a result, they may rupture, resulting in an intracerebral hemorrhage, which may extend into the ventricular system, causing an intraventricular hemorrhage (IVH) and, in some cases, obstructive hydrocephalus.

Preterm infants are very prone to IVH, usually occurring during the first few days after birth. Survivors commonly present with hydrocephalus, cerebral palsy, and developmental delay. Predisposing factors include hypoxia, hypercarbia, hypernatremia, fluctuations in arterial or venous pressure, low hematocrit, over transfusion, and rapid administration of hypertonic fluids, e.g., sodium bicarbonate and dextrose.

In preterm infants, airway manipulations, including awake tracheal intubation and suctioning, increase systemic blood pressure and anterior fontanelle pressure similar to coughing. Nonetheless "awake" intubation is generally avoided by providing analgesia and/or sedation, even though a definite link between "awake" tracheal intubation and IVH has never been established. If the airway is known or appears to be difficult to secure or maintain by facemask, then an "awake" or sedated tracheal intubation is a reasonable choice. If an awake tracheal intubation is planned, topical analgesia using weight-appropriate doses of local anesthetic (see Chap. 7) applied to the hypopharynx may attenuate the infant's physiologic responses.

Blood pressure fluctuations during surgery or painful procedures should be minimized by providing adequate anesthesia and analgesia. Rapid injections of undiluted hypertonic solutions, such as dextrose, sodium bicarbonate, and mannitol, should be avoided. Blood and fluid losses should be replaced 1:1, and severe anemia and/or coagulopathy corrected promptly. Periventricular leukomalacia is a major feature of persistent brain injury in preterm infants and may follow IVH or may be a consequence of prematurity, hypoxia, ischemia, inflammation, and chronic persistent hypotension. Indomethacin prophylaxis may reduce the incidence of severe IVH.

Cerebrospinal Fluid and Hydrocephalus

The CSF, whose composition is similar to interstitial fluid, is formed by the choroid plexus in the temporal horns of the lateral ventricles, the posterior portion of the third ventricle, and the roof of the fourth ventricle. Meningeal and ependymal vessels and blood vessels of the brain and spinal cord also contribute small volumes of CSF. The volume of CSF in neonates is approximately 15 mL/kg, which decreases to 2–4 mL/kg by adulthood. The rate of CSF formation is variable, increasing in the first 2 years to adult rates, 300–500 mL/d.

CSF flow is initiated by pulsations in the choroid plexus. From the lateral ventricles, CSF passes into the third ventricle via the foramen of Monro and along the aqueduct of Sylvius into the fourth ventricle, each ventricle contributing more fluid by secretion from its choroid plexus. CSF then flows through the two lateral foramina of Luschka and the midline foramen of Magendie into the cisterna magna and through the subarachnoid spaces. CSF is reabsorbed by hydrostatic filtration through the arachnoid villi into the venous system, which projects from the subarachnoid space into the venous sinuses. Hydrocephalus is an abnormal accumulation of CSF within the cranium that may be either obstructive or nonobstructive.

Obstructive hydrocephalus (blockage of CSF flow) may be communicating when the CSF pathway into the subarachnoid space is open, e.g., after chronic arachnoiditis, or noncommunicating, e.g., the fluid path proximal to the subarachnoid space is obstructed, as in aqueductal stenosis, blood clot from an IVH, or an Arnold-Chiari malformation.

Nonobstructive hydrocephalus is caused by a reduction in the volume of brain substance with secondary dilation of the ventricles; by overproduction of CSF, e.g., in choroid plexus papilloma; or by diminished reabsorption of CSF due to scarring. All causes of hydrocephalus may lead to bulging fontanelles.

Eyes

Retinopathy of Prematurity

Retinopathy of prematurity (ROP) is a leading cause of blindness in premature infants, affecting 30–50% of very low-birth-weight neonates. It is caused by retinal vessel proliferation and retinal detachment. The possible role of increased hemoglobin oxygen saturation (SaO_2) in the etiology of ROP has long been recognized, but ROP has also occurred in infants never exposed to high oxygen concentrations and in those with cyanotic heart disease. A target SaO_2 of 91–95% is currently recommended as a balance between the ROP risk at an SaO_2 > 95% and increased morbidity/mortality at <90%. On occasion, it may still be necessary to err on the side of safety and maintain the SaO_2 > 95%. Although a multi-institutional study of tight control of oxygen administration failed to reduce the incidence of ROP, we advocate adjusting the inspired fraction of oxygen in preterm infants to maintain the SaO_2 at 91–95%. Large fluctuations in the inspired oxygen concentration should also be avoided. Currently, supplemental oxygen appears to be a minor factor in the development of ROP compared with other factors such as hyper- and hypocapnia, hypotension, sepsis, RBC transfusions, chronic lung disease, steroid administration, and increased glucose concentrations.

Respiratory System

Anatomy

There are major anatomic differences in the airways among neonates, infants, and adults:

1. In the neonate, the occiput is relatively large; the head is in the "sniffing position" naturally. This is offset by a short neck, with a cephalad larynx. If the head is elevated, the larynx also moves anteriorly (see Chap. 4).

2. The tongue is large relative to the size of the mouth, which impairs the view of the larynx and blocks the pharynx during and after anesthesia; an oropharyngeal airway or jaw thrust is often needed.
3. The nasal passages are narrow and easily blocked by secretions, edema, or a nasogastric tube. Neonates are "obligate nose breathers," attributed in part to the immature coordination of breathing and swallowing. This coordination rapidly matures after birth, although some may fail to convert to mouth breathing if their nasal passages are obstructed, which may lead to asphyxia, e.g., choanal atresia. Upper airway obstruction is more likely to occur when the infant's neck is flexed; the neck should be extended after extubation until the infant completely recovers from anesthesia.
4. The larynx is more cephalad (mid-C3 level in preterms, C3–C4 in full terms, and C4–C5 in teenagers).
5. The cricoid ring (the only solid circumferential cartilage in the airway), which lies just below the vocal cords, is the narrowest part of the airway. With airflow being turbulent in the upper airway, i.e., Reynold's number > 2100, where $R \propto 1/r^5$ and where R is the resistance and r is the radius of the airway, any narrowing of the lumen increases the resistance to airflow and work of breathing to the fifth power. Pseudostratified, ciliated epithelium that is loosely bound to the underlying tissue lines the cricoid ring. If trauma, e.g., a tight tracheal tube (TT); infection, e.g., croup; or an inhalation injury causes the epithelium to swell and the cross-sectional area of the cricoid ring to narrow. Insertion of a TT also encroaches on this space, as the internal diameter of the TT becomes the area for gas flow; hence, airway resistance increases. This is more important in neonates and the reason that uncuffed TTs, which allowed a larger ID tube to be placed, were advocated for neonates in the past.
6. The epiglottis is relatively long and stiff. It is U shaped and projects posteriorly at an angle of approximately 45° above the glottis. Often, it must be lifted by the tip of a laryngoscope blade before the glottis can be visualized. For this reason, a straight laryngoscope blade is recommended in neonates and younger infants, although a properly used Macintosh blade provides a similar view in older infants and children.

7. The trachea is short (approximately 5 cm in the neonate), so precise placement and firm fixation of the ETT are essential. The tracheal cartilages are soft and can easily be compressed by the fingers of an anesthesiologist holding a mask or collapsed at the level of the thoracic inlet (dynamic collapse) by the infant's vigorous attempts to breathe against an obstructed airway.
8. The right main bronchus is larger and less acutely angled than the left; if the TT is advanced too far, it usually enters the right main bronchus. This often occurs while taping the tube in place or with changes in position for surgery. Flexion of the head advances the tip of the tube; extension withdraws the tube; bilateral breath sounds must be verified after positioning for surgery (see Chaps. 4 and 8).
9. Because the ribs are almost horizontal, ventilation is mainly diaphragmatic. The abdominal viscera are bulky and can hinder diaphragmatic excursion, especially if the gastrointestinal tract is distended.

Table 2.1 lists the approximate airway dimensions in infants and children.

Table 2.1 Approximate airway dimensions in infants and children

Age (years)	Tracheal length (cm) (vocal cords to carina)	Trachea (AP diameter) (mm)	Diameter (mm)	
			Right bronchus	Left bronchus
<0.5	5.9	5.0	4.5	3.5
0.5–1	7.2	5.5	4.8	3.7
1–2	7.5	6.3	5.1	3.9
2–4	8.0	7.5	6.4	4.9
4–6	8.6	8.0	6.7	5.3
6–8	9.5	9.2	7.9	6.1
8–10	10	9.75	8.4	6.5
10–12	11.5	10.5	9.2	6.8
12–14	13.5	11.5	9.8	7.5
14–16	14.5	13.2	11.5	8.8

AP anteroposterior

Physiology

Breathing movements begin in utero and are characteristically rapid, irregular, and episodic during late pregnancy. Fetal breathing plays a role in lung development and provides exercise for the muscles of respiration. Monitoring fetal respirations provides fetal health information: hypoxemia leads to a decrease in fetal breathing; severe hypoxemia leads to gasping respirations. The fetal lungs are filled with fluid, which is moved by this respiratory muscle activity. Production of surface-active substances (surfactants) by type II pneumocytes begins by 23 weeks gestation and matures by ~34 weeks. Surfactant detected in amniotic fluid (lecithin-to-sphingomyelin ratio) provides a diagnostic index of lung maturity and hence neonatal prognosis.

Passage of the fetus through the birth canal compresses the thorax, expelling much of the fluid from the lungs. After delivery and when the chest expands, air is drawn into the lungs, increasing lung compliance. Peripheral (cold, touch, temperature, etc.) and biochemical (respiratory and metabolic acidosis) stimuli promote the onset of regular, continuous breathing. Other factors such as an increase in the PaO_2 or removal of central biochemical inhibitors are important contributors. The first few spontaneous breaths are characterized by increased transpulmonary pressures (>50 cm H_2O) establishing the functional residual capacity (FRC) of the neonate's lungs. Residual lung fluid is removed during the first few days after birth by the pulmonary lymphatics and blood vessels. Infants who are delivered by cesarean section are not subjected to the same thoracic squeeze, resulting in more residual fluid in the lungs and reduced lung compliance. This may result in transient respiratory distress (transient tachypnea of the newborn).

Alveolar stability depends on adequate amounts of surfactant. Lack of surfactant in preterm infants leads to collapse of alveoli, maldistribution of ventilation, impaired gas exchange, decreased lung compliance, and increased work of breathing, i.e., the respiratory distress syndrome (RDS).

Control of Respiration in the Neonate

Control of respiration, which involves biochemical and reflex mechanisms, is well developed in the healthy full-term neonate but exhibits several differences from adults. Respiration relative to body mass in the infant is greater for any given arterial carbon dioxide tension ($PaCO_2$), reflecting a greater metabolic rate. The ventilatory response to hypercapnia is preterm neonate < full-term neonate < older infants. Any increase in the work of breathing is poorly tolerated (see further). The slope of the carbon dioxide response curve is decreased in infants displaying episodes of apnea, and hypoxemia, which further attenuates the response to hypercapnia.

The neonate is sensitive to changes in arterial oxygen tension (PaO_2). Administration of 100% oxygen decreases ventilation, indicating the existence of tonic chemoreceptor activity. The ventilatory response of the neonate to hypoxia is modified by many factors, including gestational and postnatal age, body temperature, and sleep state [rapid eye movement (REM) sleep]. Preterm and full-term infants younger than 1 week of age who are awake and normothermic usually demonstrate a biphasic response to hypoxemia—a brief period of hyperpnea followed by ventilatory depression. Hypoxia depresses the ventilatory response to carbon dioxide, and it may also induce periodic breathing that may be abolished by oxygen administration. Full-term infants older than 2–3 weeks of age demonstrate hyperpnea in response to hypoxia, probably as a result of maturing of the chemoreceptor function.

Hypothermic infants and preterm infants respond to hypoxemia with ventilatory depression without the initial hyperpnea. Depressed ventilation has been attributed to the central effects of hypoxia on the cortex and medulla. The peripheral chemoreceptors, although active in neonates, do not significantly influence this hypoxic response.

Reflexes that arise from the neonatal lung and chest wall are probably more important in maintaining ventilation, possibly compensating for inadequacies in other control mechanisms. They primarily determine the rate (f) and V_t but are also important for maintaining lung volume (i.e., terminating expiration). The Hering-Breuer inflation reflex, which is active in the neonate, is even more powerful in the preterm infant. This reflex disappears during REM sleep and progressively fades during the early weeks of life. The paradoxical "Head's" reflex, a large inspiration triggered by small lung inflation, may play a role in maintaining neonatal lung volumes and may be present during anesthesia.

Periodic breathing (rapid ventilation alternating with periods of apnea lasting 5–10 s) is normal in most preterm infants but should comprise <1–3% of full-term infant respirations; a greater fraction of periodic breathing in a full-term infant is a warning sign of possible abnormal control of ventilation. It is associated with increased peripheral chemoreceptor activity. In the preterm infant, the $PaCO_2$ is greater than normal during these episodes of periodic breathing, but the heart rate does not change significantly. In the full-term infant, hypocapnia may occur during periodic breathing, which seems to have minimal physiologic consequences 46 to 48 weeks postmenstrual age. Some preterm infants demonstrate far more serious and indeed life-threatening episodes of apnea. These commonly exceed 15 s and may be accompanied by bradycardia (possibly due to chemoreceptor-mediated or vagal reflexes) and hemoglobin oxygen desaturation. Brief apnea (<15 s) may also be accompanied by significant bradycardia (<80 beats/min). The pathogenesis of apnea in preterm infants is not fully understood. Apnea may reflect an immature central respiratory control system because it tends to resolve as the brain matures. Apneic episodes may be central in origin, either without ventilatory effort or obstructive with ventilatory effort but without gas exchange. Obstruction occurs in the infant's nasopharynx, pharynx, or hypopharynx. Mixed apneas (a combination of central and obstructive) commonly occur. One type of apnea may progress to another. Many apneic episodes occur during REM sleep, associated with fatigue of the ventilatory muscles. Although neonatal apnea may be idiopathic, it may also be symptomatic of an underlying disease process, such as sepsis, intracranial bleeding, anemia, hypoglycemia, hypothermia, a patent ductus arteriosus, or a sensitivity to sedatives.

Preterm infants must be carefully monitored with both pulse oximetry and a respiratory monitor such as capnography for post-anesthesia apnea. Treatment may be as simple as tactile stimulation or require bag-mask ventilation. Aminophylline, caffeine (central stimulation), or continuous positive airway pressure (increased reflex activity of lung and chest wall reflexes and "splinting" of the airway) may attenuate the incidence of apneas. Preterm and former preterm infants up to 65 weeks postmenstrual age, particularly those with anemia, are at risk for postoperative apnea even if apnea free at the time of anesthesia. Spinal anesthesia may reduce the frequency and duration of apnea events as well as the upper age risk limit. These infants will benefit from appropriate postoperative respiratory monitoring for at least 12 apnea free hours.

Muscles of Respiration

Type I muscle fibers (slow twitch, highly oxidative, fatigue resistant) are incompletely developed in the neonatal diaphragm and intercostal muscles (preterm < full term <2-year-old) and do not achieve adult values until ~2 years of age. Thus, any increase in the work of breathing may lead to fatigue, one of the leading factors for post-anesthesia apnea. Ventilation is also affected by changing sleep states. The preterm infant spends 50–60% of sleep in REM sleep, during which time intercostal muscle activity is inhibited, and paradoxical movement of the soft chest wall occurs. The reduced intercostal muscle activity is offset in part by an increase in diaphragmatic activity.

Respiratory Mechanics

The specific lung compliance (CL) increases slowly after birth as fluid is removed from the lung. The chest wall of the infant (especially the preterm infant) is very compliant, so that total compliance approximates CL. This highly compliant chest wall provides a relatively weak force to maintain the functional respiratory capacity (FRC) and to oppose the action of the diaphragm. The

FRC of the small infant is maintained by a rapid respiratory rate, the point of termination of expiration, controlled expiration ("laryngeal braking"), and the tonic activity of the ventilatory muscles. It is not surprising that large decreases in FRC occur with apnea and during anesthesia when inhalation agents depress intercostal muscle function.

These large decreases in FRC are accompanied by airway closure during tidal breaths leading to impaired oxygenation. Intercostal muscle inhibition during REM sleep or with inhaled anesthetic agents compounds the weakness of the chest wall and results in paradoxical movement. This paradoxical chest wall movement is markedly augmented by any airway obstruction. Infants generally require controlled ventilation during anesthesia; positive end-expiratory pressure (~5 cm H_2O) maintains lung volume and avoids airway closure and pharyngeal collapse during spontaneous respirations. As the child grows through infancy and childhood, the rib cage stiffens so that it becomes better able to oppose the action of the diaphragm, thus maintaining FRC. The transpulmonary pressures needed to optimally inflate the lungs are remarkably similar in healthy infants, children, and adults. During assisted ventilation, peak inspiratory pressures of 15–20 cm H_2O are normal.

The nasal air passages contribute up to 50% of the airway resistance in infants (Caucasian neonates 49% versus African-American neonates 31%) compared with 65% in adults. In infants the majority of resistance to airflow occurs at the level of the bronchi and small airways. Insertion of a nasogastric tube (NGT) may double total airway resistance in the neonate.

Lung Volumes

In the full-term infant, total lung capacity (TLC) is approximately 160 mL; the FRC is about half this volume. The tidal volume (V_t) is approximately 16 mL (6–7 mL/kg), and dead space volume (V_D) is about 5 mL (30% of the V_t). Relative to body size, all of these volumes are similar to adult values. However, any increase in dead space in the breathing circuit is much more impactful to the small tidal volumes of the infant, e.g., a 5-mL apparatus dead space would increase the total effective V_D by 100%.

In contrast to the static lung volumes, alveolar ventilation (V_A) is proportionally much greater in the neonate (~100–150 mL/kg/min) than in the adult (~60 mL/kg/min). This high V_A in the infant results in a V_A:FRC ratio of 5:1, compared with 1.5:1 in the adult. Consequently, the FRC is a much less effective "buffer" in the infant, so changes in the concentration of inspired gases (including anesthetic gases) are more rapidly reflected in alveolar and arterial values.

The closing volume (CV) is relatively greater in infants and young children than in young adults; it may exceed the FRC to encroach on the V_t during normal respirations. Airway closure during normal respirations may explain the reduced normal values for PaO_2 in infants and neonates (Table 2.2). A decrease in FRC, which usually occurs during general anesthesia and persists into the postoperative period, further increases the significance of the large CV and increases the alveolar-arterial oxygen tension gradient (A-aDO_2). The younger the infant or child, the greater the decrease in FRC. The decrease in FRC may be partially reversed by continuous positive end-expiratory pressure.

The total alveolar surface area in infants (2.8 m^2) is small compared with adults (100 m^2). The infant's large rate of oxygen consumption and small alveolar surface area for oxygen uptake are handicaps for gas exchange. This assumes even greater importance in the presence of congenital pulmonary hypoplasia or lung damage, e.g., from meconium aspiration, since the remaining healthy lung tissue may be inadequate to sustain life.

Table 2.2 Arterial oxygen tension in healthy infants and children

Age	Normal arterial oxygen tension (mmHg) in room air
0–1 week	50–75
1–10 months	75–100
4–16 years	80–100

Work of Breathing

The muscles of respiration generate the force necessary to overcome the resistance to airflow and the elastic recoil of the lungs and chest wall. These two factors dictate an optimal rate of ventilation and a V_t that delivers a given V_A while expending minimal muscular energy. Because the time constant of the infant's lung is relatively small, efficient alveolar ventilation can be achieved at high respiratory rates. In the neonate, a spontaneous respiratory rate of ~37 breaths/min is most efficient. Full-term infants are similar to adults in that they require ~1% of their metabolic energy to maintain ventilation; the oxygen cost of breathing is ~0.5 mL/0.5 L of ventilation. The preterm infant has a greater oxygen cost of breathing (0.9 mL/0.5 L), which is greatly increased if the lungs are diseased, as in RDS or bronchopulmonary dysplasia.

Ventilation-Perfusion Relationships in the Neonatal Lung

Ventilation ($\dot{V}$) and perfusion ($\dot{Q}$) are imperfectly matched in the neonatal lung, in part a result of gas trapping. $\dot{V}/\dot{Q}$ mismatch is evident in the alveolar-arterial nitrogen difference (A-aDN_2), which is 25 mmHg immediately after birth and declines to about 10 mmHg within the first week. The normal PaO_2 in an infant breathing room air is about 50 mmHg just after birth and increases to ~70 mmHg by 24 h. The large A-aDO_2 in infants is mainly caused by persisting anatomic shunts (see pages 38, 39) and the relatively large CV.

Lung Surfactant

Surfactants in the alveolar lining layer, principally lecithin produced by type II pneumocytes, stabilize the alveoli and prevent their collapse during expiration. Reducing the surface tension at the alveolar tissue interface also reduces the force required for re-expansion. The quantity of lecithin in the fetal lung increases steadily beginning at 23 weeks gestation and then increasing sharply at 34 weeks as the lungs mature. The lecithin/sphingomyelin (L/S) ratio in amniotic fluid is used as a measure of lung maturity and predictor of RDS. The L/S ratio is usually <1 until 32 weeks' gestation, reaching 2 by 35 weeks, and 4–6 by term.

Preterm infants with inadequate pulmonary lecithin production develop RDS. The biochemical pathways for surfactant production are depressed by hypoxia, hyperoxia, acidosis, or hypothermia; therefore, early correction of these abnormalities in the sick neonate is vitally important. Maturation of biochemical processes in fetal lungs in utero may be accelerated by maternal corticosteroid administration. The use of exogenous surfactant to treat RDS is now standard practice, reducing severity of disease, air leaks, pneumothorax, and mortality.

Lung Growth and Development

The lungs continue to develop, particularly microvascular structures surrounding the alveoli, during the first two decades of life. The number of alveoli increases rapidly during the first 6 years, reaching adult levels (~300 million) by 8–10 years of age.

Pulmonary Function Testing in Children

Children older than 6 years of age may cooperate sufficiently to enable standard tests of pulmonary function, although they should be interpreted cautiously as they depend on patient cooperation. Maximum expiratory and inspiratory flow-volume curves help to determine the site and nature of airway obstruction; for example, they can differentiate between intrathoracic and extrathoracic obstruction. Such studies may be most useful in the preoperative assessment of children with a mediastinal mass. Spirometric studies also provide information regarding the degree of reversible airway obstruction in response to bronchodilators in those with reactive airway disease, assisting in preoperative planning. They may also determine the extent of restrictive disease associated with scoliosis, thereby predicting the likelihood of postoperative pulmonary insufficiency. Forced oscillometry is a useful method to assess lung function in children, as this test is independent of patient cooperation.

Respiratory System Changes with Anesthesia

1. Inhaled anesthetic agents decrease tidal volume and increase the respiratory rate during spontaneous ventilation. These changes are explained by a combination of effects of anesthetic drugs on the central chemical control of respiration and the muscles of respiration. Intercostal muscle activity is inhibited by inhaled anesthetic agents; consequently, diaphragmatic breathing dominates, and the chest wall may move paradoxically, even if the airway is only partially obstructed. Surgical stimulation tends to increase ventilation back toward normal levels. Most intravenous agents with the exception of ketamine depress respiration.
2. Inhaled anesthetics reduce the FRC by loss of chest wall stability and elevation of the diaphragm with the greatest effect in infants and toddlers. As the FRC decreases, airway closure may overlap with tidal volume, leading to recommendations to use 5 cm PEEP in this cohort.
3. The ratio of physiologic dead space to tidal volume (V_D:V_T) remains constant in children breathing spontaneously but may increase in those whose ventilation is controlled. During controlled ventilation, major increases in $\dot{V}/\dot{Q}$ mismatch within the lungs result from changes in the action of the diaphragm. Apparatus dead space, especially in infants and toddlers, may assume considerable importance during spontaneous respirations.
4. Compliance changes minimally and airway resistance is generally reduced by the bronchodilator action of inhaled anes-

thetic agents. A TT increases the total flow resistance, especially in neonates and toddlers.

5. The efficiency of gas exchange may also be impaired by the effects of anesthetic drugs or hypoxia on the regional distribution of blood flow through the lungs.
6. Laryngospasm and bronchospasm occur more frequently in children compared with adults, especially those with an active or recent upper respiratory infection (URI) (see Chap. 4). Laryngeal closure results from apposition of the aryepiglottic, vestibular, and vocal folds.

Cardiovascular System

The Fetal Circulation

The fetal cardiovascular system perfuses the low-resistance placental circulation, directing 36–42% of the combined ventricular output to this organ; only 5–10% goes to the lungs. The high pulmonary vascular resistance limits flow to the fetal lungs, resulting in blood bypassing the lungs via the foramen ovale and the ductus arteriosus. Most of the blood returning from the placenta bypasses the liver via the ductus venosus. The pattern of flow from the inferior vena cava into the right atrium (RA) ensures that about one-third of the oxygenated placental blood is directed through the foramen ovale into the left atrium. This blood, which combines with the limited venous return from the lungs, is pumped by the left ventricle into the ascending aorta and thence to the coronary, cerebral, and forelimb circulations with a hemoglobin saturation of ~65–70%. Blood returning via the superior vena cava (saturation ~ 40%) passes through the RA into the right ventricle, from which most of the output flows through the ductus arteriosus into the descending aorta (combining with blood from the left ventricle). Thus, blood supplied to the heart and upper body has a greater oxygen content than that supplied to the abdominal organs, lower limbs, and placenta. In utero, the right ventricle pumps about 66% of the combined ventricular output, and the left ventricle pumps the remainder.

Circulatory Changes at Birth

At birth, pulmonary ventilation is quickly established, with blood flow to the lungs increasing dramatically as placental flow decreases precipitously. While the lungs expand and fill with air and the pO_2 increases, pulmonary vascular resistance (PVR) decreases suddenly as a result of the decrease in pulmonary vasomotor tone. PVR decreases by ~80% within minutes after initiation of breathing. As the PVR decreases, blood flow to the lungs and the left atrium increases, thereby increasing left atrial pressure above that in the RA, closing the flap valve foramen ovale.

Simultaneously, as flow to the placenta ceases because of clamping or umbilical artery constriction, a large, low-resistance vascular bed is excluded from the systemic circulation. This results in a large increase in systemic vascular resistance (SVR) and a decrease in inferior vena cava blood flow and RA pressure. The increase in SVR and the simultaneous decrease in PVR increase aortic pressure above that in the pulmonary artery, reversing blood flow through the ductus arteriosus, i.e., becomes left to right, filling it with oxygenated blood. The increased ductal pO_2 constricts the muscular wall of the ductus secondary to a prostaglandin-mediated response, and the ductus closes. Flow through the ductus is usually insignificant by 15 hours after birth with permanent closure occurring within 5–7 days, although in some cases, closure may take ~3 weeks.

The ductus venosus, which communicates between the umbilical veins, the portal vein, and the inferior vena cava, also remains patent for several days after birth. This channel provides a shunt past the hepatic circulation and therefore may reduce the clearance of drugs metabolized in the liver.

The Transitional Circulation

During the early neonatal period, the circulation may revert to the fetal pattern during hypoxia or hypercarbia. In these cases, PVR increases, which in turn increases the RA pressure, opening the flap valve of the foramen ovale, resulting in a right-to-left shunt away from the lungs. The ductus arteriosus may also reopen with a significant proportion of blood bypassing the (now high-resistance) pulmonary circulation, causing a rapid decrease in arterial oxygenation. Impaired tissue oxygenation results in acidosis which may further increase PVR, establishing a vicious cycle of hypoxemia → acidosis → impaired pulmonary blood flow → greater hypoxemia. Reversion to a fetal pattern of circulation may complicate any condition that causes hypoxemia, hypercarbia, or acidemia. In most cases, hyperventilation with 100% oxygen reduces $PaCO_2$ and thus pulmonary artery pressure, thereby facilitating closure of the foramen ovale.

The Neonatal Cardiovascular System

In healthy neonates, the wall thickness of the right ventricle exceeds that of the left. This is reflected in the ECG, which shows an axis of up to +180° during the first week of life. After birth, the left ventricle enlarges disproportionately leading to an adult ratio of ventricular size by 3–6 months (axis approximately +90°). During the immediate neonatal period, the rhythm is regular between 100 and 170 beats/min. As the child grows, the heart rate gradually slows (Table 2.3). Sinus arrhythmia is common in children; all other irregular rhythms are abnormal.

Table 2.3 Normal heart rate

	Heart rate (beats/min)	
Age	Average	Range
Neonate	120	100–170
1–11 months	120	80–160
2 years	110	80–130
4 years	100	80–120
6 years	100	75–115
8 years	90	70–110
10 years	90	70–110
14 years	80–85	60–105
16 years	75–80	55–100

In the full-term neonate, the normal blood pressure is 60/35 mmHg. These pressures vary considerably, 10–15 mmHg greater if clamping of the umbilical cord is delayed or the cord is "stripped," causing an increase in circulating blood volume. In either case, they decrease to normal values within 4 h after birth. Preterm infants have reduced arterial pressures, as low as 45/25 mmHg in a 750-g infant (Table 2.4).

The myocardium of the neonate contains less contractile and more supporting tissue than the adult heart. Consequently, the neonate's ventricles are less compliant, limiting stroke volume and rendering cardiac output more dependent on the heart rate. Bradycardias invariably reduce cardiac output. The infant heart has a normal Frank-Starling response to volume loading, but the response peaks at a much lower filling pressure in the neonate (~8–10 mmHg) versus the adult (~13–15 mmHg). Thus, cardiac output is both rate dependent and volume dependent. Reduced ventricular compliance and contractility predispose the infant heart to failure with increased volume load; failure of one ventri-

Table 2.4 Normal blood pressure[a]

	Blood pressure (mmHg)		
Age	Systolic	Diastolic	Mean
Neonate			
Preterm (750 g)	44	24	33
Preterm (1000 g)	49	26	34.5
Full term	60	35	45
3–10 days	70–75	45	57
Infants			
6 months	95	55	67
Children			
4 years	98	59	73
6 years	110	60	81
8 years	112	60	82
12 years	115	65	85
16 years	120	65	87

[a]Reported awake blood pressure values for infants and children must be considered in light of the method of determination. These values should serve as a guide only

cle rapidly compromises the function of the other leading to biventricular failure.

The reduced contractility of the neonatal heart is also secondary to the immaturity of the myofibrils and the less developed sarcoplasmic reticulum. Cyclic calcium flux within the neonatal myocardium depends more on exchange across the cell membrane (sarcolemma) than on the function of the sarcoplasmic reticulum, thus depending more on blood ionized calcium levels. As the infant grows, the myocardial sarcoplasmic reticulum assumes the dominant role in myocardial calcium regulation, typical of the adult heart. This immaturity of calcium regulation within the myocyte may explain the greater sensitivity of the neonate to myocardial depression from inhalational anesthetics, which block calcium channels. This may also explain the severe cardiac depressant effects associated with the sudden reduction in ionized calcium concentrations during the rapid administration of citrated blood products such as fresh frozen plasma or platelets.

Autonomic innervation of the heart in the neonate is incomplete, and there is a relative lack of sympathetic elements. This may further compromise the ability of the less contractile neonatal myocardium to respond to stress. The differences in the neonate's myocardial function are all particularly marked in the preterm infant.

In neonates, cardiac output averages 2–3 times greater than in adults reflecting an increased metabolic rate. Systemic vascular resistance is less in neonates than in adults, reflecting the greater proportion of vessel-rich tissues in neonates (~18%), double that in adults. Vessel-rich tissues have a relatively reduced systemic arterial pressure despite the large cardiac output.

The Pulmonary Circulation

The changes in the pulmonary circulation that occur at birth continue over the subsequent 3 months with a slower progressive decrease in PVR. This is associated with a parallel regression in the thickness of the medial muscle layer of the pulmonary arterioles. During the neonatal period, PVR remains increased, and the muscular pulmonary vessels are highly reactive. Hypoxia, acidosis, and stress, e.g., from suctioning the tracheal tube, may all further increase the PVR. If an increase in the PVR is sustained, right-sided intracardiac pressures may exceed those on the left, opening the foramen ovale that results in a right-to-left shunt. This is known as persistent fetal circulation; without intervention, this may lead to right ventricular failure that rapidly progresses to biventricular failure.

In some, the muscular layer of the pulmonary vessels may not regress, and PVR may not decrease. Continued hypoxemia, caused, for example, by continued high altitude or excessive pulmonary blood flow as a result of left-to-right shunts, e.g., ventricular septal defect, may lead to persistently increased PVR into childhood and beyond. Initially, this increased PVR is reversible, e.g., with pulmonary vasodilators; however, over time, it stimulates structural changes in the pulmonary vascular bed that are irreversible, resulting in pulmonary vascular obstructive disease.

Nitric oxide, an endogenous free radical produced in normal lung tissue that regulates pulmonary vascular tone, is known as endothelium-derived relaxing factor. It is commonly administered exogenously to treat "pulmonary hypertension of the newborn."

Blood Volume

Blood volume varies considerably during the immediate postnatal period, the primary determinant being the amount of blood drained from the placenta before cord clamping. Delay in clamping or stripping the cord at delivery may increase the blood volume by more than 20%, resulting in transient respiratory distress. Conversely, fetal hypoxia during labor may vasoconstrict the cord, shift blood to the placental circulation, and cause hypovolemia in the already asphyxiated neonate. Blood volume decreases with increasing age (Table 2.5).

Table 2.5 Estimated normal blood volumes of children by age

Age	Blood volume (mL/kg)
Micropremie (≤800 grams)	110
Premature Neonate	100
Term Neonate	90
6 weeks to 1 year	80
>1 year to puberty	70

The Response to Hypovolemia

The changes in arterial blood pressure in the neonate are proportional to the degree of hypovolemia. The ability to restore intravascular volume from capacitance vessels is limited, and baroreflexes, especially in the preterm infant, are inactive during anesthesia, further compromising the response to hypovolemia. Since the infant's systolic arterial blood pressure is closely related to the circulating blood volume, systolic blood pressure is an excellent guide to the adequacy of blood replacement.

The Response to Hypoxia

Oxygen consumption in neonates (4–6 mL/kg/min) is greater than in adults (2–3 mL/kg/min) and even greater in preterm infants (up to 10 mL/kg/min), explaining the rapidity of desaturation in neonates and infants. Any episode of unexplained bradycardia should be attributed to hypoxia and treated immediately with 100% oxygen. Hypoxemia causes pulmonary vasoconstriction, increasing pulmonary artery pressure and thus right atrial pressure, which opens the foramen ovale, shunting blood right-to-left. The same holds for the ductus arteriosus, and both sources of shunting further decrease SaO_2. Neonates experiencing hypoxemia rapidly become bradycardic with a decreased cardiac output; rapid intervention (usually hyperventilation to reduce $PaCO_2$) is necessary to prevent progression to cardiac arrest.

Oxygen Transport

The blood volume in neonates varies by age and is considerably greater in premies and micropremies (Table 2.5). The hematocrit (Hct) may be as great as 60% and the hemoglobin (Hb) 18–19 g/dL. The values for blood volume, Hct, and Hb vary from infant to infant, depending on the time of cord clamping. These values change little during the first week of life, after which the Hb level starts to decrease. The decrease in Hb level occurs more rapidly in preterm infants.

Most (70–90%) of the Hb present at birth in a full-term infant is fetal hemoglobin (HbF). The affinity of HbF for oxygen is greater than that of adult hemoglobin (HbA), primarily because of a lack of effect of 2,3-DPG on the HbF–O_2 interaction. HbF combines with more oxygen but releases it to tissues less readily than HbA. The pO_2 at 50% Hb saturation (P_{50}) for HbF is ~20 mmHg, in contrast to 26–27 mmHg for HbA. Adequate oxygen transport to tissues in the neonate therefore requires a greater Hb concentration. An Hb less than 12 g/dL constitutes anemia, and even greater levels are desirable in chronic hypoxic states such as cyanotic congenital heart disease. Despite a remarkable improvement in transfusion safety, administration of any blood product should be carefully considered. In general, correction of anemia by blood transfusion may be indicated to maintain the Hct greater than 40% in cases of severe cardiopulmonary disease, 30% in moderate cardiopulmonary disease or major surgery, and 25% in symptomatic anemia (apnea, tachycardia, lethargy, poor growth).

During the first weeks after birth, the Hct and Hb levels decrease steadily, in part because of a progressive increase in blood volume and suppression of erythropoiesis caused by improved tissue oxygenation (see Table 6.4). Physiologic anemia of infancy in full-term neonates reaches a nadir at 2–3 months of age with Hb levels of 9–11 g/dL and in preterm infants less than 1500 g at birth earlier than 2 months with Hb levels of 7–8 g/dL. Physiologic anemia has been attributed to a short erythrocyte life span, rapid growth, and decreased erythropoietin production. This is further exaggerated in NICU patients who require frequent blood testing. The early "physiologic" anemia in preterm infants is often followed by a continuing "late" anemia, which is secondary to nutritional deficiencies. Severe anemia may lead to tachycardia, tachypnea, poor feeding and growth, diminished activity, and apnea. In severe states, congestive heart failure may occur. At the nadir, most HbF has been replaced by HbA. Thus, oxygen delivery to tissues is improved. Provided that nutrition is adequate, the Hb level subsequently increases over several weeks to 12–13 g/dL, which is maintained throughout early childhood.

Metabolism: Fluid and Electrolyte Balance

Glucose Homeostasis

The term neonate has stores of glycogen that are located mainly in the liver and myocardium. These are used during the first few hours of life until gluconeogenesis becomes established. Small-for-gestational-age and preterm infants may have inadequate glycogen stores and may fail to establish adequate gluconeogenesis. Hence, they often depend on IV infusions to prevent hypoglycemia.

Hypoglycemia is common in the stressed neonate (Table 2.6). Blood glucose levels should be measured frequently in sick neonates, and if they decrease to <45 mg/dL (2.2 mmol/L), they

Table 2.6 Factors associated with hypoglycemia in neonates

Prematurity
Perinatal stress
Sepsis
Small for gestational age
Polycythemia
Hypoxia
Excess insulin
Infant of diabetic mother
Beckwith-Wiedemann syndrome

should be corrected by a slow continuous infusion of 10% dextrose at 5–8 mg/kg/min (0.05–0.08 mL/kg/min). Symptoms of hypoglycemia (jitteriness, convulsions, and apnea) should be treated immediately by slow injection of 10% dextrose (1–2 mL/kg). Neurologic damage occurs in up to 50% of infants with symptomatic hypoglycemia (usually with values ≤30 mg/dL). Infants of diabetic mothers and those with Beckwith-Wiedemann syndrome must be treated with particular care because a bolus dose of intravenous glucose may precipitate hyperinsulinemia and rebound hypoglycemia; a slow glucose infusion is recommended. Older infants and young children rarely become hypoglycemic even during an excessively long preoperative fasting period. Current pediatric practice minimizes preoperative fasting (see Table 1.1).

Hyperglycemia is a common iatrogenic problem of small infants receiving intravenous glucose therapy, probably as a result of inadequate insulin release and continued hepatic glucose production. The effects of hyperglycemia can be serious. Osmotically induced cerebral fluid shifts may lead to cerebral hemorrhage, and glycosuria may cause diuresis, resulting in water and electrolyte depletion. Hyperglycemia (glucose values >200 mg/dL) may also increase the extent of neurologic damage during a cerebral hypoxic-ischemic event. It is essential that glucose therapy be carefully controlled to avoid hyperglycemia. We recommend using a continuous infusion pump to maintain glucose levels and a separate infusion of balanced salt solutions to replace intraoperative losses.

Calcium Homeostasis

Calcium is actively transported across the placenta to meet the needs of the fetus. This transport accelerates in the near term and may cause a decline in maternal calcium levels. After birth, the infant depends on its own calcium reserves even though parathyroid function is not fully established, and vitamin D stores may be inadequate. As a result, hypocalcemia must be anticipated in preterm infants, after birth trauma, neonatal asphyxia, any severe neonatal illness, or blood transfusion (especially fresh frozen plasma or platelets). Continuing hypocalcemia may be a sign of parathyroid dysfunction and is typically present in DiGeorge syndrome (see Chap. 15).

Symptoms of hypocalcemia include twitching, increased muscle tone, and seizures (hypocalcemia is not always easily distinguished from hypoglycemia). The Chvostek sign may be present, but confirmation depends on laboratory test results (total and ionized calcium). Infants prone to hypocalcemia are treated with continuous calcium infusions. Symptomatic hypocalcemia requires a slow infusion of either 10% calcium chloride (10–30 mg/kg) or 10% calcium gluconate (30–90 mg/kg), with continuous ECG monitoring. Calcium-containing solutions may cause severe skin damage, leading to sloughing if they leak into adjacent tissues; they should preferably be given through a central line.

Magnesium Homeostasis

Magnesium and calcium metabolism are closely related: an imbalance in one may affect the other. Magnesium levels affect parathyroid hormone secretion; the renal excretion of calcium and magnesium are interrelated. Chronic hypomagnesemia is commonly accompanied by hypocalcemia secondary to the effect on parathyroid function.

Hypomagnesemia is more common in preterm infants, small-for-gestational-age infants, infants of diabetic mothers, and infants with intestinal disease. It may also complicate massive blood transfusions. Hypomagnesemia results in abnormal muscle activity, tremors, seizures, cardiac arrhythmias, and sensitivity to muscle relaxant drugs.

Hypermagnesemia may complicate renal failure, or, in the neonate, it may be a consequence of the administration of magnesium sulfate to the mother. It may result in depression of the central nervous and respiratory systems, hyporeflexia, and hypotension.

Bilirubin Homeostasis

During the first week after birth, unconjugated hyperbilirubinemia (physiologic jaundice) occurs secondary to an increased bilirubin load in full-term neonates, limited hepatic cell uptake of bilirubin, and deficient hepatic conjugation to the water-soluble glucuronide. Serum bilirubin levels seldom exceed 7 mg/dL (103 μmol/L). In preterm infants, greater levels (10–15 mg/dL) are commonly reached. These persist for a longer period, owing to a greater bilirubin load and delayed maturation of the hepatic conjugation pathway. The preterm infant may sustain neurologic damage (kernicterus) at reduced serum bilirubin levels (~6–9 mg/dL) compared with the full-term infant (~20 mg/dL). This predisposition is a result of the preterm infant's less effective blood-brain barrier and may be exacerbated by hypoxia, acidosis, infection, hypothermia, or a low level of serum albumin and, hence, decreased binding sites. The preterm infant must be monitored for increased serum bilirubin levels and specific treatment (phototherapy, possible exchange transfusion) as required. Some drugs, e.g., diazepam, sulfonamides, and furosemide, that compete with and displace protein-bound bilirubin, e.g., "acidic" binding sites for albumin, as well as hypoxia, acidosis, hypothermia, and hypoalbuminemia, increase the risk of neurologic injury.

Composition and Regulation of Body Fluids

Body Water

Total body water in neonates and infants is relatively greater than in adults. Its distribution also differs, as the proportion of water in the extracellular fluid (ECF) is greater in neonates and young children than in adults. In preterm infants, the ECF exceeds the intracellular fluid (ICF), whereas in older children and adults, the ECF is only half the volume of the ICF (Table 2.7). Thus, the volume of distribution for water-soluble medications is greater in neo-

Table 2.7 Approximate extracellular and intracellular fluid compartments

Fluid	Preterm neonate	Full-term neonate	Infant (7–8 months)	Adult
ECF	65	45	30	20
ICF	25	35	35	40

Data are percent body weight

Table 2.8 Normal blood chemistry values

Parameter	Preterm neonate	Full-term neonate	2 years to adult
Serum chloride (mEq/L)	100–117	90–114	98–106
Serum potassium (mEq/L)	4.6–6.7	4.3–7.6	3.5–5.6
Serum sodium (mEq/L)	133–146	136–148	142
Blood glucose (mg/dL)	40–60	40–80	70–110
Total protein (g/dL)	3.9–4.7	4.6–7.7	5.5–7.8
$PaCO_2$ (mmHg)	30–35	33–35	35–40

nates and toddlers, necessitating a larger initial loading dose (See Chap. 3). Normal levels of serum electrolytes in the neonate are listed in Table 2.8.

Neonatal Renal Function and Water Balance

In neonates, renal function is limited by immaturity of tubular function and an increased renal vascular resistance, which reduces renal blood flow and glomerular filtration rate (GFR). During the first few weeks after birth, renal vascular resistance decreases and renal function matures rapidly. GFR (mL/min/1.73 m^2) rapidly increases as renal blood flow increases: ~20 mL/min/1.73m^2 in preterms, ~40 in term neonates, ~55 at 2 weeks of age, ~60 at 3 months, ~80 mL/min/1.73m^2 by 6 months, and adult values at ~1 year of age. The neonate has a limited capacity to readily handle an excessive water load and may be unable to excrete excess electrolytes (especially sodium) or other substances that depend on glomerular filtration for elimination. Several factors including hypoxia, hypothermia, congestive heart failure, increased intrabdominal pressure, e.g., pouch closure of gastroschisis, and mechanical ventilation decrease GFR.

The immature tubular function impairs the infant's ability to modify the glomerular filtrate for conservation or excretion. For this reason, sodium losses may be large, especially in the preterm infant, and must be balanced by intake. These losses are further increased if the GFR is increased by a high fluid intake, hence, the tendency of the neonate to hyponatremia. Glucose reabsorption is limited in the preterm infant, and glycosuria may occur. In the child with marked hyperglycemia, the resultant osmotic diuresis may lead to severe dehydration. The ability of the tubule to excrete acid is reduced in the preterm infant, thus impairing renal compensation during acidosis. The capacity to excrete hydrogen ions increases with gestational age. The renal threshold for bicarbonate excretion is less in infants than adults, leading to reduced serum bicarbonate levels. Immature renal function necessitates careful fluid and electrolyte replacement therapy to match losses. Additionally, renally excreted medications require increased intervals between dosing but may require larger loading doses (Table 2.9).

Fluid loss and hence the required fluid replacement are related to insensible fluid losses, urine output, and metabolic rate. Insensible fluid losses are relatively great during infancy, major factors being the increased alveolar ventilation and the thin skin especially in low-birth-weight infants. Fluid losses are markedly

Table 2.9 Recommended loading dose and intervals for gentamicin administration to neonates

Gestational age	Loading Dose (mg/kg) Gentamicin	Interval between doses (hours)
25 weeks	5	48
32 weeks	5	36
40 weeks	4	12
44 weeks	2–2.5	8

increased by the use of radiant heat and/or phototherapy. Because of the infant's proportionally greater water turnover and the limited ability to concentrate urine and conserve water, dehydration rapidly develops when intake is restricted or losses occur.

Maintenance Requirements

Although maintenance requirements are directly related to the metabolic rate and caloric expenditure and are more accurately expressed in milliliters per square meter of surface area, it is most convenient clinically to relate them to body weight. Fluid requirements for full-term neonates are reduced (40–60 mL/kg per 24 h) during the first few days of life as excess fluid present at birth is being excreted. By 1 week of age, the requirements are increased. Table 2.10 shows the volumes of fluid required during the period of great metabolic activity in infants weighing 4–20 kg.

Table 2.10 Daily maintenance requirements for fluid, electrolytes, and carbohydrates in relation to weight

Weight	H_2O (mL/kg)	Na^+ (mEq/kg)	K^+ (mEq/kg)	Carbohydrate (g/kg)
Neonate[a]				
1000 g	≤200	3.0	2.0–2.5	≤10
1000–1499 g	≤180	2.5	2.0–2.5	
1500–2500 g	≤160	2.0	1.5–2.0	≤8
>2500 g	≤150	1.5–2.0	2.0	≤5
Infants				
4–10 kg	100–120	2.0–2.5	2.0–2.5	5–6
Children				
10–20 kg	80–100	1.6–2.0	1.6–2.0	4–5
20–40 kg	60–80	1.2–1.6	1.2–1.6	3–4
Adult	30–40	50 mEq total	50 mEq total	100–150 g total

[a]Adjust according to postnatal age, exposure to phototherapy, reduced insensible losses with assisted ventilation, etc.

(From The Hospital for Sick Children: Residents' Handbook of Pediatrics, 6th Ed. Toronto, Canada, 1979, with permission)

Intraoperative fluid management in the neonate must include replacement of fluid deficits, third-space losses, blood loss, and maintenance fluids. Deficits and losses are generally replaced with a balanced salt solution, whereas maintenance therapy is replaced with an infusion of 5% glucose and one-half to one-fourth normal saline, containing 20 mEq of K^+ per liter. If a high-concentration glucose solution (D-10 or D-20) is infusing preoperatively, the rate may be reduced by half during anesthesia; however, the serum glucose concentration should be monitored during anesthesia where possible. In critically ill neonates, colloid solutions or plasma may be indicated for volume expansion, as hypoproteinemia is common.

Physiology of Temperature Homeostasis

Because of their large surface area relative to body weight and their lack of heat-insulating subcutaneous fat, infants lose heat rapidly via four routes in order of importance: radiation (~39%) > convection (~34%) > evaporation (~24%) > conduction (~3%). Evaporative heat is lost into the respiratory tract and through the skin which is especially increased by the thin skin in preterm infants. When heat loss occurs, endogenous heat production must increase to maintain a normal core temperature. In adults and older children, heat production is principally a function of involuntary muscular activity (shivering) accompanied by increased oxygen consumption, both of which are precluded by neuromuscular blocking drugs. However, infants rely primarily on non-shivering thermogenesis which occurs mainly in the brown adipose tissue that surrounds the scapulae, the kidneys, the adrenal glands, and the mediastinum. Brown fat comprises 2–6% of the full-term infant's body weight and less in the preterm infant. The cells of the "brown fat" have many mitochondria and fat vacuoles, with a rich blood and autonomic nerve supply. Brown fat activity is initiated by norepinephrine released at the sympathetic nerve endings. Hydrolysis of triglycerides to fatty acids and glycerol occurs with associated increased VO_2 and heat production.

Brown fat deposits decline during the first weeks of extrauterine life.

Exposure to a cool environment together with a decrease in central temperature normally triggers thermoregulatory vasoconstriction in awake infants and children. This vasoconstriction tends to limit further heat loss from the body surface. These compensatory temperature mechanisms are well developed in full-term neonates, although core temperature may decrease if the compensatory heat production cannot match the heat losses. On exposure to a cool environment, increased metabolic activity is initiated in the brown fat to maintain the core temperature. This is accompanied by a progressive increase in oxygen consumption as the temperature gradient between the skin and the environment increases. Oxygen consumption is minimal when this gradient is less than 2°C, i.e., neutral thermal environment. Exposure to a cool environment also leads to increased glucose consumption and acid metabolite formation.

The physiologic responses to cooling lead to increased oxygen and glucose consumption, which may cause an acidosis, further compromising the sick infant. The infant with chronic hypoxemia, e.g., cyanotic congenital heart disease, is unable to compensate if exposed to a cool ambient temperature and cools rapidly. To eliminate the need for compensatory responses, sick neonates should be maintained in a neutral thermal environment, i.e., in an ambient temperature that minimizes oxygen consumption (Table 2.11).

During anesthesia, the normal thermoregulatory response of the infant to cold stress is lost, and oxygen consumption is unchanged in response to a cool environment. In addition, thermoregulatory skin vasoconstriction is inhibited. There is also a redistribution of body heat away from the central core to the periphery. Therefore, heat loss readily increases and body temperature decreases in anesthetized infants and children. Measures that minimize heat loss and avoid cold stress (warmed OR, warmed preparation and irrigation solutions, and convective forced air warmers) should be instituted during anesthesia (see Chap. 5).

Table 2.11 Neutral thermal environment temperatures (°C)

Age	Weight			
	1200 g	1200–1500 g	1500–2500 g	>2500 g
0–6 h	34–35.4	33.9–34.4	32.8–33.8	32.0–33.8
6–12 h	34–35.4	33.5–34.4	32.2–33.8	31.4–33.8
12–24 h	34–35.4	33.3–34.3	31.8–33.8	31.0–33.7
24–36 h	34–35	33.1–34.2	31.6–33.6	30.7–33.5
36–48 h	34–35	33.0–34.1	31.4–33.5	30.5–33.3
48–72 h	34–35	33.0–34.0	31.2–33.4	30.1–33.2
72–96 h	34–35	33.0–34.0	31.1–33.2	29.8–32.8
4–12 days	–	33–34[a]	31–33.2	29.5–31.4
2–3 weeks	–	32.2–34[a]	30.5–33.0	–
3–4 weeks	–	31.6–33.6[a]	30.0–32.7	–

[a]1500 g

Suggested Reading

Al-Matary A, Abu Shaheen A, Abozaid S. Use of prophylactic indomethacin in preterm infants: a systematic review and meta-analysis. Front Pediatr. 2022;10:760029.

Dalal PG, Coté CJ, Malviya S, et al. Postanesthesia apnea in former preterm infants for inguinal Herniorrhaphy: An update of risk factors from an individual participant data meta-analysis Anesthesiology 2026;144(6):1442–53.

Hong EH, Shin YU, Cho H. Retinopathy of prematurity: a review of epidemiology and current treatment strategies. Clin Exp Pediatr. 2022;65(3):115–26.

Jane EH, Jane MA, Taygen EE, Chris JDM, Linda G. Neonatal hypoglycaemia. BMJ Med. 2024;3(1):e000544.

Loukou I, Moustaki M, Deligianni A, Sardeli O, Douros K. Forced oscillation technique for monitoring the respiratory status of children with cystic fibrosis: a systematic review. Children. 2021;8(10):857.

Odackal NJ, Crume M, Naik T, Stiver C. Cardiac development and related clinical considerations. NeoReviews. 2024;25(7):e401–14.

Ramaswamy VV, Abiramalatha T, Bandyopadhyay T, Boyle E, Roehr CC. Surfactant therapy in late preterm and term neonates with respiratory distress syndrome: a systematic review and meta-analysis. Arch Dis Child Fetal Neonatal Ed. 2022;107(4):393–7.

Segar JL, Jetton JG. Fluid and electrolyte management in the neonate and what can go wrong. Curr Opin Pediatr. 2024;36(2):198–203.

Williams MD, Lascelles BDX. Early neonatal pain-a review of clinical and experimental implications on painful conditions later in life. Front Pediatr. 2020;8:30.

Clinical Pharmacology 3

Routes of Administration

Intravenous The intravenous route is the most reliable route to deliver drugs to target organs. It is essential to review each drug, its concentration, and recommended directions from the manufacturer/pharmacy regarding the dose/kg, route of administration, speed of injection, and dilution before administration. For example, rapid injection of vancomycin may cause severe physiologic responses, e.g., hypotension/cardiac arrest or "red man syndrome." It is particularly important in neonates to administer drugs using tuberculin syringes or, when diluted, always double check the dilution. Flush all intravenous tubing and aspirate air from injection ports and eject all air bubbles from the syringe before administration. Critical events have occurred when muscle relaxants or opioids remained in the IV tubing and were unknowingly later flushed into the child.

N.B. Drugs should not be injected into *intralipid* or *hyperalimentation* because infection or thrombosis may ensue. However, some children may have a central line for repeated anesthesia/sedation procedures; it should be accessed using appropriate connectors under aseptic conditions. A peripheral IV may be "hep-locked" for use during repeated procedures.

J. Lerman, C. J. Coté, *Steward's Manual of Pediatric Anesthesia*,
https://doi.org/10.1007/978-3-032-24545-8_3

Intramuscular The intramuscular route of drug administration is less preferred, but drugs administered by this route are rapidly absorbed, especially in small children, but there is a risk of sterile abscess formation. Intramuscular drugs are usually administered in the lateral thigh or deltoid region of the arm. Some drugs are more rapidly absorbed from the upper than the lower extremity, e.g., succinylcholine. Intramuscular injections are much less reliable in hypovolemic children, and there is a danger that repeated doses may have a cumulative effect when muscle tissue perfusion improves. Intramuscular injections are painful and generally avoided in awake children.

Intralingual Injections into the tongue have been recommended for use in an emergency, e.g., succinylcholine, due to rapid drug absorption when IV access is limited. *However, never inject in the midline sublingually, as there is a risk of causing a lingual hematoma; we only recommend this route as a last resort.*

Intratracheal Drugs sprayed into the trachea through a tracheal tube are rapidly absorbed; this route is useful in an emergency if an intravenous route is not available, e.g., to administer atropine or epinephrine. This route is not recommended as a first choice for resuscitation; if necessary, larger drug doses are required. It is important to also either dilute the drug to a larger volume or flush the drug into the tracheobronchial tree with 3–5 mL of saline to ensure delivery to a mucosal surface. Beware that local anesthetics sprayed into the trachea are rapidly absorbed; always check to ensure that the total dose given is weight appropriate.

Rectal The use of suppositories (acetaminophen) or rectal administration of drugs, e.g., midazolam and methohexital, is accepted by children younger than 3 years of age. Absorption is less certain than with other routes, in part because of the partial first-pass effect of the liver when absorption occurs through the inferior/middle hemorrhoidal veins and the variable volume and pH of the rectal milieu. Unanesthetized children older than 3 years of age may be upset if medications are administered via this route. This route is infrequently used today.

Oral Preoperative medication and postoperative analgesics may be given by this route, but the oral route cannot be used if the child is vomiting or if other gastrointestinal dysfunction exists. Many drugs are rapidly absorbed via the oral transmucosal route.

Intranasal Some drugs are well absorbed across the nasal mucous membranes via the posterior turbinates and rapidly effective by this route, e.g., sufentanil and midazolam. Nebulized medications are increasingly utilized; absorption is markedly dependent upon particle size (larger size increases rainout prior to passage into the middle turbinate region). Absorption occurs along neurovascular structures directly into the CNS. However, many children object to having drops instilled in their nose, and there is a theoretical concern that some drugs or their preservatives, e.g., ketamine, might be neurotoxic if they penetrate the cribriform plate and enter the brain.

Intraosseous This route is recommended for resuscitation in all age groups when an intravenous route is not available or initial attempts at venous access fail (See Chap. 5); drugs are rapidly absorbed and may be given in the usual doses.

Topical Several local anesthetics may be delivered efficiently through the skin; topical anesthetics containing prilocaine should not be directly applied to mucosal surfaces, particularly in neonates, due to the risk of methemoglobinemia.

Distribution of Administered Drugs

The size of the extracellular fluid compartment in infants and young children is larger than in adults; hence, larger loading doses of hydrophilic drugs, e.g., succinylcholine, are required in infants.

The fraction of unbound drugs confers end-organ pharmacologic effects: the greater the unbound fraction, the greater the pharmacologic effect. In neonates, the unbound fraction is greater than in older children because of decreased protein binding and impaired metabolism. In neonates, protein binding is decreased because the total serum protein concentrations and concentrations of specific proteins, e.g., α_1-acid glycoprotein/albumin, are less in neonates. Immature cytochrome P450 enzymes in neonates impair drug metabolism, resulting in greater drug concentrations for greater periods.

Body composition also influences drug distribution; neonates have little fat or muscle tissue compared with older children; thus, the plasma concentrations of drugs distributed in these tissues will be increased (less uptake), and their duration of action may be prolonged.

Metabolism and Elimination of Drugs

The half-lives of drugs metabolized in the liver in neonates and infants are generally greater than in adults. Hepatic blood flow and hepatocellular enzymatic activity are the primary determinants of the rate of metabolism of many drugs by the liver. Hepatic blood flow is similar in the small infant and adult, although it may be reduced in the presence of increased intra-abdominal pressure and in children requiring vasoactive support or who have congestive cardiac failure.

In the first few postnatal days, blood may shunt past the liver via a patent ductus venosus. Phase 1 cytochrome enzymes mature during the first few years of life, some not reaching adult levels until adolescence. Phase 2 conjugation pathways for drug metabolism are immature in preterm infants and are not fully active until several months postnatally. Hence, the elimination half-life of drugs such as morphine in this age group is increased. In addition, alternative pathways for drug metabolism may accumulate metabolites, some of which may be pharmacologically active, e.g., morphine-3- and morphine-6-glucuronide. Older infants and young children demonstrate a rapid elimination of some drugs, reflecting the greater hepatic blood flow and enhanced metabolic activity in the liver.

Drug clearance (Cl) via the kidney, e.g., most antibiotics, depends on the glomerular filtration rate (GFR) or tubular secretion capacity, both of which are reduced during the first 3–6 months of postnatal life (necessitating an increased interval between drug doses). GFR increases with age, reaching adult values by ~2 years of age (See Table 2.9).

Drugs Used in Anesthesia

Inhalation Agents

The concentration (or partial pressure) of inhaled anesthetics in the alveoli increases more rapidly with decreasing age: infants > children > adults. This is the result of the increased alveolar ventilation to functional residual capacity ratio, the greater proportion of vessel-rich tissues that rapidly equilibrate with blood concentrations, and the reduced blood gas and tissue-gas partition coefficients (λ) of the inhaled anesthetics (except sevoflurane) in infants compared with adults. Therefore, induction of anesthesia is more rapid in infants and small children. The rapid increase in alveolar, blood, and tissue partial pressures of inhaled anesthetics may account in part for the precipitous decreases in blood pressure during inhalation induction when greater concentrations of inhalation anesthetics are administered to infants, particularly during controlled ventilation.

Excretion of inhaled anesthetic agents, and therefore recovery, is also more rapid in infants and small children than in adults, provided that ventilation is not depressed. The alveolar concentration of N_2O decreases to 10% within ~2 min in neonates after discontinuation of 70% N_2O, a level not reached until ~5 min in adults.

The minimum alveolar concentration (MAC) of inhaled anesthetics in preterm infants increases steadily to term and peaks in infancy for most anesthetics. Thereafter, MAC decreases with increasing age (Table 3.1); why age affects MAC in this manner is unknown. MAC values have been determined for a number of anesthetic interventions (Table 3.2).

All inhaled anesthetics depress ventilation to a similar degree as evidenced by CO_2 response curves. A dose-related decrease in V_t and minute ventilation is accompanied by an increase in $PaCO_2$.

Table 3.1 Minimum alveolar concentration (MAC) (%) of inhalational agents

Age	Halothane	Isoflurane	Sevoflurane	Desflurane
Preterm neonate	Not available	1.3–1.4	Not available	Not available
Full-term neonate	0.87	1.6	3.3	9.1
Infant	1.2	1.8	3.2	9.4
Child	0.95	1.6	2.5[a]	8.5[a]

[a]60% nitrous oxide reduces the MAC values ~25%

Table 3.2 MAC for anesthesia interventions in children

	Inhalational Agent	Minimum Alveolar Concentration (MAC %)
Tracheal intubation	Halothane	1.3
	Sevoflurane	2.7
Tracheal extubation	Isoflurane	1.4
	Sevoflurane	1.70, 2.3
	Desflurane	7.7
LMA insertion	Halothane	1.5
	Sevoflurane	2.0
LMA extubation	Sevoflurane	1.84
	Desflurane	3.39 (with caudal block)
		3.56 (with fentanyl)
Tracheal intubation/ skin incision ratio[a]	Halothane, enflurane, sevoflurane	1.33
Awake	Sevoflurane	0.3
	Age: 2–5 years	0.66
	5–12 years	0.43
IV cannulation	Sevoflurane	1.32
BIS_{50}	Sevoflurane	2.83

[a]Calculated using the above MAC data
From Anderson et al. (2025), p. 126

Intercostal muscle activity is inhibited, particularly during halothane anesthesia. This contributes to the depressed ventilation and may lead to paradoxical chest wall movement, especially if airway obstruction occurs.

Inhaled anesthetics depress the myocardium in a dose-dependent manner, due to their calcium channel-blocking activity. The severity of the myocardial depression follows the order: halothane > isoflurane ≥ sevoflurane and desflurane. Halothane frequently causes bradycardia; sevoflurane frequently causes tachycardia and rarely bradycardia. Severe bradycardia should be rapidly corrected with IV atropine; hemodynamically important bradycardia may require chest compressions and epinephrine. Inhaled anesthetics may prolong the QT interval (halothane > sevoflurane > isoflurane) in some children, especially young infants. Although this may be insignificant in isolation, if combined with an increased dispersion of repolarization (defined as the difference between the maximum and minimum QT interval) (>100 ms), it may predispose to torsades de pointes. In children with long QT syndrome, medications that increase the QT interval may predispose to serious arrhythmias.

Inhaled anesthetics inhibit hypoxic pulmonary vasoconstriction, thereby disrupting the mechanism that normally redistributes perfusion away from underventilated alveoli. This increased shunt may cause a clinically important decrease in SaO_2, especially in infants with lung disease, e.g., bronchopulmonary dysplasia.

Inhaled anesthetics increase cerebral blood flow (CBF) by decreasing cerebral vascular resistance following the order from greatest to least: halothane ~ desflurane > isoflurane > sevoflurane. These effects are offset in part by decreasing the cerebral metabolic rate for oxygen consumption. The net effect for each anesthetic is described below.

All of the inhaled anesthetics reduce the requirements for non-depolarizing neuromuscular blocking drugs (NMBDs) to produce a standard degree of neuromuscular blockade. This relaxant enhancing effect may be useful in reducing the total dose of NMBDs administered and facilitate antagonism of the blockade.

All inhaled anesthetics are capable of triggering malignant hyperthermia (MH) and should be avoided in children at risk for MH.

Nitrous Oxide (N_2O)

N_2O is commonly used to speed and facilitate induction and to provide analgesia/amnesia during maintenance. It may also be administered to sedate and to provide analgesia to facilitate IV catheter placement before an intravenous induction. N_2O is odorless and insoluble [blood gas partition coefficient ($\lambda_{b/g}$) is 0.47] with a MAC of 104% in adults. In large concentrations, it enhances the rate of uptake of the inhaled anesthetics, accelerating induction (second-gas effect). The analgesic and amnesic effects of N_2O may complement the anesthetic regimen during maintenance. The effects of N_2O on ventilation appear to equal those of equipotent concentrations of halothane. N_2O mildly depresses cardiac output and systemic blood pressure in infants, but it has little effect on pulmonary artery pressure or pulmonary vascular resistance, even in those with pulmonary vascular disease. In infants and small children, the cardiovascular effects of N_2O combined with either halothane or isoflurane to 1.5 MAC are similar to those of equipotent (1.5 MAC) concentrations of either halothane or isoflurane in oxygen. N_2O rapidly diffuses into any gas-containing space within the body (being 34 times more soluble in blood than nitrogen); this contraindicates its use in children with lung cysts, pneumothorax, lobar emphysema, necrotizing enterocolitis, bowel obstruction, and any other gas-filled cavity. N_2O (70%) doubles the size of a pneumothorax in 12 min and that of gas-containing bowel in 120 min. The tenfold difference in doubling time is the result of compromising the blood supply to the bowel as the bowel expands and unchanged blood flow to the chest wall/pleura as the pneumothorax expands. N_2O also diffuses into the middle ear and may displace the graft during tympanoplasty. In some children with a normal ear and an intact eardrum, postoperative absorption of N_2O from the middle ear results in atelectasis of the drum and a later complaint of earache. N_2O does not appear to increase postoperative vomiting in children. However, when treating adolescents for procedures that are associated with PONV, it may be prudent to limit the exposure to nitrous oxide. Clinicians have decreased fresh gas flows as they become increasingly concerned about global warming and ozone depletion (with N_2O having a

125 year half-life in the atmosphere); the sources of N_2O in the atmosphere include natural and anthropogenic sources, the latter being primarily agriculture and industrial.

Sevoflurane

Sevoflurane, a fluorinated methyl isopropyl ether with a low solubility in blood ($\lambda_{b/g}$ is 0.68), a pleasant odor, and non-irritating to the airway, has become the preferred anesthetic for inhalational inductions in children. Induction can be most rapidly achieved by administering the maximum deliverable initial concentration (8%) in a single step, from 0 to 8%. Slowly increasing the inspired concentration of sevoflurane prolongs the excitement period. To mask the odor of 8% sevoflurane, the facemask may be flavored with a lip balm and/or the child allowed to breathe 70% N_2O in oxygen. For older, cooperative children, a single breath induction, i.e., a vital capacity breath, through an anesthesia circuit primed with 8% sevoflurane with (or without) 66% nitrous oxide in oxygen provides a rapid and smooth induction. The effect of age on the MAC of sevoflurane differs from that of the other anesthetics: it is 3.2% in infants 1 to 6 months of age and 2.4% in children 6 months to 10 years. The large MAC values limit the effectiveness of the overpressure technique with an 8% vaporizer. The addition of 60% N_2O to sevoflurane in children only decreases the MAC by 25%. Attempts at intravenous cannulation should not be made until the child is adequately anesthetized and unresponsive. Satisfactory conditions for tracheal intubation without neuromuscular blocking agents can be achieved quite rapidly as anesthesia is deepened, especially if a single dose of propofol is administered before intubation or ventilation is controlled for a brief period.

Minute ventilation decreases ~50% during 8% sevoflurane as a result of a decrease in tidal volume, despite a compensatory increase in respiratory rate. Surgical stimulation reverses in part the decreased minute ventilation. In practice, the addition of nitrous oxide to sevoflurane decreases the MAC of the latter and offsets in part the respiratory depression in the spontaneously ventilating child. Sevoflurane is a potent bronchodilator and effective for relaxing the airways in children with reactive airway disease.

Sevoflurane causes less myocardial depression than halothane, isoflurane, or desflurane and infrequently causes arrhythmias, even in the presence of epinephrine-containing solutions. Heart rate increases and blood pressure decreases minimally with induction of anesthesia. Occasionally, bradycardia occurs during induction in infants, particularly in children with trisomy 21. This may be prevented by pretreating with an anticholinergic. Compared with halothane, sevoflurane causes less hypotension in children with congenital heart disease.

Sevoflurane has similar effects on CBF and oxygen consumption as isoflurane. Sevoflurane increases CBF, although cerebral autoregulation is maintained up to 1.5 MAC. Like isoflurane, prior hyperventilation restores autoregulation during sevoflurane anesthesia and attenuates the increase in CBF. Sevoflurane decreases the cerebral metabolic rate for oxygen the most of all inhalational anesthetics. The net effect is that sevoflurane provides the optimal ratio of CBF/oxygen consumption, and like isoflurane, sevoflurane has a minimal effect on ICP, particularly if preceded by hyperventilation. Both sevoflurane and isoflurane decrease the dose requirement for non-depolarizing relaxants.

Epileptiform EEG activity and myoclonic jerking movements have been rarely reported during sevoflurane anesthesia. The combination of large concentrations of sevoflurane and hyperventilation increases EEG epileptiform activity, although frank seizures are exceedingly rare. Epileptiform EEG activity during sevoflurane may cause paradoxical readings on processed electroencephalogram monitors, e.g., the bispectral index monitor, suggesting that the depth of anesthesia appears to lessen as the inspired concentration exceeds 3%. Caution should be exercised when interpreting processed electroencephalograms in the presence of high concentrations of sevoflurane.

Emergence from sevoflurane anesthesia is smooth and rapid, although emergence delirium may occur in some infants and children, especially preschool-age children (see Chap. 20). This transient phenomenon (lasting <15 min in most) is characterized by restless and inconsolable behavior, inability to establish eye contact, lack of purposeful movement, and lack of interaction with their surroundings. Antinociceptive strategies, including a regional block or systemic analgesics combined with propofol, an $alpha_2$ agonist, e.g., dexmedetomidine, or an opioid during emergence, may reduce the risk of emergence delirium.

Sevoflurane is metabolized (5%) in vivo by CYP2E1 releasing inorganic fluoride; maximum plasma concentrations occur within 2 h of terminating the anesthetic. Although nephrotoxicity after methoxyflurane was attributed to large blood concentrations of inorganic fluoride, evidence pinpointed the mechanism of nephrotoxicity to the affinity of renal CYP2E1 for the ether anesthetics, which release inorganic fluoride in the renal medulla impairing renal tubular function. The affinity of CYP2E1 for sevoflurane is only 20% of that of methoxyflurane; hence, nephrotoxicity does not occur after sevoflurane despite plasma concentrations of inorganic fluoride similar to those after methoxyflurane.

Sevoflurane is also degraded in vitro, in the presence of some carbon dioxide absorbents (soda lime ≫Amsorb Plus). The degradation yields five compounds, the most common being compound A, a vinyl compound that is nephrotoxic in rats. The production of compound A increases in parallel with the child's weight. In some countries, a minimum fresh gas flow (2 L/min) and concentration-time exposure have been recommended for sevoflurane in the presence of soda lime absorbents, although there is no evidence that fresh gas flows <2 L/min present any risk to humans. Absorbents that are free of potassium hydroxide and sodium hydroxide such as lithium-based absorbents do not degrade sevoflurane and have no recommended minimum fresh gas flows. Amsorb is an example of a lithium-based absorbent, which does not degrade sevoflurane. To date, neither sevoflurane nor its degradation products have been proven toxic to humans. If a soda lime absorbent is used, the extent of sevoflurane degradation increases as the fresh gas flow decreases and the soda lime becomes desiccated.

Desflurane

Desflurane, an isomer of isoflurane, is a fluorinated ether with a boiling point of 23 °C and the smallest $\lambda_{b/g}$, 0.42. It is the least soluble anesthetic. It is a very stable compound, with less than 0.02% metabolized in vivo, although it is degraded to carbon monoxide in vitro, in the presence of some desiccated absorbents, e.g., soda lime. However, carbon monoxide is not produced in the presence of lithium-based absorbents, e.g., Amsorb. Desflurane is the least potent ether anesthetic agent with a MAC of 7–9.5% in children. MAC increases with decreasing age, peaking in infants 6–12 months of age, and decreasing thereafter and in neonates. The MAC of desflurane, like sevoflurane, in children decreases only 25% in the presence of 60% nitrous oxide. The MAC of desflurane is subject to pharmacogenomic variation; in adults, the MAC in redheads (homozygous for a variant in melanocortin 1 gene) is 20% greater than in non-redheads. It is not known if the same holds true in redheaded children. The effects of 1 MAC desflurane on the cardiovascular system are similar to those of other ether inhalational anesthetics, although bradycardia is very rare. When desflurane is the sole anesthetic agent, sudden increases in the inspired concentration can lead to a profound central sympathetic discharge, resulting in clinically important increases in blood pressure and heart rate. This may be prevented by prior administration of opioids.

Desflurane is very pungent and causes upper airway irritation when administered by mask; breath holding and laryngospasm are very common (~50%). Thus, desflurane is not recommended for inhalational inductions in children. It can, however, be safely used to maintain anesthesia in children whose airways are intubated. Desflurane is not approved for maintenance in children whose airways are not instrumented; adverse respiratory responses are increased when administered with an LMA in children <6 years. Emergence from anesthesia is very rapid as a result of its low solubility. Airway reflex responses are infrequent after extubation during desflurane anesthesia; however, caution should be exercised when LMAs are removed during deep desflurane anesthesia. In this case, airway reflex responses are more common than when the LMAs are removed when the children are awake. To prevent the sudden onset of acute surgical pain after desflurane, analgesics should be administered before emergence. Emergence delirium has also been reported after desflurane.

Desflurane increases ICP more than isoflurane and sevoflurane, although this effect may be attenuated in part, if hyperventilation precedes its introduction. As a result, it is not the preferred inhalational anesthetic for children with increased ICP.

Desflurane decreases the dose of non-depolarizing relaxants and delays recovery after neuromuscular blockade similar to isoflurane.

Desflurane is less convenient to use than other agents because its low boiling point demands a specially designed, electrically heated vaporizer. A greater concentration is required to maintain anesthesia (because of its greater MAC), necessitating small fresh gas flows to limit the cost.

Isoflurane

Isoflurane, a polyhalogenated methyl ethyl ether anesthetic, irritates the upper airway (with coughing, laryngospasm, and breath holding), and, like desflurane, it is unsuitable for inhalational inductions in children. The molecule itself is stable with less than 0.2% metabolized in vivo, although it is degraded to carbon monoxide in the presence of some desiccated CO_2 absorbents. It is eliminated almost completely unchanged via the lungs; therefore, recovery should be very complete.

The $\lambda_{b/g}$ of 1.43 dictates that wash-in to the alveoli is slower than that of sevoflurane. Nonetheless, isoflurane can be successfully administered for maintenance after an intravenous induction, provided the concentration is increased slowly. Isoflurane depresses the respiratory system to a similar extent as sevoflurane. Recovery after isoflurane anesthesia is slower than after sevoflurane, with a similar frequency of emergence delirium. The incidence of laryngospasm during extubation and emergence is similar to that with halothane (see later discussion).

During isoflurane anesthesia, blood pressure decreases although heart rate does not change substantively. The decrease in blood pressure is due in part to myocardial depression but also to peripheral vasodilation; hence, intravenous fluids usually restore the blood pressure. Isoflurane depresses the baroreflex in the neonate, thus impairing the ability to compensate for changes in arterial blood pressure and for hypovolemia. Isoflurane does not sensitize the myocardium to the effects of catecholamines or theophylline.

As with the other ether inhalational anesthetics, isoflurane decreases cerebral vascular resistance and therefore increases CBF. At the same time, isoflurane decreases the $CMRO_2$, increasing cerebral volume up to ~1.5 MAC in adults. The effects in children are likely similar to those in adults. Nonetheless, with prior hyperventilation, isoflurane, like sevoflurane, increases ICP the least of the current inhalational anesthetics.

Isoflurane potentiates non-depolarizing neuromuscular blocking drugs to a greater extent than sevoflurane or halothane; the neuromuscular effects of isoflurane reverse as isoflurane is withdrawn, thereby facilitating antagonism of neuromuscular blockade.

Halothane

Halothane was considered the ideal anesthetic for children, although it has become all but extinct since the introduction of sevoflurane. Halothane is inexpensive making it attractive in many parts of the world. Pediatric anesthesiologists familiar with halothane consider that it offers advantages over sevoflurane when a more prolonged induction or emergence is needed to facilitate endoscopy with spontaneous ventilation, e.g., laryngoscopy, bronchoscopy, or to manage a difficult airway.

With a $\lambda_{b/g}$ of 2.3, the wash-in of halothane is slow compared with sevoflurane. Halothane provides a smooth inhalation induction without irritating the airways. However, with a 5% maximum inspired concentration and a MAC in children of approximately 1%, the overpressure technique is more effective with halothane than with sevoflurane. However, many more MAC multiples may be administered with halothane vaporizers compared with sevoflurane, leading in part to anesthetic overdose. The MAC in children who are cognitively challenged is 25% less than in children who are not challenged.

Halothane is a potent bronchodilator that depresses respiration in a dose-dependent manner. Its bronchodilator properties make it very useful in children with reactive airway disease. Minute ventilation decreases during halothane anesthesia primarily by a decrease in tidal volume as the respiratory rate increases.

Respiratory depression prevents an anesthetic overdose as long as respirations remain spontaneous (see later discussion). Minute ventilation returns toward normal during surgical stimulation. Ventilation is predominantly diaphragmatic during halothane as it inhibits intercostal muscle activity. This often leads to paradoxical movement of the chest wall. Halothane severely depresses the ventilatory response to hypoxia even at very low concentrations in children of all ages. Laryngospasm may occur during light planes of halothane anesthesia, especially during extubation of the trachea. This effect can be minimized by extubating the trachea while the child is either deeply anesthetized or wide awake. Lidocaine (1–2 mg/kg IV) before extubation may reduce coughing but will not prevent laryngospasm.

Halothane depresses myocardial contractility and heart rate, especially in neonates, thereby decreasing cardiac output. Severe hypotension may ensue if large concentrations of halothane are administered, particularly with controlled ventilation. The combination of a rapid wash-in and decreased cardiac output speeds the increase in the partial pressure of halothane in the child's myocardium, leading to electromechanical dissociation/cardiac arrest.

Administration of atropine prevents bradycardia, which reverses in part the myocardial depression in neonates. Atropine does not affect myocardial contractility in neonates. However, in infants (>3 months) and children, atropine not only increases heart rate but triggers a calcium-dependent, force-frequency response that increases myocardial contractility and restores cardiac output.

The infant's blood pressure is very sensitive to changes in cardiac output. However, vasoconstriction is less effective than in the adult, and halothane also depresses reflex baroresponses. Accordingly, the blood pressure should be carefully monitored and the inspired concentrations limited to 0.5–1% during controlled ventilation to prevent profound hypotension. In children with cardiac failure, the myocardial depressant effects of halothane are prominent, and severe hypotension may occur.

Arrhythmias and ventricular premature beats are common during light planes of halothane anesthesia, especially during spontaneous ventilation and in the presence of hypercarbia or increased endogenous catecholamines. If arrhythmias occur, ventilation should be assisted or controlled, the pCO_2 decreased, and the depth of anesthesia deepened; if they persist, then halothane should be discontinued and replaced, e.g., with sevoflurane. Junctional rhythm and wandering pacemaker may also occur during halothane anesthesia.

Halothane increases CBF to the greatest extent of the inhalational anesthetics (see above) and therefore may increase ICP. At small concentrations, however, this effect is minimal, and if hyperventilation precedes exposure, the increase is limited even in those with space-occupying intracranial lesions.

Halothane is metabolized 15–20% in adults but less in children. Rare instances of hepatic failure have been reported in children, despite its wide and often repeated use. Halothane hepatitis, confirmed by the presence of halothane-related antibodies, generally runs a less fulminant course than in adults. The reason for the reduced susceptibility of children to halothane hepatitis is unknown. Contraindications to halothane include a history of unexplained postoperative jaundice.

Summary

1. The MAC values of inhalational anesthetics increase with decreasing age from adults to peak in infancy. MAC decreases steadily as age decreases from infancy to neonates and preterm infants.
2. The smaller the child, the more rapid the wash-in of inhalational anesthetics.
3. Large concentrations of inhalational anesthetics can cause serious hypotension in infants and young children, particularly when ventilation is controlled. *Beware*: *overdose of inhaled agents is a leading cause of serious complications.*
4. Sevoflurane is currently the most commonly used induction agent in infants and children; it is well tolerated by face mask, a respiratory bronchodilator, and with limited cardiovascular depression (in part because of the limited MAC multiples of the sevoflurane vaporizer).

5. All inhalational anesthetics may be used for maintenance, although recovery is more rapid with those of reduced solubility: desflurane < isoflurane ~ sevoflurane < halothane.
6. Emergence delirium occurs most commonly in preschool-age children after all ether anesthetics; analgesics, propofol, and α_2 agonists attenuate its frequency.

Miscellaneous Gases

Oxygen

Oxygen toxicity is rare, but two groups of children are vulnerable to large oxygen concentrations: premature infants and those treated with bleomycin and several other chemotherapeutic agents:

1. Preterm infants are vulnerable to the effects of reactive oxygen species produced by large concentrations of oxygen through two pathways. First, high inspired oxygen concentrations have been associated with retinopathy of prematurity (ROP). Although this association is far more complex than simply administering excess concentrations of oxygen, limiting the oxygen concentration to SaO_2 of 90–95% reduces severity without increasing mortality. Second, exposure to excess oxygen at delivery increases oxygen free radicals and oxidative stress, which may increase perinatal mortality. This has led to the practice of resuscitating neonates with room air, provided the preductal SaO_2 is >93%. If, however, the infant remains hypoxic on room air, then supplementary oxygen must be added to achieve the target SaO_2.
2. Children with cancer treated with bleomycin are at increased risk for pulmonary oxygen toxicity by the promotion of free radical formation in the presence of excess oxygen. Oxygen toxicity develops 4–10 weeks after >400 mg bleomycin. Risk factors for pulmonary toxicity include a cumulative dose of >400 mg, poor pulmonary reserves, radiotherapy, uremia, greater inspired oxygen concentrations, and multiple chemo-

therapeutic agents. Limiting the risk of toxicity is most effectively achieved by restricting the dose of bleomycin and the concentration of oxygen.

Nitric Oxide

Nitric oxide, a selective pulmonary vasodilator, has a primary role treating infants with acute or chronic pulmonary hypertension as a result of congenital heart disease, persistent fetal circulation, congenital diaphragmatic hernia, and meconium aspiration. It has a very brief half-life, necessitating continuous administration. To maximize the delivery to the lungs in patients with tracheal tubes, the delivery tubing is "y"ed. into the breathing circuit as close to the patient as possible. Nitric oxide is most commonly delivered with the assistance of respiratory therapists.

Helium

Helium is a rare, noble gas with a molecular weight (MW) of 4. It has two roles in anesthesia: (1) to decrease the density of gases to reduce the work of breathing in the presence of small airways and (2) as a nonoxidizable, nonflammable carrier gas. Gas flow in the upper airway and in the presence of a narrowed airway is turbulent (Reynold's number > 2100). Under these conditions, gas flow is inversely proportional to the square root of the density of the gas. Since density is directly proportional to the MW of an ideal gas, substituting 100% helium (MW 4) for 100% oxygen (MW 32) increases airway flow by $\sqrt{8}$ or 2.65-fold. Changing from 100% oxygen to an 80:20 mixture of helium-oxygen (with a MW of 9.6) increases the gas flow 1.83-fold. If the oxygen requirements increase, the incremental improvement in gas flow decreases by the square root of the MW ratio of the gases, reducing helium's therapeutic benefits.

Intravenous Agents

Propofol

Propofol (2,6-diisopropylphenol) is a short-acting general anesthetic with a very rapid onset and offset of action with antiemetic properties. Since propofol is hydrophobic, it is suspended in an emulsion of soybean oil to increase its solubility. All formulations in the USA contain an antibacterial agent (EDTA, sodium metabisulfite, or benzyl alcohol) to preclude bacterial contamination, and each vial must only be used for one patient. Benzyl alcohol may trigger bronchospasm in asthmatic children and may be toxic in neonates. Anaphylactoid reactions have been reported after the use of the metabisulfite formulations. Unused propofol should be discarded after the vial has been opened or in a syringe for >12 h. The dose of propofol to induce anesthesia ranges from 1–5 mg/kg; larger doses may be required for younger infants and unpremedicated children, although the dose in neonates remains undetermined (Table 3.3). The respiratory and cardiovascular effects of a sleep dose (2.5–3.5 mg/kg) are similar to those of thiopental; a brief period of apnea may occur, and blood pressure may decrease transiently. An LMA may be inserted after a dose of 3.5 mg/kg. During induction of anesthesia with sevoflurane, 1.5–2 mg/kg of propofol facilitates laryngoscopy and tracheal intubation without prolonged apnea.

N.B. The ED_{95} values are ~50% larger than the ED_{50}.

Propofol depresses airway reflexes and oropharyngeal muscle tone, facilitating airway instrumentation, e.g., LMA, intubation without muscle relaxant, and difficult airway. The hypertensive response to airway instrumentation is less after an induction sequence with propofol and a muscle relaxant than after thiopental and a muscle relaxant. In the presence of a difficult airway, incremental doses of propofol may be used to facilitate tracheal intubation after an inhalational induction. The advantage of repeated doses of propofol is that spontaneous respirations return

Table 3.3 Effect of age on the effective dose (ED_{50}) for induction of anesthesia or loss of corneal reflex

Age	Thiopental (mg/kg)	Propofol (mg/kg)
Neonate	3–4	
Infant	6–7	3–5
Child	4–5	1–2.5

quickly. Propofol is associated with extraneous limb movements during induction, especially after small doses.

Pain is common at the IV injection site, although it is less severe if propofol is injected into a free-flowing infusion in a large, e.g., antecubital vein. Pain is attributed to trace concentrations of propofol in the aqueous outer layer of the emulsion droplets that trigger nociceptive nerve endings within the vein upon contact. Administration of 70% N_2O by mask, adding lidocaine 1 mg/kg to the propofol immediately before injection, or application of a "mini Bier block" with 0.5–1.0 mg/kg lidocaine for 60 s before IV administration, eliminates or substantively reduces injection pain.

A continuous infusion of propofol may be used for maintenance of anesthesia (TIVA). This technique facilitates a rapid recovery with minimal sequelae (no PONV) and may also simplify providing anesthesia in locations with limited space. It is the drug of choice for children who are MH susceptible or if somatosensory or motor-evoked potential monitoring is required. The infusion rates for children are greater than those in adults but vary depending on concurrent medications. Propofol clearance is less in preterm and full-term neonates and infants less than 1 year of age than children; repeat doses or a large infusion rate may cause drug accumulation. Infusion rates to maintain anesthesia should be adjusted to match the predicted elimination of the drug (to maintain a constant blood level) and prevent light or excessive depth of anesthesia. The infusion may be adjusted manually or controlled by a computer, as in target-controlled infusion, as dictated by the pharmacokinetic parameters for the child's age group. These parameters vary considerably more in children than in adults, but clinically useful recommendations have been developed (Table 3.4); intermittent intravenous boluses are also both effective and efficient. Propofol infusions are commonly used outside the OR, e.g., for MRI and other radiological studies, radiotherapy, medical procedures, burn dressing changes, and endoscopies.

Propofol has a potent antiemetic effect, and it is especially useful for children with a history of PONV, motion sickness, or procedures where the risk of vomiting is substantial.

Table 3.4 Step-wise infusion regimen for propofol anesthesia in children

1. Anesthesia may be induced by inhalation (in such cases, a loading dose may be unnecessary)
2. Loading sleep dose: 2.5–5 mg/kg
3. Initial infusion rate (first 20 min)[a]: 200–300 μg/kg/min or 12–18 mg/kg/h
4. Subsequent infusion rates (next 20 min): Reduce dose by 20%; to 160–240 μg/kg/min or 9.6–14 mg/kg/h
5. Final infusion rate:[b] 50% of the initial rate; to 100–150 μg/kg/min or 6–9 mg/kg/h as indicated

[a]Increasing rates (possibly as great as 400–500 μg/kg/min) may be required to prevent movement during radiological procedures in neonates and cognitively impaired toddlers

[b]These rates must be adjusted or supplemental doses administered if signs of light anesthesia appear. If an opioid is used, these infusion rates may be reduced by 25%

Propofol has been used in neonates, e.g., before intubation in the NICU; however, isolated cases of severe hypotension and cardiac arrest have been reported. Thus small incremental doses are indicated in this cohort.

Propofol is not recommended for prolonged sedation in the pediatric intensive care unit due to reports of propofol infusion syndrome (PRIS). PRIS manifests as acute refractory bradycardia progressing to asystole, associated with severe metabolic acidosis and other metabolic derangements, after prolonged propofol infusions (>5 mg/kg/h for 48 h), although incipient PRIS has been reported even after exposures of several hours during anesthesia. Unexpected arrhythmias and metabolic acidosis herald the onset of PRIS; the infusion should be immediately discontinued. The mechanism underlying PRIS is unclear but may be due to impaired fatty acid oxidation and inhibition of electron transport among the complexes in the mitochondrial respiratory chain. Emergency treatments that have reversed PRIS include hemodialysis, plasmapheresis, partial-exchange transfusion, and extracorporeal membrane oxygenation (ECMO). There is some concern with the use of propofol in children with mitochondrial disorders, particularly those associated with fatty acid metabolism. In these children, the smallest effective dose of propofol should be used.

Thiopental

Thiopental has been supplanted by propofol as the primary intravenous induction agent in infants and children. The induction dose varies with age (see Table 3.3). Neonates are especially sensitive to barbiturates because of reduced protein binding. Transient apnea may occur after an induction dose; cardiovascular changes are usually minimal in healthy children. Barbiturates should be administered cautiously in those who are hypovolemic, have limited cardiac reserve, and with a difficult airway and should be avoided in children with porphyria. Thiopental is useful for induction of anesthesia in children undergoing ophthalmologic or neurosurgical procedures, as it reduces IOP and ICP. To prevent thiopental from precipitating when it is mixed/followed by an acidic drug. e.g., rocuronium, flush the IV tubing between the two drugs. Thiopental is no longer available in the USA.

Methohexital

Methohexital is rarely used for induction of anesthesia, although some report a more rapid recovery than after thiopental. 1% methohexital may be painful upon intravenous injection, but this can be attenuated by adding plain lidocaine (1 mg/mL). Methohexital often causes muscle twitching or hiccups—effects that can be minimized by avoiding large doses.

Rectal methohexital is most effective for sedation/induction of anesthesia in apprehensive children younger than 3 years of age, while the parent holds them, although rectal inductions are uncommon today. Doses of 20–30 mg/kg of a 10% solution or 15 mg/kg of a 1% solution induce sedation/anesthesia in 6–8 min. Methohexital is delivered through a well-lubricated No. 10 soft catheter inserted into the rectum 3–4 cm. A diaper should be placed under the child, as soiling is common. Rarely, ventilatory obstruction or depression may occur; children must be closely observed after administration.

Ketamine Hydrochloride

Ketamine, a phencyclidine derivative, has been used to sedate and anesthetize infants and children for a wide variety of situations, although less so since the introduction of propofol. Ketamine may be administered IV, IM, or orally either alone or in combination with a benzodiazepine; oral bioavailability is ~20%. Some recommend concomitant administration of an antsialagogue to block the occasional copious secretions. Recovery is achieved by redistribution from the brain to peripheral tissues. Ketamine is metabolized primarily by CYP3A4 to norketamine, which has about one-third the potency of the parent drug. Clearance is unaffected by age, when normalized to a 70-kg adult.

Ketamine 1–2 mg/kg IV induces general anesthesia within 1 min. For sedation, 3–10 mg/kg IM has a 2–5 min onset and about a 30–60 duration of action. Infants require larger doses than older children and adults. Oral ketamine (5–10 mg/kg) may be useful as a premedication or combined with midazolam (Table 1.5), although this combination should not be used when heavy sedation might be dangerous.

Low-dose ketamine has also been used for perioperative analgesia, particularly after tonsillectomy in children with OSA (see Chap. 11). Ketamine has generally been avoided in children with central nervous system diseases, although the evidence is conflicting. It produces profound analgesia, unconsciousness, a cataleptic state, and amnesia. Ketamine increases CBF, ICP, and $CMRO_2$. The airway is usually well maintained, but secretions may induce laryngospasm. Apnea is rare if other sedating medications are avoided. Ketamine increases both the heart rate and the mean arterial pressure, although it has direct myodepressant properties. In healthy subjects, cardiac output is increased, and peripheral vascular resistance is maintained. These indirect cardiovascular responses are mediated by adrenergic pathways.

Ketamine has limited gastrointestinal effects, although hypersalivation, nausea, and vomiting may occur. Aspiration is extremely rare with ketamine. Ketamine is infrequently associated with emergence phenomena, including hallucinations and nightmares, which may be reduced by concomitant administration of a benzodiazepine and recovering the child in a quiet area. The effects of ketamine on ICP and CBF remain controversial. Ketamine has no effect on visceral pain and therefore is unsatisfactory for abdominal surgery, unless regional analgesia is also provided.

Ketamine has been widely used for burn dressing changes, minor skin grafting, and superficial procedures. For prolonged procedures, the advantage of an early return to normal nutrition is outweighed by the slow emergence. Ketamine is valuable for providing anesthesia in children with right-to-left intracardiac shunts, epidermolysis bullosa, and Stevens-Johnson syndrome; for the induction of children in severe shock; and for general anesthesia when facilities are limited as in less medically advanced countries or during large-scale disasters.

Etomidate

Etomidate is not widely used in children. The recommended single induction dose is 0.2–0.3 mg/kg IV; repeat doses or infusions should be avoided. Pain on injection, random movements, myoclonus, and laryngospasm have been reported. Pretreatment with IV lidocaine may attenuate these effects. Its main advantage is cardiovascular stability in hypovolemic patients or those with cardiovascular disease, e.g., cardiomyopathy. However, a major concern which may have clinical implications in critically ill children, is suppression of adrenocortical function, which may persist for 24 h, even after a single dose.

Midazolam

Midazolam is a water-soluble benzodiazepine with anterograde amnestic properties that is an effective premedication that may be administered PO, IV, IN, or per rectum (see Table 1.5). It has an oral bioavailability in young children of 35% and an elimination half-life of ~3 h after a single oral or IV dose. IN instillation causes nasal irritation in older children. Rectal administration may be unpredictable. Ventilation and cardiovascular homeostasis are generally maintained. Midazolam does not reduce emergence delirium; its effects on postdischarge behavior are conflicting. Midazolam is the only benzodiazepine approved for use in neonates, although severe hypotension has been reported in neonates when combined with fentanyl.

A new formulation of midazolam known as Ozalin® (0.2% solution) is a midazolam γ-cyclodextrin complex. Cyclodextrin renders midazolam palatable. The pharmacology and safety profile of Ozalin® are similar to midazolam. At this time, Ozalin® is only available in the EU.

Remimazolam

Remimazolam is an ultra-short acting benzodiazepine that undergoes rapid ester hydrolysis to an inactive metabolite, resulting in abrief, 8–10 minute half-life, even after a prolonged infusion. Like midazolam, remimazolam confers anxiolysis, sedation with minimal cardiorespiratory depression, and amnesia in adults. Anecdotal reports suggest that a starting infusion rate of 5–10 μg/kg/min provides effective sedation in children, although some required larger doses. Remimazolam is approved for use in adults, but is currently used off-label in children.

Lorazepam

Lorazepam is very useful for adolescents greater than 12 years of age. In an oral dose of 1–2 mg, it produces anxiolysis with a significant degree of amnesia. There are insufficient data to recommend its use in children less than 12 years of age.

Ciprofol

Ciprofol is a new gamma-aminobutyric acid type A ($GABA_A$) receptor agonist that is similar to propofol but with 2 additional phenol groups that increase its lipophilicity requiring fewer lipids, 4-5 fold greater affinity for the $GABA_A$ receptor, and greater margin of safety. Compared with propofol, induction time is similar, pain on injection markedly less, and recovery slightly prolonged. Hypotension and apnea were less with ciprofol, although adverse event rates were similar. Limited studies in children 3–12 years demonstrated that 0.6 mg/kg ciprofol combined with rocuronium 0.3 mg/kg provided satisfactory intubating conditions in 92% (BIS <75) at 90 seconds, pain in 3.5%, and stable hemodynamics. This drug awaits FDA approval.

Benzodiazepine Antagonists

Flumazenil

Flumazenil has a rapid onset, which peaks within 5–10 min after IV administration. A dose of 2–20 μg/kg IV may be repeated as required to reverse the sedative/respiratory effects of benzodiazepines; it may also be given IM to prevent recrudescence. Children who receive flumazenil should be observed for a minimum of 2 h.

Alpha-2 Agonist Drugs

This class of drugs acts at presynaptic α-2 receptors in sympathetic nerves and postsynaptic sites in the central nervous system inhibiting the release of norepinephrine and other neurotransmitters, thus affecting the level of consciousness and perception of pain.

Clonidine

Clonidine is used in children as an adjunct to neuraxial blockade with local anesthetics and as a premedication/sedative, although these indications are not FDA approved (see Table 1.5). In children, IV clonidine has a volume of distribution (Vd) of 1 L/kg, an elimination half-life of 5.5 h, and a clearance of 4.85 mL/kg/min. With a much smaller Vd and greater clearance than in adults, the elimination half-life is approximately one-half that in adults.

When combined with local anesthetics via the epidural route, clonidine 2 μg/kg extends the duration of caudal epidural analgesia by approximately 3 h without side effects. However, there are reports of apnea, especially in infants after epidural clonidine. Hence, some limit the epidural dose to 1 μg/kg.

For oral premedication, the sedative effects of 4 μg/kg are similar to those of midazolam, although the former reaches its peak effect by 60–90 min. Some add oral atropine to prevent bradycardia; mild hypotension should be anticipated. Clonidine reduces the cardiovascular responses to tracheal intubation and decreases the MAC for inhaled anesthetics. Analgesia, sedation, and a reduced risk of delirium may persist into the postoperative period; hence, minimum doses are recommended.

Dexmedetomidine

Dexmedetomidine is eight times more specific for the α_2-receptor than clonidine with similar physiological effects. It is used in the ICU, the OR, and remote sites offering the advantage of sedation without respiratory depression. It is administered as a bolus for brief procedures or as a continuous IV infusion often after the loading dose. The elimination half-life after IV administration in children is approximately 2 h.

Various regimens have been proposed to use dexmedetomidine as a sedative. For MRI, 1 μg/kg dexmedetomidine is administered over 10 min in combination with 0.1 mg/kg midazolam and followed by an infusion of 0.7 μg/kg/h. Recovery after this regimen in children is slightly delayed when compared with propofol. It has also been used for sedation to secure a difficult airway and for cardiovascular stability during CV surgery.

As an oral premedication, it has a faster onset than clonidine. Intranasal dexmedetomidine (1–2 μg/kg) has been used for premedication, although it is not FDA approved by this route. (see Table 1.5).

Neuroleptics

Droperidol

Droperidol is a powerful tranquilizer that potentiates sedatives and hypnotics that is rarely used since the FDA issued a “black box” warning after reports of prolonged QT interval and torsades de pointes in adults. It is a potent antiemetic when administered in small doses. Although droperidol may slightly increase the QT interval in children, it does not increase the dispersion of repolarization, so arrhythmias are extremely unlikely. Thus, droperidol itself does not pose a risk for torsades in healthy children.

Opioid Medications

Morphine and fentanyl are well established as part of balanced anesthesia in children. Alfentanil, sufentanil, and remifentanil have also been used; remifentanil may be particularly useful in a TIVA protocol. In addition to providing analgesia, fentanyl and sufentanil may block the stress response to surgery in neonates and infants. Meperidine is only indicated as a single dose to treat shivering in PACU; chronic administration is contraindicated due to accumulation of normeperidine, which may cause seizures, particularly in children with impaired renal function.

Morphine

Morphine provides excellent analgesia and sedation and remains a most satisfactory agent for postoperative systemic analgesia. Morphine is used in the perioperative period through the IV, PCA, epidural, and spinal routes. A standard initial dose of morphine in children during surgery is 0.05–0.1 mg/kg IV with additional doses as indicated. Dosing regimens for postoperative morphine IV and PCA are found in Tables 20.3 and 20.4 and for the epidural/caudal and spinal routes in Chap. 7. Oral morphine with a bioavailability of 25–35% due to first-pass effect, is prescribed for postoperative analgesia, 0.2–0.5 mg/kg q4–6 h.

Neonates have been considered more sensitive to the ventilatory depressant effects of morphine than meperidine. Several factors have been postulated to account for this apparent sensitivity including differences in the permeability of the blood-brain barrier and clearance. Probably the most important factor is the relatively slower, less predictable clearance of morphine in the neonate, which may accumulate during continuous infusions or repeat dosing. The decrease in the blood concentration after discontinuation of a morphine infusion may also be delayed in small infants. Indeed, sometimes a transient increase in the blood concentration may be observed, possibly as a result of enterohepatic recirculation. Morphine can be safely administered by continuous infusion even in the neonate provided careful monitoring and small infusion rates are used. The infant should be monitored for apnea for 24 h after discontinuation of a morphine infusion.

Codeine

Codeine is a naturally occurring opium alkaloid constituting approximately 0.5% of raw opium. It may be administered by the oral, rectal, or IM route but should not be administered by the IV route; severe hypotension may occur, possibly due to histamine release. The oral or IM dose is 0.5–1.5 mg/kg.

Codeine is a prodrug, which must undergo O-demethylation via the CYP2D6 isozyme to release the active analgesic, morphine (5–15% of the administered dose of codeine). CYP2D6 is less active in the neonate, reaching adult levels of activity by 10 years of age. This may explain the relative tolerance displayed by children to codeine. However, specific populations express genetic variations in the 2D6 activity resulting in negligible analgesia in some (poor metabolizers) and opioid toxicity including respiratory arrest or death in others (ultrarapid metabolizers). Several genetic polymorphisms of CYP2D6 explain these variable responses; e.g., up to 10% of the Caucasians and 30% of Hong Kong Chinese are CYP2D6 poor metabolizers. In contrast, 29% of Ethiopians and 1% of Swedes and Germans are CYP2D6 ultrarapid metabolizers (due to duplicate wild or normal genes or a rapid conversion polymorphism). Furthermore, repeated dosing of codeine in individuals with ultrarapid metabolizer polymorphisms and in others with opioid sensitivity, e.g., children with OSA and/or obesity who desaturate at night (see Chap. 11) may be fatal. As a result, the FDA issued a black box warning against its use after adenotonsillectomy in children <18 years of age and obese children <12 years of age. Codeine is no longer on formulary at most children's hospitals.

Oxycodone

This semisynthetic opioid with potent antitussive and analgesic properties is prescribed for moderate to severe pain. The oral formulation provides ten times greater analgesia than codeine. The pediatric dose of oxycodone is 0.05–0.15 mg/kg orally 4–6 h. It is available in tablet and liquid formulations; caution should be exercised when it is combined with acetaminophen to avoid an overdose of acetaminophen in infants and young children. A sustained-release formulation, OxyContin, is available for oral use; the dose should be reduced in hepatic failure. OxyContin abuse has limited its use.

Bioavailability of the oral formulation is 40%, and protein binding is 50%. The onset time is ~20–30 min with a duration of action of ~4–5 h. The terminal elimination half-life is 4 h in neonates and infants <2 months and 2 h in infants 2 months to 8 years. It is metabolized via CYP3A4 to noroxycodone (major metabolite) and CYP2D6 to oxymorphone (minor). The dose should be reduced in children with renal impairment.

Hydrocodone

This semisynthetic μ-receptor opioid analgesic is derived from codeine, with antitussive and analgesic properties for moderate to severe pain. It is 20–50% protein bound, with an onset time of ~20 min and a duration of ~4 h. Its potency exceeds that of codeine; based on its oral bioavailability, 5 mg of hydrocodone is equianalgesic with 30 mg of codeine. Caution should be exercised if it is combined with acetaminophen to avoid an overdose of acetaminophen.

Hydrocodone undergoes hepatic metabolism via both CYP2D6 (to hydromorphone) and CYP3A4 (to norhydrocodone) pathways. Hydromorphone is a more potent analgesic than the parent compound, which could render ultrarapid metabolizers of CYP2D6 susceptible to exaggerated opioid effects. Inhibitors of CYP3A4, including clarithromycin and valproic acid, may delay the elimination of hydrocodone. Furthermore, both hydromorphone and norhydrocodone depend on uridine diphosphate glucuronosyltransferase for their elimination, rendering those with reduced activity of this enzyme susceptible to prolonged effects of these metabolites.

Fentanyl

Fentanyl is a potent short-acting synthetic opioid whose metabolism is age dependent: neonates, and especially preterm infants, metabolize fentanyl more slowly than older infants. IV dosing 1–2 μg/kg provides analgesia for brief surgery. If extubation is planned after surgery, an infusion of 2–4 μg/kg/h may be used to supplement N_2O during balanced anesthesia. However, larger doses should not be given to small infants unless they are ventilated or closely monitored postoperatively. The context-sensitive half-life of fentanyl after continuous infusion increases rapidly as the duration of the infusion increases. Rebound of fentanyl blood levels may occur and cause depression of ventilation; therefore, if large doses have been given, the child must be carefully monitored. Infants older than 3 months of age may be less sensitive to fentanyl-induced ventilatory depression and have been demonstrated to metabolize the drug more rapidly. Bradycardia may occur after fentanyl unless it is preceded by an anticholinergic agent, e.g., atropine or pancuronium. Chest wall (muscle) rigidity may infrequently occur after IV fentanyl in infants and children.

In neonates, increased intra-abdominal pressure, e.g., repaired omphalocele or intestinal obstruction, slows the clearance of fentanyl by reducing hepatic blood flow. As a sole analgesic agent in neonates, 15–20 μg/kg IV fentanyl blocks the stress response in infants undergoing intra-abdominal surgery, whereas 25–50 μg/kg blocks the stress response to PDA surgery. Supplemental fentanyl may not be required for 60–90 min.

Infants who receive large doses of fentanyl over a prolonged period may develop tolerance, and a significant number may also show signs of dependence. This effect is common in infants who have been treated with a fentanyl infusion for a period of days. Such infants subsequently require escalating doses to prevent responses to stimulation. It may then be appropriate to substitute another analgesic drug. A methadone program may be required to wean the child off opioid dependency. Neonatal abstinence syndrome may occur when fentanyl is withdrawn after continued use for as little as 7 days; it is characterized by crying, hyperactivity, fever, tremors, abdominal distention, poor feeding and sleeping, and—in the extreme case—vomiting and convulsions. These sequelae can be avoided by tapering the opioid dose slowly but may require intervention with methadone.

Remifentanil

Remifentanil, an ultrashort-acting synthetic opioid, is administered as a continuous infusion. It is supplied as a lyophilized powder that requires reconstitution. The kinetics of remifentanil are unique: its elimination half-life, which is 3–10 min, is independent of both the dose and the duration of the infusion as well as hepatic and renal immaturity. Its context-sensitive half-life is constant, approximately 4 min. Its action is terminated by hydrolysis of an ester bond by ubiquitous tissue esterase enzymes.

The intravenous loading dose is 0.5–2.0 μg/kg, and the maintenance dose is 0.05–2.0 μg/kg/min. The loading dose should be administered slowly to prevent chest wall rigidity. As an analgesic, the potency of remifentanil is 20–30-fold greater than that of alfentanil. The maintenance dose is reduced by half if a potent inhaled agent is administered. This is the only opioid with a shorter elimination half-life in neonates and infants less than 4 months of age than adults; this offers a great advantage in instances where an intense but brief opioid effect is desired in this cohort. The rapid offset of the analgesia once an infusion is discontinued requires that an alternative analgesic be administered before discontinuing remifentanil to prevent severe acute pain. This drug should only be administered by an infusion pump (with a separate carrier by pump) and should be diluted to 5 μg/mL in neonates and infants, compared with the dilution of 50 μg/mL in adults. Remifentanil is a very useful adjunctive agent in a TIVA protocol. The side effects from remifentanil are similar to those of other opioids and include bradycardia, hypotension, apnea, chest wall rigidity, and vomiting; a vagolytic agent may be indicated to prevent bradycardia. Acute tolerance after remifentanil has been reported but is dose dependent; tolerance is less likely after smaller (0.3 μg/kg/min) rather than larger (>0.6 μg/kg/min) infusion rates.

Hydromorphone (Dilaudid)

Hydromorphone is a potent mu-receptor opioid that is more lipophilic and 5–7 times more potent than morphine. It is used to treat acute pain as an IV bolus or infusion (including PCA) as well as epidurally in children. The oral dose of hydromorphone is 0.03–0.08 mg/kg/dose q3–4 h and the IV dose is 5–10 μg/kg/dose q2–4h. Hydromorphone may be used with PCA: bolus doses of 2–4 μg/kg with a lockout of 8–15 min are recommended with an optional basal infusion rate of 2–4 μg/kg/h.

Oral hydromorphone is rapidly absorbed in the duodenum (within 30–60 min) resulting in 60% bioavailability as a result of first-pass metabolism. Hydromorphone is less than 20% protein bound; 95% is eliminated as the 3-glucuronide metabolite. Although clearance in children is double that in adults, its large volume of distribution offsets the rapid clearance resulting in an elimination half-life of 1–3 h, similar to that in adults. Renal and hepatic failure delay elimination of both the parent compound and the 3-glucuronide metabolite. Although the metabolite is inactive, it may accumulate in renal/hepatic insufficiency producing neuro-excitatory side effects including allodynia and seizures.

Methadone

This racemic opioid is increasingly used in infants and children because of its prolonged duration of action, inactive metabolites, and lipophilicity. Parenteral methadone is fivefold more potent than morphine; thus, ~20 μg/kg methadone should provide equivalent analgesia to ~100 μg/kg morphine. It has a high bioavailability after oral administration. Protein binding ranges from 60 to 90%. The clearance and volume of distribution are age independent despite its dependency on CYP3A4 for 60% of its metabolism, with lesser contributions from CYP2D6 and CYP2B6. The metabolites are inactive analgesics. The elimination half-life for the racemate is ~15–60 h. Side effects are similar to those of other opioids including apnea, nausea and vomiting, and sedation. Methadone prolongs the QT interval, although there is no evidence that it increases the dispersion of repolarization. It has been associated with torsades de pointes and ventricular fibrillation in adult patients with chronic cardiac or liver disease or those abusing drugs.

Sufentanil

Sufentanil is ten times more potent than fentanyl and has a smaller elimination half-life. Clearance is slower in infants younger than 1 month of age. Sufentanil has been administered in large doses during cardiac surgery in infants, producing cardiovascular stability, minimal depression of ventricular function, and favorable metabolic and neuroendocrine responses.

Alfentanil

Alfentanil has a more rapid onset and a shorter duration of action than fentanyl and a greater incidence of vomiting than other opioids. It is less lipophilic than fentanyl and is extensively protein bound. Most of the drug is metabolized in the liver; <1% is excreted via the kidney unchanged. Clearance is slower and more variable in young infants, especially preterm infants. Otherwise, in older infants and children, the pharmacokinetics are similar to those in adults. The drug has minimal cardiovascular effects. Alfentanil, 35 μg/kg as a bolus followed by intermittent doses of 10 μg/kg every 10–15 min, has been suggested as suitable for children. A continuous infusion may be used, but remifentanil may be the preferred drug (see previous discussion).

Oliceridine

Oliceridine is a new G-protein selective agonist of the μ-receptor with limited agonism of the beta-arrestin-2 resulting in analgesia comparable to morphine but with fewer adverse effects, e.g., respiratory depression. Evidence suggests that it depends on P-glycoprotein to cross the blood-brain barrier. It was approved by the FDA for adults in 2020, although pediatric studies have not been forthcoming. In adults, dosing begins with 1.5 mg IV followed by demand doses of 0.35–0.5 mg IV.

Opioid Antagonists.

Provided opioids are carefully administered, they rarely require antagonism after general anesthesia. If the opioids have been completely antagonized, the child may experience severe pain; alternatively, if they have been inadequately antagonized, recrudescence of sedation or airway obstruction may recur.

Naloxone Hydrochloride

Naloxone hydrochloride (Narcan), an *N*-allyl derivative of oxymorphone HCl, antagonizes opioids; respiratory depression may be reversed with as little as 0.5 μg/kg IV, although larger doses (up to 100 μg/kg) may be required. Repeated small doses titrated to effect to reverse opioid-induced respiratory depression without affecting the analgesia are preferred unless apnea has occurred, in which case a full dose is indicated. The same cumulative dose that reversed the respiratory depression may also be administered intramuscularly to prevent recrudescence. Naloxone is contraindicated in children who are opioid dependent.

Neuromuscular Blocking Drugs

Neuromuscular blocking drugs are widely used to facilitate tracheal intubation and provide muscle relaxation during controlled ventilation and surgery. The pharmacodynamic effects in infants often differ compared with adults. The neuromuscular junction in infancy has less reserve than that of the adult. Fade occurs at high rates of stimulation. This has led to the suggestion that infants show a myasthenic response and would be sensitive to non-depolarizing relaxants. In fact, to produce a similar degree of block, infants and adults require similar doses of relaxants on a milligram-per-kilogram basis (due to a larger volume of distribution), but the variability in dose requirements and intervals between doses is greater (due to reduced clearance). It is prudent to monitor the degree of neuromuscular block to guide dosage.

Depolarizing Muscle Relaxant

Succinylcholine

Succinylcholine is the only depolarizing relaxant in clinical use. Its onset and offset are more rapid than those of other relaxants. Succinylcholine is metabolized, by pseudocholinesterase of which there are five major alleles: typical (E^u), atypical (E^a), fluoride resistant (E^f), silent gene (E^s), and C_5 variant (or Cynthiana). E^a, E^f, and E^s have reduced pseudocholinesterase activity, with the homozygote genotypes expressing less activity than the heterozygote genotype, thus prolonging the duration of action of succinylcholine, whereas the C_5 variant is an ultrarapid metabolizer, abbreviating the duration of paralysis.

Succinylcholine may be administered IV, IM, or intralingually. IV succinylcholine (2 mg/kg) has an onset of action of 20–30 s in children, reaching its maximum effect within 40 s. IM succinylcholine (4–5 mg/kg) has a slower onset of action compared with the IV route. Intralingual or submental succinylcholine may be emergently used when other routes are not accessible; this route could cause a lingual hematoma. Infants and children require a relatively larger dose of succinylcholine than adults (2 vs. 1 mg/kg, respectively) due to their large extracellular fluid compartment.

Bradycardia occurs commonly after a single dose of IV succinylcholine in infants and children. This can be prevented by prior administration of intravenous atropine (0.02 mg/kg) or glycopyrrolate (0.01 mg/kg). IM succinylcholine (4–5 mg/kg) changes the heart rate and rhythm minimally, even in anesthetized children who have not received atropine. There is no minimum dose of atropine.

Although myoglobinemia and myoglobinuria occur more commonly after succinylcholine in children than in adults, especially if halothane precedes succinylcholine, the incidence of strong fasciculations and muscle pain is less. Nonetheless, children who are ambulatory may benefit from pretreatment with a non-depolarizing relaxant (10% of an intubating dose) to reduce postoperative muscle pain. Serious rhabdomyolysis, severe myoglobinuria, and hyperkalemic cardiac arrest may occur in young children with myopathies (including Duchenne muscular dystrophy).

Masseter spasm has been reported in ~1% of children who received IV succinylcholine after a halothane induction. However transient masseter spasm is a normal variant and generally relaxes allowing the mandible to be opened. However a very small percentage of such cases result in masseter tetany ("jaws of steel") during which the mandible cannot be opened preventing insertion of the laryngoscope blade; generally these children can still be readily ventilated as they are otherwise paralyzed. This condition is strongly associated with MH, and the halothane-caffeine contracture test is positive in ~50%; the child should be monitored and investigated accordingly (see Chap. 8).

Succinylcholine does not decrease the gastric-esophageal barrier pressure in part, because some muscles of the crura of the diaphragm are not skeletal in origin. Intraocular pressure increases transiently after succinylcholine (~5–10 mmHg) because of greater tension in the smooth muscles lining the globe of the eye and possible dilation of the choroidal blood vessels. If intraocular pressure is to be measured, e.g., for glaucoma, or if forced duction testing is planned, e.g., for strabismus surgery, it may be best to avoid succinylcholine. If succinylcholine is considered for a child with an open globe injury, the ophthalmologist should be consulted, as pinpoint punctures of the globe are less likely to lead to extrusion of intraocular contents after succinylcholine than are large (>4 mm) lacerations. Alternatively, high-dose rocuronium (1.2 mg/kg) provides similar intubating conditions in children 30 s after administration.

Serum potassium levels do not increase in children with cerebral palsy who receive succinylcholine, but they do increase in children with burns beyond the first 24 h, crush injury, muscle and neurologic diseases (upper and lower motor neuron lesions), chronic bedridden conditions, and renal failure. These increases in K^+ may result in ventricular tachycardia. Intravenous calcium chloride (or gluconate) and other measures to treat acute hyperkalemia must be initiated immediately and repeated as needed to restore cardiac rhythm and cardiac output.

Intermediate-Acting Non-depolarizing Neuromuscular Blocking Agents

Rocuronium

Rocuronium is a steroid-based, non-depolarizing muscle relaxant that has a more rapid onset and shorter duration of action but similar hemodynamic stability as vecuronium. The rapid onset of rocuronium stems from its reduced potency, one-sixth that of vecuronium. The speed of onset of blockade is dose dependent, with an ED_{95} in infants of ~0.25 mg/kg and in children of ~0.4 mg/

kg IV. Low-dose rocuronium (0.3 mg/kg) provides satisfactory intubating conditions after 3 min and can be antagonized within 15–20 min. A dose of 1.2 mg/kg is recommended for rapid sequence intubations with an expected prolonged duration of effect (~75 min). Rocuronium may also be administered as a continuous infusion (10 μg/kg/min and adjusted up or down by 2–3 μg/kg/min according to the train-of-four response). All inhalational anesthetics potentiate the effects of rocuronium. The duration of action of an intubating dose (twice the ED_{95}), 0.6 mg/kg, in infants during nitrous oxide/opioid anesthesia is 50% greater than that in older children, 42 vs. 27 min. Recovery after similar weight-based dosing increases with decreasing age. Rocuronium is extensively metabolized by the liver (70–90%, possibly via CYP3A4 and CYP2C19) and excreted through the biliary tract. Onset time and recovery of the twitch are prolonged ~50% in liver failure due to an increased Vd. The duration of action of rocuronium is increased in adults in renal failure, but not in children after 0.3 mg/kg.

Rocuronium causes pain on injection, an effect that may be mitigated by prior treatment with propofol, lidocaine, or remifentanil. Rocuronium is devoid of cardiovascular and histamine effects. It should be noted that co-administration of thiopental and rocuronium precipitates thiopental and may block the IV cannula.

Vecuronium

Vecuronium (lyophilized powder) is an intermediate-acting nondepolarizing steroidal neuromuscular blocking agent devoid of cardiovascular effects and histamine release that has been supplanted by rocuronium. The ED_{95} in infants is 47 μg/kg; in children 2–10 years old, 81 μg/kg; and in adolescents, 55 μg/kg. Its duration of action in children is 35–45 min but prolonged in neonates, ≥70 min. The duration of action of vecuronium increases in liver disease and renal impairment. Because vecuronium has no vagal blocking effect, bradycardia may occur if vagotonic drugs are coadministered; atropine may be required. Vecuronium may also be administered as a continuous infusion in infants at ~1–2 μg/kg/min, and in older children, ~2–3 μg/kg/min.

Atracurium

Atracurium, a benzylisoquinolinium, is a non-depolarizing neuromuscular blocking agent with an intermediate duration of action (~30 min). It is a mixture of ten stereoisomers that vary in potency and side effects. It is infrequently used, having been replaced by *cis*-atracurium. Atracurium degrades spontaneously at physiologic pH to inactive compounds (Hofmann elimination) and hence has a predictable rate of elimination that is unaffected by the presence of severe disease or immaturity of hepatic or renal function. Hence, this drug is ideally administered as a continuous infusion particularly in neonates. In children, an initial bolus of 0.3–0.4 mg/kg followed by an infusion of ~9 μg/kg/min (and the adjusted ±1–2 μg/kg/min based on the train-of-four response) during TIVA and 6 μg/kg/min during an inhalational anesthetic provides satisfactory relaxation. Neonates require ~25% less. Atracurium has little effect on the cardiovascular system at normal doses, although it does release histamine, especially if administered as a rapid IV bolus, which could cause hypotension. Atracurium is best avoided in children with asthma. A rash is common, but significant hypotension is uncommon.

Cisatracurium

Cisatracurium, one of the ten stereoisomers of atracurium besylate, confers the most stable hemodynamics and least histamine release of the isomers, having largely supplanted atracurium in clinical practice. It has a relatively slow onset of action. The dose for tracheal intubation is 0.15–0.2 mg/kg, with a duration of action of ~35 min. Cisatracurium may be administered by infusion (1–2 μg/kg/min). Its action is also terminated via Hofmann elimination and ester hydrolysis. The duration of action of cisatracurium is unaffected by renal or hepatic failure and in neonates.

Long-Acting Non-depolarizing Relaxants

Pancuronium

Pancuronium is the only non-depolarizing relaxant available with a prolonged duration of action. It is excreted principally via the kidney; its elimination half-life may be quite prolonged in renal failure.

An initial dose of 0.1 mg/kg IV permits intubation in about 2 minutes. Supplementary doses should be guided using a nerve stimulator; additional doses should generally be ~10–20% of the initial paralyzing dose. Pancuronium has a vagolytic effect and causes an increase in heart rate and blood pressure, particularly when given as a rapid intravenous bolus. These effects are more pronounced in younger patients. In preterm infants, pancuronium causes a sustained tachycardia and hypertension and increased plasma epinephrine levels. In practice, if pancuronium is combined with fentanyl, their effects on heart rate offset one another resulting in stable hemodynamics. Pancuronium causes little histamine release and is the preferred relaxant for prolonged surgery and in children with asthma.

Antagonism of Neuromuscular Blockade

Non-depolarizing neuromuscular blocking agents should always be antagonized unless the child has completely recovered normal neuromuscular function as documented with a quantitative nerve stimulator. Neuromuscular blockade may not be fully antagonized in infants and in children who are hypothermic (less than 35 °C), necessitating redosing. Rarely, antibiotics, e.g., aminoglycosides, potentiate neuromuscular blocking drugs preventing them from being antagonized.

The adequacy of antagonism may be difficult to judge if a qualitative monitor is used. Hence, antagonism to 90% of the full twitch response should be sought. Muscle tone is often best judged in neonates and infants by flexion of the elbows and hips. The ability to generate a negative inspiratory pressure of −25 cm H_2O is also a useful index. When any doubt exists about the adequacy of the antagonism, controlled ventilation should continue, repeat testing with a nerve stimulator should be performed, and redosing of the antagonist should be considered.

Commonly used regimens to antagonize the non-depolarizing muscle relaxants in infants and children are as follows:

1. Neostigmine (50 μg/kg) mixed with atropine (20–25 μg/kg) is effective with the fewest cardiac arrhythmias. Glycopyrrolate (0.01 mg/kg) may not prevent neostigmine-induced bradycardia. In those in whom tachycardia is to be avoided, e.g., hypertrophic obstructive cardiomyopathy (HOCM) or aortic stenosis, it may be prudent to use sugammadex to antagonize rocuronium or vecuronium blockade.
2. Sugammadex is a cyclodextrin that irreversibly traps rocuronium and vecuronium; the complex is eliminated via the kidneys. In children with a TOF ≥2 twitches, 2 mg/kg IV is recommended but for a TOF < 2 twitches, 4 mg/kg is recommended. Quantitative monitoring identifies those whose train-of-four remains <0.9 and may receive a second dose of sugammadex. After a large dose of rocuronium or zero twitches, 8–16 mg/kg IV may be required. Sugammadex effectively antagonizes rocuronium in adults in renal failure, although recovery to TOF >0.9 may take longer than in those with normal renal function.

Nonsteroidal Anti-inflammatory Drugs

Acetaminophen

Acetaminophen is an analgesic and antipyretic without anti-inflammatory actions but is commonly grouped with the NSAIDs. It is useful as an analgesic for mild pain and is also useful as an opioid-sparing adjunct for more severe pain. Oral dosing is 10–15 mg/kg q 4–6 h with a peak effect in 10–20 min. Rectal dosing is 35–45 mg/kg followed by 20 mg/kg PR q6h with a peak after 60–180 min. The total daily dose should not exceed 100 mg/kg. *Hepatic failure may occur with an overdose and is a particular risk in the seriously ill debilitated child. When an overdose is suspected, N-acetylcysteine (NAC) must be given as soon as possible to limit the hepatotoxicity. NAC may be given by inhalation (preferred), orally, or IV. The oral route is not preferred because of the poor bioavailability; the IV route is effective, although severe anaphylactic-like reactions have been reported.*

Two formulations of IV acetaminophen are available: propacetamol and paracetamol. The former is a water-soluble parenteral prodrug of acetaminophen (1 g = 0.5 g acetaminophen) that is only available in Europe and Asia. It undergoes rapid hydrolysis by nonspecific plasma esterases to the active compound paracetamol within 10–30 min of IV administration. The latter is intravenous paracetamol (acetaminophen, OFIRMEV), which is available in the USA in a 10 mg/mL concentration. Recommended doses are: 12.5 mg/kg q6h for preterm infants ≥32 weeks gestational age max 50 mg/d; 15 mg/kg q6h up to 75 mg/kg/d children 2–12 years of age, and 15 mg/kg adolescents <50 kg q6h up to 75 mg/kg/d; patients >50 kg 1000 mg q 6 h.

Several cases of IV paracetamol overdose that led to transient hepatic insufficiency in young children and a death in a young adult have been reported. These overdoses were attributed to drug dosing errors, a dosing mix-up between the prodrug and the native drug, and a lack of knowledge of the maximum daily dose limit for IV paracetamol. Caution must be exercised when dosing IV acetaminophen to document the concentration of the acetaminophen formulation, the correct dose, and the maximum allowable daily dose.

Ibuprofen

Ibuprofen (4–10 mg/kg PO q6h max. 40 mg/kg/day) reduces postoperative morphine requirements and improves pain relief. Alternating doses of acetaminophen and ibuprofen may be a useful alternative to opioids after tonsillectomy. IV ibuprofen 10 mg/kg reduces opioid requirements in the perioperative period, including post-adenotonsillectomy without evidence of increased hemorrhage. It undergoes oxidative metabolism by CYP2C9 and CYP2C8 in the liver with the metabolites excreted renally.

Diclofenac

Diclofenac is a nonsteroidal anti-inflammatory agent that is available in oral (25–75 mg tablets), intravenous, and rectal formulations (50 or 100 mg suppositories). Outside of North America, rectal formulations as small as 12.5 mg per suppository are available. Rectal absorption is slower than oral, but bioavailability is similar. Recommended pediatric dosing is 0.3 mg/kg IV and 1 mg/kg orally and rectally every 8 h. It provides similar analgesia to IV paracetamol. Rectal diclofenac is widely used in Europe for children after minor superficial surgery. It is metabolized in the liver by CYP2C9, and the metabolites are excreted via renal and biliary routes. Its effect on platelet activity is intermediate between placebo and ketorolac.

Ketorolac

Ketorolac is a nonsteroidal analgesic racemic mixture that is available for use IM or IV. It is considered a moderately potent analgesic that is devoid of respiratory depression, vomiting, sedation, and urinary retention effects. The dose for children more than 6 months of age up to children <50 kg is 0.5 mg/kg IV (max. 15 mg/dose), repeated every 6 h (max. Daily dose of 60 mg). The dose for children >50 kg is 0.5 mg/kg IV up to 30 mg/dose or 120 mg/24 h. Ketorolac undergoes metabolism by CYP2C9 followed by renal excretion resulting in an elimination half-life in children of 4–6 h.

Ketorolac should be used only for brief periods (i.e., several days at a time) because of the risk of nephrotoxicity. Ketorolac should be administered with caution to children with impaired renal or hepatic function. Like most nonsteroidal anti-inflammatory drugs (NSAIDs), ketorolac reversibly inhibits platelet function and may cause increased bleeding, especially if it is administered before or early during the surgical procedure. Postoperatively, ketorolac does not appear to increase bleeding, although most clinicians avoid it in surgeries where bleeding may be a problem (adenotonsillectomy, cleft palate, etc.). There are limited data in animals that suggest ketorolac may impair bone healing, prompting some orthopedic surgeons to avoid this agent.

Tramadol

Tramadol is a weak mu-opioid receptor agonist that also inhibits the reuptake of noradrenaline and serotonin. The dose is 0.5–1 mg/kg with a maximum dose of 50 mg every 3–4 h. Its elimination half-life, 6–7 h, is greater than other oral analgesics. This is compounded by an active metabolite with a 10-h elimination half-life.

Tramadol is metabolized by CYP2D6 to the O-methylated metabolite, which holds 200-fold greater affinity for the mu-opioid receptor than tramadol. Both the ontogeny and polymorphisms of CYP2D6 and renal maturation may impact the analgesic potency and cause drug accumulation of tramadol. Tramadol causes less sedation and respiratory depression than opioids. It may lower the seizure threshold in children and is best avoided in those with seizures. The FDA has issued a black box warning contraindicating its use in obese children <12 years of age and in patients <18 years of age undergoing adenoidectomy or tonsillectomy.

Parecoxib

Parecoxib is a prodrug that undergoes rapid hydroxylation by CYP2C9 and CYP3A4 to the active compound, valdecoxib. It is a COX-2 inhibitor that does not inhibit platelet aggregation. Parecoxib is available for oral and IV dosing. In children, the IV dose is ≤ 1 mg/kg IV due to a ceiling effect. Parecoxib confers a morphine-sparing effect after adenotonsillectomy.

Celecoxib

Celecoxib is a COX-2 drug that is FDA approved in children for rheumatoid arthritis. An oral loading dose of 6 mg/kg preoperatively followed by 3 mg/kg twice daily for 3 postoperative days reduces post-adenotonsillectomy pain without an increase in post-tonsillectomy bleeding. The CYP2C9*3 polymorphism confers increased analgesia without increasing adverse events.

Topical Local Anesthetics

1. *EMLA*. Eutectic mixture of local anesthetics (EMLA), a combination of 2.5% lidocaine and 2.5% prilocaine, is the oldest effective topical local anesthetic for vascular cannulation in children (eutectic mixture refers to the melting point of the mixture being less than those for the individual local anesthetics). The local anesthetics numb pain receptors within 3–4 mm of the skin surface. The total dose should be limited to 0.5 gm

to intact skin in infants and 1 gm in toddlers and children; cover with a Tegaderm® for 45–60 minutes for peak effect. EMLA may cause methemoglobinemia if applied to mucosal surfaces. It has several disadvantages including vasoconstriction and blanching of the skin that could render venous cannulation difficult. The cream should be removed after 60 minutes to prevent absorbing excess drug; duration of analgesia is 2–4 hours. Young infants should be monitored, as there are reports of ingesting the cream and the Tegaderm; contact dermatitis has been reported.

2. *Amethocaine 4%.* This concentrated ester anesthetic is widely used outside the US. It has a high affinity for neural tissue. A dose of 1 mg is applied to a skin area the size of a US quarter coin and covered with a Tegaderm®. The onset time is ~30 minutes with a duration of action of 4–6 h. It should only be used in term infants >1 month of age and children. Amethocaine does not blanch the skin, but it may cause an allergic response such as a rash that may persist.
3. *ELA-MAX.* Ela-max is liposomal lidocaine in which lidocaine is encapsulated in liposomes to speed transdermal absorption and resist metabolism. It provides analgesia after a 30-minute application without an occlusive dressing. A dose of 1–2.5 g of LMX-4 cream (4% concentration) may be applied to infants (2–12 months) and children.
4. *SYNERA.* Synera is a self-heating patch that combines 70 mg lidocaine and 70 mg tetracaine. When applied to the skin for 20–30 minutes, the heat increases absorption of the local anesthetic to numb the skin. It was previously approved for children >3 years but is no longer available in the US. Side effects include redness, swelling, and skin discoloration. The patch contains iron, so it should be removed before an MRI.
5. *J-Tip.* This needleless injection system administers 2–2.5 mg of lidocaine using a carbon dioxide cartridge. Analgesia is achieved in 1–3 minutes; there is minimal pain associated with the delivery, but children should be warned about the noise it makes upon administration.

Suggested Reading

Anderson BJ, Lerman J, Coté CJ. Pharmacology of drugs used in children. In: Coté CJ, Lerman J, Anderson BJ, editors. A practice of anesthesia for infants and children. 7th ed. Philadelphia: Elsevier; 2025. p. 77–149.

Kim S, Hahn S, Jang M-j, et al. Evaluation of the safety of using propofol for paediatric procedural sedation: a systematic review and meta-analysis. Sci Reports. 2019;9:12245.

Lyseng-Williamson KA. Midazolam oral solution (Ozalin®): a profile of its use for procedural sedation or premedication before anaesthesia in children. Drug Ther Perspect. 2019;35:255–62.

Olsson EM, Lonnqvist P-A, Stiller C-O, et al. Rapid systemic uptake of naloxone after intranasal administration in children. Pediatr Anesth. 2021;31:631–6.

Thibault C, Pelletier E, Nguyen C, et al. The three W's of acetaminophen in children: who, why, and which administration mode? J Pediatr Pharmacol Ther. 2023;28:20–8.

Vanlinthougt LE, Driessen JJ, Stolker RJ, et al. Spontaneous recovery from neuromuscular block after a single dose of a muscle relaxant in pediatric patients: a systematic review using a network meta-analytic and meta-regression approach. Pediatr Anesth. 2024;34:720–33.

Yang C-Q, Yu K-H, Huang R-R, et al. Comparison of different sedatives in children before general anaesthesia for selective surgery: a network meta-analysis. J Clin Pharm Ther. 2022;47:1495–505.

Pediatric Airway

4

Anatomy

The anatomy and physiology of the pediatric airway are detailed in Chap. 2 and summarized in Table 4.1.

Table 4.1 Comparison of infant and adult airways

	Infant	Adult
Head	Large prominent occiput	Flat occiput
Tongue	Relatively large for the size of the mouth	Relatively small
Larynx	Cephalad position, opposite C2 and C3 vertebrae	Opposite C4 to C6
Epiglottis	Ω shaped, soft	Flat, flexible
Vocal cords	Short, concave, white and slanted caudally and posteriorly	Horizontal
Smallest diameter	Cricoid ring	Vocal cords
Cartilage	Soft, less calcified	Solid, calcified
Lower airway	Smaller, less developed	Larger, more cartilage

J. Lerman, C. J. Coté, *Steward's Manual of Pediatric Anesthesia*,
https://doi.org/10.1007/978-3-032-24545-8_4

Management of the Airway

Mask Anesthesia

Soft cushioned sterile masks are favored for faces of all shapes. Most masks (except masks for neonates) have an inflation port to fill the cushion, which should be partially filled so it can be sealed against the face. Most masks are clear to facilitate detecting excessive saliva and vomitus. When applied properly, the mask should fit over the nose and cover most of the mentum to effect a seal.

Mask sizes range from 0 to 6/7 depending on the manufacturer (Table 4.2).

Laryngeal Mask Airway (LMA)

The LMA Classic consists of an elliptically shaped bowl with a cuff that expands on all sides. Bars cover the stem where it enters the bowl to prevent downfolding of the epiglottis. An MRI study of infants and children demonstrated that the tip of the epiglottis is deflected posteriorly (<45°) in the majority of children, although the airways remained patent. These supraglottic airways (SGAs) have standard 15-mm adaptors and are sized by the child's weight (Table 4.3). When optimally placed, the LMA tip rests against the upper esophageal sphincter, the sides against the pyriform fossa, and the upper border against the base of the tongue, thus encircling the glottic opening. Correctly positioned, the LMA causes

Table 4.2 Facemask sizes in infants and children

Common size designations
Size 0: Premature infants and very low birth weight infants (<1.5 kg or ~3.3 lb)
Size 1: Infants (e.g., up to 1 year)
Size 2: Small children (e.g., 1–3 years)
Size 3: Older children (e.g., 4–10 years)
Size 4: Small adults or larger children
Size 5 and above: Typically for adults

Table 4.3 Guide to the selection of an LMA and the ETT and fiberoptic scope (FOB) sizes that fit in the stem

LMA size	Child's weight (kg)	Maximum cuff volume (mL)	Largest ETT[c] Classic LMA	Largest ETT[c] Unique™ LMA[a]	Largest ETT[c] ProSeal™ LMA[b]	Largest FOB ETT (mm)
1	<6.5	4	3.5	3.5	N/A	2.7
1.5	5–10	7	4.0	4.0	4.0, some manufacturers	3.5
2	10–20	10	4.5	4.5	3.5	4
2.5	20–30	14	5.0	5	4.0	5
3	30–50	20	6.0, cuffed	5.0, cuffed	4.5	5
4	50–70	30	6.0, cuffed	5.5, cuffed	5.0	
5	70–100	40	7.0, cuffed	6.0, cuffed	5.0, cuffed	
					6.0, cuffed	

[a]These sizes ETT pass easily through the LMA.
[b]Olympus Surgical Inc., Orangeburg, NY
[c]ID, mm
ETT, endotracheal tube
An Olympus LF-P (outside diameter 2.2 mm with no suction channel) will pass through 3 mm ID ETTs or larger and through a 26 Fr double lumen tube
An Olympus LF-2 (outside diameter 4 mm with 1.5 mm suction channel) will pass through 5-mm ID ETTs or larger

less resistance to inspiration than a tracheal tube in spontaneously breathing children, and it may be used with controlled ventilation without distention of the stomach, provided low peak airway pressures are maintained (<~15 cm H_2O). The Classic LMA does not protect the airway should vomiting or regurgitation occur.

A variation on the Classic LMA is the ProSeal LMA. This SGA provides a better seal around the glottis (average leak at ~25 cm H_2O peak inflation pressure) and has an esophageal conduit to vent the stomach; this device is easier to insert successfully in small children and is preferred over the Classic LMA. Newer SGAs include the i-gel®, air-Q®, and Ambu® Aura-i™. The first two of these employ a soft thermoplastic elastomer to form the bowl that molds to the walls of the hypopharynx as it warms in the pharynx; there is no inflatable cuff. In smaller children the wider conical mask of the i-gel®, designed to prevent rotation after placement, may become displaced after positioning. The Ambu® Aura-i™ is similar to the Classic LMA but has a smaller cuff to better fit in infants. The air-Q® and Ambu® Aura-i™ are rigid to prevent rotation, and the air-Q® was specifically designed with a shorter, wider tube and a detachable 15-mm connector for fiber-optic intubation.

The cuff should be leak checked (if it is an inflatable cuff) and lubricated before insertion. SGAs may be inserted using any of several methods:

(a) After deflating and lubricating the cuff, insert it following the curve of the palate into the pharynx with the aperture positioned anteriorly until resistance is felt. If the LMA becomes “hung up” on the posterior pharyngeal wall, a finger should be inserted into the mouth to lift the tip of the inflated cuff, reorient the tip caudad, and continue inserting using gentle pressure. Correct placement is usually confirmed by observing the LMA rise slightly out of the mouth when the cuff is inflated. Generally, a leak will occur at ≥~15 cm H_2O peak inflation pressure.
(b) A second method is to partially inflate the cuff and insert the LMA with the device facing posteriorly. The LMA is then rotated 180° as it enters the pharynx. It may also be inserted with the cuff partially inflated but in the recommended orientation with the mask facing anteriorly.
(c) A third method is to insert the mask partly inflated into the mouth with the bowl facing the angle of the mouth and then rotate it 90° as it passes into the correct orientation.
(d) The ProSeal™ LMA may be “railroaded” into correct position over a suitable catheter advanced via the conduit in the mask into the esophagus.

The black guideline on the stem of the SGA should lie against the central incisors when the device is correctly placed. Coughing and laryngospasm may occur if the SGA is inserted under a light plne of anesthesia, especially in infants and small children.

Difficulty inserting SGAs occurs in up to 25% of infants with the Classic LMA; this is more likely in the smaller child who requires a size 1 or 1.5 LMA. The suitability of the Air-Q in small infants may be superior to other SGAs. If it is impossible to correctly position the LMA, alternate airway strategies are indicated.

When correctly positioned, the SGA provides a stable airway, avoids instrumenting the glottis, and frees the anesthesiologist from holding a facemask. It is particularly useful during imaging procedures, radiotherapy, and for other short procedures where mask anesthesia with spontaneous ventilation might be used but the operator is remote from the head of the patient. Some use SGAs during adenotonsillectomy, suggesting that a lighter depth of anesthesia is required, fewer airway reflexes are triggered during anesthesia and emergence, and aspiration of blood is less frequent than with an uncuffed endotracheal tube. In practice, we prefer tracheal intubation with a cuffed tracheal tube during adenotonsillectomy.

SGAs have established a special role in managing the child with a difficult airway. The SGA may be inserted in infants, e.g., with Pierre Robin sequence, after inhalation of nebulized lidocaine and light sedation, providing a safe method to deepen anesthesia and provide a conduit to intubate fiberoptically. The SGA is also useful when ventilation proves to be difficult in a child after multiple failed laryngoscopies. It may also be advantageous in infants with tracheal stenosis, in whom passage of a tracheal tube would severely reduce an already compromised airway. It must be remembered that the SGA does not guarantee a secure airway as does an ETT, and it does not protect against aspiration. However, the ProSeal LMA provides a superior seal allowing peak inflation pressures >20 cmH_2O and with the added advantage of having a gastric drainage channel.

We recommend measuring the cuff pressure since excessively high pressures (>60 cm/H_2O) may increase the leak and cause postoperative sore throat or, in rare cases, nerve injury. If the LMA is inserted with the cuff inflated, it may require partial deflation to avoid excessive pressure after positioning.

At the end of the procedure, the LMA may be left in place until protective reflexes have returned, or it may be removed while the child is still deeply anesthetized. Removal during a deep level of anesthesia may result in fewer airway complications, but a facemask should be applied until the child is able to maintain a safe airway. The incidence of postoperative sore throat is similar whether an SGA or a tracheal tube is used.

Laryngoscopy

In preparation for laryngoscopy, have two functioning laryngoscope handles with age-appropriate blades tested and available.

1. Ensure that the head is correctly positioned and supported.
   (a) For infants and children younger than 6 years of age, the head should be level on the table and supported in a low head ring. At this age, the larynx is positioned high in the neck, and there is no advantage to anterior displacement of the cervical spine because the relatively large occiput accomplishes this naturally. A simple extension of the neck at the atlanto-occipital joint aligns the oral, pharyngeal, and tracheal axes for optimal visualization. External pressure (the so-called optimal external laryngeal manipulation [OELM]) applied to the thyroid cartilage region of the anterior aspect of the neck (applied most effectively by the anesthesiologist using their second hand or a skilled assistant, pushing in a posterior and cephalad direction) may further improve the view of the glottic aperture.
   (b) For older children and adolescents, place a folded sheet or blanket under the head to displace the head anteriorly (sniffing position), aligning the airway axes and the view of the glottis as in adults.
   (c) Beware of conditions that may be associated with an unstable cervical spine, e.g., Down syndrome and Marfan syndrome. In such cases, note the range of spontaneous motion of the neck when the child is awake and inquire about the presence of long-track neurologic symptoms

preoperatively, e.g., wide-based gait, urinary, or fecal/urinary incontinence. There is no evidence that preoperative cervical spine X-rays are helpful in ruling out unstable cervical vertebra, and they are not recommended; however, we advise limiting neck movement during laryngoscopy and surgical positioning. Note that older children may have had prior radiologic evaluation of the cervical spine to allow participation in school sports.

2. Examine young children for loose deciduous teeth. If loose teeth are present, the parents should be informed that it may be safer to remove them once the child is anesthetized. If teeth are removed, they should be retained and given to the parents after the anesthetic (along with a reward from the tooth fairy).
3. Straight or curved blades can be used in older infants and children. However, in neonates, the glottic view with the straight blade is far superior to that with a curved blade. A Wis-Hipple blade is particularly useful since it has a flat flange allowing better control of the tongue.
4. The paraglossal approach is preferred when undertaking laryngoscopy with the Miller straight blade. With this approach the blade is inserted at the right commissure of the mouth with the tongue completely displaced to the left of the blade. The tip is advanced into the hypopharynx, aiming it medially until the epiglottis is visualized. With the tip under the epiglottis, lift the epiglottis to view the glottic inlet.
5. In neonates and small infants, the epiglottis can slip off the laryngoscope blade obscuring the view. To prevent this, advance the blade into the cricopharyngeal muscle area of the hypopharynx and slowly withdraw it until the glottis slips off the blade and the base of the epiglottis is firmly held. Alternatively, a straight blade may be used, as would a curved blade, and slowly advanced along the dorsal surface of the tongue. As the tip of the blade enters the vallecula, lift the base of the tongue to avoid trauma to other laryngeal structures. Do not press the tip of the Miller blade into the lingual-epiglottic fold, as the tip is not rounded like the Macintosh blade.
6. Insufflating oxygen into the pharynx during laryngoscopy in neonates/infants with a difficult airway to maintain the SaO_2

during prolonged/repeated laryngoscopies using high-flow nasal prongs, a nasopharyngeal airway, or an ETT (or RAE tube) cut 3–5 cm in length and taped in the mouth at the left commissure is recommended.

Orotracheal Intubation

A selection of suitably sized tracheal tubes should be available. In the past, uncuffed ETTs were widely used in infants and children, but these have been replaced with cuffed ETTs. The original cuffed ETTs were low compliance spherical cuffs that required large inflation pressures. However, when the Microcuff® tube was introduced, it had great appeal because the cuff is elliptical shaped, requires very low inflation pressures to seal the airway (~10 cm H_2O), the polyurethane cuff is very thin, and the lower cuff inflation pressure should reduce the potential for tracheal mucosal injury. The use of cuffed ETTs in premature and full-term infants remains controversial. If cuffed tubes are selected, use ~0.5 mm ID smaller than the corresponding uncuffed tubes. The size of the ETT and depth to mid-trachea in infants and children are listed in Table 4.4.

(a) The optimal size of the tube is the largest one that passes easily through the glottis and subglottic regions without incurring resistance. Uncuffed tubes are still recommended in preterm and small full-term infants. The presence of a leak around an uncuffed tube at ~20 cm H_2O peak pressure depends on a number of factors (including head position and muscle relaxation). A leak should be tested and achieved between 20 and 30 cm H_2O peak inflation pressure. If the leak is too large, then a similarly sized cuffed tube may be inserted. Conversely, if the tube will not pass the cricoid ring or if it does pass and there is no leak at 30 cm H_2O, then a smaller diameter tube should be considered. If a cuffed tracheal tube is used, it should also have a leak when the cuff is deflated (see later discussion).

Table 4.4 Approximate diameter and mid-tracheal depth of cuffed and uncuffed tracheal tubes in infants and children

Age of the child (years)	Internal diameter (ID) (mm)[a]	Approximate depth of insertion (cm) to mid-trachea from:	
		Teeth	Nares
Premature[b]	2.5 (for infants <1500 g) 3.0 (for infants >1500 g)	6–9	8–11
Neonate[b]	3.5	9–10	12
1	3.0–3.5	11	13
2	4.0	12	14
4	4.5	14	16
6	5.5	15	17
8	5.5	16	18
10	6.0	17	19
12	6.5	18	20
14	7.0	19	21
16	7.5	20	22

[a]Formula for cuffed tracheal tubes: (age (≥2 years) (year) ÷ 4) + 3.5 = size of tube ID (mm); for uncuffed tubes (age (year) ÷ 4) + 4 = size ID (mm). The tube diameters listed are given only as a guide
[b]Uncuffed tracheal tubes

(b) Cuffed tubes are preferred for major surgery, for patients with reduced lung compliance, and those who may be at increased risk for regurgitation of gastric contents. The use of appropriately sized cuffed tracheal tubes does not increase postoperative morbidity, reduces the need to change tubes, reduces OR pollution, and may reduce the risk of aspiration. In children with a known tendency to subglottic stenosis, e.g., Down syndrome, use a smaller size tube; incremental cuff inflation is always preferred. In infants and small children when a cuffed tube is used, the tube may make a tight seal without inflating the cuff.

(c) When using a cuffed tube, positioning the cuff below the cords may place the tip of the tube very close to the carina in small infants and increase the risk of an endobronchial intubation or occlusion of the right upper lobe bronchus. Hence, a Murphy eye was added to the distal end of the ETT. However, the Microcuff® tube lacks a Murphy eye and as such should be positioned with the thick black semicircular line on the shaft at the level of the vocal cords. It should be noted that an in vitro study reported that a portion of the inflated Microcuff® tube cuff may rest at the lower limit of the cricoid ring in cadaver infants. This underscores the need to limit the inflation pressure of the cuffs in Microcuff® ETTs to 10 cm H_2O to prevent mucosal ischemia.

(d) The correct positioning of the tracheal tube should be immediately confirmed by observing bilateral chest excursion, the presence of humidity within the lumen of the tube, the capnograph trace, and chest auscultation in both axillae. The length of the trachea of the infant and toddler is short, so the tip must be accurately placed at mid-tracheal level to minimize the risk of an endobronchial intubation or accidental extubation. Note the ETT depth numerals (cm) from the beveled tip to the teeth or alveolar ridge. An easy method to remember the correct depth of an ETT at the level of the teeth or alveolar ridge is ~1**0** cm in a neonate, ~1**1** cm for a 1-year-old, and ~1**2** cm for a 2-year-old (N.B. The second digit (bold) in this number is the child's age in years); beyond 2 years, halve the child's age and add to 12 cm (see Table 4.4). Tubes must be firmly taped preferably in the corner of the mouth on the up side of the face so that secretions do not loosen the tape.

(e) Avoid pressure on the child's face or head from anesthetic hoses and other equipment by using suitable padding.

(f) The anesthesia circuit and tube must be positioned and supported to prevent traction on the ETT that might cause it to kink or become dislodged.

(g) Remember that extension of the neck withdraws the tip of the tube proximally in the trachea, and flexion advances the tube; 1–3 cm of movement may occur between full flexion and full extension in infants. Always reassess bilateral ventilation after repositioning the child.

(h) Be aware that some neonates and infants have a congenitally short trachea, which increases the potential for endobronchial intubation (e.g., DiGeorge syndrome). Others may have complete tracheal rings with severe tracheal narrowing that prevents advancement of a standard size tracheal tube more than 6–8 cm.

Awake Intubation in the Neonate

Awake intubation is infrequently performed in neonates; our current practice is to induce anesthesia first, then intubate the trachea, as intubation is more likely to be successful and desaturation less likely. Awake intubation might be considered in neonates who are hemodynamically unstable, have micrognathia or a difficult airway, are extremely premature or in remote sites. To perform a modified awake intubation, sedate the neonate with small doses of fentanyl (0.5–1 μg/kg) and midazolam (0.05–0.1 mg/kg) before preoxygenation and IV atropine. Lidocaine (diluted, with the maximum dose predetermined; see Chap 3) may be applied to the oropharynx and palate to reduce the distress and struggling. Use a styletted ETT, and have an assistant position the neonate's arms fully abducted against the head to stabilize the neonate's head. The use of a laryngeal mask airway (LMA) to establish the airway before anesthesia may also be considered (see later discussion). After preoxygenation and topicalizing the airway, remove the facemask and intubate the trachea.

When performing a nasotracheal intubation, efforts should be used to minimize bleeding including the application of a vasoconstrictor, e.g., oxymetazoline, to the nasal mucosa; passing the ETT over a well-lubricated elastic bougie; or telescoping the tip of the TT into the flange end of a well-lubricated red rubber catheter. Warming the tip of the ETT softens it but does not reduce bleeding. The left nostril is preferred since the tip of the ETT [bevel on the left] lines up directly with the glottic opening in the hypopharynx and orients the bevel of the tube on the turbinate side of the nasal passage to minimize trauma. Once the catheter is visualized in the oropharynx, it is snapped off the ETT (either manually or with McGill forceps), and the tube is then advanced into the trachea.

Rapid Sequence Induction

Rapid sequence induction (RSI) is used to rapidly secure the airway with an ETT when there is a risk of aspiration. Undertake an RSI as follows:

(a) Prepare two age and size appropriate laryngoscopes and tracheal tubes with stylets.
(b) Predetermined weight-appropriate drug doses.
(c) Two sets of suction tubing (should one become blocked, another is immediately available).
(d) Preoxygenate with 100% oxygen.
(e) Administer atropine 0.02 mg/kg.
(f) Induce anesthesia intravenously using predetermined doses based on weight and physical status (propofol 3–4 mg/kg, ketamine 1–2 mg/kg, or etomidate 0.2–0.3 mg/kg). Follow immediately with a muscle relaxant (succinylcholine 2 mg/kg or rocuronium 1.2 mg/kg) IV.
(g) Position the child's head during induction and have an assistant apply cricoid pressure (see below); before your assistant applies cricoid pressure, ensure they know where to apply the pressure and how much force to apply. The force required to occlude the esophageal lumen and maintain the laryngeal dimensions in an infant may be as little as 5–10 Newtons or 15% of that in an adult.
(h) Once paralyzed, the trachea is immediately intubated and the ETT cuff inflated. If the glottic opening cannot be visualized, release the cricoid pressure and then intubate the trachea. A modified RSI technique allows assisted ventilation with 100% oxygen while maintaining cricoid pressure (see later discussion).

Cricoid Pressure

Cricoid pressure (Sellick maneuver) should be applied to the cricoid ring with thumb and long finger as anesthesia is induced and maintained until the ETT is confirmed to be correctly placed in the trachea and the cuff inflated. It should be noted however that there is no evidence that cricoid pressure prevents pulmonary aspiration during an RSI, and when applied to the neck of a neonate/infant, it may create difficulties in either laryngoscopy or intubation; practice has shifted to evaluating the risk/benefit ratio of using cricoid pressure in each infant/child. *We do not ascribe to the requirement that cricoid pressure must be applied in all cases.* In adults, 30–40 N (3–4 kg of force) is required to compress esophageal lumen. One pediatric study found that appropriately applied cricoid pressure prevented gastric distention up to 40 cmH_2O peak inflation pressure; however, as little as 5–10 N force compresses the diameter of the subglottic airway by 50% in neonates and young infants rendering intubation and ventilation more difficult. Thus, in some infants cricoid pressure must be released to visualize the glottic inlet to intubate the trachea. Furthermore, as cricoid pressure compresses the upper esophageal sphincter, the lower esophageal sphincter relaxes. If mask ventilation is necessary in a child with a full stomach, it is prudent to continue to apply cricoid pressure to prevent gastric insufflation and limit the peak inflation pressures. Contraindications to cricoid pressure should also be recognized (Table 4.5).

Table 4.5 Contraindications to cricoid pressure

Contraindication	Potential complication
Active vomiting	Rupture of the esophagus
Airway issues	Fractured cricoid cartilage ⇒ may be worsened
	Sharp foreign body in the airway may perforate the airway
Esophageal issues	Regurgitation from a Zenker diverticulum
	Sharp foreign body may perforate the esophagus or larynx
Vertebral/neurologic issues	Unstable C-spine may cause disruption of spinal cord
	Sharp foreign body may perforate the spinal cord
Education	Lack of knowledge, expertise, and/or ability to properly apply cricoid pressure

Difficult Tracheal Intubation

Preoperative Assessment

Preoperatively, assess the airway to determine whether upper airway obstruction during an inhalational induction of anesthesia is likely and whether metrics that have been associated with a difficult laryngoscopy and intubation are present, e.g., retrognathia, facial asymmetry, trismus, etc. If the child has a syndrome, ensure that a difficult airway is not a feature. Always review previous anesthesia records but do not be lulled into a false sense of security by a previous uneventful anesthetic; not all anesthetic difficulties are detailed in the record or child's chart, but even if they were, the ease of laryngoscopy and intubation may change as the child grows. In some cases, intubation becomes easier with age (Pierre Robin sequence), whereas in others, it becomes more difficult (Treacher Collins, Goldenhar, and Klippel-Feil syndromes).

In contrast to adults, examination of the airway in children usually provides clues that suggest a difficult airway:

(a) Assess the extent of mouth opening.
(b) Check the extent of neck flexion and extension.
(c) Check the shape and size of the mandible and maxilla (profile view).
(d) Examine the mouth, tongue size, and palate.
(e) The presence of external ear deformities.
(f) Measure the distance between the ramus of the mandible and the thyroid cartilage.

There are no indices to judge the difficulty of the airway, as they change as the child grows. Inability to fully visualize the fauces and uvula, especially if accompanied by limited mouth opening, also suggests a possible difficult intubation, although the Mallampati score does not predict a difficult laryngoscopy in children. Since successful laryngoscopy depends on the ability to displace the soft tissues of the oropharynx, any deformity that limits this space (short or shallow mandible) or increases oropharyngeal tissue (large tongue and soft tissue masses) can compromise efforts to visualize the glottic opening.

Management Strategies

Confirm that a "difficult pediatric airway cart" with all essential supplies is immediately available. Expert anesthesia assistance and a second pair of hands are invaluable (ASA "known difficult airway" algorithm). Having a surgeon with the skills and age/size appropriate equipment to establish an emergency airway present is highly recommended.

A preoperative anticholinergic drug will decrease secretions in the mouth and pharynx if sialorrhea is present. Consider an anxiolytic, particularly for "frequent fliers," using appropriate monitoring. If the child is not fasted, i.e., for emergency surgery, consider a histamine$_2$-blocker and intravenous metoclopramide.

A recommended sequence to follow is outlined in the pediatric difficult airway algorithm (Fig. 4.1).

The choice of anesthetized versus awake/sedated intubation depends on the age of the child: infants, toddlers, and young children almost always require general anesthesia, whereas adolescents may accept sedation. An exception is advised for certain small infants, e.g., Pierre Robin sequence, in whom maintaining a patent airway and tracheal intubation may be very difficult under anesthesia and who may be more safely managed by topical anesthesia of the mouth and insertion of a well-lubricated LMA while the infant is awake. The LMA can then be used as a route to induce anesthesia and, if necessary, as a conduit for fiberoptic intubation (see Table 4.3).

Standard Management

The classic approach is an inhalational induction (administer 8% sevoflurane), maintain spontaneous respirations, and then perform direct laryngoscopy once an adequate depth of anesthesia is achieved (with or without IV propofol and a muscle relaxant). This method permits determining airway patency and the potential difficulty of direct laryngoscopy. These details, along with the type of laryngoscope blade used and other data, can then be clearly recorded in the anesthesia record. *Although this procedure*

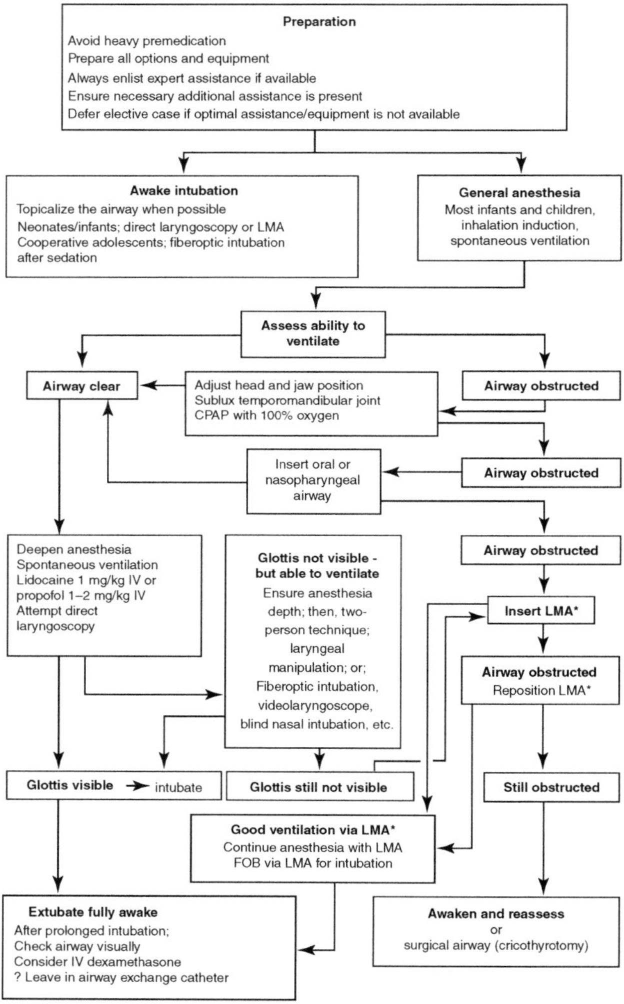

Two-person technique: the second person either inserts the ETT as the operator performs laryngoscopy and applies optimal external laryngeal pressure (OELM) or applies OELM.
*Consider ProSeal™ LMA as it allows greater inflation pressures and the ability to decompress the stomach

Fig. 4.1 Difficult airway algorithm

is still recommended as a standard basic management plan, some children may be more effectively managed by early insertion of the LMA or other techniques (see Alternative Techniques below).

Induction of anesthesia should be performed by inhalation; neuromuscular blocking drugs are generally contraindicated. Sevoflurane is preferred for a smooth, rapid induction. If halothane is available, induction of anesthesia may be slower, but its greater solubility facilitates a more prolonged laryngoscopy than is possible with sevoflurane before triggering airway responses. As anesthesia is induced, the muscles of the tongue and pharynx relax. At this time, obstruction may occur, and immediate measures may be required to reestablish a clear airway.

(a) Adjust the position of the head applying a jaw thrust to lift the tongue off the posterior pharyngeal wall and open the upper airway. A two-handed method is preferred, with one digit behind the most cephalad tip (condyle) of the ascending ramus on each side of the mandible. The finger is wedged in the triangle formed at the base of the skull between the ascending ramus of the mandible anteriorly and the mastoid process posteriorly, immediately behind the tragus. Pull the mandible toward the frontal hairline. This maneuver subluxes the mandible anteriorly and rotates the temporomandibular joint, thereby opening the mouth. At the same time, two thumbs hold the mask on the face. With this maneuver, an oropharyngeal airway is often unnecessary.

(b) If necessary, insert an appropriately sized oropharyngeal airway (measured against the outside of the face, the tip should extend just to the angle of the mandible), but be aware that if the child is too lightly anesthetized, this may trigger coughing and laryngospasm. Initiate ~10 cm H_2O CPAP to distend pharyngeal soft tissues.

(c) When an airway is established, anesthesia should be maintained with 8% sevoflurane in oxygen with gently assisted ventilation to prevent atelectasis. Before laryngoscopy, administer lidocaine (1.5 mg/kg) and/or propofol (1–3 mg/kg propofol) to ensure an adequate depth of anesthesia to permit laryngoscopy. Note: Supplemental oxygen may be insufflated into the pharynx via a catheter, nasal prongs, a shortened tracheal tube taped at the corner of the mouth, or a special laryngoscope blade (Oxyscope). If an adequate view of the glottis is obtained, tracheal intubation is performed; if not, other manipulations should be attempted:

- With the laryngoscope in place, apply posterior and cephalad pressure on the cricoid region of the neck to bring the larynx into view [Optimal External Laryngeal Manipulation (OELM)]. In children with severe retrognathia, consider pushing the larynx to the right to visualize the glottis.
- In some cases, a "two-person approach" to intubation is preferable. One person who holds the laryngoscope with one hand and also applies OELM to align the axes of the larynx and oropharynx. Once the glottis is visualized, the laryngoscopist tilts his head to the left to enable the second person to insert the ETT.
- A retromolar or paraglossal approach may be indicated. Insert a straight blade at the extreme right side of the mouth behind the bicuspid or last molar tooth while rotating the head to the left and retracting the corner of the mouth with a small surgical retractor. The epiglottis is visualized, and the tracheal tube is advanced off a stylet.
- An alternative approach after induction and confirming the ability to ventilate the lungs is to paralyze with succinylcholine or rocuronium; with the availability of sugammadex, rocuronium is the preferred relaxant. This may facilitate intubation, but it limits the time available for each intubation attempt particularly in infants and small children. N.B.: Administration of a relaxant drug might result in a "can't intubate/can't ventilate" situation with an apneic child. If rocuronium has been given, have sugammadex (16 mg/kg) immediately available for emergent antagonism of the rocuronium should ventilation become difficult/impossible.

If laryngoscopy proves impossible by direct vision, the mask should be reapplied, deep anesthesia continued, and other options considered (see Fig. 4.1). Repeated and prolonged attempts at direct laryngoscopy are discouraged because of the increasing risk of trauma and bleeding, thus compromising the chances of success with other methods or by other individuals.

Alternative Techniques

(a) *Videolaryngoscope*. Videolaryngoscopes incorporate a camera at the tip of either Macintosh or Miller blades to visualize the glottis on a monitor. Some videolaryngoscopes include preformed curved stylettes to align the tip of the ETT with the laryngeal inlet. Palatal injuries have been reported while passing the scope through the mouth. We recommend using devices with which the anesthesiologist is most familiar.

(b) *Laryngeal Mask Airway*. The introduction of the LMA has made possible many new approaches to manage the difficult airway, provided the mouth and pharynx are of adequate size. If intubation under direct vision is impossible, an LMA may establish a patent upper airway, although a deep level of anesthesia is required to prevent laryngeal spasm. Once in place, the LMA can be used as a route for ventilation and oxygenation, to continue anesthesia, and as a conduit for a flexible bronchoscope with two tracheal tubes stacked (one to push the other into the trachea and to remove the LMA without displacing the tracheal tube) (Table 4.3).

(c) *Flexible Bronchoscope*. In some children it is impossible to insert an LMA (i.e., very small or scarred mouth), and it may be necessary to perform flexible bronchoscopy via the mouth or nose. A suction channel, present only on larger scopes, can be used to clear secretions, administer directed doses of topical anesthetic, or act as a conduit to administer oxygen.

    If the nasal route is chosen, the flexible bronchoscope should be prepared in advance by sliding a well-lubricated appropriately sized tracheal tube (without the connector) over the scope. After topicalization of the nares and measures to reduce bleeding (see above), the bronchoscope is passed to the glottis and into the trachea; the ETT is then advanced over the scope into the trachea. If the tube does not pass the cords, the tube should be rotated 90° so that the tip of the tube is midline. A useful mnemonic is *UNDO*, i.e., the tip of the tube facing *U*p for *N*asal intubation and *D*own for *O*ral intubation. Practicing flexible fiberoptic bronchoscopy in children with normal airways is essential; ~50 intubations are required to develop proficiency. When a very small endoscope is not available, an alternative method includes visualizing the glottis with a larger scope to pass an airway exchange catheter into the trachea under direct vision, over which the tracheal tube can subsequently be threaded or guiding the tracheal tube into the glottic opening under direct vison.

(d) *Light Wand Optical Stylet Intubation.* The Bonfils Optical Stylet (Karl Storz Inc., Endoscopy-America Inc., Culver City, CA) accommodates a 2.5 mm ID tracheal tube with a video camera and monitor to facilitate visualization of the laryngeal inlet. The Shikani optical stylet (Clarus Medical, Minneapolis, USA) best accommodates a 3.0 tracheal tube. However, these devices have, in general, been superseded by videolaryngoscopes. Recently, the introduction of a stylet with an adjustable tip (range up to 95°) and a video camera on the tip (ProVu™ reinforced video stylet, Flexicare Inc., Irvine, Ca.) ensures that the tip of the ETT is visualized entering the larynx. The tip can be adjusted manually using a rotor mounted on the ETT connector to align the tube with the glottic opening. Infant and toddler-sized video stylets are not yet available.

(e) *Retrograde Intubation.* This technique involves puncture of the cricothyroid membrane with a needle sufficiently large to allow retrograde passage of a guide wire through the vocal cords into the pharynx. This is potentially a dangerous technique with reduced success in infants and small children because of their compliant tracheas and the small tracheal dimensions that together increase the risk of tracheal and extratracheal tissue injury. If cannulated successfully, the wire is then retrieved in the mouth and used to guide a tube into the trachea. A modification of this technique passes the retrieved wire retrograde up the suction port of a bronchoscope. The scope is then guided into the trachea by the wire; this technique is rarely used in children.

Failed Intubation If intubation options fail, consider the following:

1. Awaken the child.
2. Can this case be done safely with mask anesthesia?
3. Can this case be done safely with an LMA for airway support?
4. Do we need a surgical airway?

Extubation of the Trachea

1. Children are prone to laryngeal spasm during extubation, especially if extubated during a light plane of anesthesia. Therefore,
   (a) Before extubation, ventilate with 100% oxygen and ensure that all airway equipment for reintubation is available.
   (b) Extubate the airway when the child is fully awake (or, if indicated, deeply anesthetized).
   (c) Some children should not cough or strain with the tracheal tube in situ during emergence, e.g., those having neurosurgery or intraocular surgery. This may be achieved with a planned "deep" extubation, preceded by careful suctioning of the stomach and pharynx. Lidocaine (1–2 mg/kg IV) or dexmedetomidine (0.2–0.3 μg/kg) administered before extubation decreases the risk of coughing and breath holding. After the tracheal tube is removed, a facemask should be applied, the airway maintained, and oxygen administered until the child is awake.
   (d) When judging whether the child is "awake" enough for awake extubation, wait until the eyes and mouth open spontaneously, all limbs are moving, and the child resumes regular spontaneous respirations.

   (e) Do not disturb the child unnecessarily during the awaking stage so as to minimize coughing and bucking on the tube before the child is fully awake.
   (f) All monitors should be left in place until successful extubation is complete.
2. Severe laryngospasm upon extubation may be followed by pulmonary edema as the laryngospasm is relieved. If this occurs, it should be treated by continued positive-pressure ventilation and a diuretic, e.g., furosemide (see Fig. 4.2).
3. The following are examples of children who should be fully awake before extubation:
   (a) Those in whom tracheal intubation was difficult (see below).
   (b) Those who have had emergency surgery and are at risk for vomiting because of a full stomach.
   (c) Those with moderate/severe OSA.
   (d) Neonates and infants.
4. Children who have had a mouth gag with tongue blade inserted by the surgeon, e.g., for cleft palate repair, are at risk for postoperative swelling of the tongue; always inspect the mouth before extubation.

Extubation of the Difficult Pediatric Airway

Extubation should only occur when the necessary equipment and personnel to reintubate the child are readily available. In selected children a trial extubation, leaving an airway exchange catheter in situ, may be indicated. Children with difficult airways should be extubated or have the LMA removed only after they have fully regained consciousness and when all danger of swelling in the region of the airway has passed. Corticosteroids (dexamethasone) have been used before extubation to decrease the likelihood of stridor.

The golden rule: If there is any doubt about the airway, leave the trachea intubated.

Airway Complications

Laryngospasm

Laryngospasm occurs most commonly during induction of anesthesia but also during emergence and occasionally during maintenance if the child is stimulated during light anesthesia. It occurs more commonly in infants (compared with older children), in preterm infants, children with recent URIs, children with reactive airways disease, after airway surgery, in those with secretions/gastric fluid in the pharynx, and in those exposed to second-hand smoke. It is more commonly associated with desflurane and isoflurane than sevoflurane or halothane and is rare during propofol anesthesia. The clinical hallmarks of incomplete laryngospasm include high-pitched sounds with inspiratory stridor that may progress to silence as the glottic aperture closes. Suprasternal and supraclavicular retractions occur with paradoxical chest wall motion and increased diaphragmatic excursions during inspiratory efforts; if the spasm persists unabated, laryngospasm may lead to severe hypoxemia, bradycardia, and asystole.

As soon as laryngospasm is suspected, the pharynx should be suctioned of secretions, blood, or other foreign material. Initial treatment includes 100% oxygen delivered with positive airway pressure (CPAP) (maximum pressure of 20 cmH_2O) without attempts to ventilate the lungs (Fig. 4.2). Pressure should be applied immediately to the condyle of the ascending ramus of the mandible using a single digit behind each pinna to sublux the mandible while the thumbs seal the facemask to the face to maintain CPAP. Applying pressure to the condylar head of the mandible is very painful, triggering respiratory efforts, which breaks the laryngospasm. Applying the jaw thrust in this manner obviates the need for an oral airway. However, if an oral airway is used, be aware that short oral airways may push the tongue into the glottic opening, thereby worsening obstruction, and longer airways may traumatize the epiglottis and displace it into the glottic opening; in both instances this results in obstructing rather than opening the

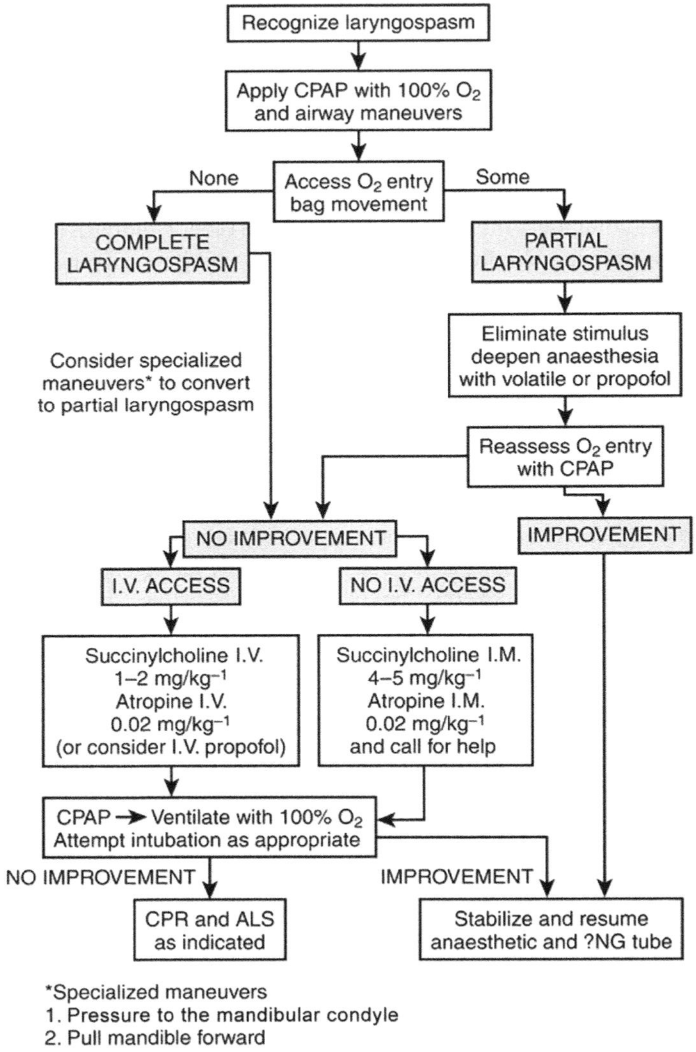

Fig. 4.2 Laryngospasm algorithm. (Modified from Hampson-Evans et al. (2008) with permission)

airway. If these measures fail and the SaO_2 and heart rate continue to decrease, administer IV atropine (0.02 mg/kg) followed by IV propofol (1–2 mg/kg) and/or succinylcholine (1–2 mg/kg IV or 4–5 mg/kg IM). If succinylcholine is contraindicated, rocuronium (1.2 mg/kg IV or 1 mg/kg IM in infants or 1.8 mg/kg IM in children) may be administered before the child is in extremis, i.e., before the onset of severe hypoxia, bradycardia, and asystole. The trachea may require intubation if a muscle relaxant has been given.

Postobstructive Pulmonary Edema

Postobstructive pulmonary edema is a complication that may occur after relief of acute (laryngospasm) or chronic upper airway obstruction (tonsillectomy). The mechanism is the generation of extreme negative intrathoracic pressure against a closed glottis and its sudden release causing a dramatic increase in pulmonary blood flow resulting in low pressure, noncardiogenic pulmonary edema. This complication should be suspected when pink frothy sputum appears in the tracheal tube. Treatment is to continue positive-pressure ventilation and administer IV furosemide (Lasix) as needed.

Postintubation Croup

Postintubation croup or subglottic edema is associated with traumatic intubation, tight-fitting endotracheal tubes, coughing on the tube, repositioning, prolonged intubation, surgery of the head and neck, a history of croup, a history of prolonged neonatal intubation, and Down syndrome. Treatment includes the inhalation of cool mist, IV steroids, and inhaled racemic epinephrine (0.5 mL in 3 mL normal saline over 10 min). This is usually effective, although its effects are temporary and its use may be followed by rebound edema. Prolonged observation or overnight admission may be required.

Airway Equipment

The ideal anesthetic circuit for children should be lightweight, with low resistance and dead space; with low compliance; adaptable to spontaneous, assisted, or controlled ventilation; and readily humidified and scavenged. These conditions were met by the T-piece systems in the past (Mapleson circuits); however, pediatric sized circle systems are now almost exclusively used for children, primarily to reduce fresh gas flows and costs. The T-piece system is generally used during patient transport and by some anesthesiologists for small patients breathing spontaneously. A fresh gas flow rate of twice the minute ventilation is required to prevent rebreathing.

Circle Absorber Systems

The circle absorber system is modified for children by incorporating a smaller diameter breathing circuit and smaller CO_2 absorbent containers. The integrity of the circle system and the correct functioning of the valves and CO_2 absorbent must be checked before each use. The use of very low flows (FGF < VE (expired minute ventilation)) delivered using a circle circuit with dessicated absorbent has been associated with the accumulation of carbon monoxide (CO) within the circuit. The CO is thought to originate from accumulated expired gases or from degradation of inhalational agents (isoflurane, desflurane). Both CO and compound A may be avoided by using a lithium-based CO_2 absorbent.

Manual Ventilation

Manual ventilation is used after induction of anesthesia, when checking proper ETT position, or when there is doubt about the adequacy of ventilation or in the event of sudden deterioration in the child's vital signs. In this situation it is wise to switch to manual ventilation allowing auscultation of the lungs, observation of chest movement, and the contour of the $PetCO_2$ waveform.

Rapid ventilation with small tidal volumes provides optimal results in the neonate because this pattern of ventilation tends to maintain the functional residual capacity and prevent airway closure. $PetCO_2$ levels should be monitored continuously because it is very easy to over-ventilate the lungs of small infants. Hyperventilation (and consequent respiratory alkalosis) causes significant adverse physiological changes including reduced cerebral blood flow and should be avoided.

Spontaneous Respirations

Respirations during the maintenance phase of anesthesia have traditionally been managed by facemask, e.g., during myringotomy and tube placement or after instrumentation of the airway with an SGA or ETT. With induction of anesthesia, lung compliance decreases resulting in atelectasis and decreased FRC and intrapulmonary shunting. To offset these effects, PEEP is recommended, but this maneuver may only partially restore adequate lung volumes. Thus, pressure support ventilation (PSV) may be advantageous in spontaneously breathing patients, improving gas exchange and decreasing the work of breathing. PEEP is set to ~4–5 cmH_2O and the flow trigger is set to the lowest value that will avoid auto-triggering, usually about 0.4 L/min. The pressure should be set to achieve a V_t of approximately 6–8 mL/kg; greater pressures may be required in younger patients. Evidence supports better gas exchange if pressure-assisted ventilation is used rather than spontaneous respirations and PEEP.

Techniques

Mechanical Ventilation

Current anesthesia workstations with compliance compensation incorporate circuitry and ventilators capable of delivering appropriate tidal volumes to even the smallest infants. However, it is also important to apply patterns of ventilation ("lung protective") that will avoid causing ventilator induced lung injury (VILI). This is essential in the critically ill neonate. Lung injury may be caused by excessive pressures (barotrauma) or tidal volumes (volutrauma). Volume targeted ventilation (VTV) with at least 5 cm of positive end-expiratory pressure (PEEP) is often preferred for small infants. V_t in the range of 4–6 mL/kg with PEEP is recommended for the sick preterm infant. The use of VTV avoids the possibility of volutrauma to the lungs, and the use of PEEP will maintain the FRC and optimize gas exchange. The use of a flow detector between the tracheal tube and the anesthesia circuit greatly facilitates this process. The adequacy of ventilation must be constantly monitored. Mild degrees of hypercapnia are preferred to hypocapnia in the neonate since extreme hypocapnia may reduce cerebral blood flow and cause cerebral ischemia. The application of PEEP is essential to prevent a decrease in FRC below the closing volume, which inevitably accompanies anesthesia. In infants whose lungs are already being ventilated in the NICU, similar ventilator settings should be applied in the OR. In some cases, a neonatal ventilator may be used in the OR, or the decision may be to operate in the NICU, the latter especially for those infants who require high-frequency oscillatory ventilation (HFOV). Older children's lungs may be ventilated applying the principles that are effective in adults; current recommendations suggest smaller tidal volumes with PEEP may be optimal in those with lung disease.

HFOV prevents volutrauma due to repetitive lung expansion and permits selection of a mean airway pressure that is optimal for gas exchange yet minimizes lung damage. While it has often been used in children failing conventional ventilation methods, it has a role as primary therapy in those at risk of significant lung damage. Use of such ventilation management under anesthesia mandates a TIVA approach.

Humidification of Anesthetic Gases

Humidification of inspired gases during anesthesia has been recommended to prevent damage to the respiratory tract by dry gases and to minimize heat loss via the respiratory tract and thereby assist in maintaining normothermia. Dry gases inhibit ciliary activity and lead to the accumulation of inspissated secretions, which may, in the extreme, progress to obstruct the tracheal tube. Degenerative changes in cells exfoliated from the trachea after exposure to dry gas have been described, but an increased incidence of postoperative morbidity from pulmonary complications remains unproven. Gases should be humidified during very prolonged surgery and in the intensive care unit to reduce the risk of tube blockage from inspissated secretions.

Humidified anesthetic gases significantly reduce heat loss during surgery, particularly in neonates and infants. However, heated humidifiers are no longer recommended, as accumulated water may plug the capnogram tubing. Alternatively, a heat and moisture exchanger (HME) may be inserted at the connection of the tracheal tube to the circuit. The HME conserves approximately 50% of the water normally lost via the respiratory tract and thus reduces heat loss. The HME is most efficient with smaller tidal volumes and greater respiratory frequency, so it is quite useful in pediatric cases. These normally are very low resistance devices, but if blocked by secretions, they will significantly increase airway resistance; always monitor ventilation when an HME is used. Use of low fresh gas flow in circle systems will also help to reduce water loss.

Suggested Reading

Galvez JA, Acquah S, Ahumada L, et al. Hypoxemia, bradycardia, and multiple laryngoscopy attempts during anesthetic induction infants. A single-center, retrospective study. Anesthesiology. 2019;131:830–9.

Hampson-Evans D, Morgan P, Farrar M. Pediatric laryngospasm. Pediatr Anaesth. 2008;18:303–7.

Huang AS, Sarver A, Widing A, et al. The design of the perfect pediatric supraglottic airway device. Pediatr Anesth. 2020;30:280–7.

Kaplan RF, Uejima T, Lobel G, et al. Intramuscular rocuronium in infants and children: a multicenter study to evaluate tracheal intubating conditions, onset, and duration of action. Anesthesiology. 1999;91:633–8.

Koo B-W, Oh A-Y, Hwang J-W, et al. Comparison of standard versus 90° rotation technique for LMA flexible™ insertion: a randomized controlled trial. BMC Anesthesiol. 2019;19:95.

Larson PC Jr. Laryngospasm-the best treatment. Anesthesiology. 1998;89:1293–4.

Lerman J. On cricoid pressure: "may the force be with you." Anesth Analg. 2009;109:1363–6.

Li L, Zhang Z, Yao Z, et al. The impact of laryngeal mask versus other airways on perioperative respiratory adverse events in children: a systematic review and meta-analysis of randomized controlled trials. Intl J Surg. 2019;64:40–8.

Miller RA. A new laryngoscope for intubation of infants. Anesthesiology. 1946;7:205–6.

Rocha ADS, Habre W, Albu G. Novel ventilation techniques in children. Pediatr Anesth. 2022;32:286–94.

Veyckemans F. Tracheal extubation in children: planning, technique, and complications. Pediatr Anesth. 2020;30:331–8.

Walker RW, Ravi R, Haylett K. Effect of cricoid force on airway calibre in children: a bronchoscopic assessment. Br J Anaesth. 2010;104:71–4.

Weiss M, Balmer C, Dullenkopf A, et al. Intubation depth markings allow an improved positioning of endotracheal tubes in children. Can J Anesth. 2005;52:721–6.

Monitoring and Vascular Access

5

Routine Monitoring

Monitoring during anesthesia must always include the following:

1. Pulse oximeter: The oximeter probe should be applied before induction of anesthesia; oxygen saturation should be monitored throughout the perioperative period and during transfer to the PACU or PICU. The light source and sensor must be positioned to transilluminate a part of the body (earlobe, finger, toe, palm of hand, or sole of foot in a neonate or infant). With the probe placed on the earlobe or buccal angle, the initial response time during acute desaturation may be slightly faster than when it is placed on the finger or foot. In infants with a possible patent ductus arteriosus, the oximeter probe should be placed at a pre-ductal site (head or right hand). In those patients, a second post-ductal oximeter probe is useful to detect shunting. Pulse oximetry provides an early warning of developing hypoxemia; failure of the oximeter to detect and/or record a pulsatile flow may provide a warning about the child's circulatory status (severe hypotension, anaphylaxis, hypovolemia, and anesthetic overdose). If the pulse oximeter fails, first check the child's color (mucus membranes or nail beds), breath sounds, heart rate, and blood pressure (BP); second, troubleshoot the equipment.

J. Lerman, C. J. Coté, *Steward's Manual of Pediatric Anesthesia*,
https://doi.org/10.1007/978-3-032-24545-8_5

The pulse oximeter measures the amount of red (660 nm) and infrared (940 nm) light from diodes that pass through to calculate the ratio of oxygenated to deoxygenated hemoglobin. The SpO_2 accurately reflects the oxygen saturation in extracted blood (SaO_2) for values between 80% and 100%, with an accuracy of ~±2%. However, in the critically ill patient, changes in SpO_2 do not necessarily track changes in SaO_2 especially at SaO_2 values <80% and particularly in children with cyanotic congenital heart disease. SpO_2 may be overestimated in these children. Fetal hemoglobin, sickle cell hemoglobin, and hyperbilirubinemia do not significantly affect pulse oximeter measurements.

Nail polish (blue or green), intravenous methylene blue or cardio green, and severe anemia may underestimate the oximeter reading; increased skin pigmentation overestimates the SaO_2 oxygen saturation and may delay the diagnosis of hypoxemia. High skin temperatures can overestimate the SaO_2, an effect that is further exaggerated at low saturations. Methemoglobin and carboxyhemoglobin (COHb) affect the accuracy of readings depending on the particular oximeter algorithm: the former has a nonlinear effect, either underestimating or overestimating saturation, whereas the latter increases the SpO_2 1:1 with the increase in COHb concentration. The photoplethysmography signal may be distorted by a number of external factors (see Table 5.1).

Table 5.1 Factors that impact the accuracy and interpretation of pulse oximeter readings

Factors affecting pulse oximetry accuracy		
SpO_2 Underestimation	SpO_2 Overestimation	Waveform distortion
Peripheral perfusion	Skin pigmentation	Motion artifacts
States of low perfusion	Hemoglobinopathies	Light contamination
Cold skin temperature	Warm skin temperature	Heart rate of more than 150 beats per minute
Nail polish or tattoos		Electromagnetic interference (EMI)
Hypoxemia, anemia		Sensor placement
Training at high altitude or hypoxia		Henna dye, cardiogreen, methylene blue

Modified with permission from León-Valladares et al. (2024)

An arterial saturation of 90–95%, which reflects a PaO_2 of 30–67 mmHg in infants <29 weeks, is a safe range for the preterm infant. However, because of the slope of the Hb/O_2 dissociation curve, pulse oximetry is less precise in the assessment of hyperoxia than it is in hypoxia. If deemed necessary, an arterial blood sample should be obtained to compare the PaO_2 with the level of saturation. This level of saturation can then be maintained by varying the fraction of inspired oxygen (FIO_2).

The complications of pulse oximetry are few, but severe burns have occurred when an incorrect sensor from a different manufacturer has been substituted. Burns may also occur when a non-MRI-compatible pulse oximeter is used in the magnetic resonance imaging suite (see Chap. 19).

2. Stethoscope, precordial, or esophageal: heart and breath sounds should be monitored throughout anesthesia. Despite the trend away from using precordial stethoscopes, this is an essential aid should the equipment fail. If the monitors fail, check the child before checking the equipment.
3. Blood pressure cuff of suitable width: the cuff should occupy two-thirds of the upper arm. If the cuff is too narrow, the BP readings are falsely high; if it is too wide, they are falsely low. A width of 4 cm is recommended for full-term neonates. A non-invasive blood pressure device may be used, but ensure that it is set to provide readings at a maximum of 5-min intervals. Non-invasive BP measured in the upper extremity correlates more closely with invasive pressure measurements than those measured in the leg; measurements in the forearm and at the ankle in children are unreliable.
4. Electrocardiogram: The ECG should be monitored throughout every anesthetic. Most arrhythmias that occur in children are benign—most commonly, occasional premature ventricular contractions (PVCs); bradycardia; and rarely, supraventricular tachycardia. Bradycardia is often a very late sign that the child is in extremis. The ECG is particularly valuable in children with underlying cardiac conduction defects or repaired and unrepaired congenital heart disease.
5. Thermistor probe (axillary, esophageal, or rectal) (see Management of Body Temperature).

6. Capnometer (end-tidal carbon dioxide [$etCO_2$]). The adequacy of ventilation and pulmonary perfusion is assessed by measuring exhaled carbon dioxide tension. It also provides the most reliable indicator of successful tracheal intubation. Two types of continuous monitors are available: "sidestream" that aspirates gas from the breathing circuit, and "in-line" that measures the concentration within the breathing circuit. The former monitor is more common clinically; the latter is a bulkier addition at the elbow of the circuit. When using a sidestream analyzer with a partial rebreathing circuit, for example a T-piece, $etCO_2$ accuracy is greatly improved by sampling from within the lumen of the tracheal tube for infants <12 kg. When a circle circuit is used, proximal sampling with the sidestream analyzer at the elbow of the tracheal tube yields valid results even in small infants. The presence of a leak around the tracheal tube may also affect $etCO_2$, especially when positive end-expiratory pressure is applied.

   Partial pressure of $etCO_2$ ($PetCO_2$) is the peak (plateau) $etCO_2$ displayed on the capnogram. Normal $etCO_2$ readings are 35–45 mmHg. The $etCO_2$ estimates the alveolar PCO_2 and the arterial $PaCO_2$ accurately in healthy children. In contrast, $PetCO_2$ correlates poorly with the $PaCO_2$ in children who have severe pulmonary disease or congenital heart disease with a right-to-left shunt or mixing lesion; the lower the saturation, the greater the $PaCO_2$-$PetCO_2$ gradient. In those with left-to-right shunting, $PetCO_2$ readings accurately reflect the $PaCO_2$.

   A sudden decrease in the $PetCO_2$ provides an early indication of reduced pulmonary blood flow or cardiac output and may be diagnostic of a pulmonary embolism, air embolism, anesthetic overdose, or anaphylaxis. This may be a useful metric for early diagnosis of cyanotic spells in the child with tetralogy of Fallot. During CPR, an $PetCO_2$ of 10–20 mmHg indicates adequate chest compressions and pulmonary blood flow; comparable values less than this indicate inadequate compressions.
7. Peripheral nerve stimulator: should be used whenever nondepolarizing muscle relaxants are administered. Despite the

availability of sugammadex to antagonize steroidal muscle relaxants, residual muscle weakness continues to be reported. In neonates and infants, technical limitations may prevent serial monitoring (lack of access to an extremity) of the train-of-four and the lack of criteria to interpret the response limit the clinician's decision-making, although in all instances, attempts should be made to obtain objective readings. In children, the train-of-four response and post-tetanic count are most widely used, with double burst stimulation used less commonly to detect residual muscle weakness. Newer, pediatric-designed equipment that permits quantitative assessment of neuromuscular blockade including mechanomyography, electromyography, and kinemyography offers advantages over the current qualitative assessments, although their accuracy remains problematic in neonates and small infants.

8. Arterial catheter: should be inserted for direct measurement of BP and to provide for intermittent blood gas analysis when indicated. The radial or femoral artery is usually cannulated (see later discussion); rarely, the axillary artery may be used. We recommend checking for collateral flow from the ulnar artery when cannulating the radial artery (Allen test). The brachial artery has poor collateral vessels but may be canulated with ultrasound guidance in extreme cases (see Precautions with Arterial Lines). Cannulation of the superficial temporal artery is also feasible, but this site introduces the possibility of retrograde intracranial embolization. Children with Down syndrome may have a single (median) artery in the wrist, in which case arterial cannulation in the forearm should be avoided; always check the wrist vessels in Down syndrome children before attempting cannulation.
9. Urine output: record this at regular intervals for all children undergoing major surgery and prolonged surgery, hypovolemic patients, or those with impaired renal function.
10. Central venous pressure (CVP): CVP is a direct, invasive measure of the pressure in the right atrium that reflects filling volume in most cases. A normal CVP is 2–8 mmHg in the

neonate and 8–12 mmHg in adolescents. Factors that affect the CVP are primarily the fluid status, cardiac function, and type of ventilation. CVP decreases with hypovolemia but increases with heart failure, pulmonary hypertension, pneumothorax, cardiac tamponade, and right-sided valve incompetence or stenoses.

The internal jugular vein (IJV) is the most common site to insert a CVP catheter, although the femoral and external jugular veins are alternative sites. The CVP should be monitored in children in whom major blood loss, air embolism, and/or impaired cardiac performance are anticipated.

Ancillary Monitors

1. Non-invasive Hb monitoring.

   Continuous Hb monitoring is available using either occlusion spectroscopy or pulse co-oximetry. In the former, a digital sensor transiently obstructs blood flow in a digit, whereas, in the latter, infrared spectrophotometry is used to detect light absorption through the finger to quantify real-time monitoring of Hb. These devices may be helpful as trend monitors but are less reliable than actual blood sampling methods.

2. Depth of anesthesia monitors.

   Several depth of anesthesia monitors are available with the bispectral index (BIS) being the most common in North America. This monitor interprets a processed EEG based on a "black box" algorithm from a strip with four electrodes fixed to the forehead. The dimensionless BIS readings range on a scale from 0 to 100; lack of recall at values <75, sedation from 65 to 85, and general anesthesia from 45 to 60. The veracity of BIS assessments in younger patients, particularly neonates or infants, is a concern because the EEG algorithm was not based on pediatric EEG patterns. Interestingly, when the inspired concentration of sevoflurane exceeds 3.5%, the BIS reading increases; a similar response is observed with increasing doses of ketamine. Some studies reported different BIS measurements when the probes were placed on the right and left sides of the head, as the depth of neuromuscular blockade changed, and with different patient positions raising questions about the reliability of the BIS reading.

The BIS is a useful monitor particularly in adolescents during total intravenous anesthesia (TIVA) anesthesia to ensure that an adequate depth of anesthesia is maintained, for example, during scoliosis repair, and to facilitate a more rapid recovery, although there is little evidence for the latter.

3. Near-infrared spectroscopy.

   Near-infrared spectroscopy (NIRS) is a non-invasive monitor that measures real-time regional tissue oxygen saturation (a mixture of both arterial and venous blood) using near-infrared light (wavelength 660–940 nm). Probes placed on the skin (usually forehead) transmit light 2–3 cm below the skin's surface or 10–15 mm into the cerebral cortex in neonates (a depth three-fold greater than in adults) to quantify the relative concentrations of oxy-Hb and deoxy-Hb. The normal cerebral oxygen saturation in neonates ranges from 55% to 85%, reflecting predominantly venous oxygen saturation due to the ratio of venous to arterial blood contributions (3:1). NIRS is commonly used to monitor brain tissue oxygenation in neonates undergoing cardiopulmonary bypass and in critically ill neonates with hypoxic-ischemic encephalopathy and intraventricular hemorrhage. Several factors affect the NIRS readings including the location of the sensor pad, type of sensor, gestational age, skin pigmentation, and conjugated bilirubin concentration. The most important physiologic factor affecting NIRS is ventilation, as an increased PaO_2 increases NIRs and hypocarbia decreases NIRS. Currently, NIRS is not considered "standard of care" as the threshold below which an adverse event will occur has not been defined nor have randomized controlled trials demonstrated the benefit of NIRS to long-term neurocognitive outcomes. However, many centers use NIRS routinely for neonates undergoing congenital heart surgery requiring cardiopulmonary bypass.

Vascular Access

Venipuncture for Induction of Anesthesia

1. The ability to perform a venipuncture painlessly and to cannulate small veins successfully is essential for the pediatric anesthesiologist. Apply a topical local anesthetic cream 45–60 min in advance whenever possible (see Appendix C). Alternatively, nitrous oxide may be administered (50–75% inspired concentration) to sedate and provide analgesia while a skilled assistant steadies the hand for cannulation. Distraction is very effective in young children during venous canulation.
2. A vein on the dorsum of the hand or the foot is usually most suitable.
3. Do not attempt venipuncture unless the vein is well-filled and the site prepared with an antiseptic (chlorhexidine is preferred except in neonates).
4. Use an age-appropriate IV canula, but keep the canula away from the child's view. Ultrasound guidance is particularly useful in obese children or the Veinfinder in graduates of the NICU or PICU who have had many prior attempts at IV access.
5. Be aware that canulating veins in the antecubital fossa, anatomical snuffbox, or scalp may unknowingly result in an arterial puncture/canulation; inject medications only after assuring that the access is venous.
6. Label the date and time the IV canula was placed.

Intraosseous Infusions

When venipuncture is impossible and urgent fluid or drug therapy is indicated, the intraosseous route should be employed. Any drug or solution that can be given intravenously can also be given by this route. In "shock" or "arrest" states, absorption from the intraosseous site may be more rapid than from a peripheral intravenous line.

The usual insertion sites for intraosseous access are the distal femur (midline 1 cm above the patella) and the proximal tibia (medial on the tibial plateau 1 cm below the tuberosity); accidental injections into the epiphysis do not usually cause harm. A bone marrow needle, a strong large-bore spinal needle, or a specifically designed intraosseous device such as the EZ-IO is advanced through the bone until a "give" is noted and the needle stands rigidly. At this point, bone marrow can be aspirated and fluid can be injected with little resistance and with no swelling or extravasations. The EZ-IO battery-powered drill-like device limits the depth of insertion of a specifically designed needle and provides a low profile connection for the IV fluid.[1]

Cannulation Techniques

Radial Artery Cannulation

The radial artery in the non-dominant hand is the preferred site to access:

1. Locate the artery by palpation; ultrasound guidance is now considered the standard of care.
2. Use an aseptic technique preparing the skin with chlorhexidine.
3. Make a small skin incision over the artery with an 18-gauge needle. This prevents damage to the tip of the catheter during skin puncture.
4. Perform the ultrasound-guided arterial puncture; as soon as blood is seen rising into the hub of the needle, turn the needle so that the bevel faces down and advance the cannula gently into the artery (Fig. 5.1).
5. If the catheter will not advance, withdraw the needle until blood flows freely and carefully insert a fine guide wire, then advance the cannula over the wire.

[1] Arrow® EZ-IO® Intraosseous Vascular Access System, Teleflex, Shavano Park, TX.

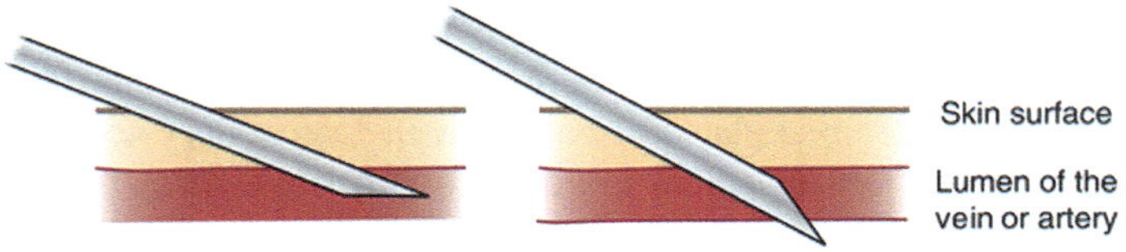

Fig. 5.1 Cannulation of small veins or arteries. *Hints*: Success may be improved if the bevel of the needle is turned down as in (**a**) so that the entire breadth of the end of the needle is intraluminal versus the situation in (**b**) where the tip may be through the distal wall and prevent advancing the catheter off the needle. Alternatively, when a flashback of blood is seen in the hub of the cannula, a fine guide wire may be advanced through the needle to guide the cannula into the vein. (Image adapted from: Filston and Johnson 1971; Steward 1999)

6. If the artery cannot be cannulated, re-evaluate the site with ultrasound.
7. If pulsations are visible on ultrasound or a pulse is palpable, reattempt cannulation more proximally.
8. After successful cannulation, apply an antibiotic ointment and cover the puncture site with a tight sterile dressing.
9. Place a red label indicating that this is an arterial line at the site of insertion and all connections to prevent confusion with a venous line. Label the date and time of placement.

Femoral Artery Cannulation

In some children, the radial artery cannot be cannulated or is inappropriate, for example, after surgery of the aortic arch. In such cases, the femoral artery may be used.

1. Place a low pad under the child to elevate the pelvis.
2. Palpate the femoral artery *below* the inguinal ligament. If the artery is difficult to palpate, ultrasound may facilitate identification of the artery.
3. Use an aseptic technique preparing the skin with chlorhexidine.

4. Using the Seldinger technique, puncture the artery *below* the inguinal ligament using an appropriate-sized thin-walled needle. Punctures superior to the inguinal ligament introduce the risk of a retroperitoneal bleed.
5. Avoid needling the head of the femur; aseptic necrosis may result in infants and young children.
6. When the artery is entered, pass the guide wire and use it to introduce an appropriate size catheter. Secure the catheter and cover it with antibiotic ointment and a clear plastic dressing.
7. Place a red label indicating that this is an arterial line at the site of insertion and all connections to prevent confusion with a venous line. Label the date and time of placement.

Other Precautions with Arterial Lines

1. Secure all connections, using Luer-Lok fittings, to reduce accidental disconnections. Plug sampling taps when not in use. Tape stopcocks in the "line-open" position if they will be hidden under the drapes and inaccessible. Clearly indicate all access ports with red tape or label as "arterial line" to avoid accidental arterial drug administration.
2. For radial lines, immobilize the forearm and wrist on a padded splint to prevent accidental decannulation.
3. Use a continuous flush device, but beware of accidental fluid overload. Use 1 N or 0.5 N saline with heparin (1000 IU/500 mL); do not use dextrose because of the increased risk for bacterial growth in the line.
4. Beware of embolization.
   (a) Return blood removed during arterial sampling to an IV line, NOT to an arterial line.
   (b) Do not use high pressure to clear a blocked cannula.
   (c) Intermittently and slowly flush small volumes of flush solution after each sampling; in small infants, volumes of only 0.5–1.0 mL injected rapidly into the radial artery may flow retrograde into cerebral vessels and cause an ischemic event.

5. Remove the arterial line as soon as it has served its purpose. Complications especially thrombosis and sepsis increase with the duration of vessel cannulation.

Internal Jugular Vein Cannulation

The use of ultrasound greatly improves the success rate and decreases the incidence of complications.

1. Position the child—head to slightly leftward, 20° Trendelenburg, with a rolled towel under the shoulders to reduce concavity of the neck.
2. Locate and mark the position of the internal jugular vein (IJV) using ultrasound. It is located at the apex of the triangle consisting of two bellies of the sternocleidomastoid muscle and the clavicle, usually at the level of the cricoid cartilage. Note the relation of the IJV to the carotid artery.
3. Prepare skin and drape, gown, and glove.
4. Using the Seldinger technique, insert the thin-walled needle through the skin at 45° over the marked course of the IJV (or under direct ultrasound guidance) until the vein is punctured: a flow of venous blood is usually obtained as the needle is being slowly withdrawn.
5. Pass the guide wire; there should be no resistance to passage. The presence of premature ventricular beats indicates successful venous cannulation and passage of the guide wire into the right ventricle; withdraw the wire several centimeters. Remove the needle, make a skin nick with a scalpel blade, and complete the cannulation after advancing and removing the dilator. Note that gentle pressure on the liver will greatly increase the size of the IJV and facilitate cannulation.
6. Suture the catheter in situ.
7. Apply antibiotic ointment with an occlusive dressing; label with the date and time of placement.

If ultrasound is not available, cannulation may be performed using anatomic landmarks; after positioning the child as described in (1) previously:

1. Palpate the carotid pulse lateral to the medial belly of the sternocleidomastoid muscle and identify the triangle formed by the two bellies of the sternocleidomastoid muscles and the clavicle.
2. Introduce the needle at the apex of the sternocleidomastoid triangle aiming toward the ipsilateral nipple. Gradually fan medially until the vein is found and use the Seldinger technique for catheter placement (see above).

N.B. It is advisable to attach the needle or cannula to a transducer and confirm that the pressure is venous before dilating the vessel, especially in children with cyanotic heart disease.

The optimal position is that the catheter tip is at the junction of the superior vena cava and right atrium.

Always check the position of the tip of the catheter if it is to be left in place postoperatively. Catheters that extend into the right atrium or whose tip is against the side wall of the SVC may perforate a vessel or the heart.

If IJV puncture cannot be performed and the external jugular vein is visible, it may provide a useful alternative route for CVP monitoring. The subclavian vein is another useful alternative.

External Jugular Vein Cannulation

1. Use the same technique as for internal jugular vein cannulation described above.
2. Feed a J-wire through the catheter and advance it centrally, rotating as necessary. A J-wire with a 3-mm radius of curvature at the J is most likely to pass into the subclavian and

toward the heart. The wire must be manipulated gently to avoid the possibility of puncturing the vein. It may be advantageous to abduct the child's arm to direct the wire toward the heart.

3. When the wire has advanced, a dilator may be gently inserted, taking care not to pass it more than 1–2 cm into the external jugular vein, otherwise it might tear the vein at the junction with the subclavian.
4. Advance the soft central venous catheter over the guide wire until it is sited at the junction of the superior vena cava and right atrium.
5. Confirm correct position if it is to be left in situ postoperatively.
6. Apply antibiotic ointment with an occlusive dressing; label the date and time of placement.

Management of Body Temperature

Monitoring

Continuous monitoring of body temperature with a thermistor probe is essential for all children undergoing general anesthesia. In larger children having minor surgery, the temperature is usually recorded from the axilla with the tip of the probe in close proximity to the axillary artery and the child's arm adducted. Adhesive skin temperature sensors, for example, on the forehead, do not accurately measure core temperature. In infants and children undergoing major surgery, core temperature is best monitored in the distal esophagus or tympanic membrane. Esophageal temperatures should be recorded at the lower third of the esophagus to avoid falsely low readings caused by gases flowing into the trachea. When inserting an esophageal stethoscope with a thermistor, continue to insert the probe until the heart sounds are loudest; the thermistor is then optimally placed behind the left atrium.

Tympanic membrane probes closely follow lower esophageal temperature, but care must be taken not to damage the ear.

Conservation of Body Heat in Neonates

The goal of body heat conservation is to prevent cold stress and avoid hypothermia. Hypothermia delays recovery from anesthetic and relaxant drugs, impairs coagulation, and increases postoperative oxygen consumption.

The sources of body heat loss are radiation (39%) > convection (34%) > evaporation (24%) > conduction (3%). Preheating the OR and wrapping the child reduce radiation heat loss; the use of a forced-air warmer decreases convection and conduction heat loss. The use of an heat moisturizer exchanger (HME) reduces evaporative losses.

(a) *Preoperatively*. Adjust the OR ambient temperature to 24 °C (75 °F) or greater. Select an appropriate size forced-air heating mattress. Keep the infant in the heated transport incubator until you are ready to induce anesthesia.
(b) *Intraoperatively*. Neonatal forced-air blankets should be positioned under the patient. They are placed on the table before the infant arrives and warmed to 43 °C. If the room is warmed and the forced-air blanket used, an infrared heating lamp is not needed. However, the forced-air blanket is usually turned off just before surgical prep and turned back on after the infant is covered by surgical drapes. If there is concern that this interval will result in heat loss, then an infrared heating lamp may be useful. Cover the infant's head whenever possible. Use warmed intravenous solutions when large volumes will be infused. Warmed (40 °C) skin preparation solution should be used, and excess fluids should be dried from the skin to prevent cooling by evaporation. The use of plastic drapes creates a "warm tent" around the infant.
(c) *Postoperatively*. Use the forced-air warmer during extubation and other procedures after the anesthetic ends. Alternately, the infrared heater may be used. Place the infant in a warmed incubator or, if the incubator is an open transport, apply a warm pack under the blanket and return the infant promptly to the post-anesthesia care unit or the NICU.

Hyperthermia During Surgery

Hyperthermia sometimes develops during surgery if heat-conserving procedures are followed. If this occurs, the forced-air heater should be set to ambient temperature until the infant's temperature begins to decrease and then discontinued. Other causes for hyperthermia during surgery include pyrexial reactions, for example, from manipulation of an infected organ or a blood transfusion reaction, infants with arthrogryposis multiplex congenita or osteogenesis imperfecta, and very rarely, with malignant hyperthermia (see Chap. 5), cocaine overdose, or thyroid storm.

Suggested Reading

Al-Beltagi M, et al. Pulse oximetry in pediatric care: balancing advantages and limitations. World J Clin Pediatr. 2024;13:9650.

Annalyn NSL, et al. Effectiveness of near-infrared light devices for peripheral intravenous cannulation in children and adolescents: a meta-analysis of randomized controlled trials. J Pediatr Nursing. 2024;75:e81–92.

De Silvestro AA, Kruger B, Steger C, et al. Cerebral desaturation during neonatal congenital heart surgery is associated with perioperative brain structure alterations but not with neurodevelopmental outcome at 1 year. Eur J Cardiothorac Surg. 2022;62(5):ezac138.

Filston HC, Johnson DG. Percutaneous venous cannulations in infants and children: a method for catheter insertion without cutdown. Pediatric. 1971;48:896–901.

Kowshik S, et al. Heparin vs. saline infusion to maintain patency of arterial catheters in children: a randomized, double-blind, noninferiority trial. Indian Pediatr. 2024;61:132–8.

Lai L-L, et al. Significant factors influencing inadvertent hypothermia in pediatric anesthesia. J Clin Monitor Comput. 2019;33:1105–12.

León-Valladares D, et al. Determining factors of pulse oximetry accuracy: a literature review. Rev Clin Esp (Barc). 2024;224:314–20.

Martin D, et al. Effect of skin tone on the accuracy of the estimation of arterial oxygen saturation by pulse oximetry: a systematic review. Br J Anaesth. 2024;132:945–56.

McIntosh AL, McLeod C. Accuracy of non-invasive hemoglobin (nHgb) monitoring in an AIS population. JPOSNA. 2023;5(2):598.

Moreira L, Engelman E, Estruch-Pons I, et al. Non-invasive vs. biological blood determination of haemoglobinemia for perioperative management: a systematic review with meta-analysis. J Clin Monit Comput. 2025; 39(6):1113–5.

Naik VM, et al. Vascular access in children. Indian J Anaesth. 2019;63:737–45.

Nemeth M, Miller C, Brauer A. Perioperative hypothermia in children. Intl J Environ Res Pub Health. 2021;18:7541.

Ozgen ZSU. Neuromuscular blockade monitoring in pediatric patients. Anesth Pain Med. 2024;19(Suppl 1):S12–24.

Pfeiffer D, et al. Factors influencing the success and complications of intraosseous access in pediatric patients-a prospective nationwide surveillance study in Germany. Front Pediatr. 2023; 11:1294322.

Rao A, et al. Near-infrared spectroscopy monitoring in pediatric anesthesiology: a pro-con discussion. Cureus. 2021;13(3):e13875.

Steward DJ. Venous cannulation in small infants: a simple method to improve success. Anesthesiology. 1999;90:930–1.

Templeton TW, Alex G, Eloy JD, et al. BIS guided titration of sevoflurane in pediatric patients undergoing elective surgery: a randomized controlled trial. Pediatr Anesth. 2025;35:277–86.

Vyas V, et al. Infrared vein visualization devices for ease of intravenous access in children: hope versus hype. Anaesthesiol Intens Ther. 2021;53:69–78.

Fluid and Blood Product Management

6

General Principles

It is highly recommended to insert a Buretrol® or similar graduated reservoir between the intravenous bag and the administration set for all infants and children <20 kg to prevent accidental fluid overload and to accurately measure infused volumes.

1. In preterm and full-term neonates, always use an infusion pump.
2. For major abdominal surgery and lower extremity surgery, intravenous access should be secured in the upper limbs.
3. Before surgery commences, ensure that the intravenous line is patent and infusing; do not embark on any procedure with a doubtful intravenous line.
4. Do not be lulled into security if the child has a multi-lumen central venous pressure (CVP) catheter, as resistance to flow may be so great that rapid infusion of packed red blood cells (PRBCs) or whole blood is impossible. It is also unwise to rapidly infuse blood into CVP lines in neonates and infants, as both the low temperature and high K^+ content of stored blood may cause serious arrhythmias.
5. A neonate's insensible water loss decreases by 30–35% when nursed in a high-humidity atmosphere or ventilated with humidified gases. Insensible water loss is increased by crying, sweating, hyperventilation, and the use of a radiant heater or "bili" lights. Pyrexia increases water loss by ~12% per 1 °C.

J. Lerman, C. J. Coté, *Steward's Manual of Pediatric Anesthesia*,
https://doi.org/10.1007/978-3-032-24545-8_6

Preoperative Fluid Replacement

Children undergoing elective surgery are usually instructed to ingest unlimited clear oral fluids 2 h preoperatively (Table 1.1); however, in many instances, children remain nil per os (NPO) for much longer, even >12 h. This prolonged fasting is often due to unclear, contradictory instructions or parental fears that surgery may be canceled. Some reports suggest that reducing the fasting interval to 1 h (after ingesting 3–5 mL/kg of clear fluids) reduces the frequency of but does not eliminate prolonged fasts. One study found a 92% compliance with preoperative oral fluid instructions when parents received a text message the day before surgery instructing them to give preoperative unrestricted oral fluids 2 h before their child's admission time to hospital. Enhanced recovery after surgery protocols in adults instruct patients to ingest clear fluids up to 2 h preoperatively. The same should be adopted for children undergoing elective surgery: ingest clear fluids up to 2 h preoperatively. Infants with chronic fluid depletion secondary to their diseases should have their deficits corrected perioperatively; Table 6.1 classifies the dehydration in infants.

Restoring euvolemia in dehydrated infants should follow three phases:

PHASE 1 *Treatment of overt or impending shock* (severe dehydration and hypovolemia): Start with a balanced salt solution (lactated Ringer's solution or normal saline—20 mL/kg); administer PRBCs (10 mL/kg) if anemia is present in the presence of dehy-

Table 6.1 Dehydration in infants

Mild dehydration: 50 mL/kg (~5% body weight loss) normal wet mucous membranes, tears present, flat anterior fontanel, normal skin turgor, and normal to slightly increased heart rate.
Moderate dehydration: 100 mL/kg (~10% body weight loss) dry mucous membranes, normal to reduced tears, possible sunken anterior fontanel, slightly increased skin turgor, tachycardia, and oliguria.
Severe dehydration: 150 mL/kg (~15% body weight loss) parched mucous membranes, absent tears, sunken anterior fontanel, sunken eyeballs, increased skin turgor, tachycardia, hypotension, and anuria.

dration, as the severity of the anemia will be greatly under estimated. About 20 mL/kg of 5% albumin may be administered as an alternative if anemia is not present. Fluid boluses are repeated as indicated by clinical responses (slowing of HR, improved BP, improved perfusion [less vasoconstriction], and increased urine output).

PHASE 2 *Replacement of extracellular water and sodium:* Half the estimated fluid deficit should be replaced over the initial 6–8 h with 0.3 N saline; if the deficit is very severe, give an initial infusion of 1 N saline (20 mL/kg). The following formula is useful in correcting sodium deficiency:

$$\text{Na}^{+}\text{deficit (mEq)} = \left[\text{normal Na}^{+}\text{(mEq)} - \text{measured Na}^{+}\text{(mEq)}\right] \times 0.6 \times \text{weight(kg)},$$

where 0.6 = volume of distribution.

Severe metabolic acidosis should be treated simultaneously, using the formula:

$$\text{Dose required}\left(\text{mEq of HCO}_3\right) = \text{base deficit} \times 0.3\left(0.4 \text{ for infants}\right) \times \text{weight (kg)}$$

where 0.3 (or 0.4) is the volume of distribution. Give half the calculated deficit, then reassess the acid-base status.

PHASE 3 *Replacement of potassium:* Potassium (K^+) replacement should begin only when a good urinary output has been established, according to the following:

1. Replace a maximum of 3 mEq/kg of potassium per 24 h
2. The rate of administration should not exceed 0.5 mEq/kg/h
3. Complete correction of severe K^+ deficiency may take 4–5 days

These rates are estimates and should be adjusted for changes in metabolic activity, clinical conditions, and extrarenal losses, for example, gastric suction.

Intraoperative Fluid Management

The volume and type of fluid for infusion and replacement strategies have evolved with the latest recommendations focusing on the prevention of perioperative hyponatremia. Preoperative estimates must consider:

1. Dehydration present *before* preoperative fasting
2. Fluid deficit incurred *during* preoperative fasting
3. Estimated extracellular third space fluid loss related to surgical trauma
4. Replacement of blood loss
5. Insensible fluid losses due to an increase in body temperature or exposed body surfaces

For brief surgical procedures in healthy children, intravenous fluids are not usually needed if the preoperative deficit is small, blood loss or tissue trauma minimal, and oral intake likely to be reestablished early, for example, myringotomy and tubes. Intravenous access should, however, be available and ready to use should an emergency develop.

For prolonged surgeries and/or when reestablishment of oral intake may be delayed:

1. Intravenous access should be established.
2. A balanced salt solution, for example, lactated Ringer's, should be administered until oral intake is reestablished.
3. The goal is to replace fluid deficits and ongoing losses to restore euvolemia. Antidiuretic hormone (ADH) is normally upregulated in the perioperative period as a result of many perioperative stimuli (Table 6.2). To prevent perioperative hyponatremia, ADH must be suppressed, and restoring euvolemia is the most effective means to suppress it. To that end, Holliday and Segar revised their perioperative (4:2:1 rule, 4 mL/kg for the first 10 kg, 2 mL/kg for the second 10 kg, and then 1 mL/kg for >20 kg) fluid strategy for the perioperative period by recommending 10–40 mL/kg of a balanced salt solution infused over several hours (10–20 mL/kg in the first hour) for most simple, non-blood loss surgical procedures. An addi-

Table 6.2 Perioperative causes of increased ADH release

Non-osmotic	Osmotic
Pain	Fasting
Inflammation	Hypovolemia
Stress: catecholamines	Hypertonicity
Surgery: laparoscopic surgery	Hypotension
Vomiting	Renal insufficiency
Hypoxia	Hepatic insufficiency
Hypercapnia	
Medications (e.g., opioids, amiodarone, vincristine)	
Respiratory diseases (e.g., asthma, pneumonia, atelectasis)	
Central nervous system disorders (e.g., head injury, tumors)	

tional benefit from restoring intraoperative euvolemia is reduced postoperative nausea and vomiting.

4. However, for neonates and infants <6 months, we continue to recommend following the 4:2:1 rule for maintenance fluid management (see below).
5. For those who were fasted for a prolonged period and others at risk for hypoglycemia, for example, premature infants, a glucose-containing solution may be indicated to prevent hypoglycemia. A 1–2.5% dextrose solution in lactated Ringer's, delivered using an infusion pump at maintenance rates, may be piggybacked into the main IV line. Check the plasma glucose concentrations as indicated.
6. For extensive surgery in preterm and term neonates, it is essential to separate the administration of dextrose-containing fluids from other fluid therapy. If the infant is receiving total parenteral nutrition, intralipids should be stopped (to minimize infections from using the IV line), and the clear electrolyte/glucose fluids continued. Current evidence recommends halving the glucose infusion during laparotomies in neonates to

reduce the frequency of postoperative hyperglycemia events and decreasing the rate by ~25% in most other surgeries. If no glucose was infused preoperatively, an infusion of 5 or 10% dextrose at 5–8 mg/kg/min (using an infusion pump) minimizes the risk of perioperative hypoglycemia. Blood glucose levels should be checked serially. Generally, older otherwise healthy children do not require intraoperative glucose infusions.

7. For surgical procedures causing extensive tissue trauma and/or blood loss, additional fluids are indicated to replace extracellular fluid lost in blood or sequestered into damaged tissue. These losses should be replaced with a balanced salt solution, for example, lactated Ringer's solution, with electrolyte concentrations similar to those in extracellular fluid (Table 6.3). Prolonged superficial or extremity surgery (associated with minimal fluid loss) requires only ~5 mL/kg/h fluid replacement, moderate procedures, for example, spine surgery, require ~10 mL/kg/h, and major procedures, for example, laparotomy, require ~15 mL/kg/h. Thoracotomy is associated with much less translocation of fluid and surgical manipulation of the lungs may trigger interstitial pulmonary fluid sequestration. Hence, administer smaller fluid volumes during thoracic surgery.
8. When replacing blood loss with balanced salt solutions, the volume required is 3 mL for every mL of blood lost. We recommend assessing the coagulation status after replacing one blood volume. If blood has been replaced with PRBCs only, fresh frozen plasma (FFP) should be considered after one blood volume loss. Platelet replacement is generally indicated after 2–3 blood volumes unless the platelet count was low (≤100,000/mm^3) at baseline (see massive transfusions, Chap. 18). Adequacy of fluid replacement is best judged by continuous monitoring of the cardiovascular indices and urine output. If urine output is less than 0.5–1 mL/kg/h, the fluid infusion rate should be increased. Postoperative hyponatremia is usually associated with the intraoperative and postoperative use of hypotonic solutions or occasionally inappropriate secretion of ADH. Holliday and Segar recommended postoperative

Table 6.3 Composition of electrolyte solutions

	Concentration (mEq/L)					Concentration of HCO_3^- (mEq/L)			
Solution	Na^+	K^+	Mg^{2+}	Ca^{2+}	Cl^-	Acetate HCO_3^-	Gluconate	Lactate	Osmolarity
Lactated Ringer's solution[a]	130	4	–	3	109	–	–	28	276
Normal saline (0.9 %)	154	–	–	–	154	–	–	–	308
Plasma-Lyte 148	140	5	1.5	–	98	527	23	–	294
0.3 N saline in D_5W	51	–	–	–	51	–	–	–	
0.2 N saline in D_5W	34	–	–	–	34	–	–	–	
Normosol-M	40	13	3	–	40	16	–	–	
Normosol-R	140	5	3	–	98	27	23	–	280

Magnesium sulfate (2 mL amp., 50% w/v (where w/v is weight/unit volume)): 4.0 mEq Mg^{2+}/ml
Sodium bicarbonate (50 mL amp., 7.5% w/v): 0.9 mEq HCO_3^-/mL
Calcium gluconate (10 mL amp., 10% w/v): 0.447 mEq Ca^{2+}/mL
Calcium chloride (10 mL amp., 10% w/v): 1.36 mEq Ca^{2+}/mL
D_5W, 5% dextrose in water

[a]Or Hartmann's solution

infusion rates for balanced salt solutions of 2:1:0.5 (2 mL/kg/h for the first 10 kg, 1 mL/kg/h for the second 10 kg, and 0.5 mL/kg/h for >20 kg) to prevent hyponatremia while avoiding salt overload when using a balanced salt solution. This strategy is recommended for the first 12 h post-surgery and then reversion to the 4:2:1 rule thereafter, until oral intake is resumed. Serum electrolytes should be monitored serially after all major surgery to ensure that electrolyte concentrations remain normal.

Blood Replacement

Preoperative Assessment

Although minor surgical procedures are commonly performed in children who are mildly anemic with no problems, a normal Hb level (Table 6.4) is desirable for *major* elective surgery; elective surgery may be delayed until the anemia has been investigated and treated. For more urgent surgery, anesthesia must be adjusted with considerations for their anemia (see Chap. 8). When surgery cannot be delayed despite a very low Hb, for example, 5–7 g/dL, and blood loss is expected, packed red blood cells (PRBCs) should be administered either preoperatively or before incision. Approximately, 4 mL/kg of packed cells and 6 mL/kg of whole blood increase the

Table 6.4 Normal hemoglobin concentrations with age

Age	Hb conc. (g/dL)
First day of life—full-term infants	20 (18–22)
Second week	17
2–3 months	10–11[a]
2 years	11
3–5 years	12.5–13.0
5–10 years	13.0–13.5
10+ years	14.5

[a]This Hb concentration nadir in full-term infants results from increased oxygenation (reduced erythropoietin), shorter red cell lifespan, and slower red cell production. In preterm infants, the physiologic nadir is less, 7–9 g/dL

Hb concentration ~1 g. If no or minimal blood loss is expected, then have packed cells available for possible transfusion.

When significant blood losses (15% of the estimated blood volume [EBV] or greater) are expected, the child's blood group should be determined and an appropriate number of units cross-matched. The hemoglobin content in stored whole blood is ~12 g/dL, in PRBCs ~24 g/dL, and in buffy-coat-poor washed cells ~28 g/dL.

Perioperative Management

Before surgery, determine the child's preoperative Hb, their estimated blood volume (EBV) (Table 2.5), and calculate the maximal allowable blood loss (MABL) on the anesthesia record:

$$\text{MABL} = \frac{(\text{Starting Hct} - \text{target Hct}) \times \text{EBV}}{\text{Starting Hct}} \tag{6.1}$$

Assessment of Blood Loss

Accurate estimates of blood loss must be maintained throughout the surgery.

1. In infants, the systolic BP is the most reliable indicator of blood volume.
2. Measure blood loss from the surgical site:
   (a) All sponges must be weighed before they dry out. This method is simple and accurate (assume 1 g = 1 mL blood and subtract the known dry weight).
   (b) Measure blood from suction canisters.
   (c) Estimate blood on drapes.
3. Chart the running total continually.
4. Be aware that blood losses may be hidden in body cavities, for example, peritoneum, pleura, or on the floor.

Blood Transfusion

The decision to transfuse blood must be based on the preoperative Hb level, the estimated blood loss, and the child's cardiovascular responses. As a rough guide, in otherwise healthy children, blood replacement should be considered with ongoing bleeding once ~15% of the EBV has been lost. The need for blood transfusion can be determined more accurately from serial hematocrit (Hct) measurements. Normally, the Hct should be maintained ≥30–40% in infants and in those children with significant cardiac or respiratory disease, and at ~20–25% in otherwise healthy children.

Check each unit of blood against the child's identity bracelet. Blood should be warmed to no greater than 37 °C before administration; more than 38 °C may cause hemolysis. PRBCs are often diluted with normal saline before administration. Massive blood transfusions in smaller children may require that the PRBCs be diluted in fresh frozen plasma (FFP) to prevent a dilutional coagulopathy (see Chap. 18). Calcium supplementation may be indicated if the rate of infusion of FFP or reconstituted blood exceeds 1 mL/kg/min (See below). Avoid direct and rapid transfusion of cold blood products into a central vein or right atrium in infants, as life-threatening arrhythmias may ensue.

Massive Blood Transfusion

If a massive blood transfusion is developing and anticipated to worsen, consider instituting a massive transfusion protocol (see Chap. 18) and assess coagulation indices. Platelet counts, prothrombin time, and partial thromboplastin time together should be repeated at least after every 0.5–1 blood volume is replaced; assessments of fibrinolyis by measuring fibrin split products should be made as indicated. A baseline preoperative platelet count should be obtained if a massive transfusion is possible. A low baseline platelet count (<100,000/mm^3) may necessitate an early platelet transfusion. Platelet counts of less than 50,000/mm^3 in otherwise healthy children are associated with the onset of clinical bleeding and should be corrected. In practice, if platelets are monitored during a continuing massive replacement, platelets should be ordered as the count decreases to <100,000/mm^3. As a rule, the original platelet count decreases ~40% after the first blood volume loss, decreases a further ~20% after the next blood volume, and another ~10% by the third blood volume. Thus, if the starting platelet count was 200,000/mm^3 at baseline, by the third blood volume lost, one could anticipate a count of

Table 6.5 Common initial doses of blood components and expected effects in children

Component	Dose	Effect
Packed red blood cells	10–15 mL/kg	Increase hemoglobin by 2–3 g/dL
Platelets	5–10 mL/kg	Increase platelet count by 50,000–100,000/mm^3
Fresh frozen plasma	10–15 mL/kg	Factor levels increase by 15–20%
Cryoprecipitate	0.1–0.2 units/kg	Increase fibrinogen by 60–100 mg/dL
Fibrinogen concentrate	70 mg/kg	Increase in fibrinogen level of 120 mg/dL

From Coté CJ, Grabowski EF, Sloan SR: Strategies for Blood Product Management, Reducing Transfusions, and Massive Blood Transfusion. Table 10.7. In: A Practice of Anesthesia for Infants and Children, seventh Ed. Coté CJ, Lerman J, Anderson BJ eds. Philadelphia, Elsevier 2025

~60,000/mm^3. Infusion of 5–10 mL/kg of platelet concentrate increases the platelet count by 50,000–100,000/mm^3 (see Table 6.5). Platelets must be stored at room temperature, not refrigerated, and should be rocked periodically. Platelets should not be infused through any mesh filters.

Other deficiencies that become apparent should be dealt with by appropriate therapy; see Table 6.5 for doses of blood components and the expected responses in children. Anticipate that FFP will be required after one blood volume is lost and in a volume of at least one-third of each subsequent blood volume lost; FFP should not be needed if the blood loss does not exceed one blood volume. Be aware that clinically important hypocalcemia possibly associated with cardiac dysfunction may accompany infusions of FFP, because it has the greatest concentration of citrate per unit volume of any blood product. If the FFP transfusion is ≥1 mL/kg/min, then ionized hypocalcemia is likely, and exogenous calcium should be administered through a separate IV site during the transfusion (5 mg/kg calcium chloride or 15 mg/kg calcium gluconate, repeat as needed). In severely shocked children who require rapid massive transfusion, be prepared to also give sodium bicarbonate if indicated by serial acid-base determinations.

Prothrombin complex concentration is a plasma-derived product that contains the Vitamin K clotting factors II, VII, IX, and X, as well as proteins C and S for IV administration for severe bleeding conditions. It serves a particular role in the absence of FFP or in the presence of warfarin, offering greater concentrations of the clotting factors than those found in FFP. It does not require cross-matching but does require reconstitution. There are limited studies of its use in children, but an initial dose of 25 IU/kg (maximum single dose 3000 IU) has been suggested with an INR target of <1.5. For those whose INR is >3, 40–50 IU/kg is indicated.[1]

Alternatives to Blood Transfusion

The risk of infection, transfusion reaction, lung injury, and others has prompted the search for alternatives, many of which may be applicable in children:

1. *Autologous transfusion of blood donated preoperatively:* Suitable size donations may be collected at 4- to 5-day intervals, preoperatively. If blood donation is combined with measures to increase erythropoiesis (oral iron and Vitamin C 6–8 weeks in advance, erythropoietin 3–4 weeks in advance), significant volumes may be collected. These techniques are most applicable to teenagers.
2. *Blood conservation*: Blood losses are minimized by proper positioning, infiltration of vasoconstrictors, induced moderate hypotension, and meticulous surgical technique.
3. *Acute normovolemic hemodilution:* Blood is withdrawn after anesthesia induction but before surgery commences, and each mL removed is replaced with 3 mL of warmed lactated Ringer's solution. Hemodilution to a Hct of 25% is acceptable in otherwise healthy children. Blood is then reinfused as the surgery proceeds, saving the first collected unit of blood to be transfused last. The volume to be collected can be calculated from the following formula for estimating the MABL (see Eq. 6.1).

[1] See NACblood.ca for further dosing guidelines and contraindications.

4. *Intraoperative autotransfusion of shed blood using a "cell saver":* This technique has limited application, but it may be useful in orthopedic surgery. Shed red cells may be collected by suction, washed, and reinfused. However, coagulation factors are discarded in the washing process, and extensive reinfusion of washed cells may lead to clotting factor dilution and coagulopathy.
5. Pharmacologic strategies to reduce blood loss during surgery have focused on the use of antifibrinolytics. Two antifibrinolytics in use are tranexamic acid and e-aminocaproic acid (Amicar). To prevent fibrinolysis during surgery, the loading dose of the antifibrinolytic should be completed before skin incision. The loading dose of tranexamic acid is 10 mg/kg IV infused over 15 min followed by an infusion during maintenance at 1–5 mg/kg/h. The loading dose of Amicar is 75 mg/kg IV followed by an infusion of 15 mg/kg/h. These infusions should continue until leaving the operating room; some will continue these infusions postoperatively.

Jehovah's Witness Patients

For Jehovah's Witness patients and others who refuse allogenic blood transfusions, a perioperative protocol should be prepared. Preoperatively, the child should be assessed for Hb concentration, coagulopathies, and vitamin deficiencies. A preoperative regimen of oral iron and Vitamin C as well as replacing deficient vitamins should begin 6–8 weeks before surgery. Weekly IV or sc erythropoietin (300–600 IU/kg) should be administered to increase the Hb concentration preoperatively up to a maximum value of 18–20 g to ensure that sufficient hemoglobin is available for either intraoperative hemodilution or sequestration. Intraoperatively, antifibrinolytics should be administered to minimize blood loss. After induction but before incision, a large bore peripheral IV and arterial access are established to infuse and collect blood, respectively. Whole blood should be sequestered in blood bags while the appropriate volume of balanced salt solution maintains euvolemia. The sequestered blood should be maintained in series with the patient continuously until it is reinfused.

Suggested Reading

Coté CJ. Depth of halothane anesthesia potentiates citrate-induced ionized hypocalcemia and adverse cardiovascular events in dogs. Anesthesiology. 1987;67:676–80.

Coté CJ, Liu LMP, Szyfelbein SK, Goudsouzian NG, Daniels AL. Changes in serial platelet counts following massive blood transfusion in pediatric patients. Anesthesiology. 1985;62:197–201.

Coté CJ, Drop LJ, Daniels AL, Hoaglin DC. Calcium chloride versus calcium gluconate: comparison of ionization and cardiovascular effects in children and dogs. Anesthesiology. 1987;66:465–70.

Goobie SM, Faraoni D. Perioperative paediatric patient blood management: a narrative review. Br J Anaesth. 2025;134:168–79.

Goobie SM, Staffa SJ, Meara JG, et al. High-dose versus low-dose tranexamic acid for paediatric craniosynostosis surgery: a double-blind randomised controlled non-inferiority trial. Br J Anaesth. 2020;125:336–45.

Hickey KS, Smith M, Karam O, et al. The effect of prophylactic use of antifibrinolytics during pediatric non-cardiac surgeries on bleeding and transfusions: a systematic review and meta-analysis. Pediatr Anesth. 2025;35:668–83.

Holliday MA, Friedman AL, Segar WE, et al. Acute hospital-induced hyponatremia in children: a physiologic approach. J Pediatr. 2004;145:584–7.

Holliday MA, Ray PE, Friedman AL. Fluid therapy for children: facts, fashions and questions. Arch Dis Child. 2007;92:546–50.

Joshi GP, Abdelmalak BB, Weigel WA, et al. 2023 American Society of Anesthesiologists practice guidelines for preoperative fasting: carbohydrate-containing clear liquids with or without protein, chewing gum, and pediatric fasting duration-a modular update of the 2017 American Society of Anesthesiologists practice guidelines for preoperative fasting. Anesthesiology. 2023;138:132–51.

Kolesky SE, Nyshadham S, Williams HO, et al. Intraoperative dextrose rate during exploratory laparotomies in neonates and the incidence of postoperative hyperglycemia: a retrospective observational study. Pediatr Anesth. 2021;31:197–204.

Reeves C, Sribnick EA, Tobias JD. Prothrombin complex concentrate to treat coagulation disturbances in pediatric patients with intracranial pathology including traumatic brain injury. Int J Clin Pediatr. 2024;13:8–13.

Roberts K, Brindle M, McLuckie D. Enhanced recovery after surgery in paediatrics: a review of the literature. BJA Educ. 2020;20:235–41.

Stricker PA, Zuppa AF, Fiadjoe JE, et al. Population pharmacokinetics of epsilon-aminocaproic acid in infants undergoing craniofacial reconstruction surgery. Br J Anaesth. 2013;11:788–99.

Thomasseau A, Rebollar Y, Dupuis M, et al. Observance of preoperative clear fluid fasting in pediatric anesthesia: oral and written information versus text message information. A before-and-after-study. Pediatr Anesth. 2021;31:557–62.

Regional Analgesia Techniques

7

Local Anesthetic Drugs

Clinical Pharmacology

Local anesthetic drugs are either amino esters (procaine, chloroprocaine, and tetracaine) or amino amides (lidocaine, bupivacaine, and ropivacaine). They primarily interrupt nerve conduction by inhibiting the influx of sodium but also bind to K^+ and Na^+-K^+ ATPase channels.

The pharmacokinetics in infants differ from those in older children and adults:

1. Absorption is rapid, the cardiac output and regional tissue blood flows are greater, and the epidural space contains less fat tissue to buffer uptake. Drugs sprayed into the airway are very rapidly absorbed. The pK_a of local anesthetics is >7.4; hence, they exist in a quaternary, water-soluble form at physiologic pH.
2. Plasma levels of local anesthetics injected into the epidural space in infants are less than in young children and adults due to a greater volume of distribution, which then prolongs the elimination half-life.

J. Lerman, C. J. Coté, *Steward's Manual of Pediatric Anesthesia*,
https://doi.org/10.1007/978-3-032-24545-8_7

3. Protein binding in neonates is less than in children because the plasma concentrations of proteins are less; hence, the free fraction of local anesthetics is greater. Local anesthetics bind primarily to α_1-acid glycoprotein and, to a lesser extent, to albumin. Bilirubin binds to the acidic sites on albumin, but it does not interfere with the protein binding of bupivacaine or ropivacaine, as these anesthetics only bind to the basic sites.
4. The rate of metabolism of local analgesic drugs is reduced in infants:
   (a) Plasma cholinesterase activity is immature, prolonging the duration of action of ester type drugs.
   (b) The hepatic pathways (cytochrome P450) for metabolism of amide local anesthetics (CYP450 3A4 and 1A2) are immature. CYP450 3A4, which metabolizes bupivacaine, matures to adult levels by 9 months, whereas 1A2, which metabolizes ropivacaine, matures by 7 years. Hence, to avoid toxicity, the infusion rates of bupivacaine and ropivacaine should be reduced from 0.4 mg/kg/h in children to <0.2 mg/kg/h in neonates and infants <6 mos. and for no longer than 48 h.
5. The metabolism of prilocaine may result in methemoglobinemia. This is important in neonates and infants because the enzyme methemoglobin reductase, which converts methemoglobin to hemoglobin, is reduced. If a large volume of EMLA cream is applied to the skin of an infant, methemoglobinemia may occur. Limit the drug dose and area EMLA is applied as described in the manufacturer's recommendations (Table 7.1).

Table 7.1 EMLA dosing according to age, from neonates to adolescents

Age (weight)	Maximum dose	Maximum area	Maximum time
0–3 months (<5 kg)	1 gram	10 cm^2	1 h
3 to ≤ 12 months (>5 kg)	2 grams	20 cm^2	4 h
1–6 years (>10 kg)	10 grams	100 cm^2	4 h
7–12 years (>20 kg)	20 grams	200 cm^2	4 h

Package insert accessed 6/23/2026 from https://www.accessdata.fda.gov/drugsatfda_docs/label/2018/019941s021lbl.pdf

Local Anesthetic Drugs

(a) Lidocaine

Lidocaine is commonly used for local infiltration. Total dose should not exceed 4.5 mg/kg of a plain solution or 7 mg/kg if epinephrine is added. Epinephrine prolongs the block and decreases the peak serum concentration by ~40%.

(b) Bupivacaine

Bupivacaine is a racemic mixture; the levo enantiomer is the clinically active form, whereas the dextro is the more toxic form. Bupivacaine has been widely used for peripheral and epidural blocks. It has the disadvantage that overdosing or accidental intravascular injection may lead to severe myocardial depression that may be prolonged and difficult to reverse (use intralipid see Appendix C). Bupivacaine metabolism is reduced in small infants, thus requiring close attention to dose, particularly with infusions (see above). The addition of epinephrine to bupivacaine is less effective in prolonging the block and decreasing peak serum concentrations than with lidocaine. However, epinephrine extends the duration of action of bupivacaine in infants and young children more than in older children.

(c) Ropivacaine

Ropivacaine is also a levo enantiomer, which is less cardiotoxic than bupivacaine and produces an equal sensory block with a more rapid onset, less motor block, and a similar duration of effect. Compared with bupivacaine, ropivacaine is less rapidly absorbed from the caudal epidural space, and peak plasma levels are less after an ilioinguinal nerve block. *Ropivacaine should not be used for penile or digital nerve blocks, as vasoconstriction and ischemia could theoretically occur.* Epinephrine does not prolong the duration of epidural or other blocks with ropivacaine.

(d) Chloroprocaine

With its small risk of toxicity, caudal/epidural infusions of 3-chloroprocaine are particularly suited for neonates and infants. This ester local anesthetic proffers two distinct advantages over other local anesthetics: a small risk of toxicity and an extremely short duration of action (plasma half-life is 20 s in adults and 40 s in neonates). With such a brief half-life, there is little risk of toxicity. It is metabolized by plasma cholinesterase. 2-Chloroprocaine contains EDTA as a preservative. Some recommend maximum loading doses of 14–20 mg/kg for regional blocks, although other practitioners exceed this dose in neonates and infants. For example, for caudal/epidural use, a loading dose of a 3% solution of 2 mL/kg followed by a continuous infusion of 2 mL/kg/h in infants has been recommended for both upper and lower abdominal surgery.

(e) Levobupivacaine

Levobupivacaine is the levo enantiomer of bupivacaine. It is less cardiotoxic, approximately 20% more potent than bupivacaine, and may be more suitable for prolonged infusions.

Toxicity

Maximum doses of local anesthetics are recommended to prevent overdoses (see Table 7.2). *N.B.* The potential for toxicity is related to total dose and the drug uptake from the injection site. The order of local anesthetic absorption with different blocks is easily remembered by the acronym "*ICE Blocks*": *I* = intercostal

Table 7.2 Maximum doses of local anesthetics[a]

Maximum local anesthetic dose	Without epinephrine (mg/kg)	With epinephrine (mg/kg)
Bupivacaine	2.5	3.0
3-Chloroprocaine	10–20	
Levobupivacaine	2	3
Lidocaine/mepivacaine	5	7
Prilocaine	6	8
Ropivacaine	3	3

[a]Maximum dose depends on the site of administration

>*C* = caudal, >*E* = epidural, >*B* = peripheral nerve blocks. Intravenous lidocaine in normal doses may produce toxic effects in children with CHD and right-to-left cardiac shunting because the normal first-pass absorption within the pulmonary circulation is bypassed. The dose should be reduced by ~50% in these children.

Compared with adults, neonates may exhibit signs of central nervous system toxicity (jitteriness and seizures) at smaller blood concentrations of local anesthetics. Blocks in children are most commonly performed during general anesthesia, which may mask signs of toxicity but, depending upon the anesthesia agent used, might increase the risk of cardiac toxicity. If seizures occur, 100% oxygen should be administered, the airway secured, and medication to stop the seizure administered immediately: intravenous benzodiazepine, i.e., midazolam (0.05–0.2 mg/kg), propofol (1–2 mg/kg), or thiopental (2–3 mg/kg) in repeated doses as required.

N.B.[§] Acute intravascular (intravenous or intraosseous) injection of bupivacaine (and less likely ropivacaine or levobupivacaine) resulting in local anesthetic systemic toxicity (LAST) may cause persistent ventricular tachycardia resulting in a low cardiac output state. If asystole or pulseless electrical activity (PEA) occurs, follow the PALS algorithm; a prolonged code should be anticipated. Cardiopulmonary bypass or ECMO may be needed for rescue. The most effective treatment in animals and anecdotal reports in humans is intravenous intralipid (20%) at a 1.5 mL/kg loading dose, followed by 1 mL/kg every 3–5 min (for 3 doses) and then an infusion of 0.25–0.5 mL/kg/min for at least 10 min until return of spontaneous circulation. The mechanism of rescue is believed to be elution of the local anesthetic from the myocardium by the lipid (lipid sink). *N.B.* Propofol is not indicated for rescue and should *not* be substituted for Intralipid. The American Society of Regional Anesthesia also recommends avoiding vasopressin, calcium channel blockers, β blockers, or additional local anesthetics and reducing the dose of epinephrine to <1 μg/kg for those with cardiac dysfunction but not asystole or PEA.

Adjuvant Drugs

Epinephrine

Epinephrine is added to local anesthetics to extend their duration of action and limit absorption. It also acts as a marker for intravascular injection; peaked T waves and ST-segment elevation are more reliable signs of intravascular injection than tachycardia. Epinephrine may interact with halothane and precipitate arrhythmias, but doses up to 10 μg/kg by infiltration are considered safe. Note that test dose ECG changes are unreliable in infants anesthetized with propofol and remifentanil and that an increase in blood pressure is a more sensitive marker of an intravascular injection.

Clonidine

Clonidine (1–2 μg/mL) is a widely used adjuvant to local anesthetics for caudal/epidural blocks. It prolongs the duration of the block approximately 3 h but has inconsistent effects on the rate of elimination of the local anesthetic from the epidural space.

Apnea has been reported after epidural clonidine in preterm infants, although three toddlers who received a 100-fold overdose of clonidine experienced only prolonged postoperative sedation and no respiratory distress/apnea. Clonidine may cause postoperative sedation (usually at doses >2 μg/kg), and this may be undesirable in outpatients.

Other Adjuvants

Numerous adjuvant medications including opioids, dexamethasone, dexmedetomidine, midazolam, ketamine, and neostigmine have been administered caudally/epidurally. Opioids, specifically fentanyl and morphine, are deemed to be safe from neurotoxicity, whereas many others are proscribed. Most are proscribed due to anecdotal reports of experimental neurotoxicity in animals and are not FDA approved for caudal/epidural use.

Regional Analgesia for Pain Control

Regional analgesia techniques alone are of limited value during pediatric surgical procedures; the overall nonacceptance and lack of cooperation in the awake young child result in the need for such large doses of sedatives that general anesthesia is preferable. However, regional analgesic techniques have become an indispensable part of perioperative pain management in children. Rarely, regional blocks are also indicated for chronic pain therapy and/or diagnostic purposes.

1. Spinal and/or epidural anesthesia techniques are useful for small infants, especially for the preterm infant (with or without lung disease), for herniorrhaphy repair, circumcision, or lower abdominal surgery. This may reduce, but not eliminate, the probability and duration of postoperative apnea events.
2. Epidural analgesia may be a suitable alternative to general anesthesia in some older children, e.g., those with cystic fibrosis, that may be continued through the postoperative period.
3. Some older children (5 years of age and older) can be "charmed" or sedated into cooperation and have their upper limb fractures reduced under a regional block.
4. Intravenous regional analgesia (Bier block) can be used in selected older children having surgery for superficial lesions on distal limbs or for some fracture reductions.
5. The possibility of using regional or local infiltration analgesia should also be considered for any minor procedure in a high-risk patient, e.g., skeletal muscle biopsy in a child with cardiomyopathy or a lymph node biopsy in a child with a mediastinal mass.

Clinical Management for Regional Analgesia

1. If the block is inserted while the child is awake, apply topical anesthetic cream over the needle insertion site in advance (see Chap. 3).

2. Evidence supports performing regional blocks under general anesthesia in infants and children as a safe practice. The risks of inserting a block under general anesthesia in children are considered less than the risks of inserting a block in a crying and struggling child.
3. The maximum allowable weight-based dose of the local anesthetic should be calculated and not exceeded for each child.
4. Use as much of the allowable dose as needed to ensure a successful block.
5. Glove and use sterile technique to prepare the skin; aspirate frequently to prevent intravascular injections.
6. Ultrasound (US) is very effective to accurately place the local anesthetic solution, improve success rates, reduce complications, and reduce drug doses. Success is optimized by planning ahead and allowing sufficient time for the block to become well established before commencing surgery.
7. Children are generally upset by paresthesias; it is best to use techniques that do not rely on eliciting paresthesia, e.g., use US.
8. Additionally supplementing the regional technique with age-appropriate sedation, e.g., oral midazolam; systemic analgesics, e.g., fentanyl; and/or distraction, e.g., video player or iPad and earphones, is exceedingly helpful.
9. If regional analgesia proves unsatisfactory, be prepared to supplement with sedation and/or general anesthesia.
10. When a choice exists, peripheral nerve blocks are generally safer and have fewer side effects than neuraxial blocks.
11. Do not use epinephrine in areas with limited collateral blood supply (digits, penis).
12. Do not administer sedatives to former preterm infants who have a spinal or epidural block, as this may increase the risk of postoperative apnea.
13. Always be prepared to deal with the complications of regional analgesia. Prepare the drugs and equipment needed to induce general anesthesia, secure the airway, and ventilate the lungs. Intralipid should be immediately available to treat an intravascular injection of local anesthetic (see toxicity).

An Outline of Procedures for Regional Blocks in Infants and Children

Regional blocks in children have found ever expanding roles, particularly with US-guided selective nerve blocks, thereby reducing local anesthetic doses, motor blockade, and the risk of toxicity as well as increasing block effectiveness. For more detailed descriptions of regional nerve blocks, the reader is referred to Regional Anesthesia, Polaner (2025).

Neuraxial Blocks

Spinal Anesthesia for Infants

Awake spinal anesthesia is most commonly indicated in infants, particularly former preterm infants, for surgery at or below the umbilicus to avoid intubating the airway and reduce the incidence of post-anesthesia apnea. Spinal anesthesia maintains stable blood pressure in infants and children aged less than 6 years. Sedatives such as ketamine or midazolam are avoided as the risk of perioperative apnea after such is similar to that after general anesthesia.

Special Considerations

1. The spinal cord may extend rostrally as far as L3 in the infant <1 year (compared with L1–2 in the older child or adult); therefore, it is safest to perform the lumbar puncture at L4–5 or L5-S1.
2. The dural space extends to S3–4 in the neonate.
3. The volume of cerebrospinal fluid (CSF) in infants (4 mL/kg) is double that in adults (2 mL/kg).

Contraindications

1. Sepsis or infected lumbar puncture site
2. Coagulopathy
3. Lack of parental consent

Anesthetic Management

Preoperative

1. The child should be fasted as for general anesthesia.
2. No premedication is necessary for small infants.

Perioperative

1. The anesthesia workstation, monitors, age and size appropriate airway equipment, and all ancillary equipment should be checked.
2. A sweetened soother is often useful to settle the infant; glucose may have analgesic properties of its own in neonates.
3. Establish intravenous access using local analgesia in the lower extremity so that the infant does not feel it once the spinal is placed.
4. The blood pressure cuff is also applied to the contralateral lower extremity.
5. Instruct your assistant to gently but firmly restrain the child in the chosen lateral or sitting position while avoiding neck flexion, which may compromise the airway.
6. Using an aseptic technique, drape the child and infiltrate the skin at the L4–5 or L5-S1 interspace with 1% lidocaine.
7. A neonatal spinal needle (e.g., 22 or 25-gauge, 1 in. [26 mm]) is preferred.
8. Prepare 1 mL of hyperbaric spinal bupivacaine, 0.75% bupivacaine in 8.25% dextrose, at 0.1 mL/kg (or 0.75 mg/kg). Some use isobaric bupivacaine 0.5% at 0.2 mL/kg (or 1 mg/kg).
9. Insert the needle with the bevel oriented laterally until CSF is obtained.
10. Slowly inject the local analgesic solution; rapid injection may result in a high or total spinal.
11. Return the infant to the supine position; keep the infant supine while applying the Bovie® pad to prevent a high spinal. Motor function in the lower limbs usually ceases immediately.

12. Duration of anesthesia is usually about 1.5 h.
13. *N.B.* Total spinal anesthesia in infants is heralded by cessation of crying or apnea with blood pressure and heart rate relatively unchanged. Treat with controlled ventilation until spontaneous respirations resume.

Perioperative

1. Keep the child horizontal until motor function returns.
2. Monitor the former preterm infant for apnea; post-anesthesia apnea is less common than after general anesthesia but may still occur.

Caudal Block

A caudal block is very useful in infants and children; it provides good postoperative analgesia after abdominal, lower limb, or perineal surgery. In young infants, the contents of the epidural space offer little resistance to the spread of local anesthetic solutions. Epidural blockade is accompanied by minimal changes in blood pressure or cardiac output in children <6 years. Continuous caudal catheters have been used for more prolonged surgery and postoperatively for extended analgesia; they may safely be threaded as cephalad as T6. Catheters have been left in situ for up to 3 days without adverse events.

Caudal morphine (maximum single dose 20–30 μg/kg) in combination with local anesthesia provides analgesia for thoracic and abdominal procedures for a median of 12 h and reduces the need for systemic analgesics. However, caudal opioids are associated with side effects that include nausea, vomiting, pruritus, urinary retention, and rarely respiratory depression that are dose related; hence, caudal opioids are unsuitable for outpatients and infants.

Preferred Technique

For postoperative analgesia, the block should be performed after induction of anesthesia but before surgery begins. This provides time for the block to become established, provides possible preemptive analgesia, and reduces the dose of general anesthetics, all facilitating rapid recovery.

The child is placed in the lateral decubitus position with the knees and hips flexed. The landmarks are then identified (Fig. 7.1): the tip of the coccyx in the midline and the sacral cornua bounding the sacral hiatus. These lie at the apex of an inverted equilateral triangle, the base of which is a line drawn between the posterior superior iliac spines. The child is prepared and draped, and the operator wears sterile gloves and a mask. The skin over the sacral hiatus is nicked with an 18-gauge needle (to avoid tracking epidermal tissue into the caudal canal), after which an IV catheter (22 gauge for children <2 years, 20 gauge for those >2 years) is advanced cephalad at an angle of 45° to the skin with

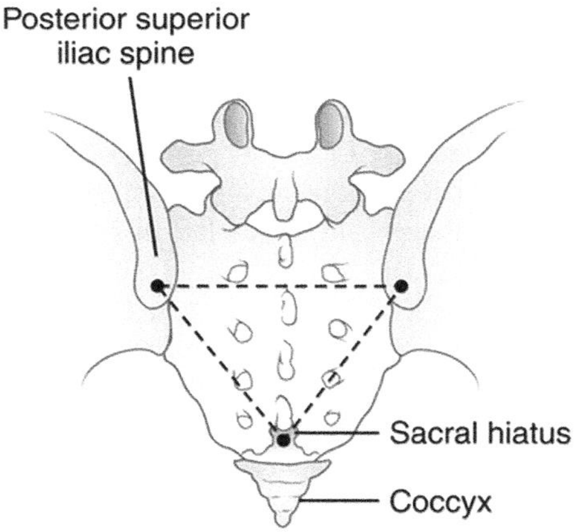

Fig. 7.1 Caudal block: surface landmarks. The sacral hiatus and posterior superior iliac spines form an equilateral triangle, with the caudal apex at the sacrococcygeal ligament

the bevel facing anteriorly. A distinctive sudden "give" is felt as the needle passes through the sacrococcygeal ligament. At this point, the angle of the needle against the skin is reduced, and the catheter is advanced off the needle into the caudal canal. The needle is then withdrawn, leaving the intravenous catheter in the caudal/epidural space. The catheter should be observed for passive reflux of blood or CSF. If neither is present, the local anesthetic is injected in incremental doses (there should be no resistance to injection; if resistance is met, then the catheter is either kinked or misplaced and should be removed) while the electrocardiogram is observed. ST-segment elevation and/or peaked T waves may be an early sign of intravascular injection during inhalational anesthesia; an increase in blood pressure is the most reliable change during TIVA. During injection of local anesthetic, a finger should be placed over the sacrum to detect inadvertent subcutaneous injection. Advancing an intravenous catheter rather than a needle diminishes the risk of an intravascular or intraosseous injection. The use of US has been advocated to improve the success rate of caudal blocks.

Drugs, Concentrations, and Volumes (see Tables 7.2 and 7.3)

Bupivacaine For single-shot caudal analgesia in outpatients, we administer 1 mL/kg of a 0.175% solution of bupivacaine with epinephrine, which provides comparable analgesia as that of 0.25% bupivacaine with less motor block. This concentration is ideal for outpatients who walk; by the time surgery and recovery are complete, children can stand without leg weakness and discharged home. (A 0.175% solution is prepared by combining 6 mL of preservative-free saline with 14 mL of 0.25% bupivacaine with epinephrine [100 μg, total volume 20 mL]). For infants who do not walk, we use a 0.2% solution as this provides slightly greater duration of block without leg weakness. (A 0.2% solution is prepared by combining 4 mL of preservative-free saline with 16 mL of 0.25% bupivacaine with epinephrine.)

Table 7.3 Dosing regimens for epidural/caudal blocks

Bupivacaine	
Loading dose (0.25%)	0.5 mL/kg
Infusions[a]	
Children	0.4–0.5 mg/kg/h for (0.125% at 0.3 mL/kg/h)[b]
Infants	0.25 mg/kg/h for (0.125% at 0.2 mL/kg/h)[b]
Neonates[c]	0.2 mg/kg/h (0.1% at 0.2 mL/kg/h)
Ropivacaine	
Loading dose (0.2%)	0.5 mL/kg
Infusions[a]	
Children	0.4 mg/kg/h
Neonates-6 mos.	0.2 mg/kg/h
PCEA (0.1 or 0.2%)	
Bolus dose	0.1 mg/kg
Lockout interval	10 min
Background infusion	0.1 mg/kg/h
Levobupivacaine	
Loading dose (0.25%)	0.5–1.0 mL/kg
Infusion[a] (0.0625–0.125%)	0.3 mL/kg/h[b]
2-Chloroprocaine	
Loading dose (1–3%):	10–20[d] mg/kg
Infusion[a] (1–3%)	0.3–1[d] mL/kg/h
Morphine	
Single dose	0.030[e] mg/kg (range of 0.01–0.10 mg/kg) preservative-free morphine in up to 15 mL preservative-free saline
Fentanyl	
Infusion	1–2 µg/mL @ 0.3 mL/kg/h without local anesthetic
PCEA	
Loading dose	1.4 µg/kg
Bolus dose	0.5 µg/kg
Lockout interval	15 min
Background infusion	0.5 µg/kg/h

[a]Start infusion immediately after the loading dose
[b]No benefit adding fentanyl to this solution
[c]Limit infusions to 48 h
[d]Maximum dose recommended is 60 mg/kg
[e]Most effective and commonly used dose; larger doses generally increase side effects
PCEA; patient-controlled epidural analgesia

Ropivacaine Ropivacaine 0.2% provides similar analgesia and duration of action as bupivacaine with less risk of cardiotoxicity. For lower abdominal surgery, use 1 mL/kg of 0.2% ropivacaine; for genital surgery, e.g., hypospadias repair, use 0.5–1 mL/kg.

The addition of clonidine (1–2 μg/mL) to bupivacaine (where 1 mL/kg local anesthetic solution is instilled) extends analgesia for ~3 h. Other drugs that prolong caudal analgesia include preservative-free midazolam, dexmedetomidine, and preservative-free ketamine; however, approved preparations are not currently available in the United States.

Awake Single-Shot Caudal Analgesia for Lower Abdominal Surgery in Small Infants

Awake caudal analgesia is an effective alternative to awake spinal anesthesia in infants for lower abdominal surgery. This block can affect motor blockade with bupivacaine 0.75 mL/kg of a 0.375% or 1 mL/kg of a 0.25% solution with a duration of analgesia up to 90 min. The dose of bupivacaine given when this technique is used may reach 3 mg/kg (to prevent leg movement), but has been considered acceptable because it is a single dose, the volume of distribution is large in the very small infant, and this dose has a proven safety record. Alternatively, an equal volume of 0.2% ropivacaine might have a better safety profile with a similar duration of anesthesia and motor blockade. A sugar-coated soother may help to calm the infant during the surgery; sedation should be avoided in former preterm infants as described above.

Continuous Caudal Analgesia

In neonates, infants, and children up to 5 years of age, prolonged intraoperative and postoperative analgesia can be provided using a continuous caudal block (see Table 7.3). Using aseptic precautions, a 20-gauge epidural catheter may be threaded through an 18-gauge IV cannula and advanced to the desired level. In most infants, it is possible to pass the catheter to the thoracic level. If resistance is felt and is not relieved by rolling the catheter or slight flexion or extension of the child's spine, do not advance the catheter further. Threading catheters, particularly those <20 gauge, to the lumbar and thoracic levels is not always possible. However, if a wire styletted catheter is used with a nerve stimulator (<0.6 mA stimulation), intercostal muscles contract tracks the location of the catheter tip as it advances. Once the catheter is positioned, apply tincture of benzoin to the skin around the puncture site and a transparent occlusive dressing. A second barrier drape is applied with benzoin to separate the rectal area from the catheter insertion site; the site should be regularly inspected. Some practitioners obtain an epidurogram to verify the correct position of the catheter tip.

Although the risk of fecal contamination is very small, some tunnel the catheter subcutaneously to further reduce the infection risk. This is achieved by inserting a Tuohy needle into the skin several centimeters lateral and cephalad to the catheter insertion site and tunneling the catheter subcutaneously such that the tip of the needle emerges at the catheter insertion site. Care must be taken to avoid severing the catheter with the tip of the Tuohy needle as it passes through the catheter site. The catheter is then passed retrograde through the tip of the Tuohy needle emerging from the upper end of the needle. The Tuohy is removed, both sites are covered, and the catheter is secured.

Continuous caudal (and epidural) infusions of local anesthetics require ongoing vigilance. Trained nurses experienced in managing infants and children with caudal/epidural catheters are essential. If such skilled nurses are not available, the child should be monitored in an ICU or similar advanced monitoring setting. The addition of opioids to a continuous epidural infusion increases the risk of perioperative apnea as well as the risk of urinary retention, and other adverse side effects (see above). Morphine may spread more rostrally than fentanyl, being less lipophilic than fentanyl, predisposing to a greater risk for apnea particularly in infants with multisystem diseases, respiratory compromise, or those who are neurologically impaired.

Neonates and infants <6 mos. metabolize bupivacaine and ropivacaine much more slowly than adults; hence, their infusion rates should be much smaller (maximum infusion rate $\leq$ 0.2 mg/kg/h), not exceeding >48 h in duration to preclude toxicity (see Table 7.3).

Some centers infuse lidocaine in their continuous epidurals to serially measure the plasma concentration of lidocaine to prevent toxicity. 2-Chloroprocaine is also used for continuous infusions particularly in neonates, because it is rapidly metabolized by tissue esterases into inactive metabolites.

Lumbar and Thoracic Epidural Blocks

Lumbar epidural blocks have been widely used for postoperative pain relief. The technique used is similar to that for adults; the "loss of resistance method" using saline is recommended to identify the epidural space. Air should not be used to test for loss of resistance because an intravascular air embolism may occur.

Thoracic epidural blocks may be performed using a technique similar to that used in adults. A midline approach is preferred, and the needle advanced at an angle determined by the configuration of the vertebral spine at the level selected. (Examination of the lateral chest radiograph is helpful before performing this block.) Thoracic epidural catheters are generally limited to adolescents who are sedated but not anesthetized during catheter placement so that paresthesias can be identified.

Special Considerations

In children who weigh more than 10 kg, the distance from the skin to lumbar epidural space (in millimeters) is approximately the child's weight in kilograms, i.e., the distance in a 20-kg child is about 20 mm.

A 19-gauge (5 cm) Tuohy needle and a 21-gauge catheter are usually used in children younger than 5 years of age. In older children, an 18-gauge Tuohy needle and a 20-gauge epidural catheter are used. US guidance improves success rate and reduces the risk of dural puncture and the number of needle passes.

Initial Volume to Be Injected

For a lumbar epidural block, bupivacaine 0.125% with 1:200,000 epinephrine or 0.2% ropivacaine is used in a dose of 1 mL/kg up to 20 mL, supplemented with a dose of 0.2 mL/kg to achieve the level of block required. For a thoracic epidural, the loading dose is 0.05 mL/kg × the number of dermatomes to be blocked. Dexamethasone 0.1 mg/kg may be added to prolong the block.

Continuous Infusion Epidural Analgesia

Solutions of 0.125% bupivacaine or 0.1% ropivacaine are widely used in combination with fentanyl (0–3 μg/mL), morphine (5–10 μg/mL), hydromorphone (3–7 μg/mL), or clonidine (0.5–1 μg/mL) (see Table 7.3). The maximum bupivacaine or ropivacaine infusion rate is 0.2 mg/kg/h in neonates and young infants <6 mos. and 0.4 mg/kg/h for infants >6 mos. and children, for up to 48 h.

Toxic concentrations and sequelae of local analgesics may occur in infants and children receiving continuous infusions, especially when the duration of the infusion is >48 h. Recognize that children may not report the early symptoms of tinnitus, lightheadedness, and visual effects. Children may find common side effects such as numbness (pins and needles) or weakness in their legs upsetting and disturbing but should be reassured. The concentration of local anesthetic may be reduced to attenuate the side effects. Some practitioners feel that intermittent "top-up" doses may be safer than continuous infusions in young children. Patient-controlled epidural analgesia (PCEA) has been effective in children as young as 5 years with both bupivacaine (0.1% with fentanyl 5 μg/mL) and ropivacaine (0.2%). The optimal dosing for PCEA in children has not been determined (see Suggested Reading). Sequelae are more common after epidural opioids in children than in adults. Vomiting may be treated with round-the-clock ondansetron and pruritus treated with a background infusion of low-dose naloxone (0.25–1 μg/kg/h) or nalbuphine

(0.025 mg/kg q6h). Urinary retention, a consequence of including opioids in the epidural solution, can be relieved with a urine catheter but may also respond to reduced opioid concentration and/or a naloxone infusion at the same rate as for treating pruritus. *Note*: *Be aware that respiratory depression is always possible and is generally heralded by a slowing of respirations; therefore, rescue orders for naloxone and narrow parameters for monitoring respiratory rate are essential.*

Peripheral Nerve Blocks

Head, Neck, and Upper Limb Blocks

(a) Supraorbital and Supratrochlear Nerve Blocks

These nerves are easy to block in children; the supraorbital nerve exits the supraorbital notch, which is readily palpated in children as one palpates the orbital rim from medial to lateral. The supratrochlear nerve exits the orbital rim several millimeters medial to the supraorbital notch.

Preferred Technique For both blocks, a 27-gauge needle is positioned as described above and 1 mL bupivacaine 0.25% with epinephrine or 0.2% ropivacaine is injected. These blocks anesthetize the ipsilateral frontal region of the scalp for superficial surgery in this region, e.g., a frontal ventriculoperitoneal shunt.

(b) Infraorbital Nerve Block

The infraorbital nerve block is also simple to perform and provides good analgesia following cleft lip repair or for children undergoing endoscopic sinus procedures. The infraorbital foramen can be palpated 1–1.5 cm below the infraorbital rim in line with the supraorbital notch and the pupil. With one technique a needle can be inserted at this point and 1–1.5 mL of local analgesic injected. However, in order to reduce the potential for a hematoma, the preferred technique is subcutaneous through the mouth.

Preferred Technique The upper lip is retracted, and a long 25 or 27 g needle is advanced through the buccal mucosa and directed subcutaneously toward the infraorbital foramen. A finger is placed on the infraorbital foramen, and the needle progress is palpated to reduce the risk of orbital puncture. After aspiration, 1 mL of 0.25% bupivacaine with epinephrine or 0.2% ropivacaine is injected.

(c) Greater Occipital Nerve Block

A greater occipital nerve block may be performed by injecting 1–3 mL of 0.25% bupivacaine with epinephrine 1:200,000 or 0.2% ropivacaine as the nerve exits the skull next to the great occipital artery at the level of the superior nuchal line. This will provide analgesia for superficial surgery involving the back of the head, e.g., a posterior ventricular peritoneal shunt.

(d) Superficial Cervical Plexus Block

The nerves of the superficial cervical plexus may be readily blocked at the posterior aspect of the sternocleidomastoid muscle. A block of the greater auricular nerve and the lesser occipital nerve may be very useful in the child who has an incision behind the ear for mastoid surgery, tympanoplasty, or cochlear implant (Fig. 7.2).

(e) Brachial Plexus Blocks

There are several approaches to block the brachial plexus; the most commonly used are the axillary, supraclavicular, and infraclavicular routes.

Axillary Approach The axillary approach is often recommended because of its simplicity and lack of serious complications, e.g., pneumothorax; it is easy to perform if the child can abduct the arm and is further simplified by placing the hand behind the head. It is useful for forearm fractures, plastic surgery procedures, and insertion of shunts for dialysis, but the block does not include the area of the upper arm and sometimes not the area supplied by musculocutaneous nerves.

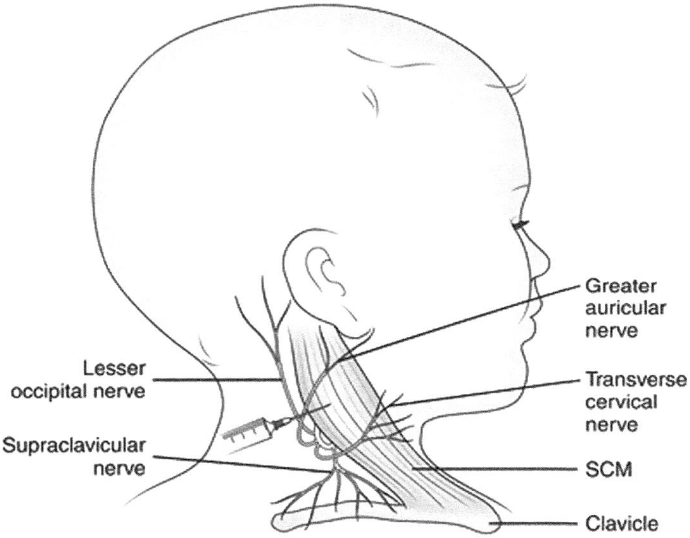

Fig. 7.2 A profile view of the right side of an infant's neck and head, highlighting four key nerves, the lesser occipital nerve, greater auricular nerve, transverse cervical nerve, and supraclavicular nerve that comprise the cervical plexus, where a needle marks the site to subcutaneously infiltrate local anesthetic; at the midpoint of the posterior border of the sternocleidomastoid muscle (SCM). Reproduced with permission: Polaner DM, et al. 2025

Preferred Technique US guidance is preferred (Fig. 7.3a). After donning gloves, sterilizing the skin, and infiltrating with local anesthesia, advance a short-beveled needle cephalad, at a 45° angle to skin, alongside and parallel to the axillary artery (Fig. 7.3b). A slight "give" or "pop" should be felt as the neurovascular sheath is entered, and the arterial pulsations will be seen rocking the needle. With a nerve stimulator, a motor response should be detected in the ulnar, radial, or median nerve with 0.2 mA stimulation. The needle is supported gently, the plastic extension and syringe are connected to the needle, and after aspiration the drug is carefully injected with periodic aspiration. Pressure distally over the axillary artery may encourage proximal spread of the local analgesic solution and a more complete block.

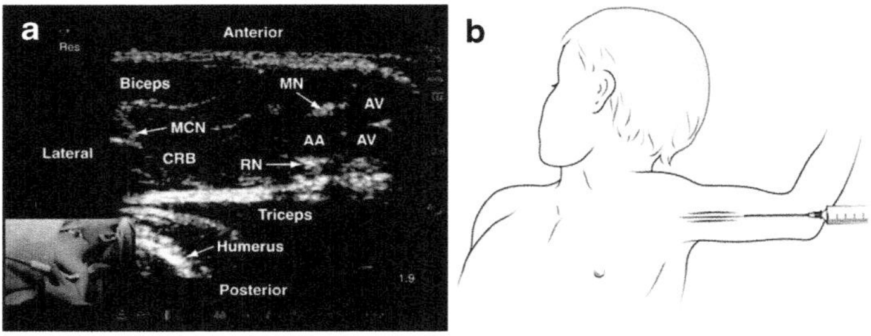

Fig. 7.3 Axillary block. (**a**) Transverse ultrasound view of the left axilla. Biceps muscle, humerus, and triceps muscle are identified. AA; Axillary artery, AV; axillary vein, CRB; coracobrachialis muscle, MCN; musculocutaneous nerve, MN; median nerve, Res; resolution, RN; radial nerve (photo). The US probe is positioned in the left axilla. (Reproduced with permission, *Regional Anesthesia*, Polaner et al. (2025) (**b**) Approach to injecting the brachial plexus in the axilla: the needle is directed parallel to axillary artery

Volume to Be Injected Use 0.2–0.3 mL/kg of any local anesthetic (Table 7.2 for maximum doses); for older children, a maximum volume of 20 mL is sufficient.

Lateral Infraclavicular Approach This block may have advantages over the axillary block by providing more reliable analgesia in the musculocutaneous nerve distribution; however, pneumothorax is a potential complication. US guidance is strongly encouraged to reduce this risk.

Preferred Technique The block is performed inferior to the clavicle adjacent to the coracoid process of the scapula, which can readily be palpated in the child. The needle is inserted slightly caudal and slightly medial to the coracoid process and advanced vertically in a posterior direction. The use of US permits a high success rate, reduces the total volume of local anesthetic required, allows each of the three nerves to be individually blocked, and facilitates catheter insertion if a continuous brachial plexus block is indicated. A nerve stimulator may be used in the anesthetized child when US is not available to position the tip of the needle adjacent to the cords of the plexus. Wrist or forearm extensor movements, i.e., from posterior cord stimulation, when stimulated with 0.5 mA, are predictive of success.

Volume to Be Injected Inject 0.2–0.3 mL/kg of local anesthetic (Table 7.2 for maximum doses).

Supraclavicular Approach This block can be performed in children for surgery involving the upper arm and forearm. With US guidance, there are few complications, but if nerve stimulation is used alone, there is a risk of vertebral artery injection and pneumothorax.

Preferred Technique US is preferable. If stimulation is used, the plexus is located above the clavicle using a short bevel stimulating needle (1 mA). After piercing the skin, movement of any muscles of the upper extremity is accepted as correct placement, and the local anesthetic is deposited.

Volume to Be Injected Inject 0.15–0.2 mL/kg of local anesthetic (Table 7.2 for maximum doses).

Intercostal Nerve Blocks

Intercostal nerve blocks may be performed to relieve pain after thoracotomy or some upper abdominal procedures.

Special Considerations

1. Systemic absorption of local analgesics is the most rapid of any block from the very vascular intercostal space with a commensurate risk of toxic effects; take care not to exceed a total dose of 2 mg/kg of bupivacaine or ropivacaine. To limit this absorption, epinephrine (1:200,000) in the local anesthetic is recommended.
2. The risk of pneumothorax is substantial, especially in small children, in whom the distance from nerve to pleura is very small.
3. The intercostal nerves are sheathed in a dural layer posteriorly; injection near their origin can result in a total spinal block.

Preferred Technique

In infants and small children, the nerve in the intercostal space is approached by placing the needle at 90 degrees to the rib. Palpate the lower margin of the rib, pull the skin upward, and advance until contacting the rib. The skin is released and the needle "walked" off the rib margin. A volume of 1–5 mL/rib of 0.25% bupivacaine or 0.2% ropivacaine with epinephrine 1:200,000 not exceeding a total of 2 mg/kg is then injected while advancing the needle in 1–3 mm increments and aspirating frequently.

Abdominal and Inguinal Peripheral Nerve Blocks

TAP Block

The transversus abdominal plane (TAP) block reduces pain and opioid use in children undergoing abdominal surgery intra and postoperatively. This block involves local anesthetic infiltration into the fascial plane between transversus abdominis and internal oblique muscles in the anterior axillary line subcostal, usually in a single dose, bilaterally for midline or unilateral surgeries (Table 7.4, Fig. 7.4). Although there is conflicting evidence as to whether this block is superior to local infiltration, ilioinguinal-iliohypogastric block, or epidural blockade for specific surgeries, it is an effective alternative with very few complications. Dosing is independent of whether high concentration/small volumes or low concentration/high volumes of local anesthetics are used.

Table 7.4 Surgeries supported with TAP blocks

Pyloromyotomy
Umbilical hernia
Gastrostomy tube insertion
Nissen Fundoplication
Laparotomy
Ureteral reimplantation
Colostomy and closure of colostomy
Appendectomy
Herniorrhaphy
Orchiopexy

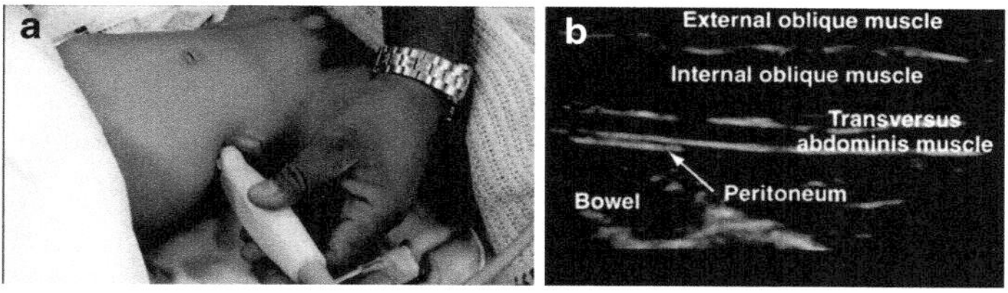

Fig. 7.4 Posterior transverse abdominis plane (TAP) block. (**a**) The US transducer is positioned between the iliac crest and the costal margin along the right midaxillary line. (**b**) The three layers of the abdominal musculature. Needle approach is directed toward the US probe in the fascial plane between the IOM and the TAM, depositing local aesthetic yielding a hypoechoic distention of the plane. (EOM; External oblique muscle, IOM; internal oblique muscle, TAM; transversus abdomen muscle). (Reproduced with permission. Regional Anesthesia. Polaner et al. (2025))

Dosing regimens include 0.25% bupivacaine (0.2 mL/kg) or 0.2% ropivacaine (0.5 mL/kg) bilaterally. The total dose of bupivacaine should be limited to 2 mg/kg in neonates, 3 mg/kg in children, and 4 mg/kg in adolescents.

Ilioinguinal and Iliohypogastric Nerve Block

The ilioinguinal and iliohypogastric nerve block provides skin analgesia over the inguinal region providing postoperative analgesia after herniotomy. The block is preferably performed immediately after induction of general anesthesia and before the operation commences; alternatively, it can be placed by the surgeon following repair. The nerves run beneath the internal oblique muscle just medial to the anterior superior iliac spine and may be blocked by a fan-shaped infiltration of the abdominal wall in this region (Fig. 7.5). US guidance improves success, decreases the volume of drug required, and reduces the potential for intra-abdominal puncture. Bupivacaine or ropivacaine 0.2–0.5% (up to 2 mg/kg) with epinephrine (1:200,000) may be used; more complete analgesia is obtained with the 0.5% solution, but occasionally this concentration produces a transient femoral nerve block with leg weakness.

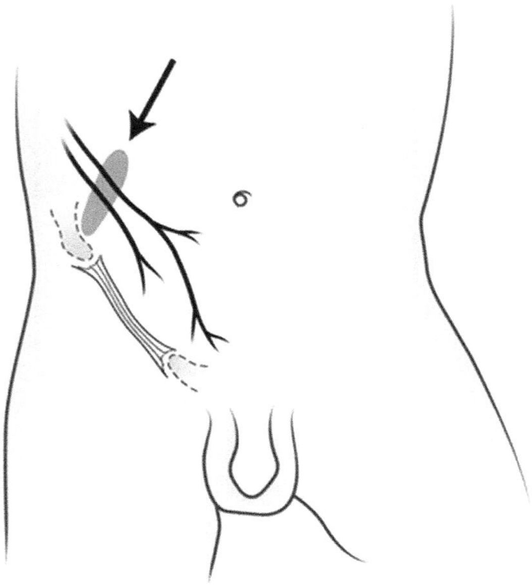

Fig. 7.5 Ilioinguinal-iliohypogastric nerve block: area to be infiltrated with local anesthetic

Penile Block

The paired dorsal nerves pass inferior to the pubic bones on either side of the midline and supply the dorsal aspect of the penis and foreskin. A block of these nerves provides good pain relief after circumcision but does not provide adequate analgesia after hypospadias repair. Epinephrine-containing solutions should not be used because vasoconstriction might result in damaging ischemia to the penis. Complications have been very rare after properly performed penile blocks.

Volume to Be Injected

Up to 2 mg/kg of 0.5% bupivacaine *without epinephrine* is injected to a maximum volume of 1 mL in the small infant or 6 mL in the large child.

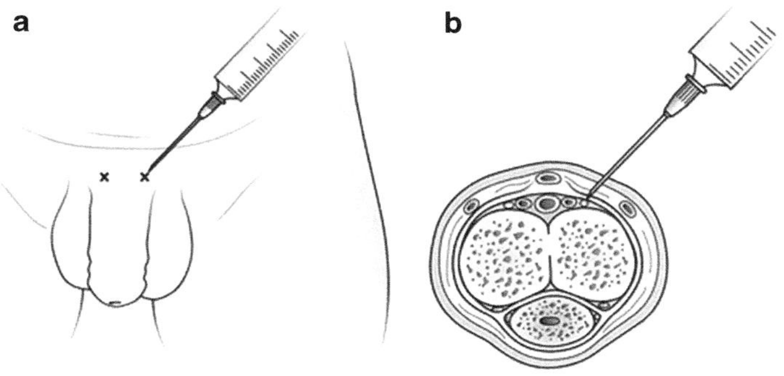

Fig. 7.6 Block of the dorsal nerves of the penis. (**a**) Injection sites. (**b**) Position of nerves at base of penis

Preferred Technique

Using an aseptic technique, bilateral injections are made beneath the pubis at the base of the penis at the 11 o'clock and 1 o'clock positions (Fig. 7.6). The needle should be felt to pass through Buck's fascia to deposit an equal volume adjacent to each nerve. In infants, it is possible to anesthetize both nerves by inserting the needle in the midline of the dorsal surface of the penis.

Alternatively, a subcutaneous ring block at the base of the penis may be performed; one study suggests that epinephrine added to the local anesthetic is safe with a subcutaneous ring block at the base of the penis.

Lower Limb Blocks

Femoral Nerve Block

The femoral nerve block is useful for fractures of the shaft of the femur and for muscle biopsy in patients with suspected myopathy (in which case it should be combined with a lateral femoral cutaneous nerve block). For children with a fracture of the femur, a continuous femoral nerve block provides continuous analgesia and relieves muscle spasms.

Preferred Technique The femoral artery is identified by palpation just below the inguinal ligament. After skin analgesia has been established, a 1-in., 22-gauge short bevel needle is advanced slowly just lateral to the artery at an angle of 45° to skin (Fig. 7.7). Slight resistance should be felt at two separate levels, the fascia lata and the fascia iliaca, after which the needle lies within the femoral sheath. The needle should then be gently supported, aspirated, and injected with periodic aspiration.

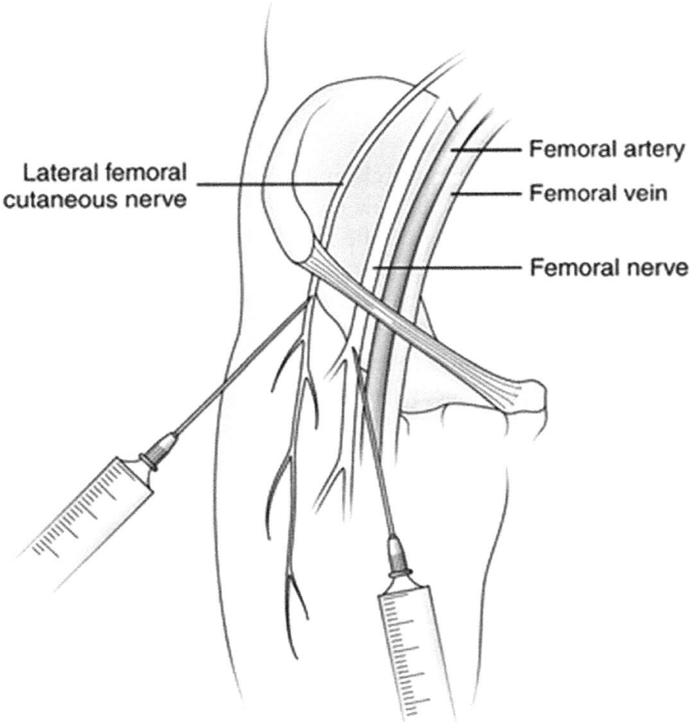

Fig. 7.7 Femoral nerve block and block of the lateral femoral cutaneous nerve of the thigh

Volume to Be Injected Use 0.2–0.3 mL/kg of local anesthetic with 1:200,000 epinephrine.

Continuous Femoral Nerve Block

Using an aseptic technique and skin analgesia, a Tuohy needle with an obturator is advanced, as outlined previously, through the two identified layers of resistance. The needle is positioned with the opening facing cephalad, and a standard epidural catheter is advanced proximally for 5–10 cm within the femoral sheath. When the Tuohy needle is correctly placed, the catheter should advance easily with little resistance. The Tuohy needle can then be withdrawn and the catheter left in situ, as when inserting an epidural catheter. Never attempt to withdraw the catheter through the needle because the tip may be sheared off and remain in the child. US guidance will improve success rate.

Volume to Be Injected Intermittent top-up doses of long-acting local anesthetic or a continuous infusion may be used at a rate of 0.1 mL/kg/h.

Lateral Femoral Cutaneous Nerve Block

Block of the lateral femoral cutaneous nerve provides analgesia over the lateral aspect of the thigh.

Preferred Technique The needle is inserted medial and inferior to the anterior superior iliac spine, just superior to the inguinal ligament, and advanced superiorly and laterally until it impinges on the iliac bone. The local analgesic solution is injected as the needle is slowly withdrawn.

Volume to Be Injected Use 2–5 mL of local anesthetic with 1:200,000 epinephrine injected in a fanlike manner.

Sciatic Nerve Block

The sciatic nerve in children may be blocked via an anterior, lateral, or posterior approach; the latter approach is considered to be the easiest and likely to be the most successful.

Preferred Technique The child should be anesthetized and placed in a semi-prone position with the side of the nerve to be blocked elevated. The needle should be inserted at right angles to the skin at the midpoint of a line between the sacrococcygeal membrane and the greater trochanter of the femur, i.e., just lateral to the ischial tuberosity, until it is adjacent to the sciatic nerve. Confirm by US or by electrical stimulation (0.5 mA) using a sheathed insulated needle.

If a catheter is needed for a continuous infusion, insert the needle just inferior to the gluteal fold and angle the needle slightly cephalad to approach the same site; the catheter will then be easier to secure and protect.

Volume to Be Injected For a single dose, 0.2–0.3 mL/kg of local anesthetic with epinephrine 1:200,000. For a continuous block, use 0.1 mL/kg/h of local anesthetic.

Popliteal Fossa Block of the Sciatic Nerve

The sciatic nerve may also be blocked as it approaches the popliteal fossa. This block is useful to provide analgesia for foot surgery. Just proximal to the popliteal fossa, the nerve divides into the tibial nerve, which innervates the posterior calf and plantar area, and the peroneal nerve, which supplies sensation to the anterior leg. To be successful, the block must be performed above the division site; this is 3–7 cm above the popliteal crease in children under 8 years but slightly more cephalad (within 3.5–8 cm) in older children. The approximate site to make the injection is 1 cm proximal to the popliteal crease for each 10 kg of body weight; the needle should be angled at 45° to the skin surface pointing cephalad. The injection is made just lateral to the midline to avoid vascular structures. The block may be performed with the child in a lateral, supine, or prone position. Successful block can be achieved using a nerve stimulator (0.2–0.5 mA) to locate the main sciatic nerve or preferably by US. Continuous popliteal nerve blocks are becoming increasingly popular to replace caudal/epidural blocks for lower extremity surgery; a single dose of 5–10 mL of local anesthetic or a 20-gauge catheter is threaded 3–5 cm into the fossa, and local anesthetic is infused at 0.1 mL/kg/h.

Adductor Canal Block

This block is a completely sensory block that reduces postoperative pain after reconstructive knee surgery or patella dislocation. Under US guidance, the subsartorial canal, which lies lateral to the belly of the sartorius muscle, is visualized mid-thigh. The canal contains the superficial femoral artery and two hyperechoic structures, the saphenous nerve and the nerve to vastus medialis, that may rest on either side of the artery (Fig. 7.8). A single dose of 20 mL ropivacaine 0.5% (with 5–10 mg dexamethasone) is deposited in the canal watching hydro expansion of the canal as the local anesthetic encircles the superficial femoral artery to block both nerves. The duration of this block after a single dose is 12–24 h.

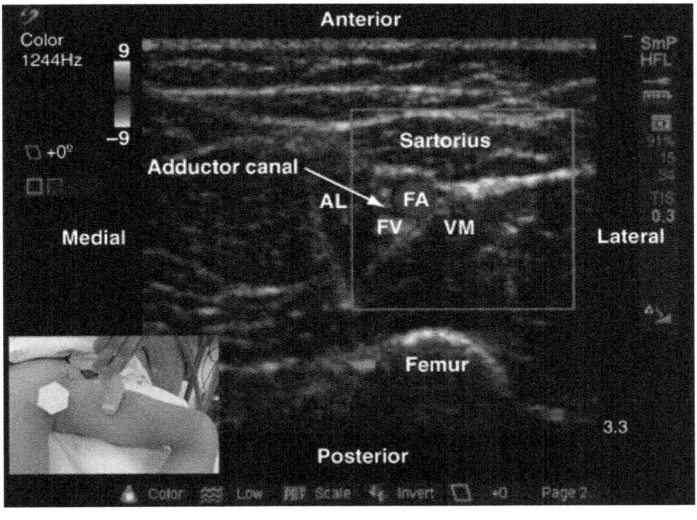

Fig. 7.8 US of the left adductor canal block for knee surgery at mid-thigh (lower left photo). The subsartorial canal (identified) mid-screen is flanked by the sartorius, adductor, and vastus medialis. The canal contains the femoral artery and vein and several nerves; the saphenous nerve, nerve to vastus medialis and two branches of the obturator nerve. AL; adductor longus muscle, VM; vastus medialis muscle. Inset depicts application of the US probe to the medial aspect of the left thigh in an anesthetized child. (Reproduced with permission. *Regional Anesthesia*, Polaner et al. (2025))

Ankle Block

Blocks of the branches of the sciatic nerve at the level of the ankle are very easy to perform and require only small doses of local anesthetics. An ankle block provides excellent analgesia following club foot repair. It is necessary to block the deep peroneal nerve alongside the anterior tibial artery, the saphenous nerve which lies alongside the saphenous vein, the posterior tibial nerve alongside the posterior tibial artery, and the sural nerve, which is just lateral to the Achilles tendon. Infiltration of the skin over the lateral aspect of the anterior tibia will block any branches of the superficial peroneal nerve supplying the dorsum of the foot.

Intravenous Regional Analgesia

The “Bier” (intravenous) block may be useful in older children with forearm fractures.

Preferred Technique

Insert a small intravenous cannula in the hand or foot. Use a reliable *double* pneumatic tourniquet. The success of the block varies with the degree of limb exsanguination, which can be achieved before injection of the local analgesic; use an Esmarch elastic bandage or elevate the limb if wrapping is too painful. Inflate the proximal cuff to 1.5–2 times the systolic pressure and inject the local analgesic solution. Do not exceed 5 mg/kg of 0.25–0.5% lidocaine (1 mL/kg). *Bupivacaine or ropivacaine should never be used for an intravenous block.* The addition of a very small dose of an intermediate-acting muscle relaxant (~10% of the usual intubating dose) will provide paralysis and perhaps improve surgical conditions by eliminating movements. When the block is established (~5 min), inflate the distal cuff and then deflate the proximal cuff. Do not release the remaining cuff until at least 30 min have elapsed, even if the operation is finished sooner.

This technique has been successfully used in children with forearm fractures requiring reduction and casting. The tourniquet should not be released until the fiberglass cast had been applied. Only a very small percentage of these patients experienced subsequent problems with a tight cast.

Suggested Reading

Barnett NR, Hagen JG, Kattail D. Pediatric regional anesthesia and acute pain management: state of the art. Best Pract Res Clin Anaesth. 2024;38:135–44.

Ecoffey C, Bosenberg A, Lonnqvist PA, et al. Practice advisory on the prevention and management of complications of pediatric regional anesthesia. J Clin Anesth. 2022;79:110725.

Guay J, Suresh S, Kopp S. The use of ultrasound guidance for perioperative neuraxial and peripheral nerve blocks in children. Cochrane Database Syst Rev. 2019;2(2):CD011436.

Mahrous RSS, Ahmed AAA, Ahmed AMM. Comparison between ultrasound-guided caudal analgesia versus peripheral nerve blocks for lower limb surgeries in pediatrics: a randomized controlled prospective study. Local Reg Anesth. 2022;15:77–86.

Polaner DM, et al. In: Coté CJ, Lerman J, Anderson BJ, editors. A practice of anesthesia for infants and children. 7th ed. Philadelphia: Elsevier; 2025. Chap 40.

Sola C, Menacé C, Bringuier S, et al. Transversus abdominal plane block in children: efficacy and safety: a randomized clinical study and pharmacokinetic profile. Anesth Analg. 2019;128:1234–41.

Wiegele M, Marhofer P, Lonnqvist P-A. Caudal epidural blocks in paediatric patients: a review and practical considerations. Br J Anaesth. 2019;122:509–17.

Xu W, Wie H, Zhang T. Methods of prolonging the effect of caudal block in children. Front Pediatr. 2024;12:1406263.

8 Special Medical Conditions

Upper Respiratory Tract Infection (URTI)

Many children have or are recovering from a runny nose or other manifestations of an URTI when evaluated before general anesthesia. Indiscriminate cancellation is unwarranted and causes emotional and financial problems for children and their families; each case must be carefully evaluated. Some children have a runny nose most of the time because of allergies or a chronic nasal infection; these children should be distinguished from those with an acute URTI.

Children have frequent URTIs, up to 6–8/year, which means once every 6–8 weeks. Although in theory, airway irritability may last for 6–8 weeks, delaying surgery more than approximately 2 weeks after a URTI does not reduce morbidity for most viruses, e.g., rhinovirus. Since COVID19, however, more children are swabbed for the cause of the URTI, e.g., streptococcus and RSV, which prompted modification of the management algorithm (Fig. 8.1). In contrast, children with an asymptomatic URTI can proceed without delay (see Fig. 8.1). Clear rhinorrhea may be treated with 1–2 drops of either Neo-Synephrine (0.25%) or oxymetazoline per nostril to dry secretions. Anticholinergics do not affect the incidence of perioperative airway complications.

Proceeding with anesthesia in otherwise healthy children within 2 weeks of having a symptomatic URTI (see Fig. 8.1)

J. Lerman, C. J. Coté, *Steward's Manual of Pediatric Anesthesia*,
https://doi.org/10.1007/978-3-032-24545-8_8

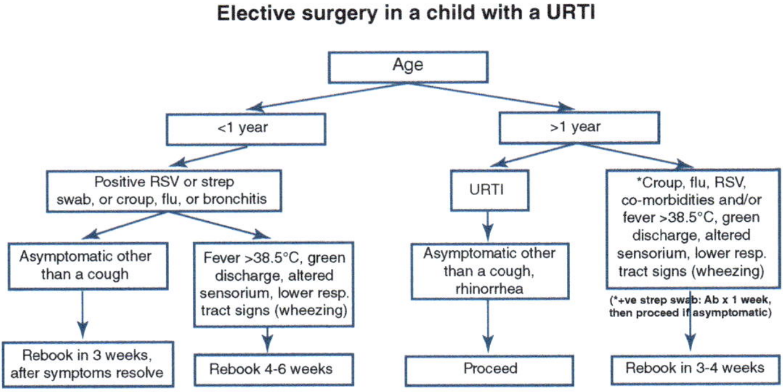

Fig. 8.1 Decision-making algorithm for children with an URTI. *Ab;* antibiotics, *RSV*; respiratory syncytial virus

poses an increased risk of perioperative respiratory events including oxyhemoglobin desaturation, bronchospasm, and laryngospasm, which may delay discharge home or result in an overnight admission. Although these complications can be disturbing, most are easily managed (see Chap. 4). Infants <1 year of age, infants who were born premature, children exposed to second-hand smoke, and children with reactive airway disease with a concomitant URTI may have more serious and more frequent airway problems in the perioperative period and should be managed more conservatively (Fig. 8.1). Children with a URTI within the past 2 weeks experience more frequent pulmonary complications if they undergo major, e.g., cardiac, surgery.

Children with reactive airway disease, i.e., asthma, benefit from their usual bronchodilators; bronchodilators and a vital capacity cough may resolve mild bronchospasm and airways plugged with mucus. Tracheal intubation is avoided if the airway can be managed with an LMA; this reduces the incidence of bronchospasm. However, evidence suggests that the incidence of laryngospasm increases when LMAs are used in children with recent URTIs (where possible a face mask may be preferable).

Rebook ≥3 weeks after an URTI because the start date of the infection is often vague. J. Lerman 2025.

1. Elective surgery

   Children with a mild URTI without systemic or pulmonary symptoms may proceed with minor surgery (see Fig. 8.1) because evidence suggests no increased risk of complications. The decision to proceed should be discussed with the parents and the surgeon. Anesthesia via a face mask or laryngeal mask airway (LMA) and the use of sevoflurane may reduce airway complications. Avoid tracheal intubation when practical.

   (a) Children >1 year who present for elective surgery with croup, positive throat swab for flu, RSV, or any of the symptoms listed in Fig. 8.1 should be rescheduled after 4 weeks.

   (b) Children with a history of asthma complicating a URTI demand special attention; nonurgent surgery should be deferred for at least 4 weeks when possible.

   (c) Infants <1 year are at increased risk of perioperative respiratory complications even after a mild URTI, and their surgery should be delayed (see Fig. 8.1).

2. Emergency or urgent surgery: When designing the anesthetic prescription, the presence of a full stomach takes precedence over the URTI; an RSI and tracheal intubation should be performed. Perioperative airway problems and laryngospasm must be anticipated.

Asthma

Asthma affects 4–13% of children in North America. The disease is characterized by variable cough, wheezing, and breathlessness, which are episodic and seasonal in many. The symptoms result from bronchoconstriction, mucosal edema, and tenacious secretions in the small airways. Severe attacks may occur throughout childhood and may be life threatening. Acute exacerbations are associated with URTIs, allergens, irritants, exercise, cold induced, or emotional stress. The treatment for mild asthma is inhaled β-adrenergics for bronchodilation and improved mucociliary clearance; more severe asthma may require inhaled corticosteroids to control inflammation. Rarely, oral steroids are prescribed, but their use suggests a recent exacerbation. Severe asthmatic attacks may require systemic corticosteroid therapy and ICU admission. The disease often improves as the child ages. The severity of asthma is usually judged by the therapy required to control the symptoms.

When a child with asthma presents for elective surgery, it is most important to determine whether the child's current status is optimal. The following are important considerations:

1. During an asthma attack, airway reactivity is increased, and mucosal edema and secretions may impair pulmonary function; if possible, surgery should be delayed for at least 1 month after the last acute attack.
2. Elective surgery should be deferred if there is any evidence of an active URTI, which might precipitate and exacerbate symptoms.
3. The frequency of the asthma exacerbations and the symptoms between attacks should be assessed. Has admission to an intensive care unit or ventilator therapy ever been needed? If so, repeated severe attacks are likely.
4. What medications is the child taking, and are they controlling the child's symptoms? Have systemic corticosteroids been necessary? If so, in what dose and when was the last dose (stress dose steroids may be indicated)? Has the child taken all the usual asthma medications today?
5. A focused physical examination is important to detect bronchospasm and exclude other current pulmonary pathology. If wheezing is present, the child should be encouraged to cough deeply. If the wheezing is unresolved, a trial of bronchodilator therapy should be administered. If the bronchospasm clears, then elective surgery that does not require intubation may proceed. If the signs do not resolve, then elective surgery should be deferred.
6. The results of recent pulmonary function tests and especially any response to bronchodilator therapy should be noted.
7. A chest radiograph should be ordered for any child with significant symptoms.

Anesthesia Management

Preoperative

1. Administer routine asthma medications on the day of surgery; oral medications can be taken with a sip of water and inhalation medications repeated, if necessary, just before transfer to the OR.
2. A stress dose of steroids (IV hydrocortisone [1–1.5 mg/kg]) should be administered at induction of anesthesia to those taking the equivalent of greater than 5 mg prednisone per day (adult dose), oral steroids within 3 months, or high-dose inhaled steroids.
3. Administer a premedication if indicated. Atropine, if considered necessary, may be given intravenously to decrease secretions and provide bronchodilation.

Perioperative

1. Propofol is the preferred induction agent. Alternatively, ketamine may be used since it is a bronchodilator and may protect against bronchospasm; however, atropine may be indicated to limit secretions.
2. Inhalation induction with sevoflurane is preferred.
3. Avoid agents known to release histamine and cause bronchospasm, e.g., atracurium, morphine. Desflurane is not recommended as it increases airway resistance in children with asthma. Nitrous oxide, halothane, sevoflurane, fentanyl, rocuronium, and vecuronium are preferred drugs.
4. Tracheal intubation should be performed under deep anesthesia to avoid bronchospasm. Lidocaine (1.5 mg/kg IV) may decrease the potential for bronchospasm. If possible, use an LMA for minor or brief procedures.
5. For surgery >1 h in duration, use a heat and moisture exchanger with a circle circuit.
6. Treat intraoperative wheezing by deepening anesthesia and give bronchodilator aerosols via the tracheal tube, e.g., albuterol. Exclude non-asthmatic causes for wheezing, e.g., a partially obstructed tracheal tube, endobronchial intubation, or

pneumothorax. Albuterol may be delivered through an ETT by inserting it stem down into a 60 mL syringe (after the barrel is removed) and then reinserting the barrel. The syringe is screwed onto the capnography port of the elbow of the breathing circuit, and the barrel is compressed. Only 3–8% of the aerosol delivered using this technique reaches the trachea. To improve delivery a long catheter may be inserted to the distal third of the tracheal tube. In this manner, the majority of the aerosol reaches the tracheal mucosa. Alternatively a specially designed spacer with 15 and 22 mm connections can be placed at the ETT, and puffs coordinated with inspirations.

7. At the end of surgery, antagonize the muscle relaxants as necessary. Sugammadex is preferred, as neostigmine may increase bronchomotor tone. Deep extubation is preferred to minimize precipitating bronchospasm. If awake extubation is planned, intravenous lidocaine or propofol may be administered beforehand to reduce laryngeal and bronchial reflexes.

Postoperative

1. Administer humidified oxygen.
2. When practical, regional analgesia is ideal for pain relief; for major surgery, continuous regional analgesia or patient-controlled analgesia (PCA) may be planned (see Chaps. 5 and 7).
3. Postoperative wheezing may require additional bronchodilator and appropriate adjustment of other medications.

Cystic Fibrosis

Cystic fibrosis (CF) is an inherited disorder that results from a genetic defect on chromosome 7. Abnormal chloride and sodium transport on all epithelial surfaces affects many body systems; it may present in neonates as meconium ileus. During childhood, malabsorption due to pancreatic insufficiency predominates. In the second decade, increasing pulmonary problems (↑functional residual capacity (FRC), ↓forced expired volume at 1 s (FEV_1), and severe pulmonary ventilation-perfusion ($\dot{V}/\dot{Q}$) mismatch) occur because of abnormally viscous secretions and chronic infection. CF-induced diabetes is common in teenagers. Respiratory failure usually develops by the second or third decade of life secondary to retained secretions and chronic infection.

Surgeries for children with CF most commonly include nasal polypectomy, functional endoscopic sinus surgery (FESS), antral lavage, and bronchoscopy for removal of retained secretions and treatment of atelectasis. Children with advanced disease may present for lung transplantation; transplanted lungs do not appear to be affected by CF.

Special Anesthesia Problems

1. Copious, extremely viscous secretions are present in the respiratory tract. Violent coughing and laryngospasm may occur.
2. Because of the $\dot{V}/\dot{Q}$ disturbances:
   (a) Hypoxia may develop rapidly.
   (b) Inhalation induction is prolonged because of $\dot{V}/\dot{Q}$ mismatch; this is exacerbated with less soluble anesthetics such as sevoflurane.
3. Lung compliance is reduced. In severe cases, high airway pressures may be required to adequately ventilate the lungs; a cuffed tracheal tube is recommended.
4. Malnutrition and underweight for age result from malabsorption and chronic infection. Liver function may be reduced in older children. In such cases, drug dosages should be adjusted accordingly.
5. Many children with advanced CF suffer all the emotional upsets of those with chronic disease; they require considerate handling and much reassurance.

Anesthesia Management

Preoperative

1. Assess the child's condition and ensure that the pulmonary status is optimized by means of postural drainage, physiotherapy, and inhalation therapy with nebulized hypertonic saline (7%)

to mobilize secretions and inhaled aminoglycosides to reduce infection shortly before induction.
2. Pulmonary function is usually at its worst early in the morning. If possible, schedule surgery after chest physiotherapy and clearing of secretions.
3. Avoid anticholinergic medications that thicken secretions. Administer opioid premedication and midazolam judiciously, as oxygenation may be compromised.
4. Ensure optimal hydration; fluids must not be withheld for prolonged periods.

Perioperative

N.B. Whenever possible, use local or regional anesthesia.

1. Place an IV for hydration and emergency drug administration.
2. After preoxygenation, inhalational induction may be protracted in those with serious $\dot{V}/\dot{Q}$ mismatch. Alternatively, induce anesthesia with propofol, low-dose opioid, and a muscle relaxant as indicated.
3. Intubate with a cuffed tracheal tube.
4. Suction the trachea using saline lavage to facilitate removing inspissated secretions.
5. Use humidified gases; children with severe CF may require 100% O_2.
6. TIVA (propofol/remifentanil) may be preferred over sevoflurane as the latter impairs mucociliary function (in healthy adults) and attenuates hypoxic pulmonary vasoconstriction.
7. Minimize the use of long-acting medications, plan to extubate as soon as possible, and use a technique that ensures rapid recovery.

Postoperative

1. Give IV fluids until the child is drinking.
2. Administer humidified oxygen and additional hypertonic saline nebulization. Whenever possible place the child in a semi-recumbent position that increases respiratory comfort.

3. Provide optimal analgesia. Use regional analgesia and NSAIDs for postoperative pain whenever possible.
4. Encourage early chest physiotherapy and ambulation and rapid discharge.

Latex Allergy

Latex allergy can cause a severe, life-threatening intraoperative immunoglobulin E-mediated anaphylactic reaction. Urticaria, bronchospasm, and/ or circulatory collapse may occur. Children become sensitized after a history of repeated exposure to latex, e.g., after frequent catheterizations for neurogenic bladder (most current catheters are no longer made of latex), repeated surgery, and/or exposure to rubber balloons or dental dams. Up to 40% of children with spina bifida may have a latex allergy. Latex allergy is especially likely to develop if the child has had >5 surgeries (where latex gloves were used) and has atopy. Cross-reactivity to bananas, avocado, kiwi fruit, and chestnuts may be elicited. Skin-prick testing or radioallergosorbent testing (RAST) to latex may confirm the allergy.

Latex allergy has been the most common cause of anaphylaxis in children during surgery when anaphylaxis is not temporally related to drug administration. However, the frequency of latex anaphylaxis in the OR has diminished substantively in the past 20 years with the elimination of all latex products in the OR. When latex anaphylaxis occurs, it usually begins 30–200 min after induction of anesthesia, after the surgeon inserts their latex gloves into the abdominal cavity or examines mucosal surfaces. The initial signs include the triad of respiratory, cardiovascular, and dermatologic signs: increased peak airway pressure, bronchospasm, decreased oxygen saturation, flushing and/or urticaria, hypotension, and tachycardia.

Rapid, aggressive intervention including ventilation with oxygen, rapid infusion of warmed intravenous fluids to expand the blood volume, and epinephrine 1–10 μg/kg IV bolus followed by an infusion of 0.1–0.3 μg/kg/min may be required until symptoms abate. Supplementary treatment may include antihistamines (diphenhydramine, 1 mg/kg); histamine$_2$ (H_2) receptor-blocking drugs (cimetidine, 5–10 mg/kg); and corticosteroids (hydrocortisone 2 mg/kg).

Refractory anaphylaxis may reflect under-resuscitation with fluids as fluids rapidly migrate to third spaces. Second-line vasopressor therapy (noradrenaline, vasopressin, or dopamine) is anecdotal. Rarely, a phenylephrine infusion supplementing the epinephrine, may be required to support circulatory collapse.

Some practitioners suggest pretreatment before surgery with corticosteroids (prednisone, 1 mg/kg) and H_1- and H_2-blocking drugs (diphenhydramine, cimetidine); however, pretreatment does not prevent a latex reaction. The most important method to avoid such reactions is to maintain a latex-free environment for those at risk for developing a latex allergy or with a known history of latex allergy. It is most important that all members of the surgical team use non-latex gloves and that all latex materials be excluded from the surgical and anesthesia equipment (Table 8.1).

Table 8.1 Anesthesia equipment that may contain latex

Anesthesia circuit and bag; airway or bite block
Intravenous fluid bag
Plastic syringes; vial
IV set (ports)
Catheters
Adhesive tape
Tourniquets
Face mask
Endotracheal tube
Anesthesia circuit and bag
Ventilator bellows
Blood pressure cuff
Gloves

Down Syndrome

Down syndrome (DS) (trisomy 21) is common (1.5/1000 live births). Developmental delay is invariably present but varies in severity; many DS children are capable of relatively independent function in a protected environment.

Associated Conditions

1. Congenital heart disease (CHD) occurs in approximately ~40–50%, particularly atrioventricular canal, ventricular septal defect, patent ductus arteriosus, and tetralogy of Fallot.
2. Respiratory infections, chronic sinusitis, and ear infections are common.
3. Generalized hypotonia and joint laxity are present. Atlantoaxial joint instability occurs in ~15% that infrequently leads to cervical spinal cord injury. The neck is particularly unstable in the flexed position; minimize excessive movement during intubation and positioning.
4. Congenital subglottic stenosis is common. Ensure that the tracheal tube is not too large and that there is an audible leak when positive pressure is applied.
5. Adenotonsillar hypertrophy is often present with obstructive sleep apnea (OSA) (see Chap. 11).
6. Hypothyroidism is common as the child ages (~0.7% infants, ~12% adults); about 1/60 will eventually develop diabetes.
7. Polycythemia may occur in ~15–33% of DS neonates; some may necessitate phlebotomy to relieve circulatory failure. Leukemia develops in ~2% of children with DS.
8. Duodenal atresia is common in the neonate, as is umbilical hernia, renal malformations, undescended testis, and hypospadias.
9. Radial artery abnormalities, i.e., single median artery, are common and may make percutaneous cannulation difficult or impossible.

Special Anesthesia Problems

1. Airway: Anticipate that the large tongue and small nasopharynx will predispose to respiratory obstruction, particularly during induction and recovery. Congenital subglottic stenosis predisposes to postoperative stridor; assure that there is a leak around the tracheal tube.
2. Lungs: Is there an acute infection that requires treatment? Is there a history suggestive of OSA?
3. Problems of associated cardiac disease: endocarditis prophylaxis may be required (see Chap. 12).
4. Ask the parents for any signs or symptoms suggestive of C-spine compression due to potential joint instability (neck pain/tenderness, gait disturbances, hand weakness, dizziness, bowel and bladder dysfunction). Gently examine the range of motion of the neck and perform a CNS examination. Routine neck X-rays are not warranted in the absence of signs or symptoms.
5. Excessive neck movement should be avoided (especially flexion) during laryngoscopy and surgical positioning. An LMA is preferred in place of an ETT if possible (to avoid laryngoscopy), but consider a videolaryngoscope if neck stability is questioned.
6. Cognitively challenged children often benefit from parental presence during induction.

N.B. Children with DS are not overly sensitive to the effects of atropine.

Obesity

The pandemic of childhood obesity impacts pediatric anesthesia in many ways. The diagnosis of obesity in children is more challenging than in adults because of the need to account for growth and development. Thus, accepted definitions for obesity in children are based on their growth curves (based on sex, weight, and height):

Overweight: BMI >85 percentile
Obesity: BMI >95 percentile
Super (morbid) obesity: BMI >99 percentile

Obesity negatively affects many organ systems. Respiratory problems include a restrictive respiratory pattern and an increased incidence of asthma and obstructive sleep apnea. Cardiovascular problems may include systemic hypertension (possible left ventricular hypertrophy), pulmonary hypertension (possible right ventricular hypertrophy), and dyslipidemia. Obesity leads to insulin resistance and type II diabetes mellitus. Other clinical implications include an increased incidence of gastroesophageal reflux, nonalcoholic steatohepatitis, and pseudotumor cerebri. Orthopedic and general surgeries are most common in this condition; bariatric surgery is increasing in frequency.

All medical conditions should be optimized preoperatively. Anticipate possible difficult venous access; ultrasound guidance may be extremely helpful. Obese children undergoing elective surgery are not at increased risk from pneumonitis should aspiration occur; standard fasting intervals should be followed. However, obesity is an independent predictor of difficult mask ventilation; they are considered "difficult airways" because extensive fat deposits across their upper back raise the larynx relative to the axis of the oropharynx. To optimize their airway, obese patients should be ramped at ~25–30° head-up (this increases the functional residual capacity and oxygen reserves) with the head elevation greater than routine. This aligns the tragus at or above the sternal notch (lateral view), providing a direct view of the vocal cords during laryngoscopy. Basal atelectasis and oxygen desaturation occur commonly during brief apneas.

The pharmacokinetics of drugs depends on the their hydro- and lipophilicity. To estimate the kinetics of drugs in obesity, it is instructive to consider the "fat mass" (FM) (as a compartment distinct from their "fat-free mass" (FFM)) as the compartment into which lipophilic drugs distribute; this may be simply defined as:

$$\text{FM} = \text{total body weight}(\text{TBW}) - \text{the lean body weight}(\text{LBW})(\text{all in kg})$$

LBW is the ideal body weight (IBW) plus the added muscle mass to carry the FM or:

$$\text{LBW} = \text{IBW} + 0.3 \text{ (some use } 0.4)(\text{TBW} - \text{IBW})$$

IBW is the ideal body weight for the sex, age, and height of the child. Several formulae may be used to estimate the IBW in children. One such example is:

For those <8 years: IBW (kg) = 2 × Age (years) + 9.
For those 8–12 years: IBW (kg) = 3 × Age (years).

The dosing of anesthetics drugs in obese children based on these formulae still falls short of reliably predicting responses. Obese children have an increased cardiac output, increased extracellular fluid volume, increased LBW, and increased FM. The choice of which scalar (TBW, LBW, or IBW) best predicts the drug dose in obese children varies according with the drug. For example, the doses of propofol (per kg) should use the LBW, nondepolarizing relaxants and morphine IBW, and succinylcholine boluses and propofol infusions TBW.

The uptake (and washout) of inhalational anesthetics in obesity vary with the anesthetic solubilities. In terms of the uptake, the greater FFM in obesity slows the wash-in of more soluble anesthetics. In terms of the washout, after intermediate duration surgery (<200 min) the washout is slowed because of the increased muscle mass and after prolonged surgery (>200 min), it is slowed because of the FM with soluble compared with less soluble anesthetics. Therefore, the use of less soluble anesthetics is preferred in obesity (desflurane > sevoflurane ~ isoflurane > halothane), the benefit of which is more apparent after surgery of greater duration.

Postoperative complications including respiratory issues (airway obstruction, desaturation), prolonged stay in PACU, obstructive sleep apnea with associated opioid sensitivity, and unplanned admissions are common in obese children.

Malignant Hyperthermia

Malignant hyperthermia (MH), a potentially fatal abnormal response to inhaled anesthetic agents and succinylcholine, is a pharmacogenetic disorder of skeletal muscles. All potent inhalational anesthetics including sevoflurane and desflurane, but not nitrous oxide, may trigger MH. It is characterized by a rapid increase in $PetCO_2$, heart rate, and respiratory rate and generalized muscle rigidity. Subsequently, body temperature and oxygen consumption may increase. If untreated, profound biochemical changes will develop.

MH is a rare condition, occurring in fewer than 1 in 100,000 cases in which general anesthetics are given, although the quoted incidence in children is 1 in 15,000. Children and young adults have most frequently been affected, and it has been reported in an infant as young as 2 months of age. Increased awareness of MH and consistent operative monitoring of expired carbon dioxide have led to earlier diagnosis and prompt institution of treatment; the availability of a specific therapy (dantrolene) has reduced mortality from >70 to ~5%.

The pathophysiology of MH is associated with altered calcium homeostasis in skeletal muscle. Malignant hyperthermia-susceptible (MHS) patients demonstrate an increased calcium ion concentration in skeletal muscle, and studies in MHS swine show a marked increase in the intracellular calcium concentration on exposure to triggering agents. This increased calcium level has been linked with a potential defect in the "calcium-induced calcium release" mechanism within the cell, now further linked with a defect in the calcium release channel of the sarcoplasmic reticulum. The mechanism of the disease process in the cell produces a sustained contracture of skeletal muscle, causing increased muscle metabolism with associated heat production. The further manifestations of the acute syndrome are secondary to the acceleration of metabolic processes within skeletal muscle, which is accompanied by large increases in oxygen consumption and CO_2 production. If the acute reaction persists, cellular energy substrates become depleted, with consequent failure of cellular functions, including those regulating the intracellular and extracellular chemical composition. Substances released by damaged cells (potassium, creatine phosphokinase [CPK], myoglobin, etc.) trigger the continuing manifestations of the acute crisis, including coagulopathy and renal failure.

Detection of Susceptibility

There are still no simple, reliable screening tests to identify MHS individuals. CPK levels may be increased, but this test is nonspecific. Many MHS children have local or generalized muscular disease; however, most with a muscle disease are not MHS. Although a positive family anesthetic history of MH is the most reliable clue, its absence does not guarantee an individual's nonsusceptibility to triggering agents. Even uneventful previous anesthetics do not preclude an MH crisis during a subsequent anesthetic.

At present, MHS patients can be identified with reasonable certainty only by in vitro study of fresh living muscle tissue obtained at biopsy. Caffeine- and halothane-induced contracture of the biopsy specimen is usually diagnostic, but a relatively large biopsy specimen is required, so the test is generally recommended only for children older than 10 years. Genetic evaluation has demonstrated that MH susceptibility is linked mostly to chromosome 19. ~30/400 ryanodine R1 gene mutations have been associated with MH, with at least 5 other mutations have also been associated with MH. If the genetic blood test is positive, then no muscle biopsy is required, and, more importantly this method can be used to define the proband's family tree of susceptibility. This test will be positive in ~50–70% of susceptible patients, but that means that it is negative in 30–50%. Thus there are no noninvasive methods to diagnose MH susceptibility with certainty; if genetic testing is negative, then a biopsy is still needed.

Clinical Manifestations

Nonspecific, early signs include:

1. The hallmark of an evolving MH event is simultaneous and marked increases in expired carbon dioxide, tachypnea in non-paralyzed patients, and severe tachycardia. Other signs include sweating, desaturation, cyanosis, and overheating of the CO_2 absorbent. MH is most commonly triggered by the combination of inhalation agents and succinylcholine; each can trigger MH individually.
2. Hypertonus of skeletal muscles, particularly large muscle groups, may be evident.
   (a) It may occur immediately after the administration of succinylcholine.
   Failure of skeletal muscle to relax, the so-called jaws of steel, where one is unable to open the mouth for several minutes despite complete neuromuscular blockade. This is an indication to postpone surgery and reevaluate.
   Tightness of large muscle groups such as upper arm, thigh, and calf muscles. This should arouse suspicion.
   (b) It may also occur many hours later during anesthesia, after the use of potent inhalational anesthetics.
3. A rapid increase in body temperature (more than 1 °C) is a late sign.

The prognosis is much more favorable if the reaction is recognized early and dantrolene administered before a significant increase in the body temperature occurs.

A venous blood gas obtained soon after the development of hypercarbia and tachycardia will generally demonstrate a pure respiratory acidosis ($PvCO_2$ >80 mmHg) with an abnormally low PvO_2 (<40 mmHg). If the reaction progresses before treatment is commenced, then a combined respiratory and metabolic acidosis will occur (base deficit >25 mEq/L). *Venous desaturation is the hallmark of a hypermetabolic state and nearly pathognomonic of*

MH. Early diagnosis and intervention with dantrolene will prevent the late manifestations of hyperkalemia, generalized muscle rigidity, ventricular arrhythmias, cyanosis, and increasing body temperature associated with a full-blown MH crisis.

Therapeutic Regimen[1]

1. Discontinue all inhalational anesthetics and convert to TIVA; inform the surgeon of the diagnosis; insist that surgery be urgently terminated. *Send for help*!
2. Hyperventilate with high-flow 100% O_2. Either remove the patient from the anesthesia circuit and control respirations by an alternate means or change the circle absorber system and add Vapor-Clean agent filters to inspiratory and expiratory limbs of the circle circuit (Dynasthetics, Inc., Salt Lake City, UT).
3. Immediately give the following:
   (a) *Dantrolene*: The initial dose is 2.5 mg/kg, given as a rapid IV infusion. If necessary, repeat 2.5 mg/kg IV every 3–5 min until the reaction abates as evidenced by a return to normal heart rate and expired carbon dioxide tension. If the child's temperature is increased, it too should normalize. There is no reported maximum dose of dantrolene; up to 30 mg/kg has been required to treat an MH reaction. Do not delay giving dantrolene; each 2 °C increase in body temperature increases complications three-fold and each 30 min delay in starting dantrolene increases complications 1.6-fold. If a recrudescence occurs, then repeat IV dantrolene until the clinical metrics improve. The sooner after the suspected diagnosis and initiation of dantrolene, the better the outcome. *N.B.*: The new injectable form of dantrolene (Ryanodex, Eagle Pharmaceuticals, Woodcliff Lake, NJ) is reconstituted with 5 mL of sterile water for a final concentration of

[1] Further advice can be obtained in North America from the MHAUS hotline.

50 mg/mL and contains only 1/25th the amount of mannitol that was contained in the original formulation. Infant dosing may require use of a tuberculin syringe.

(b) Dantrolene is a muscle relaxant so patients who require large doses may be weak and require respiratory support.

(c) *Sodium bicarbonate:* 1–2 mEq/kg IV may be indicated for severe metabolic acidosis and repeated as indicated, with blood gas analyses. Be aware that if alveolar ventilation is already maximized, bicarbonate may cause a transient respiratory acidosis.

(d) *Mannitol*: 0.5 g/kg; mannitol is present in small quantities in Ryanodex so supplemental mannitol may be required to maintain an adequate urine output (>1 mL/kg/h).

(e) **Do not use calcium channel blockers** as *calcium channel-blocking agents may interact with dantrolene to produce profound myocardial depression and their use has been associated with hyperkalemia and sudden death. They do not have a therapeutic role in MH.*

(f) Use standard drug therapy to treat dysrhythmias.

(g) Use standard therapy to treat hyperkalemia.

4. *If dantrolene is unavailable*, commence active cooling. Symptomatic cooling should occur in cool/tepid water; iced temperature immersion may cause cutaneous vasoconstriction preventing heat loss. Place the child on a rubber sheet and use fans. Intragastric cooling and cold enemas may also be necessary. Infuse refrigerated saline solution intravenously at 10 mL/kg/h as necessary.

5. Continue monitoring the child closely:

    (a) Monitor $PetCO_2$, oxygen saturation, and ECG.

    (b) If the reaction is not aborted immediately after the first dose of dantrolene, an arterial line should be inserted to measure pressure and easily obtain blood samples.

    (c) Insert a CVP to monitor volume status and venous oxygen extraction.

    (d) Insert a urinary catheter and monitor urine output.

(e) Attach a multichannel thermometer (rectal, esophageal, skin, and muscle leads). Beware of overtreatment leading to hypothermia.

6. Obtain frequent arterial or mixed venous blood samples for the following studies:
   (a) Blood gas and acid/base determinations (repeat every 10 min until stable).
   (b) Serum electrolytes (Na, K, Cl, Ca, inorganic phosphate).
   (c) CPK (obtain immediately at the onset of a reaction). Its concentration peaks at 12–18 h; a CPK > 10,000 IU is a presumptive sign of rhabdomyolysis, and steps to prevent renal damage should be instituted (see below).
   (d) Coagulation studies.
7. Correct any electrolyte imbalance on the basis of biochemical indices.
8. Collect urine samples for myoglobin determinations (reddish-brown discoloration is suggestive of myoglobinuria from rhabdomyolysis). Maintain urine output at 1 mL/kg/h or greater; use mannitol or other diuretics as necessary to prevent myoglobin-induced renal failure; alkalinize the urine.
9. In severe reactions, coagulopathy may develop.
10. Admit and monitor the child in the intensive care unit with continuous $PetCO_2$:
    (a) Recrudescence may occur in up to 25% of those who have had an MH reaction; IV dantrolene may be repeated as required to treat recrudescence. Various recommendations include: observe closely; dantrolene 1 mg/kg q4–6 h; or an infusion of 0.25 mg/kg/h for the first 24 h after an event.
    (b) Pulmonary edema may occur because of fluid overload or myocardial dysfunction.
    (c) Coagulopathy and renal failure may require continued care.

Anesthesia Regimen for Patients with Known Susceptibility to Malignant Hyperthermia

All personnel concerned in the care of an MHS patient must be fully acquainted with a suitable treatment protocol (drugs and equipment). Often the clinician must assume possible MH susceptibility on questionable evidence, i.e., a family history of "anesthetic difficulties" but no positive MH testing. The simple course is to provide a trigger-free anesthetic.

Children at Risk

(a) Survivor of an MH crisis (proband).
(b) Children with a positive muscle biopsy.
(c) A blood relative of a proband or family member known to be MHS, i.e., positive muscle biopsy, genetic testing, or survivor of an MH crisis.
(d) Those with muscle abnormalities and/or an increased serum CPK level, in whom MH may be suspected.
(e) Children with central core disease or King-Denborough syndrome.
(f) A child with "jaws of steel" response to succinylcholine (see further).

Preoperative Investigation

A preoperative investigation should be done for children with a positive or strongly suggestive family or personal history.

1. Review in detail the family and personal anesthetic history, noting especially muscle disease and drug- or anesthesia-induced reactions. Deaths under anesthesia are particularly worrisome and require further exploration. There is no evidence for a relationship between mitochondrial disease or muscular dystrophy and MH susceptibility, although succinylcholine can induce rhabdomyolysis in children with the dystrophies.

2. An increased serum CPK may indicate an unrecognized muscle disorder but is not diagnostic of MHS.
3. If the history indicates a strong possibility of MH susceptibility, genetic screening is possible in young patients, but if negative, then for the child >10 years of age, it may be advisable to arrange for a muscle biopsy. A medical alert bracelet is advised for any patient with a documented family history of MH.

Preoperative Preparation

1. Schedule MH cases as first cases of the day since the concentration of inhaled anesthetic in the OR will be minimal at this time.
2. Oral midazolam may reduce preoperative anxiety.
3. Place topical local anesthetic cream on several possible IV sites.
4. Dantrolene pretreatment is not recommended for MHS children. However, dantrolene should be present in the OR prior to intravenous induction.
5. *If diagnostic muscle biopsy is to be performed, dantrolene must not be given (it impacts the test results).*
6. Ensure that all necessary drugs and equipment have been prepared:
   (a) Drugs for anesthesia—all intravenous induction agents, non-depolarizing relaxants, opioids, nitrous oxide, ketamine, atropine, and muscle relaxant antagonists are safe.
   (b) Drugs for emergency use if MH develops including dantrolene, refrigerated lactated Ringer's solution, normal saline, 7.5% sodium bicarbonate, warmed 20% mannitol and 50% glucose solutions, calcium chloride and/or calcium gluconate, furosemide, soluble (regular) insulin, and heparin.
   (c) Equipment: The possibility of trace inhalation agent in the anesthesia machine and its components must be addressed. If a "vapor-free" workstation for MH is available, it should be swapped for the workstation in the OR. If not, then the CO_2 absorbent should be replaced, a clean disposable circuit added, and an oxygen/air fresh gas flow at 10 L/min should flush the workstation for 20–40 min (while the ven-

tilator is cycling) to flush most residual inhaled anesthetic from the workstation, although the success of this process is variable, depending on the workstation. Once these steps are completed, insert a charcoal filter (Dynasthetics, Inc., Salt Lake City, UT) into the inspiratory and expiratory limbs to reliably reduce the anesthetic concentration to <5 ppm within several minutes. Note that these absorbent filters may cease absorbing inhaled anesthetics after approximately 1 h. Appropriate temperature probes and a device to cool the child may also prove useful.

(d) If possible, remove all vaporizers from the machine or tape over the top to prevent accidental exposure; remove succinylcholine from the O.R.

Induction of Anesthesia

1. Induce and maintain anesthesia using only non-triggering agents; these include propofol, thiopental, nitrous oxide, opioids, benzodiazepines, non-depolarizing muscle relaxants, and local anesthetics.
2. For all major procedures, insert arterial and CVP lines and bladder catheter as appropriate for the surgery (not simply because the patient is MH susceptible).
3. Closely observe the expired CO_2 level, heart rate, and respiratory rate [if breathing spontaneously]) for early signs of MH.

Postoperative (After Uneventful Anesthesia)

1. Transfer the patient to the PACU, with monitoring equipment, invasive monitoring lines, and intravenous cannulas in place.
2. Ensure that *all* PACU staff are aware of the possibility of a delayed MH reaction and know what to do if one occurs.
3. Vital signs should be recorded at 5-min intervals initially.
4. Continuously assess large muscle groups for rigidity (upper arm, thigh, calf).
5. Do not transfer the child to the ward or home until vital signs have been stable for 4 h and the results of any laboratory tests are satisfactory.
6. If the child is admitted, vital signs will be recorded hourly for the first 4 h and then q4h.

7. Instruct the nursing staff to call for anesthesia or critical care staff if clinically important increases in HR or respiratory rate occur or if muscle rigidity develops.
8. Immediately administer dantrolene (2.5 mg/kg IV) and repeat at 3–5 min intervals as needed if the child develops tachycardia and tachypnea unrelated to pain; once the reaction is controlled transfer to ICU for further monitoring and continued treatment.

Masseter Spasm

Masseter spasm may occur after IV administration of succinylcholine. Many children (~1%) respond with transient increased masseter tone, which generally lasts for a brief period of time (10–15 s); this is probably a normal response. However, rarely the response is so severe that one is unable to open the mouth, and the patient actively bites down ("jaws of steel") despite the nerve stimulator demonstrating complete paralysis. Such a response should be considered an early sign of MH. If there are no other signs of MH, we recommend discontinuing MH-triggering agents (change to TIVA) and obtaining serial CPK concentrations with a heightened vigilance for signs of MH. CPKs >1000 IU/L is suggestive of rhabdomyolysis, and >10,000 IU/L is suggestive of MH. A "jaws of steel" response warrants admission for further observation for a possible full-blown MH event and appropriate interventions to prevent renal injury should the CPK values become excessively elevated.

Muscular Dystrophy

Pathophysiology

Duchenne's muscular dystrophy (DMD) is an X-linked recessive genetic defect in which there is a lack of dystrophin (<3% of normal) in the cytoskeleton of muscle; the secondary increased intracellular calcium renders the muscle unstable, weak, and susceptible to rhabdomyolysis and life-threatening hyperkalemia and myoglobinemia after succinylcholine or inhalation agents. Skeletal muscle fragility becomes apparent between 2 and 6 years of age and continues to ~10 years of age; muscle atrophy in general and "pseudohypertrophy" of the calves occur, the latter due to fatty infiltration of muscles. Weakness and contractures are characteristic of this early phase as evidenced by Gower's sign. Thereafter, skeletal muscle instability wanes and smooth muscle (myocardial) involvement dominates as evidenced by electrocardiographic (conduction defects) and echocardiographic changes (cardiomyopathy is present in 100% by 18 years). There is no cure for DMD, although treatments to improve the quality of life are targeting gene therapy, exon skipping agents, and calcium regulation interventions. Most children are wheelchair bound by adolescence with life expectancies reaching the fourth decade.

Becker muscular dystrophy is a milder form of DMD that also affects primarily males but has a later onset, in the second decade. Dystrophin is reduced, but not as severely as in DMD. Proximal muscle weakness is progressive but very slow. Cardiac involvement is rare in those <16 years of age.

Emery-Dreifuss muscular dystrophy is a disorder that affects the muscle proteins emerin or lamin A or C. Muscle weakness is usually apparent by 10 years of age and progresses slowly with age. However, cardiac conduction defects are predominant and syncope is common, whereas cardiomyopathy is infrequent.

Management Dystrophies are unrelated to MH; remove inhalational anesthetics to prevent rhabdomyolysis. For anesthetic management, see Appendix A.

Mitochondrial Myopathy

Mitochondrial myopathies (MM) are a heterogeneous group of inborn errors of the respiratory chain (RC) in mitochondria that attenuate energy production. The RC consists of 5 enzymes complexes (cytochrome oxidase I-V) that are comprised of 80 polypeptides, which are under bigenomic control: (1) nuclear genomic control (most adult defects) yields 85% of the polypeptides and follow a Mendelian inheritance pattern; and (2) mitochondrial genomic control (childhood defects) yields 15% of the polypeptides and follows maternal lines of inheritance. Each cell contains thousands of mitochondria, each requiring about 100 genes to generate energy. The variable presentation (phenotype) of MM depends on the ratio of mutated to normal genes in the mitochondria in each organ throughout the body. In infancy, the signs may be nonspecific, e.g., feeding difficulties, hypotonia, involving extraocular and skeletal muscles, and abnormal laboratory tests, e.g., lactic acidosis. Other organs including brain, heart, eyes, endocrine glands, nerves, and others may also be involved. Five common MM that begin in childhood affect multiple organ systems (see Table 8.2).

Table 8.2 Mitochondrial myopathies

Mitochondrial disorder[a]	Age of onset	Clinical manifestations
Leigh encephalopathy *(Complex I, IV)*	Perinatal, early infancy	Nonspecific encephalopathy
		Hypotonia, dysphagia
		Central respiratory insufficiency
Pearson's Syndrome	Infancy, early childhood	Exocrine pancreatic dysfunction,
		DM, sideroblastic anemia, pancytopenia
		Nephropathy, hepatopathy, fatal
MERRF (myoclonic epilepsy with red-ragged fibers)	Childhood, young adult	Short stature, myopathy, neuropathy (peripheral and central incl. seizures), lactic acidosis (like KSS)
Kearns-Sayre Syndrome (KSS)	5–15 years	Short stature, myopathy, diabetes, retinitis pigmentosa and ophthalmoplegia, neuropathy, cardiac conduction defect, cardiomyopathy, sideroblastic anemia, and Fanconi's disease
MELAS (mitochondrial encephalopathy, lactic acidosis and stroke-like episodes) *(Complex I)*	Late childhood, adulthood	Short stature, lactic acidosis, DM, myopathy, neuropathy, nephropathy, cardiac defects (conduction and cardiomyopathy), Fanconi's syndrome

DM; insulin-dependent diabetes mellitus

[a]All are red-ragged fiber disorders on histologic staining except Leigh's disease

Management All anesthetics suppress the RC complexes to varying degrees. Propofol infusion syndrome has NOT been associated with any perioperative complications in children with MM. Avoid prolonged fasting intervals. Preoperatively, it is essential to measure and stabilize the plasma glucose, lactic acid, and electrolyte concentrations. MELAS (see Table 8.2) is associated with lactic acidosis (>90% of children); lactated Ringer's solution should be avoided and a dextrose or saline solution substituted. All anesthetics have been used in these children safely; specifically, adverse events have not been reported after dexmedetomidine, opioids, midazolam, and nitrous oxide. The response to neuromuscular blocking agents is unpredictable. The ideal anesthetic prescription for children with MM has not been determined; however, no anesthetic is contraindicated.

The Child with Cerebral Palsy and/or Seizure Disorder

Cerebral palsy (CP) is a collective term for a variety of clinical conditions resulting from a nonprogressive neurologic insult early in life. The clinical state varies from mild local weakness with normal intelligence to severe spastic quadriplegia with gross cognitive and motor developmental delay. Common procedures in these patients include correction of scoliosis, rotation osteotomies, and baclofen pump insertion. Some with refractory seizures may require neurosurgery. Diagnostic procedures such as GI endoscopy and MRIs are common. It is important to obtain a careful history characterizing the severity, type, and frequency of seizures so as to know what to look for postoperatively, e.g., staring spells or tonic/clonic activity. Determine if the child is on a ketogenic diet for seizure control. Communicate with the child's pediatrician or neurologist to develop a plan for managing antiseizure medications postoperatively should the child be unable to take oral medications.

Special Anesthesia Problems

1. Communication with the child may be difficult or impossible, compromising the assessment of pain and making establishment of rapport with the patient difficult. In these circumstances, the parents or other caregivers should be co-opted and relied upon for assistance.
2. Many children have undergone repeated procedures and are extremely sensitized to the hospital environment. Careful planning is required to prevent further stresses.
3. Gastroesophageal reflux disease (GERD) is common and together with increased salivation may predispose to chronic pulmonary aspiration and recurrent pneumonia. These children might benefit from drugs to treat GERD the morning of surgery.
4. Spasticity and contractures may make intravenous access and positioning difficult; carefully position and pad the child to prevent skin damage or nerve injury.
5. Baclofen (an agonist at $GABA_{\hat{a}}$ receptors in the dorsal horn) is commonly used to treat pain and contractures in CP.
6. Antiseizure medications are continued perioperatively; review the plan for postoperative management if oral medications cannot be administered. Be aware that older antiseizure medications such as carbamazepine, phenytoin, and valproic acid are associated with thrombocytopenia and bone marrow suppression. Some children will be on a ketogenic diet; in this situation, glucose and lactated ringers must be avoided and normal saline fluid therapy substituted and blood sugar measured periodically.
7. Latex allergy is common in children with CP; the history should be assessed and appropriate precautions taken (see above).

Anesthesia Management

Preoperative and Intraoperative Care

1. Preoperative evaluation of comorbidities is essential to determine whether acute disease is present, especially the potential for pulmonary aspiration, atelectasis, or pneumonia.

2. The parents or other caregivers should be questioned about previous anesthesia experiences and their child's responses. Sedative premedication should be considered except for those who are severely obtunded or have a suspected difficult airway; a reduced dose may be appropriate in some cases. Anticholinergic premedication may be useful to decrease the sialorrhea and airway secretions.
3. If intravenous induction is planned, a suitable site should be selected and a topical local anesthetic (see Chap. 3) applied at the appropriate time. If the child is vasoconstricted, application of local warming may produce venodilation and improve success.
4. Propofol may be useful as it decreases airway and bronchial reactivity; otherwise, sevoflurane is appropriate for an inhalational induction.
5. The need for an RSI must be assessed for each child. Succinylcholine does not induce hyperkalemia in children with CP; the ED_{50} for succinylcholine may be slightly less than in non-affected children. Children with excessive secretions should have the tracheal tube suctioned and sputum sent for culture for those with pulmonary disease.
6. The MAC of the inhalational anesthetics in children with CP is ~20% less than in unaffected children for unknown reasons.
7. Resistance to non-depolarizing relaxants as well as sensitivity have been observed in some children with CP and might be a result of interactions with anticonvulsant drug therapy or alterations in the neuromuscular acetylcholine receptors; a NM block monitor is highly recommended. Assure appropriate recovery from neuromuscular blockade prior to extubation.
8. Children with CP are prone to hypothermia; temperature monitoring and measures to maintain normothermia are recommended.
9. Endoscopic surgery is preferred to reduce postoperative pain.
10. Increased blood losses occur with extensive surgery, e.g., spinal instrumentation, attributed to changes in vasomotor control and platelet and clotting factor deficiencies.

Postoperative Care

1. Regional analgesia or epidural/peripheral nerve catheters are ideal for postoperative pain control. The addition of clonidine to the infusion may reduce spasticity.
2. Parents or other caregivers should be present in the postoperative area to assist in the assessment of the child's discomfort.
3. Antiseizure medications should be continued and managed in consultation with the child's neurologist; fosphenytoin may be administered to those who remain NPO.
4. Children with casts should be carefully monitored, especially when epidural analgesia is employed. Compartment syndrome may follow osteotomies and is difficult to detect; consultation with the orthopedic surgeon is essential.

Atypical Plasma Cholinesterases

The genetically determined abnormal cholinesterases may result in prolonged apnea after the administration of muscle relaxants, e.g., succinylcholine. Five alleles of pseudocholinesterase found on chromosome 3 comprise the majority of phenotypes: normal, atypical, fluoride resistant, silent gene, and E Cynthiana (or Neitlich or C5 variant); further study added the H, J, and K variants. Atypical, fluoride resistant, and silent gene may significantly prolong recovery after succinylcholine for several hours, particularly in the homozygote state (5–6 h) (incidence 1:2500) but go unrecognized in the heterozygous state (5–25 min, incidence 1:30). The E Cynthiana variant rapidly degrades succinylcholine.

Management of Prolonged Apnea

If muscle activity fails to recover after succinylcholine:

1. Continue to ventilate the lungs and provide sedation/anesthesia.
2. Confirm persistence of the neuromuscular block, using a nerve stimulator.

3. Allow the child to recover completely before ventilation and sedation/anesthesia are discontinued (this may take up to 3–6 h).

   N.B. Prolonged apnea after succinylcholine due to an atypical cholinesterase is not serious provided the above steps are followed. Do not attempt to modify the neuromuscular block by giving drugs that antagonize muscle relaxants.

Three blood samples should be obtained to confirm the cholinesterase deficiency:

1. Cholinesterase activity (normal range is 60–200 units but varies with the individual laboratory).
2. Dibucaine number (DN; normal range, 75–85).
3. Fluoride number (FN; normal range, 55–65).

Characteristically, children with the atypical enzyme have a low DN (15–25) and a low FN (20–25). Those heterozygous for the condition have intermediate values (DN, 50–70; FN, 40–50). The results of these tests may not be available for some days and are of no value during immediate management.

Other Considerations

When the diagnosis is confirmed, the child's family should have blood tests and be informed of their status. Those having homozygous atypical states should be advised to carry a warning card or wear a medical alert bracelet.

Hematologic Disorders

Anemia

Children requiring surgery may be anemic. The hemoglobin (Hb) concentration, normally 18–20 g/dL at birth in full-term neonates, decreases to a nidus of about 10–11 g/dL by 3 months of age, and thereafter increases to 12–14 g/dL by 6 years (see Chap. 2 & Table 6.10). This is known as physiologic anemia of the newborn. This nadir is lower and occurs earlier after birth in former preterm infants.

Anemia discovered before elective surgery should be investigated and corrected before surgery. Most children with a chronic Hb level of 7–9 g/dL, e.g., renal failure, can be safely anesthetized provided no further blood loss takes place. If, however, the Hb is less than 7 g/dL, the physiologic consequences of anemia may significantly compromise the margin of safety during anesthesia, particularly if substantial surgical bleeding is expected.

The following considerations are relevant for children with anemia:

1. The major compensation of oxygen transport is by increased cardiac output; a shift of the Hb-O_2 dissociation curve, caused by increased 2,3-diphosphoglycerate (2,3-DPG), contributes minimally. At a Hb <8 g/dL, cardiac output increases to compensate for the decreased oxygen-carrying capacity.
2. Coronary sinus blood is normally very desaturated; therefore, in anemia, oxygen transport to the heart muscle is maintained only by increased coronary blood flow. At Hb levels <5 g/dL, myocardial oxygen needs are compromised resulting in subendocardial ischemia; high-output congestive cardiac failure may result.
3. Children with cyanotic cardiac or respiratory disease compensate with a greater concentration of Hb than normal children but hyperviscosity may be an issue.
4. Anemic preterm infants are more prone to perioperative apnea, but transfusion is not recommended.

The following plan of action is suggested for routine elective surgery:

1. If significant anemia is discovered, delay elective surgery until the cause of anemia has been diagnosed and corrected; children with iron-deficiency anemia are generally corrected after 3–4 weeks of oral iron and vitamin C.

2. If surgery cannot be delayed, a decision must be made to proceed despite the anemic state or to transfuse packed cells to correct anemia. This decision depends on many factors, such as the overall health of the child, expected surgical blood losses, and severity of anemia.
3. Use an anesthetic technique that is optimal for the anemic state:
   (a) Avoid excessive preoperative sedation.
   (b) Oxygenate the child before induction.
   (c) Use increased concentrations of inspired oxygen during anesthesia.
   (d) Use a tracheal tube.
   (e) Control ventilation and maintain normocapnia.
   (f) Be cautious with myocardial depressant drugs.
   (g) Maintain intravascular volume: assure stable, cardiac output.
   (h) Extubate when the child is fully awake.
   (i) Administer oxygen during transport to and in the postanesthesia care unit (PACU).
   (j) Keep the child normothermic.

Sickle Cell States

In sickle cell states, an abnormal Hb (sickle cell hemoglobin [HbS]) is present. When deoxygenated, sickle hemoglobin forms a gel, distorting the shape of erythrocytes, which then occlude vessels, causing infarction in lungs (acute chest syndrome), bones, spleen and brain. Additionally, erythrocyte life span is reduced with increased hemolysis and increased bilirubin levels. Cholelithiasis is common. The course of the disease is one of many crises: sickling, hemolytic, or aplastic. Sickling crises result in ischemic pain and acute chest syndrome (see below); hemolytic crises result in further anemia; and aplastic crises may cause death. Ischemia due to sickling may involve many different organs. The disease is mainly confined to persons of African and Mediterranean descent.

In the USA, all neonates are screened at birth for sickle cell disease (SCD); however, those born outside the USA may not have been screened. SCD becomes evident during infancy (after 6 months of age) as HbS replaces fetal hemoglobin (HbF); the latter offers some protection against sickling. Hence, performing a Sickledex test in the first 6 months of life may not detect the presence of HbS. Infants with HbSS should receive pneumococcal vaccine and penicillin prophylaxis up to 6 years of age.

The severity of the disease depends on the percentage of HbS and the presence or absence of other abnormal forms of Hb (see Table 8.3):

1. Sickle cell trait (mild form, i.e., Hb AS-heterozygous) occurs in ~8% in the African-American population. Sickling is unlikely to occur without severe hypoxemia.
2. SCD (severe form, i.e., Hb SS-homozygous) occurs in ~0.3–1.3% of the Africa American population and sickling may cause serious perioperative complications such as stroke, acute chest syndrome, and in severe cases a chronic lung disease.
3. The presence of another abnormal Hb may modify the disease. For example HbC, the second most common abnormal Hb, also promotes sickling. Children with HbSC have a normal Hb concentration but an increased risk for sickling. Similarly, HbD promotes sickling when combined with HbS. On the other hand, HbF, if it is present, as in thalassemia, may protect by reducing hemolysis and sickling. It is important to know the results of the Hb electrophoresis.

Table 8.3 Hemoglobin electrophoresis in older children

Syndrome	HbA (%)	HbS (%)	HbF (%)	HbC (%)
Sickle cell anemia	0	80–95	2–20	0
Sickle C disease	0	45–50	1–5	45–50
Sickle β-Thalassemia	0–30	65–90	2–15	0
Sickle cell trait	50–60	35–45	1–2	0
Normal	95–98	0	1–2	0

4. Neonates who have a large percent of HbF are not usually anemic or considered at risk for sickling. However, sickle cell crises have been reported in severely stressed neonates. Usually, the clinical signs appear by the time the child is a few months old.
5. Splenic function is impaired, serious infections may occur, and prophylactic antibiotics are indicated. Later, autosplenectomy may occur as a result of vaso-occlusive events.
6. Renal impairment (hyposthenuria) may occur in young children, leading to increased obligatory urine output and consequent increased risk of dehydration.
7. Acute chest syndrome, consisting of chest pain, respiratory distress, fever, and multilobe lung infiltrates, is common and may lead to severe hypoxemia. Therapy includes antibiotics, fluid therapy, transfusion, and pain control (PCA, NSAIDs, and possibly epidural analgesia). Often these children will present with "pneumonia" 1–3 days postsurgery.
8. In later life, pulmonary infarction leads to pulmonary fibrosis, pulmonary hypertension, and cor pulmonale. Stroke may develop in 10% of children (before 20 years of age).

Special Anesthesia Problems

1. A sickling crisis may be precipitated by general or local hypoxemia.
2. Sickling is more likely if the child is anemic, acidotic, hypotensive, dehydrated, septic, and/or hypothermic or if the child's blood contains Hb C or D.
3. If the child has SCD, previous vascular occlusive crises may have permanently impaired cardiac, hepatic, and/or renal function.
4. Serum cholinesterase activity may be reduced.

Anesthesia Management

Perioperative management of SCD requires the assistance of a hematologist in deciding which measures are appropriate for each child.

Preoperative

1. All children of African-American descent who require anesthesia must be screened for sickle cells:
   (a) Neonatal screening using Hb electrophoresis is routine in the USA but children from other countries may not have been screened; parents generally know the results for their child.
   (b) Results of solubility tests (Sickledex, Sickleprep) are available in 5 min but do not differentiate SCD from trait for those who have not been screened.
   (c) Screening tests are unreliable in infants less than 6 months of age because HbF masks the results.
   (d) Hb electrophoresis provides the most accurate diagnosis.
2. In general, a severe form of the disease is less likely if anemia is absent, but a Hb electrophoresis is still essential to exclude any other abnormal Hb, e.g., Hb C and D, and to assess the severity of the condition. Children with Hb SC disease may have a normal Hb concentration but are still at risk for sickling.
3. If the child has sickle cell trait (less than 50% HbS):
   (a) Avoid preoperative dehydration; encourage clear fluids until 1–2 h before surgery or start intravenous fluids during the fasting period.
   (b) Avoid excessive preoperative sedation.
4. If the child has SCD (70–90% HbS):
   (a) Assess the child for sequelae of previous sickling crises, e.g., CNS strokes occur in up to 10% of children (peaking at ages 6–10 years), cardiac, pulmonary, or renal infarction). Review previous pain management strategies and drug doses.
   (b) Preoperative transfusions may be indicated to reduce perioperative complications; the most common approach is the following:
      (i) Transfuse packed cells to bring the hemoglobin up to 10 g/dL.
      (ii) Hydrate the child preoperatively with 1–1.5 × maintenance balanced salt solution.

   (iii) Each blood transfusion raises the potential for developing new antibodies in the recipient, which could make it more difficult to find compatible blood in the future.
  (c) Those who require cardiopulmonary bypass with hypothermia should have packed cell infusions or exchange transfusion to reduce the HbS level to less than 5%.
  (d) In an acute emergency, exchange transfusion may be performed.

Perioperative

1. Use high concentrations of inspired oxygen (at least 50%) to maintain 100% saturation and control ventilation.
2. Maintain normal acid-base status.
3. Maintain normal body temperature.
4. Maintain fluid balance to avoid dehydration.
5. Beware of regional ischemia:
   (a) Position and pad the child carefully to avoid any regional vascular stasis.
   (b) Do not use a tourniquet unless it is essential. If one is used, exsanguinate the limb well and use the tourniquet for a minimal time.

Postoperative

1. The child must be awake before extubation.
2. Continue supplemental oxygen and monitor SpO_2 during transport to and in the post-anesthesia care unit (PACU); continue supplemental oxygen for up to 24 h.
3. Hydration and warmth must be maintained.
4. Be alert for the possibility of pulmonary complications; they are common in children with SCD.
5. Provide effective pain management.
6. Early mobilization.
7. Incentive spirometry may be indicated.

Hemophilia

Factor VIII Deficiency (Classic Hemophilia Type A)

Classic hemophilia is inherited as an X-linked recessive disorder (1:10,000 incidence) characterized by episodes of bleeding, either spontaneous or after minimal injury. The presenting sign may be bleeding from the umbilical cord in neonates or after circumcision in infants. The diagnosis is confirmed by factor VIII assay. During childhood, many sites may be involved, hemarthrosis is common, and retroperitoneal bleeding may occur. Hemophilic children require special care during any operation, especially dental extractions.

Surgical Management Children with hemophilia should undergo elective surgery only in hospitals with facilities to care for this condition. Team care by the hematologist, surgeon, and anesthesiologist is essential. If an emergency operation is necessary but the facilities of a hematology department are not available, give fresh frozen plasma (FFP) (20 mL/kg) preoperatively and consult with a hematologist.

Preoperative

1. If there is any doubt about the diagnosis, factor concentrations should be assessed. Preoperative investigation should also include screening for factor VIII inhibitors (found in 5–10% of children), even if inhibitors were not detected previously.
2. One hour before surgery, an infusion of factor VIII concentrate or recombinant factor VIII is given under the guidance of a hematologist. Most surgery can proceed if factor VIII activity is greater than 50%; some procedures such as CNS or trauma require corrections to 80–100%. In mild cases, desmopressin (1-deamino-8-D-arginine vasopressin, DDAVP) may be effective.

Perioperative

1. Exercise great care during airway instrumentation; avoid trauma that might provoke submucosal hemorrhage.
2. A continuous infusion of factor VIII (3–4 units/kg/h) may be advisable during major surgery (consult the child's hematologist).

Postoperative

1. Depending on the nature of the surgery, factor VIII levels may need to be maintained under the guidance of the child's hematologist for 1–14 days.
2. In some cases, especially after dental extraction, ε-aminocaproic acid (Amicar) may help to inhibit fibrinolysis of formed blood clots.

N.B. When factor VIII inhibitors are present, therapy presents a major challenge that requires ongoing consultation.

Factor IX Deficiency (Christmas Disease, Hemophilia Type B)

This disease is similar to hemophilia A. Children with factor IX deficiency are treated as for factor VIII deficiency except that factor IX levels are assayed and factor IX or recombinant factor IX (rFIX) infusions are given.

Von Willebrand Disease

Von Willebrand disease (VWD) is the most common congenital bleeding disorder affecting ~1% of children, with an incidence that varies widely among ethnic groups. Congenital and acquired forms of the disease exist. It may occur secondary to another disease, e.g., chronic renal failure, congenital heart disease, Wilms tumor, and may resolve with treatment of that disease. The basic defect present in VWD (on chromosome 12) is the lack of a plasma cofactor that is a carrier protein for factor VIII and is necessary for platelets to adhere to damaged endothelium. VWD is generally divided into types 1, 2, and 3 with many subtypes, but in practical terms they are grouped as mild, moderate, or severe depending upon bleeding history and factor values.

Type 1 is the most common (60–80%) with slightly reduced von Willebrand factor but often normal prothrombin (PT) and partial thromboplastin times (PTT). Most are asymptomatic until they undergo a dental extraction or surgery.

Type 2 accounts for 20–30% of cases and there is a qualitative rather than a quantitative defect of von Willebrand factor (normal levels).

Type 3 is the most severe form (fewer than 1%) in which von Willebrand factor is absent and factor VIII values are extremely low, leading to confusion with hemophilia A.

The clinical manifestations depend on the severity of the disease. Cutaneous and mucous membrane bleeding are common, but deep tissue bleeding may also occur. A history of easy bleeding or failure to clot after dental extraction should alert the anesthesiologist. In type 1 and type 2a disease, DDAVP is usually effective, through the secretion of autologous factor VIII and von Willebrand factor into plasma, but it may exacerbate type 2b and is ineffective in type 3 disease. The latter types may require prophylactic treatment with fibrinolysis inhibitors, e.g., ξ-aminocaproic acid or tranexamic acid, or with cryoprecipitate, fresh frozen plasma, or recombinant rVIIa.

Consultation and advice from a hematologist is advised.

Diabetes Mellitus

Diabetes mellitus (DM) is the most common endocrine disorder of childhood, 0.35% of those <20 years. Children with symptomatic DM are mostly insulin dependent, although the prevalence of type 2 DM in obese children and adolescents is increasing exponentially and in parallel with the obesity epidemic. About 33% of adolescents 12–17 years old have prediabetes.

Young children typically have weight loss, polydipsia, and polyuria. However, the onset may be very abrupt, and the child may have ketoacidosis. The presentation may be accompanied by abdominal pain, leukocytosis, and mimic appendicitis. Vascular complications seldom occur in diabetic children, so the renal, cardiac, or peripheral vascular effects of the disease need not be anticipated.

The current approach to juvenile DM is to maintain blood glucose levels as close to normal as possible throughout the day by the use of twice- or thrice-daily insulin doses; some children may be using an insulin infusion pump. In some cases, control is difficult, and childhood diabetics are often unstable; the anesthesiologist should consult the medical team to plan insulin management. Oral hypoglycemics (e.g., metformin) are increasingly prescribed for adolescents (>10 years) with type 2 DM and for weight loss. More recently, glucagon-like-peptide-1 receptor agonists (GLP-1) (e.g., semaglutide) and sodium-glucose cotransporter 2 protein inhibitors (SGLT2i) (e.g., empagliflozin) are being prescribed, the former for type 2 DM and weight loss and the latter for type 2 DM. GLP-1 agonists affect weight loss in part by delaying gastric emptying, which poses a risk of aspiration at induction of anesthesia if they are not withheld before anesthesia. The last dose of GLP-1 drug before surgery should be withheld, and only clear fluids should be ingested the day before surgery. SGLT2i drugs affect glucose control in type 2 DM by inhibiting proximal renal tubular absorption of glucose, but they also facilitate ketone reabsorption in the tubules. It is advised to withhold SGLT2i drugs for 3–4 days before any procedure for which an overnight fast is required to reduce the risk of perioperative euglycemic diabetic ketoacidosis. However, if the SGLT2i was prescribed to improve cardiac function, the current opinion is to NOT withhold it preoperatively.

Anesthesia Management

Perioperatively, it is essential to achieve close control of the blood glucose level. Perioperative hyperglycemia (>200 mg/dL) increases wound infection rates in adults; similar data are not available in children.

Preoperative

1. Close monitoring of blood glucose should be instituted several days before elective major surgery to permit stabilization.
2. Minor elective surgery for children with well-controlled diabetes may be planned on an outpatient basis.
3. Severe hyperglycemia and ketosis should be treated with appropriate insulin adjustments before surgery is scheduled. HbA1c should be followed to assess metabolic stability. Defer emergency surgery, if possible, until the ketoacidosis is corrected.
4. Brief procedures (less than 1 h):
   (a) Schedule as early as possible in the morning.
   (b) Determine the preoperative blood glucose level.
   (c) Give one-half to two-thirds the usual dose of insulin as intermediate-acting insulin only (NPH or Lente). No short-acting insulin should be given.
   (d) Start an intravenous infusion of 5% glucose-containing balanced salt solution and infuse at a maintenance rate (3–4 mL/kg/h) unless the blood glucose is less than 5 mmol/L (90 mg/dL), in which case the rate should be increased and the blood glucose rechecked.
   (e) Determine the blood glucose concentration hourly during surgery and immediately after the procedure.
   (f) Use an anesthesia technique that will minimize PONV and permit early return to normal oral intake.
5. Prolonged procedures (>1 h): The preferred technique is to give an infusion of insulin plus an infusion of dextrose and monitor blood glucose levels frequently. A common regimen follows below, but the child's endocrinologist may also provide management suggestions.

(a) Add 50 units of regular insulin to 500 mL of isotonic saline. (Each milliliter contains 0.1 unit of regular insulin.) Saturate the insulin-binding sites of the intravenous tubing by running 50–100 mL of the solution through the tubing.
(b) Use a Y-tube or piggyback connection to the maintenance intravenous line, and control the rate with an infusion pump.
(c) Infuse 1 mL/kg/h to deliver 0.1 units of insulin per kilogram per hour.
(d) Infuse a 5% glucose balanced salt solution at a rate to maintain blood glucose at 5–10 mmol/L (90–180 mg/dL).
(e) Assess intraoperative blood glucose levels hourly.
(f) Postoperatively, the insulin infusion may be continued as long as necessary, depending on the circumstances. The child's pediatrician should control the rate and amount of the infusion based on the blood glucose concentration.

Postoperative

1. Brief procedures:
    (a) If the child is receiving subcutaneous insulin, give appropriate doses of short-acting insulin as required based on blood glucose levels. Continue intravenous hydration until the child is taking fluids orally.
    (b) The child's usual insulin regimen can be resumed the next day if the child is able to tolerate fluids or food.
2. Prolonged procedures:
    (a) Change to subcutaneous insulin when the child's condition allows, e.g., when the child is taking fluids orally and intravenous hydration has been discontinued.
    (b) The child's endocrinologist or pediatrician should resume management postoperatively.

Children Using an Insulin Pump

1. Ensure that the subcutaneous injection site is well protected and that the infusion needle does not become dislodged.
2. Plan management in consultation with the medical team. Generally, the basal rate will be maintained, omitting bolus doses as meals are missed. Boluses may be administered depending upon the results of blood glucose determinations.

Emergency Surgery

Diabetic ketoacidosis may result from the physiologic stresses of the surgical disease, but be aware that the symptoms of ketoacidosis may mimic those of an acute abdomen.

1. Attempt to stabilize the child before proceeding to the OR. Stabilization should be undertaken in cooperation with the medical team. Ketoacidosis must be corrected, intravascular volume restored, and electrolyte defects normalized.
2. Insert monitoring lines for central venous pressure (CVP) and arterial pressure to assist in correcting hypovolemia and hyperglycemia.
3. Infuse warmed fluids to correct hypovolemia; normal saline 10–20 mL/kg over 1 h may be required, as indicated by the CVP.
4. Intravenous regular insulin will be required. A bolus dose of 0.1 U/kg followed by an infusion of 0.1 U/kg/h may be used.
5. Monitor blood glucose frequently; the objective is to decrease the concentration by a maximum of 100 mg/dL each hour. More rapid declines may result in detrimental osmotic shifts.
6. When the blood glucose concentration is less than 300 mg/dL, continue rehydration with 0.45% saline and 5% dextrose solution.
7. Monitor serum electrolytes frequently; hypokalemia should be expected. Potassium must be added to the infusion provided that renal function is satisfactory.

8. Metabolic acidosis corrects spontaneously as hypovolemia is corrected and insulin administered. Ketones are metabolized, and their production is halted. Sodium bicarbonate is unnecessary and may be deleterious except in very severe acidosis (pH less than 7.0).
9. Subclinical brain swelling occurs during the treatment of diabetic ketoacidosis, and, rarely, dangerous cerebral edema may develop. The PICU team should be aware of these potential complications and manage fluids accordingly.

Malignant Diseases

Anesthesiologists frequently care for children with malignant disease. Special problems may arise depending on the site and type of disease, but all of these children require special attention to their emotional status. Extreme care must be taken to ensure a minimum of discomfort and upset for both child and parents during painful diagnostic and therapeutic procedures, e.g., lumbar puncture, bone marrow aspiration.

Special Anesthesia Problems

The child with a malignancy:

1. Abnormal anatomy, including the airway, may be present; be especially aware of the child with enlarged hilar lymph nodes.
2. Hematologic disease may result in anemia, coagulopathy, and immune deficiency. Coagulopathy may lead to intraoperative pulmonary hemorrhage and difficulty with ventilation. Urgent bronchoscopy may be required to remove clots.
3. Increased susceptibility to infection means that strict aseptic protocols should be followed.
4. A history of long-term steroid therapy necessitates perioperative stress dose corticosteroids.
5. Nausea and vomiting may complicate radiotherapy and/or drug therapy and lead to dehydration and electrolyte distur-

bance. Check the biochemistry levels. Do not administer dexamethasone without consulting with the oncologist—tumor lysis syndrome may result.

6. Cardiomyopathy may follow total body irradiation, cyclophosphamide, doxorubicin, or daunomycin (see later discussion).
7. Hypercalcemia may accompany malignant bone tumors.
8. Nephropathy may lead to impaired renal function.
9. Increased intracranial pressure may occur with involvement of the CNS.
10. Peripheral neuropathy may occur.
11. Muscle weakness and hypotonia occur in advanced malignant disease.
12. Toxic effects of chemotherapy may be present (see later discussion).
13. Tumor lysis syndrome may occur after a single dose of IV steroids in untreated lymphomas and leukemia or after treatment of these hematological malignancies. It is characterized by hyperkalemia, hypocalcemia, hyperuricemia, hyperphosphatemia, and acute renal failure.

Adverse Effects of Commonly Used Drugs

All antineoplastic drugs can cause the following effects:

1. Bone marrow suppression, with anemia, leukopenia, and thrombocytopenia.
2. Anorexia, nausea, and vomiting.
3. Stomatitis and alopecia.
4. Decreased resistance to infection.

Some of these agents produce additional adverse effects:

1. Hepatotoxicity, e.g., methotrexate, cyclophosphamide check liver function indices.

2. Renal toxicity, e.g., cisplatin, ifosfamide, which may be increased by the use of aminoglycoside antibiotics or diuretics (furosemide).

Furthermore, specific drugs have effects on cardiac or pulmonary function:

1. Cardiotoxic effects

   ECG changes are nonspecific, but prolongation of the Q-T interval suggests toxicity. Echocardiography is the most useful index of cardiac function; recent studies should be reviewed before induction.

   (a) Both *daunomycin,* used in leukemia therapy, and *doxorubicin* (Adriamycin), used in therapy for solid tumors and leukemias, affect the heart, causing:

      Nonspecific electrocardiographic (ECG) changes, with any dose.

      Disturbances of conduction, including supraventricular tachycardia, atrial and ventricular extrasystoles, and ventricular fibrillation.

      Drug-induced cardiomyopathy in 1–2% of children, leading to congestive heart failure.

      The cardiac effects of doxorubicin are dose related. A total cumulative dose of 250 mg/m^2, or 150 mg/m^2 if combined with mediastinal radiation, must alert the anesthesiologist and is an indication for a full cardiologic assessment particularly an echocardiogram to assess cardiac contractility. Children with a history of congestive heart failure are particularly likely to experience perioperative complications.

      Myocardial depressant drugs, e.g., inhalation agents, should be used with caution or avoided and cardiac parameters should be closely monitored.

      Beta blockers and calcium channel-blocking drugs may dangerously augment the cardiotoxic effects and should be avoided.

   (b) *Mitoxantrone* may cause cardiotoxicity, especially if given after previous anthracycline therapy and with cumulative doses greater than 120 mg/m^2.
   (c) *Cyclophosphamide, cisplatin, 5-fluorouracil, amsacrine, mithramycin, mitomycin, vincristine,* and *actinomycin D* may be cardiotoxic or contribute to cardiotoxicity at large doses.
2. Pulmonary toxicity
   (a) *Bleomycin,* (testicular tumors and Hodgkin disease) causes pulmonary fibrosis in ~10% of patients and may result in death (~1%). *The effects on the lung are accelerated by hyperoxia; oxygen concentrations should be carefully controlled at all times. Fluid therapy should be strictly limited since overload may further compromise lung function by causing pulmonary edema.*
   (b) *Busulfan, carmustine, methotrexate,* and *mitomycin* may cause pulmonary fibrosis.
   (c) *Cytosine arabinoside, vinblastine,* and *mitomycin* have been associated with non-cardiac pulmonary edema.
3. Anticholinesterase inhibition.
   (a) *Cyclophosphamide* and other alkylating agents—used for lymphomas, Hodgkin disease, and leukemias—inhibit serum cholinesterase; prolonged apnea with succinylcholine may occur.

The Child with a Transplant

There are numerous children with transplanted organs; these children require special considerations:

1. These children and their families have survived extensive medical and surgical interventions; they require very considerate emotional care.
2. All of them receive a regimen of anti-rejection drugs, which may have important side effects.

(a) All of the anti-rejection drugs cause reduced resistance to infection. *Take extreme care with aseptic technique.* Insert only those intravenous and monitoring lines that are really needed, and removed them as soon as possible.
(b) Cyclosporine can cause hypertension, hyperkalemia, and nephrotoxicity; therefore, check renal function tests. In addition, it may interact with and potentiate barbiturates, fentanyl, and muscle relaxants.
(c) Azathioprine can cause bone marrow depression and hepatotoxicity; check liver function. It also has anticholinesterase effects and may prolong the action of succinylcholine and antagonize non-depolarizing relaxants.
(d) Prolonged steroid therapy may require appropriate supplementation.
(e) OKT3, usually used to treat rejection crises, can cause anaphylaxis and acute pulmonary edema, especially if fluid overload is present. It may also cause psychiatric disturbances.

3. Teenagers have a relatively high rate of noncompliance with their antirejection therapy. This may lead to problems with graft rejection.

Special Considerations for the Child with a Transplanted Heart

Children with a denervated transplanted heart have altered cardiac function.

1. Effects normally mediated via the autonomic nervous system are absent, i.e., vagal slowing and baroreceptor responses to blood pressure changes. Changes in heart rate as an index of light anesthesia or hypovolemia are unreliable.
2. Indirect drug effects that depend on autonomic pathways are absent, i.e., the chronotropic effects of atropine, pancuronium, or opioids.

3. Compensation for changes in blood volume and cardiac filling pressure is limited and delayed.
4. Small vessel coronary atherosclerosis is accelerated in transplanted hearts and may occur in children. In the denervated heart, ischemia may occur without pain, and coronary angiography is required for diagnosis. Careful intraoperative ECG monitoring is essential. *Manage anesthesia as one would for an adult with severe coronary artery disease.*

The following are considerations for anesthesia in the child with a heart transplant:

1. The child should be screened for signs of rejection, which if present may increase the risks of anesthesia and surgery. Signs include:
   (a) Poor appetite, irritability, fluid retention.
   (b) Decreased cardiac function on echocardiogram.
   (c) Low-voltage ECG.
2. Practice meticulous asepsis. Avoid unnecessary cannulation; use only essential invasive monitoring lines, and remove these as soon as is safe.
3. Maintain normovolemia; ensure adequate fluid replacement.
4. Avoid high doses of drugs that have a direct cardiac depressant effect, e.g., inhalation agents.
5. Maintain afterload; avoid agents and techniques that cause rapid changes in vascular tone.
6. If cardiotonic drugs are indicated, use direct-acting agents, e.g., isoproterenol, dopamine and epinephrine.

Most children are successfully managed using an opioid- and relaxant-based anesthetic. Despite theoretic considerations of interaction between muscle relaxants and immunosuppressive therapy, the usual doses are often required (but neuromuscular blockade must be monitored).

Special Considerations for the Patient with a Transplanted Lung

Heart and lung transplantation may be performed for children with cardiac disease complicated by pulmonary hypertension. Lung transplantation is performed in children with end-stage CF, primary pulmonary hypertension, or idiopathic pulmonary fibrosis. The transplanted lungs are prone to infection and also to obliterative bronchiolitis that progresses to respiratory failure.

Regular bronchial alveolar lavage with transbronchial biopsy is performed to monitor for infection or signs of rejection. General anesthesia is usually required; a propofol infusion with and without short-acting muscle relaxation with a tracheal tube or LMA has been satisfactory. The largest tracheal tube that can easily be passed should be used. Many of these children experience considerable dyspnea on emergence from anesthesia and are more comfortable if placed in a sitting position as they awaken. Secretions may also be troublesome.

Special Considerations for the Patient with a Transplanted Liver

After a successful liver transplantation, children can be expected to have normal metabolic functions and drug metabolism. Therefore, any suitable anesthesia regimen can be used, and no agents are contraindicated. However, these children are prone to infections, particularly by viral agents (cytomegalovirus, Epstein-Barr virus, hepatitis virus), and require very careful aseptic precautions.

Those children with abnormal liver function may have abnormal drug distribution, protein binding, metabolism, and clearance. In addition they may have a coagulopathy. The PT is considered one of the most useful tests of hepatic function because it becomes prolonged before most other tests are abnormal. In these children the anesthesia regimen should be carefully chosen; inhalational agents may be used cautiously, but the response to opioids can be unpredictable. Cisatracurium and remifentanil offer advantage since neither require hepatic metabolism.

Suggested Reading

Akrimi S, Simiyu V. Anaesthetic management of children with sickle cell disease. BJA Educ. 2018;18(11):331–6.

Arasi S, Barni S, Caminiti L, et al. Latex allergy in children. J Clin Med. 2023;13(1).

Baruchel A, Bourquin JP, Crispino J, et al. Down syndrome and leukemia: from basic mechanisms to clinical advances. Haematologica. 2023;108(10):2570–81.

Black CS, Khushnood A, Holtby H, Hepburn L. Cardiac transplantation in children. BJA Educ. 2019;19(4):105–12.

Chidambaran V, Tewari A, Mahmoud M. Anesthetic and pharmacologic considerations in perioperative care of obese children. J Clin Anesth. 2018;45:39–50.

Dalpiaz H, Masi S, Piludu S, et al. Managing glucagon-like peptid-1 receptor agonists and sodium-glucose cotransporter-2 inhibitors in clinical practice. Heart. 2026;112(8):422–30.

Frassanito L, Sbaraglia F, Piersanti A, et al. Real evidence and misconceptions about malignant hyperthermia in children: a narrative review. J Clin Med. 2023;12(12).

Hayakawa H, Pincott ES, Ali U. Anaesthesia and cerebral palsy. BJA Educ. 2022;22(1):26–32.

Hore K, Ali U. Anaesthesia for the child with trisomy 21. BJA Educ. 2024;24:440–6.

James PD, Connell NT, Ameer B, et al. ASH ISTH NHF WFH 2021 guidelines on the diagnosis of von Willebrand disease. Blood Adv. 2021;5(1):280–300.

Jarraya A, Kammoun M, Ammar S, et al. Predictors of perioperative respiratory adverse events among children with upper respiratory tract infection undergoing pediatric ambulatory ilioinguinal surgery: a prospective observational research. World J Pediatr Surg. 2023;6(2):e000524.

Kim HJ, Shin SW, Park S, Kim HY. A review of anesthesia for lung transplantation. J Chest Surg. 2022;55(4):293–300.

Ledowski T, Paech MJ, Patel B, et al. Bronchial mucus transport velocity in patients receiving propofol and remifentanil versus sevoflurane and remifentanil anesthesia. Anesth Analg. 2006;102:1427–30.

Lerman J, McLeod ME, Strong HA. Pharmacokinetics of intravenous dantrolene in children. Anesthesiology. 1989;70(4):625–9.
Mallory MD, Travers C, McCracken CE, et al. Upper respiratory infections and airway adverse events in pediatric procedural sedation. Pediatrics. 2017;140(1)
Martin LD, Rhodes ET, Quinlan CA, et al. Essentials of endocrinology. In: Coté CJ, Lerman J, Anderson BJ, editors. A practice of anesthesia for infants and children. 7th ed; 2025. p. 705–27.
Mizubuti GB, Ho AM-H, da Silva LM, Phelan R. Perioperative management of patients on glucagon-like peptide-1 receptor agonists. Curr Opin Anaesth. 2024;37:323–33.
Niezgoda J, Morgan PG. Anesthetic considerations in patients with mitochondrial defects. Paediatr Anaesth. 2013;23(9):785–93.
Otsuki S, Miyoshi H, Mukaida K, Yasuda T, Nakamura R, Tsutsumi YM. Age-specific clinical features of pediatric malignant hyperthermia: a review of 187 cases over 60 years in Japan. Anesth Analg 2022;135(1).
Parisi CAS, Kelly KJ, Ansotegui IJ, et al. Update on latex allergy: New insights into an old problem. World Allergy Org J. 2021;14(8):100569.
Pouessel G, Dribin TE, Tacquard C, et al. Management of refractory anaphylaxis: an overview of current guidelines. Clin Exp Allergy. 2024;54:470–88.
Radkowski P, Suren L, Podhorodecka K, et al. A Review on the anesthetic management of patients with neuromuscular diseases. Anesth Pain Med. 2023;13:e132088.
Regli A, Sommerfield A, von Ungern-Sternberg BS. Anesthetic considerations in children with asthma. Paediatr Anaesth. 2022;32:148–55.
Schure AY, Kussman BD. Pediatric heart transplantation: demographics, outcomes, and anesthetic implications. Paediatr Anaesth. 2011;21(5):594–603.
Schyrr F, Dolci M, Nydegger M, et al. Perioperative care of children with sickle cell disease: A systematic review and clinical recommendations. Am J Hematol. 2020;95(1):78–96.
Seidizadeh O, Eikenboom JCJ, Denis CV, et al. von Willebrand disease. Nat Rev. 2024;10:51.
Thiruvenkatarajan V, Meyer EJ, Nanjappa N, et al. Perioperative diabetic ketoacidosis associated with sodium-glucose co-transporter-2 inhibitors: a systematic review. Br J Anaesth. 2019;123:27–36.
Williamson DM, Sharma A. Cystic fibrosis in children: a pediatric anesthesiologist's perspective. Paediatr Anaesth. 2022;32(2):167–73.

Neurosurgery and Invasive Neuroradiology

9

General Principles

1. Perioperative management should be designed to minimize increases in intracranial pressure (ICP) and to ensure optimal operating conditions.
2. Light general anesthesia is adequate for most neurosurgical operations; interventions may be required to prevent or treat increased ICP. Short-acting and rapidly eliminated drugs are preferred to facilitate a prompt emergence to allow accurate and continuous postoperative neurocognitive assessment.
3. Prior infiltration of the scalp incision site with local anesthetic with epinephrine reduces blood loss, blunts responses to the initial incision, reduces the need for anesthetic drugs, and reduces postoperative pain.
4. Prophylactic antibiotics to prevent surgical site infection should be administered before skin incision. For surgeries where positioning may take time, the timing of antibiotics must be discussed with the surgeon.
5. Postoperative pain must be effectively treated, but respiratory depression avoided. For major procedures such as craniofacial reconstruction, a morphine infusion may be titrated to achieve satisfactory analgesia. For minor procedures, oral opioids, ketorolac, or acetaminophen may suffice.

J. Lerman, C. J. Coté, *Steward's Manual of Pediatric Anesthesia*,
https://doi.org/10.1007/978-3-032-24545-8_9

6. Postoperative systemic hypertension may occur after intracranial surgery, increasing the risk of bleeding and increased ICP. Aggressive treatment with antihypertensives may be indicated.
7. Some children may benefit from a period of postoperative-controlled ventilation; this is usually determined after consultation with the neurosurgeon.

Intracranial Physiology and Pathophysiology

1. Cerebrovascular autoregulation maintains constant cerebral blood flow (CBF) during fluctuations in mean arterial blood pressure (MAP). Autoregulation is present in adults and children at MAPs between 50 and 150 mmHg and in the supine infant between 20 and 60 mmHg. Autoregulation may be blunted in stressed and premature infants.
2. Cerebral blood flow (CBF) in infants and children (90–100 mL per 100 g of brain tissue/min) is greater than in adults (50–60 mL per 100 g of brain tissue/min). CBF varies directly with changes in $PaCO_2$ between 20 and 80 mmHg at ~4% per mmHg change in $PaCO_2$.
3. Vasodilation of normal reactive cerebral vessels reduces blood flow in areas that have lost autoregulation, for example, arteriovenous malformations (AVMs), vascular tumors, or areas of infection or trauma. This is known as intracerebral steal.
4. Vasoconstriction of normal reactive cerebral vessels has the opposite effect, that is, inverse intracerebral steal. Hyperventilation is a means to rapidly reduce cerebral blood volume in response to acute increases in ICP; it is only effective in the short term.
5. In older children, the total volume of the intracranial contents is fixed. However, any of its three constituents—blood, CSF, and brain tissue—can increase or decrease in volume if compensated by an equal and opposite change in the others (revised Munro-Kelly hypothesis).
6. Infants have a less rigid skull than older children; an increase in the contents may be accommodated to some extent by stretching of the dura, expansion of the fontanels, and separa-

tion of the suture lines. ICP may be estimated qualitatively by palpating the fontanel.

7. The effect of a space-occupying lesion on ICP depends on its volume and rate of expansion and the rigidity of the skull. Initially, the lesion displaces CSF and/or venous blood from within the skull, the sutures may separate in infants, and ICP increases slowly, if at all. As expansion continues, compensatory responses wane and small increases in volume cause progressively greater increases in ICP. With a rapidly expanding lesion, for example, intracranial bleeding, ICP increases rapidly without compensation.

Effects of Specific Anesthetic Drugs on Intracranial Physiology

1. All inhalation agents increase CBF and may increase ICP unless preceded by mild hyperventilation ($PaCO_2$ ~30–35 mmHg):
   (a) N_2O may cause a very small increase in CBF but has been used successfully in pediatric neurosurgery for many years. It may increase ICP if air is present within the cranium; in these cases, it is contraindicated.
   (b) The increase in CBF follows the order: desflurane > halothane > isoflurane ≥ sevoflurane.
   (c) Cerebral autoregulation during changes in arterial BP is blunted as the concentrations of inhalational agents increase, but appears to be preserved at 1 MAC isoflurane and sevoflurane. Hence, modest concentrations of potent inhalation agents (<1 MAC sevoflurane) are preferred, during which the CBF responses to changes in $PaCO_2$ remain intact. Moderate hyperventilation attenuates or reverses the effects of agents that increase CBF, for example, halothane; this effect is more rapid during isoflurane anesthesia. Prior hyperventilation minimizes the increase in ICP with inhalational agents.
   (d) The cerebral metabolic rate for oxygen ($CMRO_2$) is reduced by halothane, isoflurane, and sevoflurane.

Isoflurane and sevoflurane at greater concentrations may even provide some cerebral protection against hypoxia/ischemia.

2. Intravenous anesthetic agents (with the notable exception of ketamine) either have no effect on CBF or decrease it, but if hypercarbia is present, these effects are reversed:
   (a) Propofol reduces CBF and $CMRO_2$, preserves autoregulation, and may offer some cerebral protection. Induction doses (3 mg/kg) may cause mild hypotension but also more effectively blunt the cardiovascular responses to laryngoscopy and intubation.
   (b) Thiopental (not available in North American, limited globally) reduces ICP making it an ideal induction agent in neurosurgery. However, it does not prevent increases in BP and ICP during laryngoscopy and intubation; these may be attenuated by prior administration of lidocaine (1–1.5 mg/kg IV) and/or an opioid (e.g., fentanyl 2–5 μg/kg).
   (c) Remifentanil, fentanyl, and sufentanil have little effect on CBF provided that constant ventilation is maintained. Autoregulation and the cerebrovascular response to $PaCO_2$ are also maintained. Alfentanil increases CSF pressure in children with cerebral tumors.
   (d) In the past, ketamine was thought to increase CBF, $CMRO_2$, and ICP. Hence, it was avoided in those with head injury and increased ICP. However, recent evidence suggests that it is safe to use in these children with similar outcomes as with potent induction agents and sedatives.
   (e) Midazolam and diazepam decrease CBF, $CMRO_2$, and ICP and may control seizures. Flumazenil antagonizes their effects on CBF and ICP and should be used with caution.
3. Non-depolarizing muscle relaxants have no direct effect on CBF; vasodilation from histamine release after atracurium is a possible exception. The duration of action of vecuronium and rocuronium may be reduced in children taking chronic anti-seizure medications.

4. Succinylcholine may transiently and very slightly increase CBF and ICP in children with space-occupying lesions; this response may be attenuated by prior administration of a small dose of a non-depolarizing muscle relaxant. Hyperkalemia has been reported after succinylcholine in children with cerebral trauma and other central nervous system diseases, including paraplegia, encephalitis, and subarachnoid hemorrhage and should be avoided.
5. Sodium nitroprusside (SNP), nitroglycerin, adenosine, and calcium channel-blocking drugs impair cerebral autoregulation and may increase CBF and ICP.
6. Dexamethasone (0.15 mg/kg IV to a maximum of 8 mg) may decrease focal cerebral edema.
7. If an independent vasodilator effect is absent, drugs that decrease neuronal function decrease CBF (such as thiopental).
8. Drugs that increase neuronal function increase CBF (such as ketamine).
9. Somatosensory-evoked potentials (SSEPs) to monitor brain or spinal cord function are attenuated by inhalational anesthetics if given in more than minimal concentrations. Nitrous oxide, propofol, sedatives, opioids, dexmedetomidine, and muscle relaxants have little effect on SSEPs.
10. Motor-evoked potentials (MEPs) to monitor brain and spinal cord function are much more susceptible to depression by inhalational anesthetics than SSEPs. If MEP monitoring is planned, nitrous oxide and muscle relaxants should be withheld after intubation and inhalational agents limited to 0.5 MAC. Propofol, alpha-2 agonists, benzodiazepines, and opioids do not significantly compromise MEP monitoring.

Neuroapoptosis

NMDA receptor antagonists and $GABA_A$ receptor agonists induce apoptosis (programmed cell death) in several regions of the brain in newborn animals. Most anesthetics (except α_2 agonists and opioids) induce apoptosis that is more severe if administered in combination and for prolonged periods. Additionally, these anesthetics cause structural and neurocognitive functional changes to the nervous system in animals after anesthesia. Curiously, other medications, including acetaminophen, dexamethasone, and carbon dioxide, have also been shown to cause apoptosis in animals. The evidence that young children who received anesthesia may develop neurocognitive dysfunction is conflicting. Prospective studies to date have failed to demonstrate neurocognitive dysfunction in young children after a single exposure to general anesthesia for a brief period. Population studies have demonstrated only subtle changes in some executive brain functions after multiple exposures to anesthetics but the results too are conflicting. Parents should be reassured and informed that their decision to proceed with surgery should balance the risks of delaying or avoiding surgery with the improbable risk that the anesthesia may harm their child's brain.

Anesthesia Management

Premedication

Children with normal ICP who are undergoing elective or noncranial surgery, for example, laminectomy, may be premedicated as usual. However, those with increased ICP should not receive doses of drugs that depress ventilation, prolong recovery, or hamper postoperative assessment (see Chap. 1). Therefore, with one exception (see below), avoid sedative premedications in those scheduled for a craniotomy. If IV access has not been established, topical local anesthetic or 50% nitrous oxide will facilitate pain-free placement. Some children may benefit from a small dose of oral midazolam for anxiolysis before surgery, but they should be closely observed.

Exception Children with a vascular aneurysm or AVM, especially if there is a history of hemorrhage, may benefit from being well sedated preoperatively in order to minimize changes in venous and arterial pressures with crying or stress at induction of anesthesia or tracheal intubation.

Induction of Anesthesia

Anesthesia should be induced aiming to minimize changes in ICP and fluctuations in arterial and venous pressures. Preoxygenation followed by an intravenous induction using propofol and a muscle relaxant is preferred, although many children arrive from home for neurosurgical procedures and require an inhalational induction, followed by IV placement and then endotracheal intubation. Lidocaine (1–1.5 mg/kg IV) and fentanyl (2–5 μg/kg) may be given before tracheal intubation to attenuate possible increases in ICP.

Anesthesia for children with vascular anomalies should be induced as above but should then be deepened with an inhalation agent using controlled ventilation to prevent hypercapnia and to avoid hypertension and tachycardia during laryngoscopy, intubation, and placement of neurosurgical devices for securing the head.

Children for emergency surgery require a rapid sequence induction using succinylcholine or high-dose rocuronium (1.2 mg/kg) incorporating all precautions to prevent regurgitation and aspiration.

For surgery in the prone position and for other procedures that entail changes in position, a nasotracheal tube is preferred. An orotracheal tube may kink in the prone patient or become dislodged if saliva loosens the adhesive tape; a nasotracheal tube is less likely to dislodge and is easier to secure at a specific tracheal depth. In older children, a reinforced oral tube may be used. Glycopyrrolate may be given for sialorrhea. Bilateral ventilation should be assured after the tube is taped and the child positioned; flexion of the head (as in posterior fossa surgery) pushes the tip of the tracheal tube toward the carina whereas extension pulls the tracheal tube cephalad. (*N.B.* To determine whether the tracheal tube is positioned properly, flex the child's neck so the chin touches the chest wall after the tube is taped but while the child is supine. If wheezing or unilateral air entry is confirmed, withdraw and retape the tube. Repeat the neck flexion maneuver to ensure that the tube is optimally positioned.) Recheck bilateral air entry after the surgeons position the child prone.

Sudden preoperative apnea may indicate an acute increase in ICP. If this occurs, hyperventilate the lungs with 100% oxygen and ask the surgeon to tap the CSF immediately.

Maintenance

If inhalational anesthetics are used, administer the smallest concentrations compatible with adequate anesthesia to minimize increases in ICP and delayed emergence. N_2O, muscle relaxants, and mild-moderate hyperventilation may be used together with short-acting opioids, for example, fentanyl, remifentanil, and sufentanil. Total intravenous anesthesia may be used when MEPs are monitored; a depth of anesthesia monitor is useful to adjust the dose of propofol in older children.

Ventilation

Limited controlled hyperventilation ($PaCO_2$ approximately 30–35 mmHg) may be used to decrease brain bulk and ICP during intracranial surgery.

Monitoring

The child should be monitored as follows:

1. Pulse oximeter, automated BP cuff, and ECG.
2. $PetCO_2$ to confirm the adequacy of ventilation and to detect air embolism.
3. Continuous recording of body temperature (esophageal or rectal).
4. Esophageal stethoscope.
5. For major neurosurgery, arterial and central venous access should be considered. Arterial access is useful to rapidly assess fluctuations in BP because of traction on neural tissues, blood loss, or air embolism and for laboratory testing. Central venous

access will help assure a stable circulating blood volume, provide a means for administering vasoactive drugs (dilator or inotrope), and provide a possible route for aspirating embolized air. Central venous access is best sited in the subclavian or femoral vein to prevent obstructing cerebral venous return. Rapid blood transfusions should not be given into CVP lines in small infants as cold, hyperkalemic blood may lead to cardiac arrest.

6. Measure urinary output, especially if mannitol or other diuretics will be given.
7. A precordial Doppler flowmeter should be used for operations with potential for air embolism. These include those performed with the child in the sitting or head-up position and all major cranial reconstructions (including cranioplasty for craniosynostosis). The Doppler probe should be placed over the right atrium (second right interspace adjacent to the sternum).
8. If neurophysiologic monitoring is planned (SSEPs, MEPs, or EEGs), ensure that the anesthetic prescription is consistent with producing optimal signals. Important considerations are:
   (a) The depth of anesthesia should remain constant to allow comparison of sequential recordings.
   (b) Ventilation ($PaCO_2$) and oxygenation should remain constant.
   (c) Body temperature should remain constant.
   (d) Opioids do not affect neurophysiologic monitoring.
   (e) Muscle relaxants do not affect SSEPs but are contraindicated in MEPs.
   (f) Nitrous oxide has little effect on latency but depresses the amplitude of SSEPs; it depresses MEPs at concentrations $\geq$50%.
   (g) Inhalational anesthetics generally increase latency and depress amplitude of SSEPs; they are limited to $\leq$0.5 MAC for MEPs.
   (h) Propofol, ketamine, midazolam, and α_2-agonists exert no significant effects.

In practice, a prescription that includes 0.5 MAC of an inhalational agent in an oxygen/air mixture, an opioid infusion (remifentanil, fentanyl, or sufentanil), midazolam, and a propofol and/or a dexmedetomidine infusion provides acceptable conditions for monitoring both SSEPs and MEPs. We prefer a single dose of rocuronium or *cis*-atracurium for tracheal intubation when MEPs are planned (if succinylcholine is used and the child has pseudocholinesterase deficiency, surgery may have to be canceled as MEPs may not be detectable). If remifentanil is used, administer a long-acting opioid to control postoperative pain before discontinuing the remifentanil.

Intravenous Fluid Therapy and Control of Intracranial Pressure

Strategies for Intravenous Fluid Therapy

A reliable intravenous cannula is essential for children undergoing neurosurgery; at least 22- or 20-gauge cannulas for infants and 18-gauge or larger cannulas for older children. Small infants undergoing major surgery should have two large and well-secured IV routes as sudden bleeding can occur.

General Rules for Intravenous Therapy

1. Maintain the intravascular volume but avoid excessive fluid administration; third-space losses are minimal during neurosurgical procedures.
2. Avoid hypo-osmolar fluids because they increase brain edema; use normal saline or lactated Ringer's solution. The syndrome of inappropriate antidiuretic hormone (SIADH) may follow neurosurgical procedures and result in hyponatremia. Monitor plasma electrolytes perioperatively.
3. Avoid dextrose-containing solutions except to treat hypoglycemia. Hyperglycemia may increase the risk of neurologic damage secondary to focal brain ischemia, including that caused by surgical retraction of the brain. If hypoglycemia is a concern, that is, in infants, plasma glucose concentrations should be measured periodically and a glucose-containing solution administered using an infusion pump to maintain normoglycemia.

4. Blood loss is difficult to measure intraoperatively; use cardiovascular indices, for example, heart rate, BP, contour of the arterial wave form, and CVP, to guide the volume management. Colloid solutions and/or blood should be administered as indicated for extensive losses (see later discussion).

Control of ICP and Reduction of Brain Volume

The anesthetic prescription for neurosurgery should ensure that the surgeon has optimal intracranial operating conditions using these strategies:

1. Prevent episodes of hypoventilation, hypoxemia, coughing, or straining, during anesthetic induction.
2. Provide a clear, unobstructed airway at all times as increases in intrathoracic and airway pressures are directly reflected in ICP. The largest tracheal tube that will pass easily should be used. It should be positioned so that there is no possibility of kinking, compression, or impinging on the carina. Reinforced tubes are preferred where possible.
3. Provide mild hyperventilation to a $PaCO_2$ of approximately 30–35 mmHg.
4. A slight head-up tilt is commonly used (15°). The veins in the neck should be totally unobstructed; avoid extreme neck rotation.
5. After discussion with the neurosurgeon, administer furosemide 0.5 mg/kg IV followed by mannitol 20% (0.5–1 g/kg) infused over 20–30 min as the skull is being opened.

After administering a diuretic, the schedule of fluid therapy depends on urine output. When urine volume equals 10% of the estimated blood volume (EBV), further urine losses are replaced (volume for volume) with normal saline. Alternatively, fluid administration can be guided by the CVP; maintaining a constant CVP generally indicates a stable circulating blood volume. Subsequently, serum electrolyte concentrations should be determined to exclude abnormalities and guide fluid replacement.

Blood Replacement

Because blood loss during neurosurgery cannot be measured accurately, it must be estimated by observation and measurement of the child's cardiovascular indices and hematocrit. The systolic BP (SBP) is a valuable guide to volume status; fluid replacement should maintain the SBP ≥60 mmHg in infants and ≥70–80 mmHg in older children. (*N.B.* The latter may lose up to 20% of EBV without a significant decrease in blood pressure.) When surgery is complete but before the dura is closed, sufficient colloid or crystalloid should be given to return the arterial BP to the pre-"blood loss" level. The decision to transfuse should be based on the hematocrit and clinical estimates of blood loss.

If a massive blood transfusion has occurred (≥1 blood volume), particularly in small infants, serum Ca^{++} should be measured. Hypotension unresponsive to volume replacement should be treated with parenteral calcium gluconate (30–45 mg/kg IV) or chloride (10–15 mg/kg IV). Assess coagulation indices and replace clotting factors as indicated.

Controlled Hypotensive Techniques

Controlled hypotensive anesthesia is rarely used, even in those with large AVMs or aneurysms, because these neurovascular defects are more often managed endovascularly rather than through a craniotomy. If controlled hypotension is planned, an arterial line is essential. A safe range of mean arterial pressure in the supine position is 60–65 mmHg in children up to 10 years of age and 70–75 mmHg in older children. The arterial transducer must be zeroed at the level of the tragus in order to accurately reflect cerebral perfusion pressure.

Drugs to Induce Hypotension

1. *Isoflurane or sevoflurane*. The inspired concentration can be increased until the desired BP is achieved. This results in very

stable BP levels but is not readily reversed and not recommended.
2. *Sodium nitroprusside, even when* administered by infusion pump with carrier, may result in tachyphylaxis and wide swings in BP and cause toxic sequelae if large doses are infused. Because SNP interferes with cerebral autoregulation and may increase ICP, it should not be infused until the skull is opened.
3. Large doses of remifentanil provide moderate reductions in BP not associated with toxicity with a slower hypotensive onset than with SNP; its advantage is that the hypotension is readily reversed by slowing or stopping the infusion.

Venous Air Embolism

Venous air embolism (VAE) is a particular hazard with surgery in the sitting position; it may also occur with the child prone, or supine if the head is elevated. It is relatively common during craniosynostosis surgery and has also occurred during laminectomy. Air may be drawn in rapidly if a venous sinus is entered, or it may trickle in through veins within the bone. VAE detected by Doppler ultrasonography has a similar incidence in children and adults, but is more likely to produce cardiovascular instability in children.

VAE most often occurs during opening of the skull, but may also occur at the time of closure when the skin clips are removed. Table 9.1 presents the signs of VAE, in order of decreasing sensitivity:

Early diagnosis and rapid therapy are required to prevent a serious outcome:

1. Inform the surgeon to compress and/or flood the wound with saline to stop the entrainment of air.
2. Lower the head to increase the venous pressure at the wound and augment venous return from the legs. If the child is prone but in a head-holding device, the wound should be covered and consideration given to releasing the head and turning the child supine to perform chest compressions. Consider the Durant maneuver (left lateral decubitus with Trendelenburg) which

Table 9.1 Monitoring for venous air embolism (from most sensitive to least sensitive)

1.	Changes in Doppler ultrasound over the precordium or appearance on transesophageal echocardiogram (detects $\geq$0.02 mL/kg of air)
2.	Sudden decrease in $PetCO_2$, SaO_2, or an increase in end-tidal nitrogen level
3.	Hypotension
4.	Change in heart sounds (windmill murmur or muffled/muted heart tones)

may prevent the gas from obstructing the right ventricular outflow tract.

3. Compress the jugular veins.
4. Ventilate with 100% O_2, discontinue N_2O to prevent further expansion of air emboli, and add 5–10 cm H_2O positive end expiratory pressure.
5. Attempt to aspirate air via the central venous catheter; this is successful in fewer than 60% of cases.
6. Initiate cardiopulmonary resuscitation and other measures, for example, inotropes, as required. *N.B.* measurable $PetCO_2$ >10 mmHg indicates adequate chest compressions.

Postoperative Considerations

All children should be fully awake at completion of surgery. Extubation should be smooth, without coughing or bucking; this can be facilitated by giving lidocaine 1.5 mg/kg IV. If the child remains unresponsive or respirations are depressed, leave the tracheal tube in place and control ventilation until the cause is determined. After some procedures, it may be preferable to continue controlled ventilation postoperatively and extubate the trachea later, particularly if the surgery was in close proximity to the brain stem. Monitor BP closely during emergence; antihypertensives may be required.

An MRI is often performed immediately postoperatively to ensure that intracranial bleeding has not occurred: this may follow either directly from the OR or later from the neurosurgical

ICU. Postoperative nursing care includes neurologic monitoring and assessing the fluid status as antidiuretic hormone levels may be altered.

Hydrocephalus

Hydrocephalus in the neonate may be caused by a congenital defect, for example, Arnold-Chiari malformation, aqueductal stenosis, or by acquired disease, for example, hemorrhage, infection, and tumor. A Chiari malformation and meningomyelocele are both present in 1–3 of every 1000 live births, although the latter defect has dramatically decreased with the use of prenatal folic acid.

Surgical Procedures: Creation of Cerebrospinal Fluid Shunts

For noncommunicating hydrocephalus (CSF blocked in the ventricles, often at the aqueduct of Sylvius) (see Chap. 2), the following procedures are performed:

1. Ventriculo-peritoneal shunt (lateral ventricle to peritoneum)—most common and preferred, because it allows the most room for growth.
2. Ventriculo-atrial (VA) shunt (lateral ventricle to right atrium)—still used occasionally but may lead to long-term complications, particularly pulmonary thromboembolism and cor pulmonale, because of pulmonary hypertension.
3. Ventriculo-pleural shunt (lateral ventricle to pleural cavity)—rare.
4. Fourth ventriculostomy.

For communicating hydrocephalus (CSF blocked as it exits the ventricles) (see Chap. 2), a lumboperitoneal shunt (lumbar subarachnoid space to peritoneum) is performed.

Shunts are positioned endoscopically or using ultrasound guidance in the lateral ventricles, for fourth ventriculostomy, and for creating a connection between the ventricles. Rarely, these procedures are accompanied by considerable bleeding.

Special Anesthesia Problems

1. The frequency of shunt revisions has decreased dramatically, with 98% failing within 10 years. Fewer revisions have resulted from improved shunt technology and image-guided accurate placement. In addition, smart shunts transmit real-time pressure, flow, and potential blockages to smart devices for an intervention before sequelae develop.
2. Increased ICP may be present and is sometimes severe. Assess the child for vomiting and dehydration; check fluid and electrolyte status preoperatively.
3. Check the previous records for difficulties with venous access, intubation, technical problems with successful shunt positioning, and latex allergy.
4. Blood loss is usually minimal, but rarely, bleeding occurs from a large vessel; be prepared with adequate IV access.
5. The child should awaken swiftly at the end of the procedure to permit rapid neurologic assessment.
6. Latex precautions should always be used in these children.

Anesthesia Management

Preoperative

1. The child with increased ICP should be continuously monitored until surgery because their condition can deteriorate suddenly, for example, becoming apneic and unresponsive, necessitating tracheal intubation, hyperventilation, and immediate ventricular tap or lumbar puncture (depending on whether the hydrocephalus is noncommunicating or communicating).
2. Assess fluid status. Administer balanced salt solutions to maintain normovolemia.

Perioperative

1. Induce anesthesia while avoiding hypoventilation, hypoxia, increased central venous pressure, and systemic hypertension:

   (a) An intravenous induction with propofol or thiopental plus a muscle relaxant is preferred to rapidly secure the airway and control ventilation.
   (b) Lidocaine (1.5 mg/kg IV) and fentanyl (2–5 μg/kg) may be given approximately 3 min before induction to attenuate the hypertensive response to laryngoscopy and intubation.
2. During surgery, maintain anesthesia with N_2O and small concentrations of isoflurane or sevoflurane. Non-depolarizing relaxant drugs permit the use of minimal inhalational agent, with rapid recovery when antagonized. Controlled ventilation is preferred. Limit the use of opioids.
3. Note the following situations:
   (a) Hypotension at the time of CSF tap. If the arterial BP was increased secondary to increased ICP and if inhalational agents have been given, the BP may decrease precipitously as the ICP returns to normal, that is, at the time of CSF tap. Discontinue all anesthetic agents, ventilate with 100% O_2, and give a fluid bolus to restore the BP to a normal level. Pressors are rarely needed.
   (b) Bradycardia and other arrhythmias may occur during and after placement of the intraventricular catheter, probably as a result of shifts in intracranial contents (VA shunts). Apply controlled positive pressure ventilation to prevent VAE while the vein is open for insertion of the cardiac end of the VA shunt. The ECG may be used as a guide for positioning the atrial end of the shunt. Fill the shunt tubing with hypertonic saline and attach it by a sterile extension wire to the left-arm ECG lead. Switch the ECG to lead III. Advance the tubing; as the tip approaches the right atrium, the height of the P waves increases, but then becomes small and biphasic when it reaches its correct position in the atrium (Fig. 9.1).
   (c) Blood loss may occur when the jugular vein is opened; secure large-bore intravenous access to rapidly administer crystalloid volume.

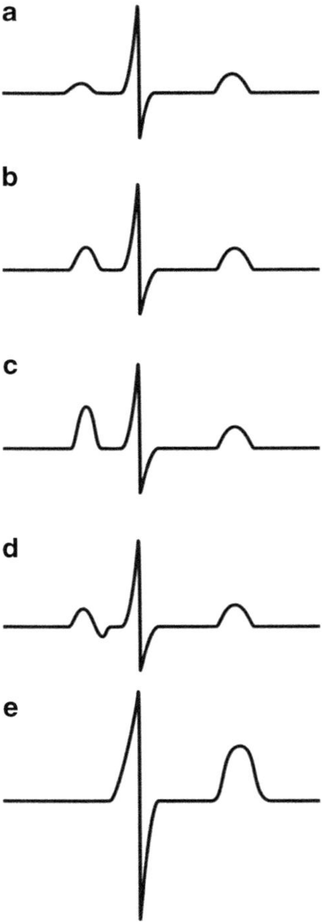

Fig. 9.1 Drawing of ECG tracings obtained as a VA shunt catheter is advanced toward the heart. (**a**), When the catheter tip is in the SVC, P waves become large as the tip approaches the right atrium (**b**, **c**), then smaller and biphasic as the atrium is entered (**d**). If the catheter is advanced too far into the ventricle, the QRS complexes become very large and the P waves disappear (**e**)

(d) Inject long-acting local anesthetic to block the supraorbital nerve for a frontal shunt and to block the posterior auricular nerve for posterior shunts.
(e) Discontinue anesthetic agents and extubate the airway when the child is completely awake and responsive before leaving the OR.

Postoperative

1. Routine post-craniotomy nursing care.
2. Analgesics as required. NSAIDs are often sufficient, if the surgical incision was infiltrated with local anesthetic and nerve blocks were placed.

Craniosynostosis

Premature fusion of a suture between bones of the cranial vault leads to this skull deformity (incidence 1:2000 births). Simple (single suture) in 75% of cases or complex or syndrome (multiple sutures) in 25%, most frequently only the sagittal suture is involved, leading to a cosmetic deformity. Fusion of more than one suture may lead to increased ICP and later to developmental delay and possibly optic atrophy. Early surgical repair (at <6 months of age) gives improved cosmetic results with less blood loss than repair at an older age.

Associated Conditions

1. Craniofacial abnormalities such as Crouzon disease and Apert syndrome may be associated with OSA (See Appendix A).

Surgical Procedure

1. Open craniectomy—division of skull along suture lines.
2. Endoscopic craniectomy.
3. Spring-assisted strip cranioplasty—less blood loss, fewer hospital days.

Special Anesthetic Problems

1. Possible increased ICP.
2. Sudden massive blood loss from damaged cerebral venous sinuses. Continued bleeding owing to the vascularity of the scalp and other membranes.
3. Difficult airway in children with craniofacial syndromes.

4. VAE is a very significant intraoperative danger.
5. Take extra care to protect the eyes in those with proptosis.

Anesthetic Management

Preoperative

1. Packed red blood cells should be immediately available in the OR.
2. Use caution with premedication if the ICP is increased.

Perioperative

1. Intravenous induction with propofol (or thiopental) and a muscle relaxant is optimal to rapidly secure the airway and prevent hypoventilation in infants with increased ICP, but a standard inhalation induction may be used in infants without increased ICP. A cuffed straight or preformed orotracheal tube should be used. Choanal atresia is occasionally associated with craniosynostosis.
2. Maintain anesthesia with N_2O/O_2, small concentrations of sevoflurane or isoflurane, and a relaxant; control ventilation.
3. Establish a secure large-bore intravenous line and have checked blood in the OR. An arterial line should be inserted if extensive surgery is planned (always discuss the surgical plan and the potential for rapid and massive blood loss with the surgeon). Monitor blood loss at scalp incision as this is the time when a massive blood loss may occur. This procedure is one of the leading causes of perioperative cardiac arrest due to hypovolemia and/or hyperkalemia during rapid blood transfusions. Avoid rapidly transfusing blood products through a central line.
4. Mild hyperventilation and possibly diuresis to control ICP.
5. Use blood conserving measures. Antifibrinolytics reduce blood loss: tranexamic acid (multiple regimens, e.g., 15 mg/kg IV loading then 5–10 mg/kg/h) or epsilon aminocaproic acid (75–100 mg/kg loading dose then 15 mg/kg/h IV infusion) until skin closed. Controlled hypotension is eschewed if increased ICP may be present.
6. A precordial Doppler probe to monitor for VAE with skull opening. Treat VAE as previously outlined.

7. Use low-dose opioids (e.g., 50 μg/kg morphine IV).
8. Extubate the airway when the child is wide awake.

Postoperative

1. Routine post-craniotomy nursing care.
2. Exercise caution when prescribing opioids. This procedure is not as painful as it seems especially if local anesthetic was used; some syndromic children may have OSA (e.g., Crouzon), and will be overly sensitive to the respiratory depressant effects of the usual doses of opioids.
3. Ensure that an open cranium is appropriately protected and padded.

Myelodysplasia: Meningomyelocele and Encephalocele

Meningomyelocele and encephalocele result from failure of the neural tube to fuse in the fetus. The incidence of meningomyelocele is approximately 1–4 per 1000 live births, with a large geographic variation. Prenatal folic acid has dramatically reduced the incidence in the last 25 years. Encephalocele is much less common. Early operation is performed to reduce the risk of infection and damage to nerve tissue. Extensive skin dissection to mobilize flaps may be needed in some cases, and this may result in considerable blood loss.

Associated Conditions

Hydrocephalus, in many cases with Arnold-Chiari malformation and aqueductal stenosis, occurs in 80% of infants with meningomyelocele or encephalocele. A short trachea is associated with meningomyelocele. Inspiratory stridor may be present secondary to cranial nerve dysfunction causing vocal cord palsy.

Surgical Procedures

Excision of the sac and repair of the defect is usually performed as soon as possible after birth.

Special Anesthesia Problems

1. Potential difficulty in positioning the child for intubation supine without compressing the defect; placing the defect in the middle of a "doughnut" will prevent pressure on the defect but also necessitates additional padding beneath the shoulders and head. Beware that children with meningomyelocele may also have a short trachea. *Ensure that the tracheal tube is not endobronchial after positioning prone for surgery.*
2. Blood loss is difficult to measure and may be considerable.
3. Body temperature may be difficult to maintain; a forced air warmer is most effective to maintain normothermia.
4. Postoperative stridor, ventilatory depression or apnea, or cranial nerve palsy is possible; ventilatory control may be abnormal.

N.B. Succinylcholine may be used as it does not cause hyperkalemia in children with this disorder.

Anesthesia Management

Observe all special precautions for the neonate.

Preoperative

1. Cover the lesion with a sterile dressing.
2. Ensure that cross-matched blood is available in the OR.
3. Ensure that the OR has been warmed to at least 24 °C.

Perioperative

1. Use all modalities for thermal homeostasis (see Chap. 5).
2. Induce anesthesia by the inhalational or intravenous route; secure the airway with a single dose of IV propofol and/or rocuronium. Administer additional muscle relaxant only after the surgeon has confirmed that a nerve stimulator will not be required to identify nerve roots. In cases of encephalocele, laryngoscopy and intubation may be easier if the child

is positioned in the left lateral decubitus, with an assistant applying forward pressure at the back of the head and backward pressure on the shoulders to prevent neck extension. If intubation cannot be performed in this position, place the infant supine, supported on a ring cushion to protect the spinal cord defect. Check the position of the tube after positioning the child prone.

3. Continue anesthesia with N_2O and isoflurane or sevoflurane, with controlled ventilation. An arterial line should be inserted if surgery is expected to be extensive.
4. For occipital defects, the infant is positioned prone on bolsters. Assure that all pressure points are adequately padded and the eyes are protected.
5. Blood loss cannot be measured accurately. Estimate the amount of bleeding and monitor the SBP and the hematocrit as guides to volume replacement.

Postoperative

1. Return the infant to a warm incubator, to be nursed prone.
2. Observe closely for signs of increased ICP, especially in cases of encephalocele. Monitor the adequacy of ventilation and for the development of stridor.
3. Do not give opioids until it is determined that there is sensory innervation of the surgical site.
4. Check hemoglobin and hematocrit on arrival in the post-anesthesia care unit.

Arnold-Chiari Malformation

The Arnold-Chiari malformation consists of an elongated cerebellar vermis that herniates through the foramen magnum with associated compression of the brain stem. Infants with this disease may have difficulty swallowing, recurrent aspiration, stridor, and possible apneic episodes. The gag reflex may be depressed or absent.

Associated Conditions

Syringomyelia is often associated with and leads to arm weakness and possible sensory deficit.

Surgical Procedure

The surgical procedure consists of decompression of the posterior fossa, enlargement of the foramen magnum with upper cervical laminectomy, opening of the dura, and lysis of adhesions. If syringomyelia is present, it is treated by drainage of the hydromyelia.

Special Anesthesia Problems

1. Control of ventilation is abnormal; stridor may require preoperative intubation, and postoperative apnea may occur.
2. Recurrent aspiration frequently impairs pulmonary function.
3. Stridor may not always improve immediately after surgery.
4. The child must be positioned prone and with the neck flexed for surgery; check the position of the tracheal tube before and after surgical positioning.

Anesthetic Management

Anesthesia management is the same as for posterior fossa exploration. The child should be monitored postoperatively, preferably in an ICU or neurosurgical unit. Rarely, the tracheal tube must be left in place postoperatively if the child cannot protect the airway. If intubation is prolonged, tracheostomy may rarely be required.

Craniotomy for Tumors and Vascular Anomalies

Intracerebral tumors are relatively common during childhood, with a peak incidence at the age of 5–8 years; about 60% are in the posterior fossa. Benign vascular lesions may also require craniotomy.

Surgical Procedures

1. Exploratory biopsy and/or excision of lesion.

Special Anesthetic Problems

1. Increased ICP and/or hydrocephalus may be present and may result in nausea, vomiting, and electrolyte disturbance.
2. Anesthesia techniques must provide optimal intracranial conditions for surgery.
3. Blood loss may be rapid, massive, and difficult to measure accurately. Appropriate invasive monitoring and peripheral venous access will be required.
4. Small infants with AVMs may have associated high-output congestive heart failure. These infants have a low diastolic blood pressure and do not tolerate further reduction in blood pressure intraoperatively (cardiac arrest may occur). Anesthesia in older children with an aneurysm or AVM includes prevention of intraoperative hypertension; controlled hypotension may be required to facilitate the surgery.
5. The child must emerge from anesthesia rapidly to permit accurate neurologic assessment and monitoring. Hypertension must be aggressively treated to prevent bleeding.
6. In a minority of cases, it may be necessary to perform intraoperative neurophysiologic studies; in others, it may be necessary to record cortical SSEPs (See above).
7. In rare cases, an awake craniotomy to map the speech area is needed after a brief period of deep sedation.

Anesthesia Management

Preoperative

1. Review and understand the pathology and the surgical procedures that will be required. Check laboratory results.
2. Confirm that several units of packed red blood cells are present in the OR.

3. Premedication is indicated for children with vascular lesions and for those with normal ICP; always establish rapport, reassure them, and explain the planned procedures.

Perioperative

1. Induce anesthesia, preferably using intravenous propofol 2–3 mg/kg (or thiopental 5–7 mg/kg), lidocaine 1.5 mg/kg, fentanyl 2–5 μg/kg, and a muscle relaxant; this permits securing the airway rapidly and prevents hypoventilation, hypoxia, coughing, or straining, and adverse hemodynamic responses associated with tracheal intubation.
2. A nasotracheal tube may be preferred for small infants and for those in whom postoperative ventilation may be required.
3. Light general anesthesia is adequate for neurosurgery. Monitor neuromuscular blockade after either intermittent doses of intermediate-acting agents or a continuous infusion; a stable degree of neuromuscular blockade (1–2 twitches) can be maintained for many hours and an infusion simplifies management. For example, commence with 10 μg/kg/min rocuronium and increase or decrease the rate by 2–3 μg/kg/min until the desired steady state has been achieved.
4. For most procedures that involve tumors and vascular anomalies, an arterial line, CVP, and urinary catheter are indicated.
5. Encourage the surgeon to infiltrate the scalp with 0.125% bupivacaine or 1% lidocaine with epinephrine 1:200,000 (maximum volume, 2.0 mL/kg) to minimize blood loss and pain.
6. The surgeon may request a diuretic to reduce cerebral edema.
7. Give dexamethasone 0.15 mg/kg IV (maximum dose, 8 mg) to minimize focal cerebral edema.
8. If extubation is planned at the end of surgery, extubate in the OR when the child is fully awake and responsive.

Special Considerations: Anterior and Middle Fossa Surgery

1. Use an armored orotracheal tube or a nasotracheal tube.
2. Position the child with a 15° head-up tilt.
3. Maintain anesthesia and monitor as previously described.

4. Arrhythmias or changes in BP may occur during dissections in the region of the pituitary gland and hypothalamus. If these occur, alert the surgeon to discontinue surgery until the situation resolves. Intravenous atropine may be required for bradycardia.

Special Considerations: Posterior Fossa Surgery (Prone Position)

1. Use a nasotracheal tube in small children as it can be precisely secured at the nostril, is less likely to kink over the palate than an oral tube, and is less likely for saliva to loosen the tape and extubate the airway. Reassess the tube position when the neck is flexed to avoid an endobronchial intubation before turning prone.
2. The child should lie prone on a frame, e.g., Relton frame, or bolsters, with a 15° head-up tilt and with the thorax and abdomen hanging free.
3. Anesthetize as for anterior or middle fossa surgery.

Special Considerations: Posterior Fossa Surgery (Sitting Position)

Many pediatric neurosurgeons use the prone position, but some still prefer the sitting position:

1. VAE is a prime concern; monitor with a precordial Doppler probe and capnograph and consider placing a CVP line at the junction of the superior vena cava and right atrium to aspirate air in the event of an embolism. May also try the Durant maneuver. (See above, Venous air embolism)
2. Zero the arterial transducer at the level of the tarsus of the ear and the CVP transducer at the level of the heart.

Postoperative

1. The child must be fully recovered from anesthesia before leaving the OR.
2. Use routine post-craniotomy monitoring and care.
3. Usually, only small doses of opioids are needed. Often, antiseizure medications are given.

4. Body temperature may increase; cool as necessary to maintain normothermia.
5. SIADH may occur with resulting oliguria and electrolyte disturbance.

Craniopharyngioma

This is the most common pituitary tumor in children, accounting for 5–10% of childhood brain tumors with a peak in children between 5 and 14 years of age. These tumors may compress adjacent structures, for example, the optic chiasm, increase ICP, and possibly cause endocrine disturbances. Recurrence is common (~10%).

Special Problems

1. These children often have hormone deficiency and tend to be obese. They often have behavior disturbances.
2. Preoperatively, corticosteroid replacement should begin; postoperatively adrenal insufficiency must be anticipated.
3. Diabetes insipidus may be present preoperatively and almost certainly will appear intraoperatively or postoperatively. Monitor CVP, urine output, and serum and urine electrolytes in the perioperative period. Be prepared to replace excessive urine losses and to administer 1-deamino-8-d-arginine vasopressin if necessary.
4. The surgical approach via a frontal craniotomy requires a relaxed brain achieved with mannitol, furosemide, and/or mild hypocapnia.
5. After excision of a craniopharyngioma, children require endocrine replacement therapy.

Aneurysm of the Vein of Galen

This uncommon disease, an AVM involving the great cerebral vein of Galen, may manifest in the neonate as severe congestive cardiac failure and a cerebral bruit; the operative risk is greatest in this age group. Current management involves neurointerventional transcatheter coil occlusion of the feeding vessels (see below) followed by surgical excision. When lesions of the vein of Galen manifest later in life, the course is more benign, and the lesion may be managed like other AVMs.

Special Anesthesia Problems

1. Neonates and very young infants are likely to present with severe congestive cardiac failure preoperatively, which may be improved by embolizing some of the aberrant vessels. Staged embolization may be needed.
2. Surgical mortality rate is high due to uncontrollable bleeding or intraoperative cardiac arrest. Meticulous monitoring of the blood loss, adequate vascular access, and timely transfusions are essential.
3. These patients become hypotensive rapidly, occasionally leading to cardiac arrest (see below).

Anesthetic Management

1. Hypovolemia or hypotension must be avoided before the vessels are clipped. The lesion's AV shunt may cause heart failure, and myocardial perfusion is threatened by low diastolic pressure. If the diastolic pressure decreases further, myocardial perfusion may become inadequate and lead to cardiac arrest. Hypotensive techniques are contraindicated; maintain BP until the aneurysm is clipped.

2. When the aneurysm is clipped, the ventricular afterload suddenly increases and decompensation may occur. Administer vasodilators and inotropic agents as needed.
3. A "cardiac anesthetic," for example, high-dose opioid or a remifentanil infusion, may be indicated for those in congestive heart failure.

Electrocorticography and Operations for Epilepsy

Many children >8 years of age cooperate adequately during awake/sedated craniotomy for electrocorticography and operations for epilepsy, that is, temporal lobectomy.

Special Anesthesia Problems

1. Drugs that modify the EEG must be avoided. A propofol or dexmedetomidine infusion, supplemented with a short-acting opioid, is preferred.
2. The child must be awake and cooperative (including being able to speak).
3. Anesthetic techniques must be designed to provide optimal intracranial conditions for surgery.
4. Blood losses are difficult to measure and may be considerable.
5. Postoperatively, the child should awaken quickly to permit a rapid neurologic assessment.

Anesthesia Management

Preoperative

1. At the preoperative visit, assess whether the child will be able to cooperate during surgery.
2. Explain to the child what will occur during the anesthetic and the reasons for it. Encourage enthusiastic cooperation in the procedure, that is, explain that in this procedure children expe-

rience a dreamy state and feel no pain, but they themselves must help make the operation a success.
3. Do not administer a premedication.
4. Omit anticonvulsant drugs on the morning of the surgery.
5. Have blood available.

Perioperative

1. Ensure that equipment is immediately available for emergency tracheal intubation and ventilation. Administer oxygen by facemask with a CO_2 sampling catheter.
2. Insert a large-bore intravenous catheter and arterial line (use local anesthesia as needed).
3. For the initial period of sedation/anesthesia, dexmedetomidine ± propofol may be used: dexmedetomidine may begin as a slow bolus of 1–2 μg/kg over 10 min followed by or simply begin with an infusion of 0.2–0.7 μg/kg/h. Alternately, a bolus of propofol 1–2 mg/kg IV followed by an infusion of 100–300 μg/kg/min may be used. A combination of propofol and dexmedetomidine has also been used. Titrate these to effect. Fentanyl 1–2 μg/kg IV may be titrated intermittently or a remifentanil infusion commenced until the skull is open. $EtCO_2$ and SaO_2 should be monitored continuously.
4. Once the child is sedated, surgeons shave the child's head and insert a urinary catheter.
5. A scalp block with local anesthesia is performed on the side of the surgery. *Effective scalp analgesia is the key to success.*
6. BP and arterial blood gases should be monitored.
7. Although the skull is open, give mannitol 1–2 g/kg or furosemide 0.5–1.0 mg/kg and dexamethasone 0.2 mg/kg IV as needed.
8. If respirations become depressed, titrate very small incremental doses of IV naloxone 0.05–0.25 μg/kg.
9. After the skull is open, the dose of sedatives should be reduced or discontinued until the child recovers, is able to respond to commands or speak, but remains still. Encourage deep respirations.

Postoperative

1. If the child remains excessively drowsy, repeat small doses of naloxone.
2. Follow routine post-craniotomy nursing care.

Spinal Cord Tumors and Tethered Cord

Spinal cord tumors are less common in children than in adults, but they can occur at any site in the spinal cord. Tethered cord, confirmed by MRI and/or computer tomography, causes bladder and bowel symptoms and weakness of one or both lower limbs. Radiological findings include a low conus, a thickened filum, and a transverse orientation of nerve roots.

Surgical Procedure

Surgical division of the filum terminal is the treatment.

Special Anesthesia Considerations

1. General endotracheal anesthesia with N_2O, low concentrations of inhalational agent, and small doses of fentanyl with controlled ventilation is preferred. Standard monitoring may be used. Check for proper tracheal tube placement after turning prone.
2. Muscle relaxants should not be used if the surgeon plans to use nerve stimulation intraoperatively. Anorectal manometry or SSEPs may be used to monitor neurologic function.
3. The child must be carefully positioned to avoid pressure on the abdomen; such pressure would increase bleeding at the surgical site.

Selective Posterior Rhizotomy for Spasticity

Some children with spasticity may benefit from rhizotomy of some of the fascicles of the posterior roots of L2 to S1 bilaterally. Intraoperative electromyography (EMG) monitoring determines which fascicles demonstrate a normal response to stimulation (brief local contraction) and which give an abnormal response (a sustained or diffuse contracture). The latter are then divided.

Management of anesthesia should be as for tethered cord (see previous discussion) *and with all considerations for the child with CP* (see Chap. 8). Non-depolarizing muscle relaxants should not be administered because they may compromise interpretation of the EMG findings. Succinylcholine may be given for intubation if required; it is safe to use in the child with cerebral palsy (CP). However, if the child has pseudocholinesterase deficiency, EMG monitoring may not be possible. Alternatively, low doses of non-depolarizing muscle relaxants will wear off before the need to interpret the EMG.

Intrathecal morphine (10–30 μg/kg), placed by the surgeon, has been successfully used for postoperative analgesia in these children.

Anesthesia for Pediatric Invasive Neuroradiology

The development of microcatheters and occlusive materials that can be delivered via microcatheters has altered the management of pediatric neurovascular lesions.

Although morbidity after the use of these methods may be generally less than after open surgery, providing anesthesia to these children in the radiology suite introduces problems for the anesthesiologist.

Special Anesthesia Problems

1. The radiology suite may be at a distance from the OR and anesthesia support services; ensure that all equipment and supplies that might be needed are available. Assure that communications to the OR are readily available so that additional equipment or help can be expeditiously obtained if needed.
2. General endotracheal anesthesia with neuromuscular block (using a nerve stimulator) is always required; it is crucial that children do not move, especially during injections of embolizing materials. Brief periods of apnea may be requested.
3. Access to the children may be limited by the radiologic equipment. Ensure that ventilator circuits, IV, and monitoring lines are routed so that they are absolutely secure during camera adjustments.
4. Maintaining normothermia may be difficult with the child on the X-ray table. Use humidified, warmed gases and forced air warming mattresses. Keep the child covered.
5. SSEPs may be monitored to guide the procedure; for this reason, inhalational anesthetics must be limited to small concentrations.
6. After the procedure, the child's neurologic status must be assessed and monitored. Therefore, a technique should be used that permits rapid and complete awakening.
7. Potential complications of the procedure include perforation of a vessel or aneurysm, accidental closure of normal vessels or draining veins (aberrant emboli), and adhesion of catheters. Some cases might need to proceed to craniotomy.

Anesthetic Management

1. Preoperative sedation is not routine, but may be preferred for some children with intracranial aneurysm or AVM.
2. Induction and intubation should be planned as for craniotomy for AVM to minimize changes in ICP and adverse hemodynamic responses.
3. N_2O with sevoflurane may be used for maintenance but does not significantly affect SSEP monitoring. Opioids (e.g., fen-

tanyl 1–2 μg/kg or remifentanil infusion IV) may minimize postoperative headache and pain. Midazolam (2 mg IV) at induction of anesthesia may confer amnesia.
4. A non-depolarizing muscle relaxant should be used and the degree of neuromuscular block monitored.
5. Special attention is required for positioning and padding to avoid pressure injuries.

Postoperative Care

1. It is desirable for the child to rest quietly but to not be obtunded, so that an accurate early postoperative neurologic assessment can be made.
2. The catheterization sites and the distal circulation should be regularly checked.
3. Suitable sedation and gentle restraint may be necessary to prevent movement that might result in bleeding or hematoma at the catheterization sites.

Suggested Reading

Alperovich M, Tonello C, Mayes LC, Kahle KT. Non-syndromic craniosynostosis. Nat Rev Dis Primers. 2025;11:24.

Costerus SA, van Hoorn CE, Hendrikx D, et al. Towards integrative neuromonitoring of the surgical newborn; a systematic review. Eur J Anaesth. 2020;37:701–12.

Fedriga M, Martini S, Iodice FG, et al. Cerebral autoregulation in pediatric and neonatal intensive care: a scoping review. J CBFM. 2024;44:1208–26.

Jimenenz DF, McGinity MJ, Barone CM. Endoscopy-assisted early correction of single-suture metopic craniosynostosis: a 19-year experience. J Neurosurg Pediatr. 2019;23:61–74.

Mazandi VM, Lang S-S, Rahman RK, et al. Co-administration of ketamine in pediatric patients with neurologic conditions at risk for intracranial hypertension. Neurocrit Care. 2023;38:242–53.

Vik SD, Torp H, Jarmund AH, et al. Continuous monitoring of cerebral blood flow during general anaesthesia in infants. BJA Open. 2023;6:100–44.

Vutskits L, Davidson A. Clinical investigations on anesthesia-induced developmental neurotoxicity: the knowns, the unknowns and future prospects. Best Pract Res Clin Anaesth. 2023;37:40–51.

Ophthalmology 10

General Principles

1. General anesthesia is almost always required because children do not tolerate sedation and local analgesia for eye surgery.
2. Intraocular surgery and surgery of the nasolacrimal duct and eyelids require a bloodless field. General anesthesia with a secure airway, proper positioning, and a quiet emergence without coughing or straining is important.
3. The oculocardiac reflex (OCR) (Aschner reflex) is a reflex bradycardia or asystole in response to sudden traction on the extraocular muscles. The afferent limb is mediated by the ciliary ganglion and ophthalmic branch of the Vth cranial nerve and the efferent via the vagus. This reflex is powerful in children. Atropine (0.01–0.02 mg/kg IV) at induction of anesthesia blocks this reflex; do not rely on IM atropine or a retrobulbar block to prevent this reflex. *Monitor the heart rate during manipulation of the eyes and extraocular muscles.* If atropine is contraindicated, remember that the OCR is more likely to be triggered by sudden traction than by gradually increasing traction on the extraocular muscles. The reflex usually fatigues rapidly, with repeated, gentle stimulation.
4. Systemic medications may have significant side effects on intraocular pressure (IOP) (Table 10.1).

J. Lerman, C. J. Coté, *Steward's Manual of Pediatric Anesthesia*,
https://doi.org/10.1007/978-3-032-24545-8_10

Table 10.1 Ophthalmic eye drops with systemic side effects

Ophthalmic medication	Indication	Side effects
Echothiophate iodide (phospholine iodide), (long-acting plasma cholinesterase inhibitor)	Glaucoma, esotropia	Nausea, vomiting, abdominal pain, prolonged apnea after administration of succinylcholine
Timolol maleate topical (β-blocking agent)	Glaucoma	Bradycardia refractory to atropine, bronchospasm, exacerbation of the disease in asthmatics
Acetazolamide (Diamox) (carbonic anhydrase inhibitor)	Glaucoma	Metabolic acidosis, and depletion of sodium, potassium, and water. It may also rarely trigger anaphylaxis, Stevens–Johnson syndrome, and bone marrow depression
Dorzolamine (carbonic anhydrase inhibitor)	Glaucoma	Bradycardia

5. Topical medications that are applied to the conjunctivas or injected into the eye may have important systemic and/or significant implications (Table 10.2).
6. The effects of anesthetic drugs on intraocular pressure (IOP) must be considered:
   (a) All inhalation anesthetics and intravenous agents, i.e., propofol, thiopental, and α_2 agonists decrease IOP ~20 % in a dose-dependent manner.
   (b) Although ketamine was presumed to increase IOP in the past, current evidence in children without eye injuries demonstrates that ketamine ≤3 mg/kg IV has no effect on IOP. Ketamine does cause nystagmus, which is generally unsatisfactory for ophthalmic surgery.
   (c) Diuretics decrease IOP, and chronic diuretic therapy may reduce the increase in IOP after succinylcholine administration.

Table 10.2 Ophthalmic medications that may have significant effects during anesthesia

Medication	Potential adverse effects and implications
Epinephrine, phenylephrine	Hypertension and arrhythmias are possible. Epinephrine eye drops are specifically contraindicated in children with tetralogy of Fallot because they may precipitate a cyanotic "tet" spell. Phenylephrine drops cause fewer problems, especially if the concentration is limited to 2.5%; 10% phenylephrine drops should not be used in children as cardiac arrest may occur. If phenylephrine is instilled on hyperemic conjunctiva, hypertension may occur. It is important to carefully track heart rate and blood pressure after topical drug instillation.
Cyclopentolate (Cyclogyl)	Ataxia, disorientation, psychosis, and seizures, especially if a 2% solution is used. A 0.5% solution should be used for infants, and a 1% solution for children
Tropicamide (Mydriacyl)	Behavior disturbance, psychotic reactions, and rarely, vasomotor collapse
Scopolamine eye drops	Excitation, disorientation, possible psychosis may be treated with physostigmine 0.01 mg/kg IV
Pilocarpine	Hypertension, tachycardia, bronchospasm, nausea, vomiting, and diarrhea
Intraocular injection of acetylcholine	Increased secretions, salivation, bronchospasm, and bradycardia. Treat with IV atropine (to produce miosis after lens extraction)
Sulfur hexafluoride (SF6), perfluoropropane (C3F8) or air may be used to tamponade a retinal reattachment	Avoid N_2O during retinal surgery if gas will be used to tamponade a retinal detachment. If N_2O is used and then withdrawn, it could damage the retinal reattachment. SF6 lasts weeks; C3F8 lasts months; avoid N_2O for long periods after using these gases

(d) Intravenous succinylcholine transiently increases the IOP (6–10 mmHg); this increase is not reliably prevented by pretreatment with a non-depolarizing relaxant but is by remifentanil 1 μ/kg IV. The increase in IOP after IV succinylcholine occurs within 1 min and returns to normal within 6 min. It has been attributed to contraction of the extraocular muscles and dilatation of the choroidal blood vessels. The increase in IOP after succinylcholine may be less in those in whom the IOP is already increased, i.e., glaucoma, but it seems prudent to omit it, especially if IOP is to be measured or the child has a penetrating eye injury. The use of succinylcholine in children with penetrating eye trauma is controversial; with puncture injuries to the globe, succinylcholine does not extrude vitreous contents whereas with lacerations ≥4 mm, extrusion of intraocular contents is possible. Alternately, use high-dose rocuronium (1.2 mg/kg) in an RSI with a penetrating eye injury. Succinylcholine may interfere with forced duction testing of the extraocular muscles and is best avoided in such cases.

(e) Non-depolarizing relaxants, opioids, and atropine have minimal effects on IOP. Atropine use is contraindicated in children with narrow (closed) angle glaucoma but not with open-angle glaucoma.

Disturbances in Physiology and Anesthesia Techniques

1. Normal IOP is 10–15 mmHg. IOP >21 mmHg is considered ocular hypertension; IOP >25–30 mmHg for long intervals can lead to vision loss. Glaucoma occurs when ocular hypertension damages the optic nerve. Aqueous humor is secreted by the ciliary body, passes the Canal of Schlemm, and exits via the pores of Fontan into the episcleral veins. Glaucoma results from a impaired drainage of aqueous humor from the eye (narrow-angle glaucoma) or excess humor production.

2. Coughing, crying, and straining all increase intrathoracic pressure, thereby increasing IOP. Hypercapnia and Trendelenburg position increase IOP, whereas their converse decrease IOP. Systolic blood pressure has an attenuated effect on IOP; IOP increases by about one-third of the increase in systolic blood pressure.
3. Direct pressure on the globe, e.g., from a facemask, increases IOP; use of a smaller-sized facemask may avoid this pressure. Laryngoscopy and tracheal intubation also may increase IOP; this effect can be modified by prior administration of lidocaine (1.5 mg/kg IV), ideally 3 min before laryngoscopy. The insertion of an LMA (Laryngeal Mask Airway) increases IOP to a lesser extent than tracheal intubation, and its removal may be associated with less coughing and straining. A smooth extubation without coughing can be achieved by prior administration of lidocaine (1–2 mg IV), a small dose of propofol (1 mg/kg) immediately before removal of the tracheal tube, or by deep extubation (contraindicated in the presence of a full stomach), although the eye is closed at this point.
4. Depth of anesthesia for ophthalmic surgery must be sufficient to ensure that the eyes are immobile and fixed centrally; during light anesthesia, the eyes often "roll upward".
5. For surgery of the eyelids and similar operations, e.g., chalazion excision, a face mask may be used. If the surgeon plans to use cautery, use the lowest FiO2 (preferably an air/oxygen blend) and avoid N_2O, which supports combustion.
6. Postoperative nausea and vomiting are common which may be decreased by using propofol as the primary anesthetic and further reduced by the intraoperative administration of intravenous ondansetron (0.1 mg/kg), dexamethasone (0.0625–0.15 mg/kg), or metoclopramide (0.15 mg/kg). Avoid dimenhydrinate if adjustable sutures are being used, as it sedates the child and may interfere with the child's ability to cooperate.
7. Pain may be troublesome after eye surgery, but nonsteroidal anti-inflammatory drugs (NSAIDs) such as preoperative oral or intraoperative intravenous acetaminophen, ketorolac, or ibuprofen may be sufficient after minor surgery. Immediately after intraocular surgery or trauma repair, a retrobulbar block

placed during anesthesia may effectively control pain. Subtenon's block with ropivacaine reduces pain after strabismus surgery. Topical analgesics, e.g., tetracaine ophthalmic drops, may reduce discomfort after anterior compartment surgery.

Correction of Strabismus

Correction of strabismus is the most common eye operation in children.

Associated Conditions

Malignant hyperthermia is very rare, but strabismus may be an associated condition.

Special Anesthesia Problems

1. OCR—Severe bradycardia and even cardiac arrest can occur with vigorous traction on the extraocular muscles (see previous discussion).
2. "Oculogastric reflex"—vomiting after eye muscle surgery is very common and should be prevented as outlined previously. The frequency of vomiting may also be reduced by only allowing children to ingest clear fluids when they express a desire to drink.
3. If adjustable sutures are used, the child must be assessable postoperatively; excessive sedation should be avoided. If a second anesthetic might be required to adjust the sutures, an intravenous line or a heparin lock should be left in place to facilitate induction of a second anesthetic.

Anesthesia Management

Preoperative

A heavy premedication should be avoided because the surgeon may wish to examine the child immediately before the operation.

Oral midazolam (0.25–0.75 mg/kg for children 1–6 years of age) is a suitable premedication.

Perioperative

1. Induction is accomplished by either an inhalational induction with sevoflurane in nitrous oxide or by intravenous propofol or thiopental followed by a relaxant.
2. Give atropine intravenously at induction or have it readily available in case the OCR is elicited.
3. Maintain anesthesia with an inhaled agent; an oral preformed or armored tracheal tube or an LMA may be placed.
4. Monitor the ECG; if bradycardia occurs, ask the surgeon to discontinue traction on the extraocular muscle, additional intravenous atropine may be given; alternatively, repeated gentle traction on the muscle may fatigue the OCR.
5. Ondansetron (0.1 mg/kg) plus dexamethasone (0.0625–0.15 mg/kg) reduces postoperative vomiting.
6. Strabismus surgery causes limited pain postoperatively in young children, which is often managed with acetaminophen or NSAIDs. In older children (>5 years of age), sub-tenon's block may be utilized. Occasionally, the pain after this surgery is much greater, warranting the use of intravenous opioids. IV ketorolac or dexmedetomidine provides effective postoperative analgesia. Tetracaine eye drops instilled by the surgeon may also provide analgesia.

Postoperative

1. In the past, deep extubation was recommended to prevent coughing and straining and possible risk of a subconjunctival hemorrhage, although most practitioners no longer consider this a priority. If the plan is to extubate the child's airway while the child is still deeply anesthetized, administer intravenous lidocaine (1.5 mg/kg) or low-dose propofol (0.5–1 mg/kg) several minutes before emergence to reduce coughing.
2. Intravenous rehydration during surgery is important to obviate the need for early oral ingestion in the PACU. Oral fluids should be ingested when the child asks for fluids to reduce the risk of vomiting. It is best to not attempt to mobilize the child

rapidly; motion sickness may also trigger PONV. Beware that vomiting may occur en route home in outpatients. It is reasonable to inform parents that their child may have double vision in the immediate postoperative period and likely will be sleepy for the rest of the day.
3. If nausea and/or vomiting occur, administer additional antiemetic therapy and continue intravenous fluids.

Intraocular Surgery and Examination under Anesthesia for Glaucoma or Tumor

Children most commonly require general anesthesia for cataract or glaucoma surgery, treatment of detached retina, or examination under anesthesia (EUA) for glaucoma or tumor.

Special Anesthesia Problems

1. The OCR (see previous discussion).
2. Anesthesia drugs, techniques, and physiological responses may increase IOP (see previous discussion).

Anesthesia Management

Preoperative

1. It is advisable to provide adequate sedation to prevent coughing and straining.
2. It is safe to give atropine to children with congenital open-angle but not narrow-angle glaucoma.
3. Explain to older children that their eye will probably be covered with a patch after surgery.

Perioperative

1. Induce anesthesia by either sevoflurane and N_2O or intravenously with propofol or thiopental.
2. Avoid succinylcholine.

3. For a brief EUA, an inhalational anesthetic via a facemask is usually sufficient, avoiding pressure on the globe. For more prolonged examinations, secure the airway with either an endotracheal tube or LMA after 2–3 mg/kg IV propofol and/or topical lidocaine to the larynx.
4. Maintain anesthesia with N_2O/O_2 and either an inhalational anesthetic or TIVA. Allow spontaneous respirations for brief EUA procedures; otherwise, support or control ventilation to prevent hypercapnia. A propofol infusion will reduce PONV.
5. Discontinue N_2O early if SF6, C3F8, or air will be injected into the eye.
6. A retrobulbar block with bupivacaine or ropivacaine will reduce postoperative pain.
7. At the end of surgery, suction the pharynx and extubate the trachea, or remove the LMA, while the child is still deeply anesthetized. Lidocaine (1.5 mg/kg IV) administered before extubation decreases the risk of coughing or straining during emergence.
8. Reapply the facemask, support the airway, and give oxygen until the child awakens.

Postoperative

1. Administer adequate sedation, analgesics, and antiemetics as required.

Probing of the Nasolacrimal Duct and Chalazion Excision

These minor procedures in infants (<12 months of age) are performed in the ambulatory setting and usually present few special challenges. The airway is usually managed with either a facemask or LMA; tracheal intubation is rarely required. Although the procedure is generally brief, insertion of a silicone Crawford tube often requires additional time. Patency of the duct is confirmed by either injecting a dilute fluorescein solution into the ducts and detecting it on a pipe cleaner in the nose or by a metal probe inserted into the duct. Either fluorescein or blood from unblocking the duct may drain into the nasopharynx and trigger laryngospasm. To prevent such an occurrence, a shoulder roll, placing the child in Trendelenburg, and a deep level of anesthesia are maintained.

For chalazion surgery, minimize the oxygen concentrations to reduce the fire risk from cautery (see previous discussion). If it appears that the procedure may be more difficult and prolonged, intubate the trachea or insert an LMA.

Penetrating Eye Trauma

Penetrating eye trauma is a relatively common injury in children.

Special Anesthesia Problems

1. Any increase in IOP in the presence of an open eye injury may cause extrusion of anterior chamber structures and/or vitreous humor. Crying, coughing, and straining should be prevented as much as possible. Although one may be tempted to sedate the child preoperatively, in most cases a full stomach is present and sedation is relatively contraindicated. Whenever a foreign body is lodged in the eye, the IV antibiotics will be prescribed preoperatively to prevent endophthalmitis, hence intravenous access will be in place. If a rapid sequence induction is indicated, then high-dose rocuronium (1.2 mg/kg) should be used to secure the airway; succinylcholine has been contraindicated in children with open eye injuries particularly with laceration injuries, although it has been used without serious sequelae (see discussion above). Nonetheless, there seem to be few indications for succinylcholine in these cases with the availability of sugammadex. Intravenous propofol or lidocaine minimizes the increase in IOP after laryngoscopy.
2. Preoxygenation may be difficult; ventilation after induction will also be a challenge if the eye is covered with a bulky dressing.

Anesthesia Management

Preoperative

1. Give light sedation and analgesics as required; avoid upsetting the child.
2. Consider giving metoclopramide (Reglan) 0.1 mg/kg IV as early as possible to expedite gastric emptying.
3. Give intravenous atropine at induction. (*N.B.* Atropine blocks the effect of metoclopramide and therefore should not be given earlier.)

Perioperative

1. Most children require a rapid sequence induction; give 100% O_2 by mask if possible before induction.
2. Inject lidocaine 1 mg/kg IV, followed by propofol (or thiopental) and rocuronium (1.2 mg/kg).
3. Have an assistant apply cricoid pressure if indicated (see Chap. 4).
4. Intubate the trachea before inflating the lungs. Aspirate fluid from the stomach.
5. Control ventilation and maintain anesthesia with N_2O/O_2 and an inhaled agent or a propofol infusion.

Postoperative

1. Administer IV lidocaine before extubation to decrease coughing.
2. Extubate the trachea when the child is fully awake and in the lateral position.

The Preterm Infant for Laser Treatment of Detached Retina

Improved management of very-low-birth-weight infants has led to an increase in the incidence of retinopathy of prematurity. The outcome of this disease is improved if laser treatment, possibly combined with intravitreal injection of bevacizumab, or cryotherapy of the detached retina is performed when the disease is at the threshold level. Attempts to manage these patients using local analgesia and sedation are often unsuccessful and accompanied by major complications. Therefore, general anesthesia is administered.

Special Anesthesia Problems

1. The infant is usually very small and subjects to all the problems of the preterm infant in the perioperative period. All precautions for the preterm infant must be observed (see Chaps. 2 and 4).
2. A heated transport incubator is required during transport to the operating room as the infant has difficulty maintaining normothermia.
3. Access to the infant during treatment is limited. Airway, ventilation, and reliable monitoring must be assured before the procedure commences. A thermoneutral environment should be provided.
4. Topical anesthetics and oral or IV acetaminophen reduce pain. Postoperatively the infant's trachea should remain intubated, and the lungs ventilated until judged stable by the neonatal team. A period of ventilation for 24–36 h is commonly required even if the infant had been weaned before the eye treatment. A period of ventilatory instability is common postoperatively. Postoperative apnea should be anticipated and the infant monitored accordingly.

Anesthesia for Retinoblastoma

This is the most common ocular tumor in children, comprising up to 4% of tumors in childhood. Two forms of this tumor exist: unilateral comprising 75% of cases (with 90% nonhereditary) and bilateral comprising 25% (inherited as the RB1 gene on 13q14). Ten to fifteen percent of children with retinoblastoma have metastatic disease. The goal of the treatment is to preserve vision and remove the tumor. Treatment depends on the extent of the disease. Enucleation is reserved for massive tumors for which conservative treatment cannot preserve vision. Anesthesia for enucleation requires a completely still infant with general anesthesia and tracheal intubation. The anesthetic prescription should follow standard management of any infant and avoid long-acting agents. The most serious, potentially fatal, complication is recession of the ophthalmic artery from the back of the orbit during dissection, resulting in massive blood loss until the artery is ligated.

Focal therapies (for tumors <6 mm in diameter) include argon laser therapy, cryotherapy, and thermotherapy; the therapy depends on the location of the tumor within the eye. Chemotherapy is reserved for metastatic disease. Radiotherapy and brachytherapy (see below) are also effective as retinoblastomas are radiosensitive, but may produce unrelated malignancies. Serial proton beam treatments may result in less potential for later malignancy.

Anesthesia for cryotherapy and laser therapy may be performed with an LMA or tracheal intubation. The goal of anesthesia is to prevent movement of the head while treatment is administered. There is no need for analgesics or antiemetics after these procedures in young infants.

Anesthesia for Radiotherapy

Infants and children with retinoblastoma may require daily repeated radiotherapy for which they must remain absolutely still; hence, general anesthesia is required. This is usually a salvage procedure when all other treatments have failed. Children who will have serial radiation therapy or proton beam treatments generally undergo a series of procedures starting with the insertion of a central access device, followed by MRI assessment, and then a CT planning session whereby a restraining facemask is constructed. During this series, it is preferable to administer anesthesia with propofol and spontaneous respirations with facemask oxygen and to assure proper positioning that maintains a clear airway. All subsequent treatments will be undertaken in a similar manner with a natural airway and supplemental oxygen. Thus, it is essential to have a proper-fitting restraining facemask created during the CT planning session. Generally, such treatments will occur 5 days per week for 20–30 treatments depending on the severity of the tumor and if it is bilateral.

Short-acting anesthetics are preferred to return the child to normal activity as soon as possible. Nasal or facemask oxygen applied to the preformed mask and capnometry combined with pulse oximetry help to assure adequate ventilation and oxygenation during the procedures.

Some institutions use the HeadFIX® Immobilization Device,[1] which applies suction to a mold of the palate, firmly supports the head, and also generally maintains a very good airway without further instrumentation. Our experience is that a propofol infusion is safe and effective in these children.

Anesthesia for Visual Evoked Potentials or Electroretinography

Visual evoked potentials (VEPs) are exquisitely sensitive to the effects of sedative and anesthetic agents because of the complex cortical pathways involved. Hence, the anesthesia technique must be carefully planned if meaningful results are to be obtained.

1. Nitrous oxide is avoided as it significantly depresses the amplitude of VEPs.
2. Potent inhaled agents decrease amplitude and increase the latency of VEPs in a dose-dependent manner: 0.5 MAC sevoflurane exerts a small effect, at 1.5 MAC, VEPs are unrecordable.
3. Propofol depresses VEP less than sevoflurane. Low-dose propofol (but not high-dose) infusions are acceptable. Dexmedetomidine does not affect VEPs so it is an excellent sedative for these cases.
4. Ketamine has a negligible effect on latency and a dose-related effect on amplitude of VEPs; fentanyl significantly decreases the amplitude.

[1]Medical Intelligence, Schwabmünchen, Germany.

5. Thiopental decreases the amplitude and increases the latency of VEPs. An induction dose of etomidate has a lesser effect.

In summary, it is difficult to provide anesthesia care for infants and small children for VEPs; low-dose propofol, dexmedetomidine, 0.5 MAC sevoflurane, or ketamine is recommended.

The results of electroretinography are less affected by anesthesia and sedative agents. These are often performed in a completely dark room in the ophthalmology department, remote from the O.R. Special screens block the light from the anesthesia monitors, necessitating close observation of the monitors. We recommend using either sevoflurane and an LMA or a propofol infusion and oxygen via nasal prongs.

Suggested Reading

Chang C-Y, Chien Y-J, Wu M-Y. Attenuation of increased intraocular pressure with propofol anesthesia: A systematic review with meta-analysis and trial sequential analysis. J Adv Res. 2020;24:223–38.

Chang C-Y, Chen H-A, Chien Y-J, Wu M-Y. Attenuation of the increase in intraocular pressure with dexmedetomidine: systematic review with meta-analysis and trial sequential analysis. J Clin Anesth. 2021;68:110065.

Halstead SM, Deakyne SJ, Bajaj L, et al. The effect of ketamine on intraocular pressure in pediatric patients during procedural sedation. Acad Emerg Med. 2012;19:1145–50.

Huang J-Y, Shih P-C, Chen C-T, et al. Effects of short-acting opioids on intraocular pressure during general anesthesia: systematic review and network meta-analysis. Pharmaceuticals. 2022;15:989.

Lewis H, James I. Update on anaesthesia for paediatric ophthalmic surgery. BJA Educ. 2021;21(1):32–8.

Pucchio A, Pur DR, Dhawan A, et al. Anesthesia for ophthalmic surgery: an educational review. Int Ophthalmol. 2023;43:1761–9.

Tanaka R, Tanaka S, Ichino T, Ishida T, Fuseya S, Kawamata M. Differential effects of sevoflurane and propofol on an electroretinogram and visual evoked potentials. J Anesth. 2020;34(2):298–302.

Thanapaisal S, Oatts J, Zhao J, et al. Effect of general anaesthesia on intraocular pressure in paediatric patients: a systematic review. Eye. 2021;35:1205–12.

Otorhinolaryngology 11

General Principles

Although many of the surgeries are simple and commonplace, ear, nose, and throat surgery has a disproportionately large potential for anesthetic and surgical complications requiring meticulous attention to all aspects of the child's perioperative care:

1. Because many of these operations involve the airway, the anesthesiologist must be prepared to provide good surgical access while ventilating and oxygenating the lungs.
2. The surgical microscope permits delicate and precise surgery for the middle ear; anesthesia for such procedures must provide optimal operating conditions, smooth emergence, and minimal disturbance postoperatively.
3. Skilled nursing care in the post-anesthetic care unit (PACU) is essential, so that signs of impending complications are detected early and appropriate interventions rapidly instituted.
4. The use of the laser to treat lesions of the larynx introduces specific additional safety issues for anesthesia management.
5. When topical vasoconstrictors are used, systemic absorption may cause hypertension and bradycardia; transient mild hypertension requires no therapy. Occasionally, severe hypertension may result in pulmonary edema; this should be treated with carefully titrated doses of direct vasodilators, e.g., sodium

J. Lerman, C. J. Coté, *Steward's Manual of Pediatric Anesthesia*,
https://doi.org/10.1007/978-3-032-24545-8_11

nitroprusside, or α-adrenergic receptor antagonists, e.g., phentolamine. Do not use β-blockers or calcium channel blockers as disastrous decreases in cardiac output and cardiac arrest have been reported.

Choanal Atresia

Complete obstruction (90% of cases) due to choanal atresia (membranous or bony occlusion of the posterior nares) causes respiratory distress immediately after birth. However, the distress is intermittent; infants are primarily nose breathers, but the obstruction is relieved whenever the infant opens the mouth and cries. The diagnosis is easily confirmed with a stethoscope by listening for air exchange over each nostril. In general, the obstruction can be relieved with an oropharyngeal airway. An orogastric tube may open the airway in some infants and facilitates feeding. Early endonasal puncture and stenting may be performed in the neonate and KTP laser to cut a hole in the bone in the preterm infant. Incomplete choanal atresia may lead to chronic nasal problems; early repair is recommended.

Associated Conditions

The "CHARGE" association consists of **C**oloboma, congenital **H**eart disease, choanal **A**tresia, growth **R**etardation, **G**enitourinary abnormalities, and **E**ar anomalies.

Surgical Procedures

1. Endoscopic transnasal puncture is preferred, especially in those with associated significant disease, e.g., the CHARGE association; KTP laser is preferred in preterm infants.
2. Transpalatal repair may be performed at age 1–2 days in the healthy, full-term infant. Stents are left for varying periods postoperatively.

Special Anesthesia Problems

The primary problem is maintaining a patent airway until completion of surgery.

Anesthesia Management

Preoperative

1. Adequate ventilation requires continued use of an oropharyngeal airway.

Perioperative

1. Observe all special precautions for neonates (see Chap. 4).
2. Leave the oropharyngeal airway in place: give 100% O_2 by mask.
3. Induce anesthesia by inhalation of sevoflurane, establish IV access, and intubate the trachea, preferably using a preformed oral tube to provide optimal access for the surgeon.
4. Maintain anesthesia with N_2O and sevoflurane or isoflurane with controlled ventilation; a remifentanil infusion may reduce the need for an inhalation agent while providing an adequate depth of anesthesia to allow the surgeon to place the necessary airway stents.
5. Suction the pharynx at the end of surgery to ensure that the stents are clear and patent.
6. Extubate the trachea when the infant is fully awake.

Postoperative

1. Deliver humidified oxygen/air. The stents must be regularly suctioned with a fine catheter to maintain their patency.
2. Constant observation is essential because aspiration during feeding commonly occurs after repair.
3. Subsequent repairs may be necessary later in childhood for restenosis, but these operations present no additional special anesthetic problems.
4. Provide appropriate analgesia.

Nasopharyngeal Tumors

Teratomas, dermoid cysts, nasal encephaloceles, and other tumors require surgical excision. Juvenile nasal angiofibroma is a rare benign but very vascular tumor that may involve the nose. Biopsy of these tumors may result in extensive bleeding that is very difficult to control; therefore, diagnosis is usually made on the basis of imaging studies. Surgical excision may result in massive blood loss requiring appropriate anticipation and preparation. The tracheal tube should be left in place until the child is fully awake since nasal obstruction and bleeding may persist.

Surgery of the Nose

The most common nasal surgical procedures are reduction of fractures, septoplasty, rhinoplasty, and excision of nasal polyps.

Special Anesthesia Problems

1. The nasal airway may be blocked. The surgeon may wish to pack the nose with gauze and a vasoconstrictor, e.g., 0.05% oxymetazoline or 1/2000 epinephrine preoperatively.
2. Children with nasal polyps usually have cystic fibrosis.
3. Functional endoscopic sinus surgery (FESS) may precipitate special problems (see later discussion).

Anesthesia Management

Preoperative

1. Assess the nasal airway.
2. If the child has cystic fibrosis, institute appropriate preoperative care (see Chap. 8).

Perioperative

1. Induce anesthesia by inhalation or intravenously, followed by a muscle relaxant.
2. If the nose is obstructed, an oropharyngeal airway may be needed to facilitate mask ventilation.
3. Perform orotracheal intubation with a preformed cuffed tracheal tube.
4. The surgeon will insert a throat pack to prevent blood pooling in the pharynx and esophagus.
5. Consider the use of bilateral infraorbital and nasociliary nerve blocks for postoperative analgesia.
6. Extubate the trachea when the child is fully awake; premature extubation may lead to laryngospasm or airway obstruction.

Postoperative

1. Administer humidified oxygen/air by mask.
2. Administer analgesics as required.
3. Postoperative airway obstruction may occur, resulting in post-obstructive pulmonary edema that will require tracheal reintubation, IPPV, and a diuretic.

Functional Endoscopic Sinus Surgery

FESS is the standard surgical treatment for chronic sinus disease. Precise endoscopic resection of diseased tissue and relief of obstruction while preserving normal mucosa to restore normal sinus function is the objective.

Special Anesthesia Problems

1. Many of these children have chronic diseases, e.g., cystic fibrosis.
2. Successful endoscopic surgery requires extensive use of vasoconstrictors. Ensure that maximal permissible doses of cocaine (2–3 mg/kg) or epinephrine (10 μg/kg) are not exceeded so as

to prevent severe hypertension. If hypertension ensues, treat it by deepening anesthesia or using vasodilators; do not use β-blockers or calcium channel-blocking agents.
3. Massive bleeding may require that the nose packing remain in place postoperatively; this requires that the child is fully awake before extubation.
4. Consider the use of bilateral infraorbital and nasociliary nerve blocks for postoperative analgesia.
5. Rarely, the surgery may encroach on the orbit or intracranial space. In the latter case, intracranial bleeding may occur. There is also a danger of pneumocephalus if positive pressure is applied via a face mask.

Tonsillectomy and Adenoidectomy

Obstructive sleep apnea (OSA) is the most common indication for adenotonsillectomy (T&A). Chronic inflammation and hypertrophy of lymphoid tissues in the pharynx are the second most common indications for T&A. Repeated middle ear infections may be improved by adenoidectomy; rarely, acute tonsillitis leads to a peritonsillar abscess (quinsy tonsil).

T&A surgery is often performed in the ambulatory unit, demanding special screening for suitable children and measured postoperative evaluation before discharge home. An efficient follow-up service must be provided to address unexpected complications. Some children may not be suitable for T&A as an outpatient. For these children (see Table 11.1), T&A surgery should be undertaken in a hospital with a planned overnight admission for observation.

Although T&A is a very safe surgery, T&A-related deaths still occur. Reported causes include excessive sedation/analgesia of children with a compromised airway, OSA with associated opioid sensitivity (see below), or a post-tonsillectomy bleed. Postoperative nausea and vomiting have become uncommon after T&A surgery because postoperative oral fluids are withheld until the child requests them, 20–25-mL/kg IV lactated Ringer's solution or equivalent is infused perioperatively, and multimodal prophylac-

Table 11.1 Indications for overnight admission post-adenotonsillectomy

1. Age <3 years
2. Those with abnormal coagulation studies or a history of increased bleeding tendency
3. Those with evidence of significant OSA (see later discussion)
4. Those with other systemic diseases that place them at additional perioperative risk, e.g., congenital heart disease, endocrine or neuromuscular disease, chromosomal abnormalities, obesity
5. Those with craniofacial or airway abnormalities, e.g., Down syndrome
6. Those with a peritonsillar abscess
7. Those who live at an excessive distance from the medical facility or whose home, social, or parental situation might preclude safe postoperative care

tic therapy with dexamethasone (0.0625–0.15 mg/kg up to 8 mg) and a serotonin-receptor antagonist (e.g., ondansetron 0.05–0.1 mg/kg up to 4 mg) is given intraoperatively.

Obstructive Sleep Apnea

Chronic obstruction due to lymphoid hyperplasia may result in OSA. Affected children may be obese (or asthenic), snore loudly, and have difficulty arousing in the morning or exhibit daytime somnolence; new onset of nocturnal enuresis and behavior problems (attention deficit disorder and limited attention span), cognitive impairment, night terrors, and nocturnal apnea and/or gasps.

Such a history strongly suggests clinical OSA, and a preoperative sleep study (polysomnogram) is recommended; if the results are significantly abnormal, admission for monitoring is advised. Polysomnographic criteria for admission post-T&A are shown in Table 11.2.

If polysomnography is unavailable, overnight oxygen saturation monitoring has been used as a valuable screening tool for OSA; resting oxygen saturations <90% and transient repeated episodes <80% are strongly predictive of severe OSA. Although the positive predictive value of overnight SpO_2 monitoring is very

Table 11.2 Polysomnographic and physiologic criteria for admission post-T&A

1. A baseline partial pressure of carbon dioxide ($PaCO_2$) ≥50 mmHg
2. A baseline awake oxygen saturation value ≤92%
3. Episodes of oxygen desaturation ≤80% (“sawtooth pattern,” during sleep, see below)
4. Apnea/hypopnea index >10

high, a negative test is less helpful and should be interpreted cautiously.

Children with OSA have reduced responses to rebreathing CO_2 and may be exceedingly sensitive to opioids (opioid dosing for analgesia may be a fraction of a standard dose), requiring dramatically reduced opioid doses or avoidance of opioids altogether. The latter is prominent in children whose nocturnal desaturation is <85% (see below). Children with mild OSA have few complications after T&A; those with moderate/severe OSA may require more intensive monitoring and postoperative care.

The child with OSA should be closely monitored before and after surgery; supervised mild sedation (oral midazolam) is generally safe preoperatively but is often omitted. Children with OSA may be at risk for desaturation at any time and should be observed closely. Either preoperative oral acetaminophen (10–15 mg/kg) or perioperative IV acetaminophen (15 mg/kg) may provide effective analgesia. In all children diagnosed with OSA, spontaneous respirations are maintained after tracheal intubation to test their respiratory responses to small incremental doses of opioid, e.g., fentanyl (0.5 μg/kg) or morphine (0.025 mg/kg). Children with upregulated opioid sensitivity (nocturnal desaturation <85%) may develop apnea after a single small dose of opioid despite surgical stimulation. In such cases, no further opioids should be administered, and postoperative opioid doses should be markedly reduced or omitted. Post-T&A, ketorolac is not routinely administered because of the risk of bleeding and reoperation, although the evidence is controversial. Diclofenac, tramadol, dexmedetomidine, ibuprofen, and celecoxib have been used to treat perioperative pain. Ketamine 0.5-mg/kg IV during surgery reduces the need for other analgesics and may be particularly useful in children with OSA. Most importantly, codeine is proscribed for postoperative analgesia in children with OSA (increased opioid sensitivity) and duplicated 2D6 isoforms (greater conversion of the prodrug codeine to morphine) as deaths have occurred. The FDA issued a black box warning (see Chap. 3) proscribing the use of codeine and tramadol in children <18 years of age after T&A surgery. It should be noted that other opioids, e.g., tramadol and oxycodone, may also have altered pharmacokinetics related to duplicated cytochromes resulting in accumulation of tramadol and greater conversion of oxycodone to hydromorphone (see Chap. 3). Alternative analgesics as described above or alternating q6h ibuprofen and acetaminophen are recommended.

Postoperative polysomnography has demonstrated that ~90% or more of those with mild/moderate OSA improve by 6 months, but only ~30% with obesity or severe OSA improve. Those whose OSA is not improved may be treated with intranasal steroids and nasal nocturnal oxygen therapy or should be investigated for residual soft tissue obstruction and evaluated for uvulopalatopharyngoplasty. In general, children do not tolerate CPAP or BiPAP devices.

Cardiorespiratory Syndrome

In very rare instances, adenoidal tissue causes severe chronic airway obstruction that may lead to pulmonary hypertension and right-sided heart failure (cardiorespiratory syndrome). This condition most commonly occurs in males of African-American heritage with a history of symptoms of ≥1 year. The child is usually febrile (due to associated adenoid or pulmonary infection), tachycardic, and tachypneic. Chest radiography reveals cardiomegaly with right ventricular hypertrophy on electrocardiogram. Children with cardiorespiratory syndrome may be critically ill and require emergency tracheal intubation to relieve the airway obstruction. Heart failure must be controlled before a T&A is performed. Postoperatively, these children often remain intubated and admitted to the PICU for further observation.

Special Anesthesia Problems for T&A Surgery

1. Sharing the airway with the surgeon.
2. Danger of postoperative bleeding (increased in obese children).
3. A history of bleeding tendency or recent salicylate therapy. If such a history is obtained, the cause of bleeding tendency must be determined, and the operation is deferred. *Salicylates should be stopped 2 weeks before* surgery.
4. A history suggestive of OSA. Such children are at risk for perioperative apnea and demonstrate increased sensitivity to opioids (see previous discussion).

Anesthesia Management

1. For children with a history of chronic infectious tonsillitis, anesthesia may be induced intravenously or by inhalation.
2. Tracheal intubation with a preformed oral tracheal tube that is positioned under the slotted tongue blade of the mouth gag is preferred. Check airway patency after the gag is positioned. Check for bilateral ventilation because the tip of the preformed tube may migrate endobronchially after the mouth gag is inserted or if the neck is flexed. Some advocate a laryngeal mask airway (LMA) in place of a tracheal tube; however, in our opinion, the very low-associated morbidity and additional security of a tracheal tube argue against using an LMA.
3. Administer standard multimodal antiemetic therapy: ondansetron (0.05–0.1 mg/kg up to 4 mg) and dexamethasone (0.0625–0.15 mg/kg, maximum 8 mg) intraoperatively and lactated Ringer's solution (20–25 mL/kg) perioperatively to reduce nausea and vomiting and improve postoperative comfort.
4. When the indication for surgery is chronic infection, maintain anesthesia with N_2O and sevoflurane or isoflurane, assist ventilation (with or without a relaxant), and supplement with opioids. When the indication for surgery is OSA, titrate opioid dosing or use alternative analgesics as described above.
5. Ask the surgeon to suction the pharynx as small residual amounts of blood may lead to laryngospasm. Extubate the tra-

chea when the child is fully awake and airway reflexes are fully restored (especially for those with OSA). Do not pass suction catheters through the nose because it may trigger adenoidal bleeding. Alternatively, the trachea may be extubated "deep" in older children. Transfer the child in the recovery position (lateral decubitus) to PACU.

Postoperative

1. For those with infectious adenotonsillitis, titrate doses of IV morphine for postoperative pain as usual. For those with OSA, titrate doses of morphine based on their intraoperative respiratory responses to IV morphine (or fentanyl) (ranging from 0% to 100% of the usual dose based on whether apnea or hypopnea occurred in response to the opioid). All children require continuous postoperative monitoring of oxygen saturation and respiratory rate. Caution: pulse oximetry is a poor measure of the adequacy of ventilation if supplemental oxygen is co-administered; use capnography in such cases.
2. Lactated Ringers' solution (20–25 mL/kg) should be infused in the perioperative period to restore euvolemia depending on the degree of dehydration. It is particularly important to hydrate children undergoing T&A on an outpatient basis before discharge.
3. Oral fluids, e.g., cola beverages and popsicles, should be offered; do not push oral fluids.
4. In the first 24-h post-adenotonsillectomy, children with OSA may have worsened airway obstruction from edema and bleeding. Such children may become apneic with opioids or sedatives and require constant and extended nursing observation and monitoring in the ICU. Some patients, e.g., those who are obese, may benefit from nasal CPAP or supplemental oxygen.
5. When ordering opioids for the restless child, restlessness may be a symptom of hypoxia secondary to obstruction and not pain. Here, opioids may produce apnea. Do not remove monitors once the child settles.
6. The outpatient should be evaluated by the surgeon for bleeding and the anesthesiologist for adequacy of ventilation before discharge. In general, we recommend observing those

post-adenotonsillectomy children without a history of OSA for at least 4 h before discharge.

7. A written analgesic regimen should be provided to the parents and discussed with them; alternating doses of acetaminophen with ibuprofen is a satisfactory alternative to opioid-based regimens.
8. A follow-up telephone call for outpatients on the first evening after surgery may improve patient/parent satisfaction.
9. Complaints of abdominal pain after T&A suggest the presence of swallowed blood, possibly from ongoing bleeding.

Reoperation for Bleeding After Tonsillectomy

Special Anesthesia Problems

1. The stomach contains blood that may be regurgitated during induction.
2. Hypovolemia may be easily underestimated since much of the blood may have been swallowed.
3. The child may also have a bleeding disorder that has not been identified; this should be evaluated.

Anesthesia Management

Preoperative

1. Ensure circulatory homeostasis with sufficient IV fluids to restore euvolemia and circulatory homeostasis; bleeding is rarely so brisk that complete restoration of blood volume cannot be achieved before the operation.
2. Obtain a type and cross; transfuse to maintain a minimum Hb of 7–8 g%.
3. Check coagulation indices.
4. In some instances, gentle restraint permits examination, insert packing, or cauterize the bleeding vessels without general anesthesia.
5. Rapid bleeding may prevent laryngoscopy; *be prepared to perform a surgical airway.*

Perioperative

1. Prepare all equipment for a rapid sequence induction (two suctions [including one tonsil tip], two functioning laryngoscope blades, and two functioning handles).
2. Confirm that the child has been adequately fluid resuscitated.
3. Give 100% O_2 by mask.
4. Rapidly inject IV atropine (0.02 mg/kg) and propofol (or ketamine or etomidate if hypovolemia is suspected), followed immediately by succinylcholine (2 mg/kg). If succinylcholine is contraindicated, use high-dose rocuronium (1.2 mg/kg). Anticipate that tracheal intubation may be difficult as edema, bleeding, and surgical tissue trauma may create a challenging view of the larynx.
5. Have an assistant immediately apply cricoid pressure if appropriate (see Chap. 4).
6. Intubate as rapidly as possible with a styletted cuffed tracheal tube. If the larynx is filled with blood despite using 2 suctions, position the child in the left lateral decubitus and Trendelenburg for intubation.
7. Maintain anesthesia as for T&A (see above); surgery for tonsil rebleeding is much less painful than the original T&A. Opioids are generally unnecessary as the previous surgical sites that are likely to bleed were already cauterized.
8. Extubate the trachea with the child in a lateral position after antagonizing neuromuscular blockade and the child is fully awake.

Postoperative

1. Monitor oxygen saturation and vital signs closely.
2. Check the Hb concentration to confirm adequacy of blood replacement.
3. Watch for further bleeding (increased in obese children).
4. Administer supplemental analgesics but be cautious:
   (a) Oversedation could result in complete obstruction of the airway.
   (b) Restlessness may indicate hypoxia rather than a need for sedation.

(c) Do not remove monitors until the child is fully awake.

Peritonsillar Abscess (Quinsy)

Special Considerations

1. Tracheal intubation may be difficult in the presence of trismus and swollen pharyngeal tissues.
2. Anticipate that the abscess may burst and flood the pharynx with pus that leads to pulmonary aspiration.

Anesthesia Management

Preoperative

1. Children with a tonsillar abscess should be closely observed for impending airway obstruction. Check the extent to which the mouth can be opened; significant trismus may be present while awake but disappears with induction of anesthesia.
2. Avoid premedication particularly in children with airway obstruction.

Perioperative

1. Ensure that suction with a tonsil tip is available. Give atropine 0.02 mg/kg IV.
2. Induce anesthesia by inhalation of sevoflurane in oxygen. Maintain spontaneous ventilation. Position the head slightly down and turned to the affected side.
3. Do not give muscle relaxants (airway obstruction may occur).
4. When the child is *deeply* anesthetized with sevoflurane in 100% O_2, give lidocaine (1–2 mg/kg) and a small bolus of propofol IV to reduce the risk of coughing or breath holding during laryngoscopy and tracheal intubation. Be careful not to rupture the abscess while instrumenting the airway.
5. Maintain anesthesia as for T&A for chronic infection (see previous discussion).
6. Suction the pharynx thoroughly and extubate the trachea when the child is fully awake and in a lateral position.

N.B. Sometimes the inflammatory swelling involves the supraglottic structures, and postextubation obstruction may occur. Dexamethasone (0.1 mg/kg up to 8 mg) IV may be indicated; close observation is essential.

Otologic Conditions

Surgery for ear conditions ranges from (minor surgery) simple bilateral myringotomy and tubes (BTT) to (major) prolonged surgery for tympanomastoidectomy and cochlear implants. The duration of BTT surgery is brief, e.g., 5 min, but is not without risk because these infants and children often have or had a recent URTI. In contrast, tympanomastoidectomy and cochlear implantation require considerations for prolonged surgery, require tracheal intubation, and are associated with PONV.

Special Anesthesia Problems

1. The child may have had repeated procedures and may be very apprehensive.
2. The child's hearing may be impaired, making communication difficult.
3. During middle ear procedures, even a small amount of bleeding may interfere with surgery; avoid anesthetic causes of bleeding, e.g., coughing, and NSAIDs. Induced hypotension is infrequently indicated.
4. If the surgeon chooses to use a vasoconstrictor drug, the dose should not exceed the maximum (see previous discussion).
5. Otologic procedures can be lengthy; if this is the case, ventilation should be controlled, with attention to positioning, padding, and using a forced air warmer.
6. If the surgeon uses a nerve stimulator, relaxants are limited to induction of anesthesia.
7. Given the frequency of postoperative PONV, multimodal PONV prophylaxis (ondansetron and dexamethasone) is indicated.

8. A great auricular nerve block before surgical incision and repeated at the end of surgery reduces pain and vomiting.

Minor Otologic Procedures: Bilateral Myringotomy and Tube (BTT) Placement

Minor otologic procedures are usually performed as outpatient procedures. N_2O has been shown to pass into the middle ear cavity if air is present and may modify findings at operation, but in general, its use is not contraindicated. N_2O does not increase the incidence of postoperative vomiting after these procedures.

Special Anesthesia Problems

1. Some children who require repeated minor otologic procedures have associated congenital deformities of the upper airway that predispose to their ear disease, e.g., cleft palate and Treacher Collins. Check previous anesthetic records for potential airway problems.
2. Many of these children present with signs of a URTI. In such instances, the decision to proceed must be based on the urgency of surgery, i.e., acute middle ear infection, compared with the severity of the URTI. If the child's behavior, eating habits, and temperature have been normal, and there are no mucopurulent secretions or chest wheezing/rales, then surgery should proceed (see Chap. 8).

Anesthesia Management

Preoperative

1. Sedation is often unnecessary. Oral midazolam will calm the very upset child, though it may delay recovery after this brief procedure. Parental presence at induction may be a suitable alternative to premedication.

Perioperative

1. Induce and maintain anesthesia by inhalation or intravenously if IV access is available or potent inhalation agents are contra-indicated.
2. Tracheal intubation is not required, but a laryngoscope and suitable tracheal tubes should be immediately available. IV access is not usually required but an IV set should be ready for urgent use if needed.
3. Keep the child's head still by resting the elbow of the hand holding the mask on the table.
4. Local anesthetic ear drops (4% lidocaine), IM ketorolac (0.5–1 mg/kg), and/or IN fentanyl (2 μg/kg) provide analgesia. Alternately, the greater auricular nerve or the nerve of Arnold block may provide effective analgesia when infiltrated with 0.2 mL of bupivacaine (0.25%).

Postoperative

1. Oral or IV acetaminophen may be administered for analgesia.

Major Otologic Procedures: Cochlear Implant, Tympanomastoidectomy, and Tympanoplasty

Anesthesia Management

Preoperative

1. Consider adequate sedation, especially for children who have had previous surgery.
2. Children should be allowed to wear their hearing aids until induction of anesthesia after which time they should be removed; they should be reinserted in PACU.
3. If the child communicates by sign language, then either a parent or health-care professional who can sign should accompany the child to the OR. If the child can lip-read, do not cover your lips until the child is anesthetized.

Perioperative

1. Induce anesthesia by inhalation or intravenously and intubate the trachea. If nerve stimulation (usually for the facial nerve) is required during surgery, only use a single low dose of intermediate-acting relaxant for tracheal intubation. We caution against using succinylcholine because a nerve stimulator will be ineffective if the child has pseudocholinesterase deficiency (1:3000 children have homozygote atypical pseudocholinesterase; see Chap. 3).
2. Topicalize the larynx with lidocaine and then insert an orotracheal tube (preferably a preformed oral tracheal tube). An extended breathing circuit is usually required as the anesthetic machine is positioned at the foot of the OR table. Ensure that ventilation is adequate for the increased compression volume and compliance of the extended breathing circuit.
3. Maintain anesthesia with N_2O/O_2 or air/O_2 and an inhalational anesthetic or a propofol infusion; anesthesia must be deep enough to prevent any possibility of bucking on the tube, which increases bleeding. Supplement with dexmedetomidine or opioids as needed, but beware that opioids may increase PONV (consider remifentanil).
4. Position the child with a 15° head-up tilt to minimize bleeding.
5. Block the greater auricular nerve (2–3 mL of 0.25% bupivacaine with epinephrine) before surgical incision and then repeat the block at the end of surgery (see Chap. 7); this will greatly reduce the need for opioids and the incidence of vomiting.
6. If epinephrine is infiltrated, ensure that the dose does not exceed the recommended maximum.
7. Prophylactic antiemetics should be given. Administer 20–25 mL/kg balanced salt solution to decrease postoperative pain and emesis.
8. For tympanoplasty, discontinue N_2O from the inspired mixture before the graft is positioned. (N_2O bubbles might float the graft off the desired position.)
9. Smooth tracheal extubation, without coughing, is essential. Therefore, administer intravenous lidocaine (1–2 mg/kg) or

propofol (0.5–1 mg/kg) 5 min before the planned time of extubation and remove the ETT while the child is still deeply anesthetized and breathing spontaneously. Maintain the airway and allow the child to awaken while administering oxygen by mask.

Postoperative

1. Administer analgesics and antiemetics as needed.

Endoscopy

Endoscopy is often indicated in infants and children for diagnosis, e.g., stridor, or for therapy, e.g., removal of a foreign body.

Procedures

1. Laryngoscopy
2. Bronchoscopy
3. Esophagoscopy

Special Anesthesia Problems

1. Existing airway problem or tracheotomy.
2. Difficulty maintaining optimal ventilation during endoscopy.
3. Possibility of complete airway obstruction during some procedures. e.g., removal of foreign body.
4. Danger of airway fire if cautery or laser is used.
5. Danger of postoperative reduction in the airway lumen by subglottic edema.

N.B. Many conditions for which endoscopy is performed can progress to complete airway obstruction under anesthesia. Always have a difficult airway cart at hand with special adjuncts such as a fiberoptic laryngoscope, videolaryngoscope, and a selection of laryngoscope blades and tracheal tubes prepared; from the start of anesthesia, ensure that the endoscopist is at hand in case surgical intervention with either a rigid bronchoscope or tracheotomy becomes urgently necessary.

General Anesthesia Management

1. *Spontaneous ventilation* is usually preferred as spontaneous respirations allows the endoscopist to examine the dynamic structures of the airway, which is particularly important when evaluating the child for airway compression, laryngeal, tracheal, or bronchomalacia; airway compression or collapse may not be adequately detected during positive pressure ventilation.
2. *Controlled/assisted ventilation* is necessary for children who are in respiratory failure and for those who cannot maintain effective spontaneous ventilation when anesthetized.

Laryngoscopy

Anesthesia Management

Preoperative

1. Avoid heavy premedication in children with airway problems but oral midazolam is useful for some older children having repeated endoscopy. Children with laryngeal papillomata present a particular risk because of possible ball-valve obstruction, airway fire, or embolism of tumor fragments distally. Discuss the optimal anesthetic prescription for the child and the planned surgery with the surgeon, e.g., spontaneous ventilation with insufflation, intermittent intubation, or paralysis with apneic oxygenation.

Perioperative

1. Apply monitors, induce general anesthesia by inhalation, and insert an appropriate-sized intravenous catheter.
2. Hydration with 20 mL/kg of lactated Ringer's solution will support the circulation during deep anesthesia.
3. When the child is deeply anesthetized, discontinue the N_2O, continue with 8% sevoflurane in O_2, perform laryngoscopy, and topicalize the larynx and supraglottic structures with lido-

caine (maximum dose, 7 mg/kg). Evidence of light anesthesia requires supplemental IV propofol.

4. Replace the mask until the lidocaine becomes effective (2–3 min). The duration of the procedure may be brief in some cases but prolonged in others. Anesthesia may be continued with either an inhalational anesthetic or TIVA.
5. Monitor ventilation.
6. Additional topical lidocaine may be applied by the surgeon as indicated.

N.B. Employing topical analgesia and an intravenous infusion of propofol with spontaneous ventilation without a tracheal tube provides the most satisfactory surgical conditions, as tracheal tubes interfere with the surgeon's field of vision.

Postoperative

1. Observe the child closely until awake.
2. Maintain NPO status until about 2 h after application of the lidocaine spray.

Special Considerations

Laryngomalacia A common cause of inspiratory stridor in the neonate, laryngomalacia can be diagnosed while the infant is awake or is awakening from anesthesia. The stridor usually disappears during deeper levels of anesthesia and with small amounts of positive end-expiratory pressure (PEEP); PEEP is especially useful in maintaining a patent airway during the initial induction. In this condition, the cartilages of the larynx are incompletely mature, and there is a tendency for the epiglottis or the arytenoid cartilages to prolapse into the glottis during inspiration, causing inspiratory stridor. The condition is self-limited and disappears as the child ages; no special therapy is usually required. However, laryngoscopy is indicated to rule out other causes of stridor, e.g., cysts.

Congenital Cysts Congenital cysts may occur near the epiglottis and aryepiglottic folds. There may be inspiratory and expiratory stridor and a poor cry. The diagnosis is usually confirmed by endoscopic evaluation and corrected by excision or marsupialization.

Congenital Webs Complete tracheal webs are generally fatal at birth. However, most webs have a single central perforation (2–4 mm diameter) through which the neonate ventilates. Respiratory distress occurs soon after birth because of the limited diameter of the perforation and the oxygen requirements of the neonate. Laryngoscopy usually reveals the presence of the web; otherwise, an appropriate-sized tracheal tube may not pass beyond the vocal cords. When the diagnosis is confirmed by bronchoscopy, laser resection of the web restores the normal airway diameter.

Subglottic Hemangioma Subglottic hemangioma may manifest with croup-like symptoms and a barking cough, usually commencing at a few months of age. This is often accompanied by other visible hemangiomas, especially on the face. The symptoms persist or recur, and diagnosis is confirmed with endoscopy. These hemangiomas are usually treated by laser ablation; subglottic stenosis may develop. Open resection of the hemangioma is advocated by some.

Laryngotracheal Cleft This embryological defect is a failure of the tracheoesophageal septum to fuse. The severity depends on the length of the defect from a type 1 cleft, which is limited to a defect from the larynx to the vocal cords to type IV, which may extend down to the carina. Type 1 cleft is managed conservatively whereas types II–IV require surgical intervention. Presentation includes swallowing difficulties, stridor, and aspiration. About two-thirds have associated anomalies, including tracheoesophageal fistula, cardiac, urologic, and craniofacial anomalies. Laryngotracheal clefts are also associated with CHARGE, VACTERL, and other syndromes. Surgical correction of types II–IV involves general anesthesia for rigid bronchoscopy and esophagoscopy for direct closure or by using tissue flaps. (see Rigid Bronchoscopy below).

Anesthesia Management

For laser resection

1. Manage as for laryngeal papillomata (see later).
2. Humidified oxygen/air should be administered postoperatively after laser therapy.

For open excision

1. An initial laryngoscopy and bronchoscopy is performed to assess the lesion. This may be managed with inhalational anesthesia plus topical lidocaine (see above discussion).
2. After the initial endoscopy, an oral tracheal tube is inserted and general anesthesia continues.
3. An anterior incision is made in the neck to open the larynx.
4. At this stage, the tracheal tube is withdrawn until the tip of the tube is exposed and a second sterile tracheal tube is passed by the surgeon distally into the trachea and secured; the first tube is removed.
5. The hemangioma on the posterior aspect of the larynx is now resected.
6. Upon completion of the resection, a nasotracheal tube is left in situ.
7. The child is returned to the ICU for postoperative ventilation, sedation, and paralysis for the initial postoperative period. Immobility of the laryngeal structures is important during the early healing period.
8. Before extubation, a postoperative endoscopy is performed several days later. If the surgical resection has been successful, dexamethasone is administered before removing the tube.
9. *Recurrent Respiratory Papillomas (RRP).* These cauliflower-like RRP, caused by the human papilloma virus (HPV), are the most frequent airway tumors in children. They can cause serious airway obstruction and, if untreated, lead to pulmonary hypertension and right-sided heart failure. There is no cure for RRP, but treatment includes cryoprobing, ultrasound, and immune sera as well as surgical resection and debulking using lasers. CO_2 lasers that only penetrate the superficial tissue layers, KTP/532 and pulsed-dye lasers, and non-laser approaches, including the microdebrider and coblation have been used successfully. The microdebrider is less expensive and a more rapid technique, although postoperative pain is similar to the CO_2 laser.

Children with this condition usually present at 2–4 years of age for increasing hoarseness and dyspnea and return for repeated endoscopies until adolescence, at which time the lesions regress spontaneously. Rarely does RRP become cancerous. A cautious approach is indicated with each endoscopy since the extent of regrowth is impossible to determine before laryngoscopy; extensive papillomas may completely obscure the glottis and create a ball-valve obstruction.

Special Anesthesia Problems

1. Acute airway obstruction may occur during induction of anesthesia; therefore, spontaneous ventilation with CPAP is preferred.
2. The glottic opening may be difficult to visualize; avoid paralytics.
3. Surgical therapy by laser demands an unobstructed view of the larynx and immobile vocal cords.
4. Instrumentation of the trachea below the glottis should be avoided because it may "seed" papillomas into the lower airways. Therefore, tracheal tubes should be avoided if possible, and tracheostomy is usually considered to be contraindicated.

Anesthesia Management for Laser Surgery

The safest and most widely used prescription includes no premedication, a smooth inhalation induction followed by laryngoscopy, and topical lidocaine spray. If obstruction develops during induction, a tracheal tube must be inserted to reestablish a patent airway. The tube can be removed when a deep plane of anesthesia is achieved and most of the papillomas have been resected. Usually, tracheal intubation is unnecessary, and laser resection can proceed once topical analgesia has been applied. Rarely, critical airway obstruction may occur necessitating an urgent rigid bronchoscopy. In this circumstance, inhaled sevoflurane anesthesia may be supplemented or replaced with intermittent boluses of propofol or a propofol ± remifentanil infusion.

Alternatively, a non-flammable tracheal tube[1] (or foil-wrapped tube) may be inserted. In this case ventilation can be controlled, but the surgeon must work around the tube. Another approach to laser

---

[1]Phycon laser shielding tube, Fuji Systems Corp., Tokyo.

surgery in the airway for lesions other than laryngeal papillomas is intermittent intubation by the surgeon with apneic oxygenation.

N.B. Jet ventilation can be very dangerous in cases of obstructing lesions of the airway. Laryngeal obstruction during jet ventilation may lead to pneumomediastinum and pneumothorax. If jet ventilation is used, extreme care must be taken to avoid barotrauma: the jet must not be advanced beyond the lumen of the laryngoscope, and peak airway pressure should be monitored and restricted to <15 mmHg.

Special Precautions for the Use of the Laser

1. Cover the child's eyes with wet gauze.
2. All personnel in the OR should wear protective goggles in case the laser beam is accidentally reflected in their direction. Post a warning sign on all doors when the laser is used.
3. N95 or charcoal-filtered face masks should be worn to protect against inhalation of vaporized viral tissue.
4. Airway fires are a real danger during laser therapy. Use the minimal FiO_2 (preferable $\leq 30\%$) in either air or helium. Avoid N_2O; it supports combustion. If a tracheal tube should ignite, it must be immediately disconnected from the anesthetic circuit and removed from the airway. Injury results both from the burn and from the products of tube combustion.

Bronchoscopy

Bronchoscopy may be performed for various indications, e.g., removal of a foreign body, diagnosis of respiratory disease, removal of secretions, treatment of atelectasis, evaluation for tracheomalacia, bronchomalacia, or airway compression by vascular structure or mediastinal tumors.

Special Anesthesia Problems

1. Difficulty maintaining adequate ventilation during the procedure, when the airway must be shared with the endoscopist.
2. Existing impaired ventilation.

Anesthesia Management

Preoperative

1. Assess the airway and the respiratory status.
2. Avoid heavy premedication if there is any doubt about the airway or ventilation.

Perioperative

Spontaneous ventilation is preferred for all children except those with respiratory insufficiency.

1. Induce anesthesia by inhalation and establish adequate venous access.
2. Discontinue N_2O; continue with 8% sevoflurane in 100% O_2 ± IV propofol.
3. When the child is deeply anesthetized, topicalize the larynx and trachea with lidocaine (maximum 7 mg/kg).
4. Resume mask ventilation and continue anesthesia with O_2 and sevoflurane until the lidocaine takes effect (2–3 min), at which time the bronchoscope can be inserted.
5. Supply O_2 and sevoflurane to the side arm of the bronchoscope and allow spontaneous ventilation ± IV propofol as needed. When the telescope is in situ with a 3.5 mm or smaller bronchoscope, the resistance to ventilation requires assisted or positive pressure ventilation. The expired carbon dioxide level may be absent or inaccurate in such cases; assess the adequacy of ventilation by observing chest expansion.
6. Ensure the audible oxygen saturation is loud enough for the surgeon to respond if the saturation begins to decrease. During bronchoscopy, position a precordial stethoscope over the lungs.
7. Consider the possibility of pneumothorax (a rare complication of pediatric bronchoscopy) if desaturation occurs.
8. If controlled ventilation is preferred, a Venturi device, e.g., Sanders injector, may be used. Note that children with severe chronic respiratory disease have reduced lung compliance so a Venturi device may be less effective. For such children, control ventilation using the anesthetic circuit connected to the side arm of the bronchoscope (Fig. 11.1).

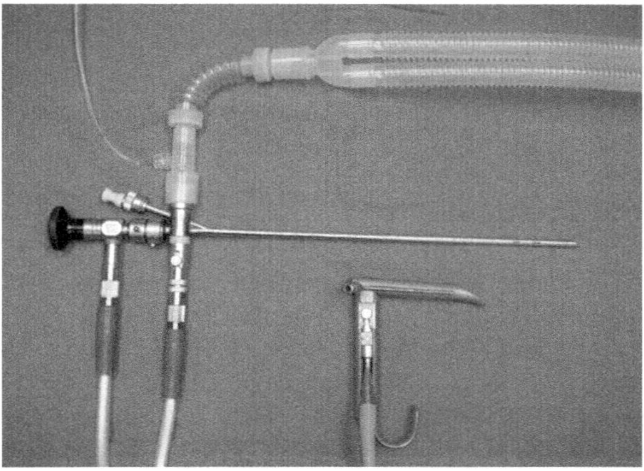

Fig. 11.1 Pediatric rigid bronchoscope with anesthesia circuit attached for controlled/assisted ventilation. Right is anterior commissure laryngoscope

Postoperative

1. Administer O_2 as needed.
2. Observe and treat stridor.
3. For persistent respiratory distress/desaturation, review a chest X-ray to rule out a pneumothorax.

Flexible Bronchoscopy

Small-diameter flexible fiberoptic bronchoscopes permit a diagnostic bronchoscopy to be performed with the child awake or with minimal sedation and topical anesthesia. In young children, however, general anesthesia is often preferred. In such cases, the bronchoscope is passed through an adapter at the elbow of an LMA or into the face mask and via the mouth or nose of the anesthetized child. An LMA is particularly useful as it ensures adequate airway patency and a means for continuing to deliver anesthesia. Alternatively, a tracheal tube can be inserted as a conduit for the bronchoscope, although the stem of the LMA is much wider than the tracheal tube that will pass the larynx; thus, a larger bronchoscope can be used with the LMA. In all cases, topical anesthesia with lidocaine as described for rigid bronchoscopy is indicated.

Rigid Esophagoscopy

In children, rigid esophagoscopy is usually performed to dilate a stricture or for removal of a foreign body.

Special Anesthesia Problems

1. The child may have undergone esophagoscopy repeatedly and therefore may be very apprehensive. Children with TEF or EA repair develop strictures and are at risk for having food, e.g., a piece of hot dog, stuck in the esophagus; anticipate possible associated subglottic stenosis.
2. In small infants, passage of an esophagoscope may compress the trachea and obstruct ventilation, even when a tracheal tube is in place.
3. Coughing, straining, or other movements can result in esophageal perforation during the procedure; anesthesia must maintain complete immobility.
4. Lower esophageal strictures or achalasia may result in esophageal dilation more cephalad. Food and secretions accumulated in the dilated segment may be aspirated during anesthesia.
5. Rarely, a sharp or potentially damaging foreign body may lodge in the hypopharynx, which may be displaced into the airway if the child coughs or strains.
6. Do not rely on a taped tracheal tube during movement of the esophagoscope; hold the tube to prevent unintended extubation.

Anesthesia Management

Preoperative

1. Administer preoperative sedation, especially for "frequent flyers."
2. Check whether the radiographs show esophageal dilation and/or retained material.
3. Discuss with the surgeon any special considerations he/she may have, and alter the anesthetic prescription accordingly.

Perioperative

1. Give 100% O_2 by mask while applying standard monitors.
2. Induce anesthesia intravenously and intubate the trachea rapidly; use cricoid pressure when there is a risk of regurgitation and aspiration—except unless contraindicated; see Table 4.5).
3. In the case of a sharp foreign body in the hypopharynx, a gentle, smooth inhalation induction of deep anesthesia is indicated.
4. Deepen the anesthesia before permitting the endoscopist to proceed.

Postoperative

1. Observe for signs of esophageal perforation, especially if difficulty was encountered. These signs include:
   (a) Tachycardia.
   (b) Hemoglobin desaturation.
   (c) Radiographic evidence of pneumothorax or mediastinal air.
   (d) Fever.
2. Order nothing by mouth until 2 h after application of the lidocaine spray.

Airway Infections

Epiglottitis

In the past, supraglottic infections, e.g., epiglottitis, were most commonly caused by *Haemophilus influenzae* B (*HiB*) bacterial infection and less frequently by *Staphylococcus* and fungi in severely immunocompromised children. Since the introduction of a *HiB* vaccine, epiglottitis has become a rare disorder in children but still occurs in adults. As the disease becomes rarer, there is an increased danger that the diagnosis may be missed. However, epiglottitis can still occur, and there is recent evidence of resurgence in *HiB* epiglottitis in non-immunized children and in those after occasionally ineffective/failed vaccines.

Epiglottitis is most common in children 3–7 years old but also in infants or adults. It is accompanied by severe systemic illness with pyrexia and leukocytosis. In addition to the epiglottis, all the supraglottic structures are swollen and inflamed, contributing to the airway obstruction. Blood cultures are almost always positive for the infective agent, which is typically *HiB*, although other bacterial and fungal infections rarely occur. The common symptoms include the triad: sore throat, dysphagia, and drooling; severe airway obstruction may develop rapidly. Typically, the child appears toxic, anxious, and in the tripod position seated forward with the chin extended and mouth open. In infants the presentation is less typical, occurring with sudden apnea during investigation of a high fever. Epiglottitis should be considered in the differential diagnosis of the infant with pyrexia and respiratory distress.

Extra-epiglottic infection may occur: pneumonia, cervical adenitis, otitis media, septic arthritis, and meningitis are described in association with epiglottitis.

Anesthesia Management

Preoperative

1. Once the diagnosis is suspected, the child should not be disturbed. Avoid venipunctures or painful injections because the child may cry and become acutely obstructed. Do not try to visualize the larynx because acute obstruction may follow. Gently apply a face mask and give O_2.
2. The child must always be attended by a physician capable of establishing an emergency airway and prepared to do so.
3. Assemble the team and transfer the child rapidly to the OR; administer O_2, allowing the child to remain in the chosen posture.
4. Do NOT send the child to the Radiology department unattended for soft tissue radiographs of the neck. Not only may they be misleading but also unnecessary to establish the diagnosis. This is a clinical diagnosis. The child should not be made to lie down for the X-ray examination. The lateral neck film will reveal a dilated hypopharynx, thickened aryepiglottic

folds, a thumb-like epiglottis obstructing the laryngeal inlet, and loss of the vallecula because of swelling of the tongue surface of the epiglottis.
5. The OR should be prepared for emergency bronchoscopy and possible tracheotomy (surgeon present, scrubbed, and ready to intervene if needed).

Apnea May Occur at any Time

1. Try to ventilate the lungs with O_2 by bag and mask and CPAP. This is usually successful.
2. If unsuccessful, proceed to an immediate attempt at laryngoscopy, intubation, or possible emergency tracheotomy.

Perioperative

1. Gently apply standard monitors.
2. Do not place the child supine. Perform an inhalational induction by placing the mask gently over the child's face while the child is seated either on the OR table or on the anesthesiologist's or parent's knee. Having a parent present may reduce the child's upset and therefore minimize dynamic tracheal collapse with crying against an obstructed upper airway.
3. After anesthesia is induced, gently lay the child supine and escort the parents out of the OR. Assisted ventilation may be necessary at this time.
4. Establish intravenous access and administer IV atropine (20 μg/kg) and 20–30 mL/kg of lactated Ringer's solution. These children are febrile and usually dehydrated.
5. Anesthetic induction is likely to be prolonged because of shallow respirations and possible $\dot{V}/\dot{Q}$ mismatch due to pneumonia. If the airway is satisfactory, there is no urgency to rush the process. Our rule of thumb is that when you think the child is deep enough to perform laryngoscopy, wait 1 more full minute or two because it is quite easy to underestimate the depth of anesthesia.
6. Administer lidocaine 1–2 mg/kg IV, supplemental IV propofol and perform laryngoscopy and orotracheal intubation with a

styletted tracheal tube. In the rare event that the glottis is obscured by swelling and distortion of the supraglottic structures, compress the chest with one brisk compression. This usually expels a salivary bubble through the larynx, identifying the glottic opening. Another useful trick is to insert the laryngoscope blade down the center of the tongue until the swollen epiglottis is observed. At this point, the tip of the blade is forced into the vallecula (which has been obliterated by the swollen tongue surface of the epiglottis). This will then apply pressure at the base of the tongue and force the epiglottis into a more favorable position to visualize the laryngeal inlet.

7. Obtain a blood culture once the airway is secured.
8. When the child is anesthetized and well oxygenated, the tube may be changed from an oral to a nasotracheal tube (one size smaller than predicted for age) provided the intubation was not difficult, as follows:
   (a) Move the oral tracheal tube to the left side of the mouth and allow an assistant to hold that tube while gently assisting respirations.
   (b) Pass a nasal tracheal tube telescoped into a red rubber catheter (to prevent bleeding) into the hypopharynx (see Chap. 12).
   (c) Perform laryngoscopy and position the tip of the tube into the laryngeal inlet using McGill forceps, in the laryngeal inlet adjacent to the orotracheal tube.
   (d) Slowly withdraw the oral tube and advance the nasal tube through the vocal cords and firmly secure the tube as accidental extubation must be avoided.
9. Very rarely, pulmonary edema occurs immediately after intubation. This has been attributed to a sudden release of the negative pressure caused by breathing against an obstructed upper airway, hypoxia, elevated catecholamines, and disturbed alveolar-capillary pressure gradient. Treat with controlled ventilation, PEEP, and diuretics.

Postoperative

1. Pediatric intensive care unit monitoring is essential. Accidental extubation must be prevented with effective sedation and tube stabilization.
2. Ensure adequate humidification of inspired gases and regular suctioning of the nasotracheal tube to prevent tracheal secretions from blocking the tube.
3. Commence antibiotic therapy with cefuroxime, a cephalosporin with a high margin of safety, and good penetration of the cerebrospinal fluid for *HiB* infections.
4. Extubate the trachea after the pyrexia has resolved (usually 12–36 h after starting antibiotics) and an audible air leak is present with the cuff deflated. Flexible laryngoscopy may be performed before extubation to verify normal supraglottic structures.
5. Observe the child after extubation for several hours. Very rarely does the trachea require reintubation for recurrent obstruction. It is reasonable to perform the extubation in the OR to facilitate reintubation if necessary.

Croup or Laryngotracheobronchitis

"Acute infectious croup" or laryngotracheobronchitis is most commonly caused by a virus in children 2–5 years of age. Do not overlook other causes including a foreign body. Inspiratory stridor is the principal symptom caused by swelling of the loose tracheal mucosa at the level of the cricoid cartilage. Symptoms are frequently worse at night.

Therapy varies according to the severity of the disease:

1. In mild to moderate cases, conservative measures (oral dexamethasone) is usually effective.
2. In more severe cases, epinephrine inhalation in addition to oral dexamethasone usually result in improvement.
3. Very rarely, nasotracheal intubation is required, generally to facilitate removal of inspissated secretions.

Epinephrine Inhalation

Inhalations of epinephrine are widely efficacious in cases that fail to respond to conservative measures.

1. The nebulizer is prepared with 0.5 mL of 2.25% racemic epinephrine added to 3.0 mL of distilled water.
2. Attach a suitable pediatric-size face mask on the face, while the child is held by the mother or father.
3. These children are usually hypoxic. Add at least 40% O_2 to the inspired gases and monitor SaO_2.
4. After ~20 min, there should be considerable improvement, if not, the diagnosis of croup should be reconsidered.
5. A single dose of IV dexamethasone (0.5–1 mg/kg) is also recommended.
6. Be aware that rebound stridor may occur. Rarely, the stridor increases rapidly, necessitating immediate establishment of an artificial airway.
7. Some children require more than one inhalational treatment; failure to respond with any improvement is an indication to review and question the diagnosis. The use of racemic epinephrine is contraindicated in infants with tetralogy of Fallot because a severe "tet" spell may be precipitated.

Nasotracheal Intubation (See Chap. 12)

If conservative measures and epinephrine inhalations with IPPB fail to relieve symptoms, an artificial airway may be required. Nasotracheal intubation with a tracheal tube of sufficiently small diameter as to provide a leak at approximately 20-cm H_2O peak inflation pressure and left in place until both oropharyngeal secretions and tissue swelling have diminished; the presence of a small tube and thick secretions renders accidental blockage very likely.

Tracheotomy

Tracheotomy may become necessary in the therapy of upper airway obstruction or to facilitate respiratory care in other conditions.

Anesthesia Management

Preoperative

1. Give 100% O_2 by mask, and assist ventilation manually as needed.
2. Avoid sedatives or opioids.

Perioperative

1. Continue 100% O_2 by mask, induce anesthesia with an inhalational induction, and assist ventilation as required (IV access must be checked for patency and replaced if necessary).
2. Deepen anesthesia and topicalize the larynx with lidocaine. The surgeon may perform a diagnostic rigid bronchoscopy before the tracheostomy to identify the area of pathology. If the surgeon performs the tracheotomy over a tracheal tube, reduce the inspired oxygen concentration to ~30 percent or less, and discontinue nitrous oxide while maintaining a deep level of anesthesia with inhalational or TIVA to minimize the risk of an airway fire. After the surgeon opens the trachea, slowly withdraw the bronchoscope or tracheal tube until the tip is above the tracheal opening. Only remove the tube or bronchoscope once the tracheostomy tube has been successfully placed. N.B. The cuff on a cuffed tracheal tube may be punctured when the surgeon makes his/her initial incision into the trachea.
3. In case of a "difficult airway," e.g., Pierre Robin syndrome, anesthesia may be induced by mask and continued after insertion of an LMA, which may then be used as a conduit to intubate the trachea.

4. Before leaving the OR, confirm that the tip of the tracheostomy tube is above the carina with a fiberoptic scope while in the position the child will be cared for postoperatively. If not, then another more suitable size should be inserted.

Postoperative

1. Obtain a chest radiograph immediately on arrival in PACU. Check that the tracheostomy tube is positioned correctly and rule out a pneumothorax.
2. Consider the possibility of an accidental extubation before the track into the trachea becomes established. If this happens, it may be very difficult to reinsert the tube. Many surgeons leave long silk sutures through the edges of the tracheal opening that can be pulled laterally to facilitate emergency reinsertion of the tracheotomy tube.

Bacterial Tracheitis

As the incidence of epiglottis has declined in the pediatric population, bacterial tracheitis has emerged as a more common cause of acute respiratory distress. The disease usually occurs with cough, hoarseness, stridor, and chest retraction. Drooling is rare, but the child is toxic and pyrexial with leukocytosis. Emergency bronchoscopy should be managed as for epiglottitis and usually reveals an inflamed, edematous trachea with purulent secretions and possible pseudomembranes. The responsible organism is usually *Staphylococcus* or *Streptococcus* pneumonia. Repeat bronchoscopy may be indicated to monitor disease recovery.

Subglottic Stenosis

Subglottic stenosis is one of the most common causes of chronic airway obstruction in infants and children. The stenosis may be congenital or acquired—with 90% acquired usually as a complication of prolonged endotracheal intubation. Neonatal and severe subglottic stenosis traditionally involve a tracheotomy followed by surgery to reconstruct the subglottic space. The surgical procedure generally involves division of the cricoid cartilage and insertion of a cartilage graft to increase the diameter. A stent is then left in place to maintain the lumen. After extensive repair, it is often preferred to sedate, immobilize the neck, and ventilate the child for several days to optimize healing. In the past two decades, advances in airway procedures have led to endoscopic balloon dilatation as the foremost intervention for acquired subglottic stenosis with 86% success in acute cases and >60% success in chronic cases. This technique offers several advantages including being less invasive, and having a reduced risk of infection and less postoperative pain, as well as shorter surgical time and hospital length of stay. Other approaches include a slide tracheoplasty and, more recently, application of 3D-designed external stents. The latter may offer greater success since there is no intraluminal suture line and therefore minimal irritation of intratracheal structures.

Subglottic stenosis, which may prevent successful extubation in neonates, may be treated by early anterior cricoid split without a preliminary tracheostomy.

Associated Conditions (Congenital Type)

1. Congenital heart disease.
2. Down syndrome.
3. Tracheoesophageal fistula.

Anesthesia Management for Cartilage Graft to Cricoid Ring

Preoperative

1. If a tracheostomy is in place, all care and monitoring of the tracheostomy is continued until the child arrives at the OR.

Perioperative

1. Anesthetize via the tracheotomy tube using sevoflurane in O_2.
2. Remove the tracheotomy tube and insert an armored tube via the stoma; suture it firmly in place. (*N.B.* The lumen of the trachea will take a larger tube than is expected.)
3. Confirm bilateral air entry.
4. Maintain anesthesia with inhalation or TIVA and control ventilation.
5. Blood loss is usually minimal.

Postoperative

1. Replace the tracheotomy tube.
2. The stent is usually removed and laryngoscopy performed 3 months later.
3. The tracheotomy is left in place until the child is able to tolerate plugging of the lumen of the tube.

For Anterior Cricoid Split (Without Tracheostomy)

This procedure is performed for neonates who cannot be extubated as a result of narrowing at the cricoid.

1. The child is anesthetized via the existing tracheal tube.
2. When the child is anesthetized, the tube may be removed and a bronchoscope inserted to examine the remainder of the airway.
3. The trachea is reintubated and the cricoid cartilage divided anteriorly.
4. An age-appropriate size nasotracheal tube is inserted into the trachea and left in place for 5–7 days.

Suggested Reading

Brown KA, Laferrière A, Lakheeram I, Moss IR. Recurrent hypoxemia in children is associated with increased analgesic sensitivity to opiates. Anesthesiology. 2006;105(4):665–9.

Dang Y, Li Y, Zhang J, et al. Comparison of short-term recovery in children with obstructive sleep apnea undergoing tonsillotomy vs. tonsillectomy. Front Pediatr. 2022;10:969973.

Feng M, Lao VF, Choby G, et al. Survey of anesthesiologists on topical vasoconstrictors and intravenous tranexamic acid for endoscopic sinus surgery. Ann Otol Rhinol Laryngol. 2022;131:59–70.

Hannam JA, Anderson BJ, Potts A. Acetaminophen, ibuprofen, and tramadol analgesic interactions after adenotonsillectomy. Paediatr Anaesth. 2018;28:841–51.

Hawksworth C, Ravury S. An audit of anesthesia safety in a pediatric cochlear implantation program. Paediatr Anaesth. 2015;25:630–5.

Hu L, He N, He S, Jiao Y. Endoscopic balloon dilatation in the management of paediatric-acquired subglottic stenosis in children. Auris Nasus Larynx. 2024;51:161–6.

Hu Y, Smith S, Coombs AT. Pediatric obstructive sleep-disordered breathing and anesthetic considerations. Curr Opin Anaesthesiol. 2025;38:272–7.

Liu H-E, He L. The performance of a post-induction fentanyl-test in predicting postoperative respiratory adverse events in children after adenotonsillectomy. J Clin Sleep Med. 2024;20:1749–54.

Martha VV, Veontela S, Calder AN, et al. Laryngeal cleft: a literature review. Am J Otolaryngol Head Neck Med Surg. 2021;42:103072.

Ohn M, Eastwood P, von Ungern-Sternberg BS. Preoperative identification of children at high risk of obstructive sleep apnea. Pediatr Anesth. 2020;30:221–31.

Polytarchou A, Ohler A, Moudaki A, et al. Nocturnal oximetry parameters as predictors of sleep apnea severity in resource-limited settings. J Sleep Res. 2023;32:e13638.

Riley B, Kawai K, Irace AL, Leung P, Adil E. Perioperative pain control and tympanostomy tube outcomes. Int J Pediatr Otorhinolaryngol. 2020;138:110337.

Schneider TA, Costeloe A, Mnatsakanian A, et al. Drug-induced sleep endoscopy for targeted sleep surgery in pediatric patients. Cureus. 2025;17(5):e84122. https://doi.org/10.7759/cureus.84122.

Wang JT, Peyton J, Hernandez MR. Anesthesia for pediatric rigid bronchoscopy and related airway surgery: tips and tricks. Paediatr Anaesth. 2022;32(2):302–11.

Dental Anesthesia 12

General Principles

1. Children do not usually cooperate well under moderate sedation unless they are highly motivated, older, and specially prepared. Consequently, most require deep sedation or general anesthesia more frequently than adults for dental procedures.
2. Many children undergoing general anesthesia have had previous failed attempts at dental treatment under local anesthesia and sedation; consequently, they are highly apprehensive.
3. Some children have behavior disorders or developmental delays and require special consideration, especially those with autism.
4. Others have medical conditions that require specific considerations, e.g., congenital heart disease.
5. Nasotracheal intubation is preferable for most children having dental surgery. Nasal intubation per se, as well as the presence of extensive caries, is associated with bacteremia. Prophylactic antibiotics are warranted for patients with heart defects at risk of endocarditis (Table 12.1).
6. Care must be taken to ensure that no foreign bodies remain in the airway at the end of the procedure (especially throat packs). Counting throat packs is essential. Direct laryngoscopy is recommended before extubation to ensure that the airway is clear.

J. Lerman, C. J. Coté, *Steward's Manual of Pediatric Anesthesia*, https://doi.org/10.1007/978-3-032-24545-8_12

Table 12.1 Indications for endocarditis prophylaxis

Patients who should receive prophylactic antibiotics include those with:
(a) Prosthetic cardiac valve, including transcatheter prostheses and homografts
(b) Prosthetic material used for cardiac valve repair, such as annuloplasty rings, cords, or clips
(c) Previous infective endocarditis
(d) Unrepaired cyanotic congenital heart defect (CHD) or repaired CHD with residual shunts or valvular regurgitation at the site of or adjacent to the site of a prosthetic patch or prosthetic device[a]
(e) Cardiac transplant with valve regurgitation due to a structurally abnormal valve
(f) Cardiac ventricular assist devices

[a]Except for the conditions listed above, antibiotic prophylaxis before dental procedures is not recommended for any other types of CHD

7. Dental procedures may be prolonged when extensive disease is present. In such instances, children should receive intraoperative intravenous fluids to restore euvolemia. It is preferable to limit the duration of general anesthesia for outpatients to a maximum of 3 h and to schedule prolonged surgery in the morning.
8. For procedures performed under sedation with local anesthesia, monitoring should be applied as for general anesthesia.
9. In rare cases, the use of air-turbine dental drills has been a cause of intraoperative subcutaneous and mediastinal emphysema, leading to airway obstruction and possible pneumothorax. If facial swelling occurs, discontinue nitrous oxide, check for pneumothorax, and prepare to support ventilation. Very rarely, these complications may present in the postoperative period after tooth extractions.

Management for General Anesthesia

Preoperative

1. A careful preoperative history and physical examination should be performed, as dentists are not authorized to perform

"medical assessments" of patient conditions in most jurisdictions. Previously unrecognized disease is often discovered in children presenting for dental surgery.
2. Special investigations and treatments should be ordered for children with other comorbidities.
3. Premedication should be tailored to the child's needs.
4. Prophylactic antibiotics should be administered before surgery.
5. It may be helpful to have the parent accompany the child to the induction area or to insert an intravenous line with the parents present.

Perioperative

1. Apply standard American Society of Anesthesiologists' monitors.
2. Induce anesthesia by inhalation if an IV is not present, or with propofol if an IV is present. Establish IV access after induction of anesthesia with an inhalational agent.
3. Nasotracheal intubation may cause a bacteremia, and endocarditis prophylaxis is recommended for those at risk.
4. To reduce the risk of a nosebleed after nasotracheal intubation, a soft catheter may be used (see below) and/or a topical vasoconstrictor (oxymetazoline). Liberal lubrication and warming the tip of the nasotracheal tube do not reduce bleeding.
5. Administer propofol and/or a non-depolarizing muscle relaxant as indicated, and preoxygenate before performing nasotracheal intubation. One approach to minimize nosebleeds is to telescope the tip of the nasotracheal tube into the flange of a soft red rubber catheter and advance the lubricated catheter tip along the floor of the nose until it is visible in the hypopharynx. Extract the tip of the catheter from the hypopharynx via the mouth with Magill forceps, and then—with a sudden jerk—pull the catheter off the tip of the tube. Then advance the tip of the tracheal tube into the larynx using Magill forceps under direct laryngoscopy. Since this technique involves several steps, oxygen desaturation is more likely if the child

is cyanotic preoperatively or has intrinsic lung disease; pre-oxygenate before commencing.

The left nostril is preferred for nasotracheal intubation since the bevels of endotracheal tubes are on the left and the turbinates are less likely to be damaged. Furthermore, as the tube enters the hypopharynx, the leading edge (tip) of the tube (which is on the right side) is in the midline, directly in line with the glottic opening.

6. The tip of the tracheal tube may fail to advance through the vocal cords despite the tube being the correct size. This occurs because the angle that the tube makes as it exits the nasopharynx is acute, directing the tip into the anterior commissure of the vocal cords. Any one of three remedies solves this problem: (A) rotate the tube so the bevel faces anteriorly and then advance the tube, (B) pick up the tube with Magill forceps 2–3 cm proximal to the distal tip and angle the distal end posteriorly so the tip passes, or (C) withdraw the tube slightly, lift the child's head, and flex the child's neck. This aligns the axes, and the tip of the tube should pass easily. If none of these approaches is successful, consider an orotracheal tube to ventilate and oxygenate.
7. Maintain anesthesia with N_2O and an inhalation agent in O_2. For brief procedures, spontaneous ventilation will suffice; for more prolonged procedures, pressure support or controlled ventilation may be more appropriate.
8. Administer a balanced salt solution at 10–20 mL/kg/h for the first 1 or 2 h.
9. Keep track of the total dose of local anesthetic administered by the dentist/oral surgeon to avoid toxicity.
10. At the end of the procedure, when all dental instrumentation has been removed, a laryngoscopy should be performed to ensure that the airway is free of debris or foreign material before extubation. Beware of throat packs that may have been forgotten.

Postoperative

1. Administer analgesics as required: nerve blocks with local anesthetic will reduce postoperative pain. Acetaminophen and NSAIDs are usually sufficient after dental surgery. Primary teeth often have short roots and do not cause pain when extracted. However, IV morphine or ketorolac may be required after multiple extractions. Ensure that analgesic instructions are provided to the parents for use after discharge.
2. Antiemetics may be required, although dental surgery is not associated with a high incidence of PONV.
3. Continue intravenous fluids until the child is ready for discharge.

Management for Deep Sedation

1. Currently, propofol is probably the most useful drug for deep sedation, allowing good moment-to-moment control of sedation and ensuring rapid recovery. Alternatives include ketamine and propofol in combination or a dexmedetomidine infusion.
2. Preoperative care and intraoperative monitoring should be as for general anesthesia, as cited in the AAP Guidelines for sedation for children undergoing diagnostic and therapeutic procedures, including dental sedation outside the hospital.
3. Preoperative medication with midazolam and prior application of a topical anesthetic cream facilitate insertion of an intravenous catheter.
4. Drugs and equipment for intubation and ventilation with O_2 should be at hand.
5. Deep sedation should be commenced with small increments of propofol (0.5–1 mg/kg as needed for induction) to avoid apnea, followed by a continuous infusion, beginning with 250 μg/kg/min (larger doses may be necessary for younger and cognitively impaired children), reducing the rate pro-

gressively to 75–100 μg/kg/min as the local anesthetic blocks become effective.
6. Oxygen may be given, and end-tidal carbon dioxide sampled by a septate nasal catheter. The airway is usually well maintained; however, close monitoring is essential.

The Child with Congenital Heart Disease

The child should be managed for anesthesia with all the necessary considerations for their cardiac disease (Chap. 15):

Table 12.2 Antibiotic dosing for endocarditis prophylaxis for dental procedures

Situation	Antibiotic	Pediatric dose	Adult dose
Oral	Amoxicillin	50 mg/kg	2 g
Unable to take oral	Ampicillin OR	50 mg/kg IV or IM	2 g IV or IM
	Cefazolin or ceftriaxone	50 mg/kg IV or IM	1 g IV or IM
Allergic to penicillin or ampicillin ORAL route	Cephalexin[a]	50 mg/kg	2 g
	OR		
	Azithromycin **or** clarithromycin	15 mg/kg	500 mg
	OR		
	Doxycycline	2.2 mg/kg < 45 kg, 100 mg > 45 kg	100 mg
Allergic to penicillin or ampicillin and unable to take by mouth	Cefazolin **or** ceftriaxone[b]	50 mg/kg IV or IM	1 g IV or IM

IM intramuscular, *IV* intravenous
Clindamycin is no longer recommended for dental procedures
[a]Or other first- or second- generation oral cephalosporin in equivalent pediatric or adult doses
[b]Cephalosporins should not be used in an individual with a documented history of anaphylaxis, angioedema, or urticaria with penicillin or ampicillin

1. *Recommendations for prophylactic antibiotics in children with congenital heart defects (CHD) having dental procedures*. The cardiac defects for which prophylactic antibiotics are now indicated are listed in Table 12.1. Antibiotic dosing, based on the recommendations of the American Heart Association (2024), is listed (see Table 12.2).
2. *Dental procedures that require prophylactic antibiotics* include all dental procedures that involve manipulation of gingival tissues or the periapical region of teeth or perforation of the oral mucosa.
3. *Dental procedures that do not require prophylactic antibiotics* include routine anesthetic injections through noninfected tissue, taking dental radiographs, placement of removable prosthodontic or orthodontic appliances, adjustment of orthodontic appliances, placement of orthodontic brackets, shedding of deciduous teeth, and bleeding from trauma to the lips or oral mucosa.

Suggested Reading

Campbell RL, Shetty NS, Shetty KS, et al. Pediatric dental surgery under general anesthesia: uncooperative children. Anesth Prog. 2018;65:225–30.

Coté CJ, Wilson S. Guidelines for monitoring and management of pediatric patients before, during, and after sedation for diagnostic and therapeutic procedures. Pediatr Dent 2025:47(6);E100-E128.

Ji YD, Peacock ZS, Resnick CM. Characteristics of national malpractice claims in oral and maxillofacial surgery. J Oral Maxillofac Surg. 2020;78:1314–8.

López-Velasco A, Puche-Torres M, Carrera-Hueso F, et al. General anesthesia for oral and dental care in paediatric patients with special needs: a systematic review. J Clin Exp Dent. 2021;13:e303–12.

Velasco AL, Carrera Huesco FJ, Silvestre FJ, et al. Pediatric morbidity after oral surgery procedures under general anaesthesia: a systematic review. J Stomatol Oral Maxillofac Surg. 2023;124:101262.

Watt S, Pickhardt D, Lerman J, et al. Telescoping tracheal tubes into catheter minimizes epistaxis during nasotracheal intubation in children. Anesthesiology. 2007;106:238–42.

13 Plastic and Reconstructive Surgery

Many children require plastic surgery to correct congenital deformities, burns, or trauma involving the head and neck which introduce special problems for the anesthesiologist.

General Principles

1. Many of these children have psychological issues that stem from both the deformity and the need for multiple surgical procedures. Previous anesthetic records will identify past experiences with premedication, venous access, difficult intubation, and adjuncts required, as well as other associated perioperative issues.
2. A smooth induction of anesthesia and a quiet emergence ensure optimal outcomes.
3. Many children undergoing reconstructive surgery need careful preoperative airway assessment and require special airway adjuncts for successful management (See Chap. 4).
4. Congenital structural anomalies commonly affect more than one body system. The child with defects requiring plastic surgery may also have diseases affecting other systems. If congenital heart disease is present, review the most recent cardiac evaluations and determine the need for SBE prophylaxis (see Chap. 12).

J. Lerman, C. J. Coté, *Steward's Manual of Pediatric Anesthesia*,
https://doi.org/10.1007/978-3-032-24545-8_13

Cleft Lip and Palate

Cleft lip and cleft palate (CLP) may present as isolated defects or in association with various syndromic combinations in ~1/1000 live births. Infants with these lesions may be malnourished and anemic as a result of feeding difficulties and may have a history of repeated respiratory infections. Treatment of CLP is optimally managed within a multidisciplinary team; the pediatric anesthesiologist is an essential member of this team.

The surgical management of CLP is evolving, with the optimal age for stages in the repair and the use of procedures such as preoperative orthodontic maneuvers to mold the bony structure of the palate are still debated. An orthodontic appliance, e.g., Latham appliance, is sometimes applied to the neonate's palate to progressively align the bony alveolar ridge before soft tissue repairs.

1. Congenital heart disease is not specifically associated with isolated cleft palate but may be present as part of a syndrome or association (see Appendix A).
2. Airway anomalies, for example, Pierre Robin sequence or Treacher Collins syndrome, may present with difficult mask ventilation and intubation. Aging affects the severity of the airway compromise, e.g., the airway in Pierre Robin sequence is difficult to intubate at birth but becomes easier with age (often resolving by 2–3 years of age), whereas the airway in Treacher Collins may be intubated easily at birth but becomes progressively more difficult with age, necessitating tracheotomy in some adolescents.
3. Syndromes associated with CLP may have other specific anesthesia implications (Table 13.1) (see Appendix 1).

The surgical care of the patient with CLP has many stages, not all of which are required by all children.

Table 13.1 Syndromes associated with cleft palate

Syndrome name	Features	Anesthetic implications
Arthrogryposis multiplex congenita	Limb contractures, CHD in 10% Stiffness of joints, GU defects	Difficult intubation due to limited mouth opening, antibiotics for CHD, position and pad carefully (see Appendix A)
Beare-Stevenson syndrome	Craniosynostosis, hydrocephalus choanal atresia, midface hypoplasia proptosis, hypertelorism, cutis gyratum	Difficult ventilation (choanal atresia), beware of tracheal stenosis, caution with neck manipulation due to cervical spine defects
Beckwith-Wiedemann syndrome	Exomphalos, macroglossia, hyperviscocity, visceromegaly, neonatal hypoglycemia	Danger of hypoglycemia, infuse glucose and monitor level, tongue reduction may be required at time of palate repair
CATCH 22	Cardiac defect, abnormal facies, thymic hypoplasia, hypocalcemia (DiGeorge syndrome)	Difficult airway. Antibiotics for CHD. Anticipate hypocalcemia. Use irradiated PRBCs
Cornelia de Lange syndrome	Short stature, developmental delay (variable), CHD in 15%	Airway obstruction, difficult intubation, antibiotics for CHD
Down syndrome	Short stature, developmental delay (variable), macroglossia, unstable cervical spine, subglottic stenosis. CHD in 50%	Difficult mask ventilation, assess neck instability, smaller ETT size, SBE prophylaxis, possible OSA
EEC syndrome	Ectrodactyly, ectodermal dysplasia, hypohidrosis Chronic respiratory infections	Malnutrition, anemia, hypohidrosis, temperature control problems. Difficult intubation, protect eyes, position and pad carefully

(continued)

Table 13.1 (continued)

Syndrome name	Features	Anesthetic implications
Kabuki syndrome	Craniofacial and skeletal defects, hypotonia anomalies, CHD, visceral and urogenital defects, increased susceptibility to infections	Difficult airway, caution with relaxants, SBE prophylaxis, asepsis
King syndrome	Congenital myopathy, MH trait. Dysmorphic features (Noonan-like)	MH precautions
Miller syndrome	Mandibular defects, limb anomalies, renal defects	Difficult airway
Multiple pterygium syndrome	Webbing of skin, syngnathia, ankyloglossia, web neck	Difficult airway—more severe with age
Nager syndrome	Malar hypoplasia, micrognathia, CHD, radial hypoplasia, absent thumbs, vertebral anomalies	Very difficult airway, limited mouth opening, cervical spine anomalies. SBE prophylaxis
Oto-palatal-digital syndrome	Skull deformity, hearing loss, cervical spine defect, Arnold-Chiari malformation, limb defects, possible thoracic hypoplasia	Possible brain-stem compression causing postoperative respiratory depression
Patau syndrome (trisomy 13)	Microcephaly, developmental delay, micrognathia, CHD, usually fatal in infancy	Difficult airway, SBE prophylaxis
Pierre Robin sequence	Micrognathia, glossoptosis, cleft palate and respiratory distress in the first 24h after birth	Difficult airway, postoperative airway obstruction
Seckel syndrome	Birdlike facies, dwarfism microcephaly, possible glottic narrowing; postop apnea reported	Difficult airway, possible smaller ETT size. Monitor for postop apnea

(continued)

Table 13.1 (continued)

Syndrome name	Features	Anesthetic implications
Smith-Lemli-Opitz syndrome	Growth failure, microcephaly, developmental delay, CHD, renal defects, hypotonia, GE reflux Thymic hypoplasia—prone to infection	Possible difficult airway, intraoperative muscle rigidity with inhalation agents, temperature control problems, SBE prophylaxis
Spondyloepiphyseal dysplasia congenita	Dwarfism, C1–C2 instability	Stabilize neck during intubation and positioning
Stickler syndrome (Pierre Robin variant)	Midface hypoplasia, cleft palate, micrognathia, "moon face" one-third of "Pierre Robin" patients	Difficult mask ventilation and intubation
Treacher Collins syndrome	Micrognathia, down-slanting eyes with colobomas, microtia with hearing loss, cleft palate, dental issues	Difficult intubation especially if right-sided or bilateral hypoplasia of mandible, postoperative hypoventilation. Airway difficulties increase with age
Walker-Warburg syndrome	Micrognathia, hypotonia, hydrocephalus, developmental delay, GU anomalies	Difficult intubation, postoperative hypoventilation
Trisomy 18	Lung hypoplasia, micrognathia, CHD	Difficult airway, ventilatory failure, SBE prophylaxis

CHD congenital heart disease, *GU* genito-urinary, *ETT* tracheal tube, *MH* malignant hyperthermia, *SBE* subacute bacterial endocarditis

Possible Surgical Procedures

1. Application of orthodontic splints or devices to the palate.
2. Cleft lip repair—usually performed at 3–4 months of age, sometimes earlier.
3. Cleft palate repair—usually performed at 12–18 months, but sometimes in younger infants.

4. Alveolar bone graft.
5. Pharyngoplasty—for velopharyngeal incompetence—usually performed at 5–15 years.
6. Maxillary advancement (Le Fort procedure) required for some adolescents.

Special Anesthesia Problems

1. Intubation with isolated micrognathia tends to be difficult in the young infant and becomes easier with age, e.g., Pierre Robin sequence, whereas in others, intubation becomes progressively more difficult with age, e.g., Treacher Collins syndrome.
2. Problems related to associated conditions (see previous discussion).
3. Blood loss during cleft palate repair is usually insignificant but rarely may require transfusion if the infant has an unrecognized coagulopathy.

Anesthesia Management

Preoperative

1. Preoperative assessment.
   (a) Special attention to the airway, lungs, and other systems that may be affected in congenital syndromes (see Appendix A).
   (b) Check for an acute upper respiratory tract infection; consider postponing surgery if there is fever, rales, or rhonchi that do not clear with coughing. Children with cleft palate have frequent and often chronic URTI symptoms; if the problem is chronic, then do not delay surgery.
   (c) Check for anemia.
2. Check for a history of bleeding as well as medications or herbal supplements associated with bleeding, e.g., aspirin, NSAIDs, gingko, garlic, or ginseng herbal medicines. In such children, a bleeding time may be indicated.
3. Blood is rarely needed for cleft palate surgery but check that the child has been typed for blood and serum saved (type and hold).

Perioperative

1. If there is concern for an abnormal airway, perform an inhalation induction and have the difficult airway cart at hand (see Chap. 4); consider starting an IV before anesthesia as tolerated.
2. For inhalation induction, deepen inhalational anesthesia until the child is adequately anesthetized for laryngoscopy and consider lidocaine (1.5 mg/kg IV) and propofol (1–2 mg/kg) before laryngoscopy to minimize the risk of coughing or laryngospasm. Some children will benefit from administration of a non-depolarizing muscle relaxant and/or assistance from a second anesthesia colleague.
3. If the cleft is large or bilateral, some recommend inserting a hard plastic "tooth guard" on the maxillary alveolar ridge to avoid trauma from the laryngoscope blade.
4. Use a preformed oral tracheal tube. Confirm bilateral ventilation after the mouth gag is placed and the child positioned. In infants, particularly those with micrognathia, preformed tracheal tubes may need to be repositioned to prevent an endobronchial intubation. Flexion of the neck during insertion of the mouth gag may advance the tip of the tube into a bronchus whereas extension may result in extubation.
5. For cleft lip repair, tape the tube to the mandible, ensuring that the upper lip is free and not distorted.
6. Reassess air entry and bilateral breath sounds each time the gag is repositioned or the child is repositioned.
7. Anesthesia may be maintained with N_2O and inhalation agent; concentrations should be tapered to ensure a prompt emergence; alternatively a TIVA regimen may be used.
8. A local anesthetic with epinephrine is often infiltrated by the surgeon for analgesia and to reduce surgical bleeding. An infraorbital nerve block (see Chap. 7) provides excellent analgesia for this procedure; consider IV acetaminophen (see Table 20.3 for infant dosing). To ensure an awake patient and a patent airway at extubation, we recommend administering low-dose opioids only at the beginning of surgery.

9. As surgery nears completion, ask the surgeon to inspect the mouth and pharynx to remove blood and clots. Extubate when the child is fully awake. After palate repair, acute swelling of the tongue causing obstruction has been reported after removal of surgical appliances; examine the mouth and if any signs of tongue swelling exist, the trachea should be left intubated.
10. A long suture is often inserted into the tongue to provide traction and facilitate immediate postoperative control of the airway in the PACU; this is usually removed when the child is fully awake but may be left in place overnight until a clear airway is ensured.

Post-operative

1. Cleft lip surgery is often performed as an ambulatory procedure because the surgery is superficial and postoperative problems are rare.
2. In contrast, cleft palate surgery is performed as an overnight admission to provide constant observation for 24 h because airway problems and/or bleeding may occur. A small percentage of children may have to return to the OR for control of bleeding and some may require reintubation.

Application of Palatal Splints or Devices in the Neonate

This is sometimes performed to mold the palate and alveolar ridge and improve the aesthetic and dental results of subsequent surgery. All provisions for neonatal anesthesia should be observed. General endotracheal anesthesia is preferred with a preformed oral tracheal tube; after the procedure only a mild analgesic, e.g., acetaminophen, is required.

Alveolar Bone Grafting

An alveolar bone graft may be required to close a gap in the bony alveolar ridge, often performed on an ambulatory basis, so that teeth may be guided into the grafted area. The bone is often harvested from the iliac crest; pre-incisional infiltration of the donor site with bupivacaine with epinephrine provides excellent analgesia and reduces bleeding. An IV opioid is usually required intra- and postoperatively. Multimodal prophylaxis to prevent PONV speeds return to normal activity.

Pharyngoplasty

Pharyngoplasty reduces velopharyngeal incompetence and improves speech. The procedure inevitably increases resistance to ventilation commonly resulting in postoperative airway problems requiring close monitoring.

Special Anesthesia Problems

1. Airway obstruction is a particular danger and may occur early in the PACU.
2. Chronic airway obstruction may persist after the operation and may lead to obstructive sleep apnea and possibly to later pulmonary hypertension.

Anesthesia Management

As for cleft palate (see previous discussion).

Post-operative

1. Observe for airway obstruction and/or bleeding in the PACU or PICU overnight.
2. A nasopharyngeal airway, placed by the surgeon intraoperatively and left in situ for 24 h, reduces serious postoperative respiratory complications.
3. Monitor for signs of obstruction during sleep; a follow up sleep study is recommended.

Fractured Mandible

Surgical Procedures

1. Interdental wiring.
2. Open reduction and wiring.

Special Anesthesia Problems

1. The child may have a full stomach.
2. Intubation may be difficult because of tissue damage, trismus, and distortion of airway anatomy.
3. Foreign bodies may be present in the airway, e.g., fractured teeth.
4. The mouth may be wired closed after the procedure; therefore, postoperative vomiting is a potentially life-threatening event. Multimodal prophylaxis is indicated and suction should be immediately available.
5. Wire cutters must be at the child's bedside at all times in case the trachea must be intubated or the airway cleared of blood and/or vomitus.

Anesthesia Management

Preoperative

1. Assess the child for trismus that may limit mouth opening and preclude a thorough examination; neither trismus nor a fractured mandible portends a difficult airway in general.
2. For children with a full stomach, delay surgery if possible and give metoclopramide 0.15 mg/kg IV to promote gastric emptying.

Perioperative

1. For emergency surgery, use an RSI (see Chap. 4).
2. Examine the pharynx quickly but carefully during laryngoscopy to search for foreign debris (radio-opaque debris such as

teeth may be visible on X-ray, consult radiographs before inducing anesthesia).

3. For elective surgery, a nasotracheal tube may be inserted initially if optimal conditions for laryngoscopy are present. For emergency surgery, use an orotracheal tube initially to secure the airway and then, after aspirating gastric contents, change to a nasotracheal tube. See Chap. 12 for nasotracheal intubation approaches to minimize nose bleeding.
4. Ask the surgeon to pack the throat with sterile gauze.
5. Maintain anesthesia with N_2O and an inhalational anesthetic or TIVA. Multimodal antiemetics should be administered.
6. Before final fixation of the jaw, ask the surgeon to remove the throat pack and to remove blood clots and other debris.
7. Antagonize neuromuscular blockade and with wire cutters present, withdraw the tube to the oropharynx and remove the tube when you are certain the child can sustain ventilation and protect the airway.
8. Leave the nasogastric tube in place.

Post-operative

1. Ensure that wire cutters remain at the bedside at all times for children whose jaws are wired closed.

Removal of Interdental Wiring

General anesthesia is usually required for removal of the wiring and arch bars when the fracture is healed. The wires holding the jaws together can be removed before induction of anesthesia. However, jaw movement remains extremely restricted because of the prolonged immobilization, possibly rendering laryngoscopy and intubation difficult.

After removal of the securing wires, anesthesia may be induced with a variety of techniques such as inhalation agents, TIVA, or ketamine until a well-lubricated soft nasopharyngeal tube can be inserted. When the depth of anesthesia and ventilation are adequate, the surgeon may remove the arch bars; have equipment for emergency intubation and/or tracheotomy immediately at hand.

Reconstructive Surgery for Burns

Children who suffer a burn injury require acute and chronic (reconstructive) burn care and surgery. Anesthesia for acute burn care is addressed in Chap. 18. Anesthesia for repeat reconstructive plastic surgery for release of contractures and hand/foot reconstruction is addressed below.

Special Anesthesia Problems

1. Contractures that result from burns to the face and neck may make laryngoscopy and tracheal intubation very difficult.
2. Extensive burns may also make it difficult to obtain reliable venous access.
3. Severe emotional problems may result from the accident, from the subsequent disfigurement, and from the repeated surgical procedures. The last problem often gives rise to fear of anesthesia, face mask, and fear of attempts at venous access; ask the child or teenager which approach is preferred.
4. Premedicate with oral midazolam; some may benefit from the addition of oral ketamine, or IN dexmedetomidine.
5. Blood loss for reconstructive procedures is generally not very extensive.
6. Temperature homeostasis is impaired, and special measures must be taken to avoid hypothermia.
7. Emergence from anesthesia should be quiet to avoid damage to recently grafted areas.

Anesthesia Management: General Endotracheal Anesthesia

General endotracheal anesthesia may be required if operating on the face or in the prone position. An LMA is usually appropriate for most other reconstructive procedures and for laser treatment of scars. Even after recovery from the acute burn, there are additional special considerations.

In adults, the induction and maintenance doses of propofol are up to a 50% greater in those with a ≥40% burn injury during the acute phase (first month) compared with non-burn adults. These pK differences have been attributed to an increased volume of distribution and clearance in burn patients, although comparable data in burn children are lacking. Some children may require IM ketamine for induction if no IV access is available. The induction dose of thiopental in children with burns several years after injury is ~40% greater than in non-burned children suggesting a pharmacodynamic (e.g., increased receptors) effect rather than pK effect.

1. Succinylcholine is contraindicated after the first 24 h after a burn and for 1.5–2 years after severe burns because it may cause a hyperkalemic cardiac arrest.
2. The dose requirements for non-depolarizing muscle relaxants are increased compared with those in unburned children for several years after the injury and the magnitude of the increase is in proportion to the size of the burn. Relaxants should be titrated to achieve the desired effect using a neuromuscular blockade monitor.
3. If the airway has been injured in the burn, subglottic stenosis may be present. Carefully select the size of the tracheal tube but prepare to use a smaller tube than expected. Some children may have a tracheostomy in place.

Preoperative

1. Conduct a standard preoperative assessment with particular emphasis on previous problems with the adequacy of premedication, a difficult airway, or difficult venous access. Often the child is able to tell you where "the best vein" is located.
2. Take time to talk with the child. Encourage questions, answer them honestly, and reassure the child about the planned procedure. Having a parent present during induction is exceedingly important to this cohort of children.

3. Have difficult airway adjuncts immediately available, e.g., video laryngoscope, fiberoptic equipment, difficult airway cart.
4. Preoperative sedation as indicated using standard routes and premedications.
5. Ensure that the OR is warmed to 25 °C or greater.
6. Confer with the surgeon regarding any special issues such as a specific route of intubation (oral or nasal, standard or preformed) ETT, eye care, positioning, site of graft harvesting, limits on local anesthetics, and postoperative surgical concerns.

Perioperative

1. If the airway is normal:
   (a) Induce anesthesia by either IV or inhalational route.
   (b) An LMA or tracheal tube as indicated by the surgery or position.
   (c) Measure blood losses and replace as needed.
2. Be prepared for a difficult airway:
   (a) If the neck cannot be extended, mouth opened, or microstomia is present, direct laryngoscopy may be difficult or impossible. Consider the following alternatives to secure the airway under sedation (midazolam, dexmedetomidine, propofol, and/or ketamine) or general anesthesia with an inhaled agent while breathing spontaneously:
      - A video laryngoscope or other advanced airway adjuncts.
      - Fiberoptic intubation.
      - Release the scar tissue (e.g., from a neck or perioral contracture) after sedation with ketamine ± dexmedetomidine, then induce anesthesia and secure the airway.
   (b) Once the airway has been secured, anesthesia can be maintained with either an inhalational anesthetic or TIVA-based technique.
3. These surgeries may be painful (particularly if a large skin graft is taken), and regional anesthesia or a field block is usually not possible. Opioids are essential adjuncts to these sur-

geries; the dose requirements are often increased because of residual tolerance from chronic use in the PICU.
4. All patients should receive multimodal PONV prophylaxis.

Postoperative

1. Emergence delirium and pain are common; low-dose ketamine is highly effective in the PACU. Some children experience severe itching (opioids and old scars); treat with an antihistamine, e.g., diphenhydramine.

Major Craniofacial and Reconstructive Surgery

Extensive reconstruction is performed to restore more normal facial features in children with severe facial deformities. The improved appearance frequently has a major beneficial effect on the child's future life; in some countries, these children cannot leave their home without restorative surgery. Surgery is often performed during infancy or early childhood to allow the child to attend school appearing as normal as possible.

External maxillary distraction osteogenesis has been applied to children requiring maxillary osteotomies. The osteotomies are performed subperiosteally and external distraction appliances attached with which the healing bone is drawn slowly apart after a short period to allow callus formation. These procedures are usually brief in duration and associated with minimal blood loss. However, external appliances may limit access to the airway.

General Principles

1. A team approach is essential.
2. Operations involving the jaw are usually delayed until dentition is complete, i.e., 13 years or older.
3. Operations not involving dentition, e.g., for craniofacial dysostosis, are usually performed at an earlier age.

Special Anesthesia Problems

1. Tracheal intubation may be difficult with severe airway deformities. Rarely, the airway cannot be secured despite the use of all adjunctive intubation techniques; in these cases, tracheotomy is performed using local analgesia and sedation.
2. Blood loss may be very extensive from the surgical and bone graft donor sites, e.g., pelvic girdle or ribs.
3. Surgery is of long duration, necessitating special precautions to protect against pressure sores, nerve compression, eye protection, and hypothermia.
4. Surgical manipulation involving the orbit and face may trigger the oculocardiac reflex.
5. Surgical manipulation may rarely damage the tracheal tube intraoperatively.
6. At the end of surgery, plan for a rapid emergence to assess cranial nerve function.
7. Extensive postoperative swelling of adjacent tissues may dictate the need for prolonged intubation.

Anesthesia Management

Preoperative

1. Preoperative assessment should focus on airway abnormalities and associated cardiopulmonary disease.
2. Associated congenital defects or other features of a syndrome may have anesthetic implications (see Appendix A). Some children may have OSA; consider reducing opioids if the SaO_2 nadir at night is <85% (see Chap. 11).
3. Check laboratory results, including coagulation indices.
4. Discuss the need for central venous and arterial lines (identify the non-dominant hand for an arterial line), a urinary catheter, nasogastric tube, and possible postoperative ventilation with the parents/child.
5. Administer preoperative sedation as warranted.
6. Have difficult airway adjuncts, e.g., video laryngoscope, fiber optic equipment, difficult airway cart, immediately available.
7. Have blood and blood products available.

Perioperative

1. Induce anesthesia:
   (a) In the absence of airway concerns, anesthesia may be induced by either IV or inhalational techniques; tracheal intubation should follow.
   (b) If a difficult airway is anticipated, anesthesia may be induced using an inhalational technique and the airway instrumented using difficult airway adjuncts as needed (see Chap. 4).
   (c) In some children with an extremely difficult airway, a tracheotomy may be performed with sedation under local analgesia or with general anesthesia with an LMA. This assures a secure airway for the procedure and postoperatively until swelling subsides.
2. The tracheal tube should be sutured or wired to structures that will remain fixed during surgery, e.g., teeth, or be so positioned in the trachea to allow for movement at its point of fixation. An armored tube is useful as it cannot be compressed during surgery, but it does not prevent the tube from being incised.
3. Maintain anesthesia with an inhalational anesthetic ± N_2O (*but if there is a risk of air embolism, substitute air for* N_2O), and an opioid. A non-depolarizing muscle relaxant may be indicated for prolonged surgery.
4. Maintain the arterial carbon dioxide pressure ($PaCO_2$) at ~30–35 mmHg.
5. Position the child with 10–15° reverse Trendelenburg.
6. Pad all pressure areas including the occiput and areas compressed by the tracheal tube, i.e., nares, lip.
7. Place protective ointment in the eyes (the surgeon often performs a tarsorrhaphy).
8. Dexamethasone IV is recommended to reduce tissue swelling and prevent PONV.
9. Monitor:
   (a) Standard anesthetic monitors.
   (b) Arterial blood pressure and central venous pressure if indicated; if reverse Trendelenburg is indicated, zero the arterial transducer at the level of the auditory canal.

   (c) Precordial Doppler ultrasound/end tidal Pco_2—for air embolism during craniectomy.
   (d) Acid-base, blood gas, hematocrit, and coagulation measures indices should be assessed serially.
   (e) Urine output.
10. Be prepared for massive blood replacement (See Chaps. 6 and 18).
11. If reduction in brain mass is required, give furosemide (1 mg/kg) or mannitol (0.5 g/kg, slowly over several minutes to avoid hypotension).
12. When indicated, moderate hypotension (SBP reduced by 10–15%) is achieved with remifentanil, dexmedetomidine, nitroglycerin, or sodium nitroprusside.
13. The child should be sufficiently awake at the end of surgery to assess vision and whether a cranial nerve injury has occurred during surgery. The child can then be re-sedated if the tracheal tube is to be left in place postoperatively.

Postoperative

1. Transfer to PICU; the ETT may be required for 48–72 h.
2. The timing of tracheal extubation depends on the return of an adequate spontaneous tidal volume, the absence of airway swelling, and the presence of a leak around the tube. The trachea may be extubated in the OR if the airway is precarious or in the PICU with an anesthesiologist and airway equipment at the bedside.
3. Caution should be exercised if an external distraction apparatus has been applied. In these cases, an airway exchange catheter may be inserted via the tracheal tube and briefly left in place after extubation to aid in reintubation should this be required. The airway exchange catheter can then be removed when it is apparent that reintubation will not be required.

Children with Mandibular Distraction Osteogenesis

Neonates and infants with severe airway difficulties and associated feeding problems, e.g., Pierre Robin sequence or Treacher Collins syndrome, may be managed by tongue-lip adhesion and a nasopharyngeal tube or a tracheostomy. Although tongue-lip adhesion maintains a patent airway while awake, it may preclude or render glottic visualization and tracheal intubation very difficult under anesthesia. Mandibular distraction osteogenesis (MDO) has supplanted the above techniques in infants with persistent respiratory distress, difficulty feeding, or a distance from the post-pharyngeal wall to the lingual root <3 mm. MDO is indicated to ensure successful decannulation of the neonate with a tracheostomy for airway difficulties. Difficulty with tracheal intubation may be anticipated based on the airway defect (see Table 13.1). The infant's airway should remain intubated (particularly if the airway was difficult preoperatively) after application of the external fixator until the infant fully recovers or the mandible has been distracted. The mandible is usually distracted 0.5 mm three times a day beginning 2–3 days after surgery, a process that continues for 4–8 weeks. If the distraction device must be modified or adjusted with general anesthesia, mask anesthesia may present challenges, although once the mandible has been distracted, tracheal intubation is usually much easier.

Tumors in the Neck: Cystic Hygroma and Congenital Cervical Teratoma

Cystic hygroma is a cystic lymphangioma that usually occurs in the neck and less commonly in the axilla. Intraoral extension of this benign tumor may cause airway obstruction. Three percent of cervical tumors extend into the mediastinum.

Teratomas may occur in the neonate, and though most occur in the sacral region, they may also involve the neck. Giant congenital cervical teratoma may cause life-threatening airway compromise. Extremely large tumors in the neck may be diagnosed antenatally by ultrasound requiring an EXIT procedure at birth (see below and Chap. 4).

Special Anesthesia Problems

1. Airway obstruction may be present.
2. Intubation may be difficult because the airway is distorted or difficult to visualize.
3. Complete removal of tumor may involve extensive dissection and repeated surgeries resulting in major blood loss.

Anesthesia Management

Preoperative

1. A focused airway examination and review of radiological investigations are essential; consider possible intrathoracic tumor extension.
2. Administer limited preoperative sedation in older infants.
3. Ensure availability of blood and blood products.
4. Have difficult airway adjuncts, e.g., video laryngoscope, fiber-optic equipment, difficult airway cart, immediately available.

Perioperative

1. Induce anesthesia using an inhalational induction, maintaining spontaneous ventilation.
2. Establish IV access.
3. Before attempting laryngoscopy, assist ventilation manually for several minutes with 8% sevoflurane in 100% O2 and administer IV propofol (1–2 mg/kg) and lidocaine (1.5 mg/kg) to ensure an adequate depth of anesthesia during laryngoscopy.
4. Intubate the trachea (consider an armored tube) and secure the tube. For some children, if intraoral dissection is planned, a nasal tube may be preferable. In the case of a difficult

intubation, insert an oral tube first and then change to a nasal tube if this is possible without risking losing the airway.

5. Maintain anesthesia with either inhaled anesthesia or TIVA and controlled ventilation.
6. For large tumors requiring extensive dissection, an arterial line and central venous access should be inserted; a urine catheter should also be placed.
7. Beware of vagal reflexes during dissection in the neck. If they occur, give a vagolytic.
8. Replace fluid and blood losses as indicated.
9. After the operation, prepare for a smooth emergence and extubation; prevent excessive coughing and bucking, which might cause bleeding at the surgical site.
10. If extensive surgery has been performed adjacent to the airway, extubation should be delayed until the extent of postoperative swelling is determined. If swelling is significant, the trachea should remain intubated until it resolves; rarely some children may require a tracheotomy.

Postoperative

1. If extubated:
   (a) Observe in the PICU or PACU overnight (because of the danger of bleeding into the surgical site or compression of the airway).
   (b) Avoid respiratory depressants, e.g., large doses of opioids.
2. If intubated:
   (a) Confirm the position of the tracheal tube radiographically.

The EXIT Procedure: Ex Utero Intrapartum Treatment

This procedure is designed to maintain the infant by means of the placental circulation until an airway can be established and pulmonary ventilation commenced (airway management on placental support). A multidisciplinary team should be convened in advance of the procedure. The team includes an obstetrician, a maternal-fetal physician, an otolaryngologist, a neonatologist, and an obstetric and pediatric anesthesiologist to identify each person's role, ensure that the necessary equipment will be present, e.g., a rigid bronchoscope and the sequence of events. A rehearsal with all participants is essential to anticipate any deficiencies. The events leading up to securing the airway are:

1. The position of the placenta is delineated to avoid damage at hysterotomy.
2. The parturient is anesthetized using general anesthesia to relax the uterus and prevent placental separation with large concentrations of inhalational anesthetics and/or nitroglycerin as tolerated. Maternal blood pressure is optimized by positioning and vasopressors as required. Massive rapid maternal blood loss is possible and a rapid infusion device should be set up and ready for use.
3. Hysterotomy is performed and the head of the fetus accessed. The airway is established by tracheal intubation, bronchoscopy, surgical tracheostomy, or initiation of ECMO.
4. Once airway and ventilation are satisfactory, the umbilical cord is clamped and the infant transferred to the NICU or another OR for further treatment as appropriate; some will require an urgent tracheostomy.

Suggested Reading

Abramowicz S, Katsneilson A, Forbes PW, Padwa BL. Anterior versus posterior approach to iliac crest for alveolar cleft bone grafting. J Oral Maxillofac Surg. 2012;70:211–5.

Alhindi N, Nukaly H, Abdulrahman L, et al. Nerve block for pain management in pediatric patients undergoing cleft lip and palate repair: a systematic review and network meta-analysis. J Plast Reconstr Anesth Surgery. 2025;105:55–64.

Coté CJ, Petkau AJ. Thiopental requirements may be increased in children reanesthetized at least one year after recovery from extensive thermal injury. Anesth Analg. 1985;64(12):1156–60.

Ferschl MB, Jain RR. Fetal and neonatal anesthesia. Clin Perinatol. 2022;49:821–34.

Hosking J, Zoanetti D, Carlyle A, et al. Anesthesia for Treacher Collins syndrome: a review of airway management in 240 pediatric cases. Pediatr Anesth. 2012;22:752–8.

Kennedy D, Novak CB, Phillips JH, et al. Catastrophic and critical intraoperative events during pediatric craniofacial surgery. Plast Reconstr Surg Glob Open. 2023;11:e4784.

Mosquera MS, Yuter S, Flake AW. Perinatal management of the anticipated difficult airway. Sem Fetal Neo Medicine. 2023;28:101485.

Pendem S, Jayakumar NK, Gopalakrishnan S, Arakeri G. Systematic review and meta-analysis of surgical approaches for improving airway stability in infants with Robin sequence: evaluating complications and outcomes. Br J Oral Maxillofac Surg. 2024;62:511–22.

Tran L, Hoffmann P, Parry S, et al. Anesthetic considerations for pediatric patients with craniofacial anomalies: an overview of key elements. Clin Plastic Surg. 2025;52:113–7.

Unal D, Hazir MS. Airway management in pediatric patients with burn contractures of the face and neck. J Burn Care Res. 2022;43:1186–202.

Zhang N, Mao Z, Cui Y, et al. Risk factors of prolonged mechanical ventilation in infants with Pierre Robin sequence after mandibular distraction osteogenesis: a retrospective cohort study. Front Pediatr. 2021;9:587147.

General and Thoraco-Abdominal Surgery

14

General Principles

1. Many children who require thoraco-abdominal procedures are neonates and preterm infants requiring special considerations.
2. Understanding the pathophysiology of the lesion and normal neonatal physiology dictates the choice of optimal anesthesia management.
3. Immediate surgery is rarely required; usually, time is available for preoperative evaluation and resuscitation as indicated. The optimal timing for surgery is decided through consultation with the anesthesiologist, neonatologist, and surgeon. Point-of-care ultrasound is used increasingly to assess the presence of food and fluids in the stomach and determine how best to proceed to mitigate the risk of regurgitation.
4. For emergency abdominal surgery, the problem of the full stomach must be considered. Even if the child has not eaten for some time, gastric emptying may be delayed as a result of bowel obstruction, ileus, or opioid administration. Children with severe gastroesophageal reflux are at increased risk.
   (a) Remember the effects of drugs on the barrier pressure, i.e., lower esophageal pressure [LES] minus intragastric pressure. Barrier pressure is reduced by atropine, midazolam, ketamine, propofol, dexmedetomidine, inhala-

J. Lerman, C. J. Coté, *Steward's Manual of Pediatric Anesthesia*,
https://doi.org/10.1007/978-3-032-24545-8_14

tional anesthetics, and cricoid pressure. It is increased by metoclopramide, rocuronium, pancuronium, and vecuronium, but minimally affected by succinylcholine.

(b) Consider administering drugs to reduce the volume and acidity of gastric contents: cimetidine, ranitidine, metoclopramide, and sodium citrate.

Possible plans of action for a full stomach:

- Neonates and small infants: aspirate the stomach contents through a vented gastric tube in the supine, right, and left decubitus positions (this may remove up to 95% of fluid gastric contents), preoxygenate, and perform a rapid sequence induction (RSI) or awake sedated intubation (see Chap. 4).
- Older children: aspirate stomach contents (if appropriate) and perform an RSI with cricoid pressure (as indicated) as anesthesia is induced. High-dose rocuronium (1.2 mg/kg), a suitable alternative for succinylcholine, has a similar onset as succinylcholine but a much greater offset. Sugammadex can antagonize high-dose rocuronium to rapidly restore neuromuscular function.
- The child should be deeply anesthetized and paralyzed before tracheal intubation. Struggling during attempts at intubation in an incompletely anesthetized and relaxed child is a common precursor to regurgitation and aspiration.

Remember: During RSI, succinylcholine does not increase intragastric pressure in children <10 years of age; pretreatment with a low-dose non-depolarizing relaxant is unnecessary (see Chap. 3).

5. During some thoraco-abdominal surgery procedures, blood loss may be considerable; be prepared for a massive blood transfusion (see Chaps. 6 and 18).
6. For major abdominal surgery, it is essential to establish intravenous access in the upper limbs or neck since the inferior vena cava (IVC) may be clamped or compressed during surgery, or lacerated during dissection or from an injury rendering transfusion via lower limb veins ineffective.

7. N_2O is generally contraindicated in bowel surgery, viscus injury, or when an air embolism is possible.
8. The airways are small and prone to plugging from bronchial secretions, necessitating tracheobronchial toilet.
9. During thoracotomy, $\dot{V}/\dot{Q}$ ratios in the lungs are disturbed necessitating an increased inspired O_2 concentration to maintain an acceptable SaO_2.
10. In infants and small children, retracting the lungs may obstruct major airways impairing ventilation, or compress the heart and great vessels leading to a precipitous decrease in cardiac output and blood pressure. Continuous monitoring of breath sounds, observing the shape of the capnogram and SaO_2 are essential. In the event of decreasing saturation, bradycardia, hypotension, or impaired ventilation:
    (a) Ask the surgeon to immediately remove all retractors.
    (b) Ventilate the lungs with 100% O_2.
    (c) Deliver large and sustained tidal volumes with high peak inflation pressures (to 30 cm H_2O as tolerated) for 30 s to re-expand areas of atelectasis (alveolar recruitment).
11. Some children who require minor surgery, e.g., herniotomy, may be preterm and/or have other conditions, e.g., renal failure, malignancy, that require special considerations (see Chap. 8).
12. Many general surgery procedures are now performed laparoscopically, which offers important advantages and requires special considerations.

Special Considerations for Minimally Invasive/ Endoscopic Surgery in Infants and Children

Advances in optical systems and instruments have greatly expanded endoscopic techniques for infants and children. Advantages are smaller scars, less postoperative pain, earlier discharge, and presumably less psychological upset. Robotic surgery via endoscopic access is becoming more common for select surgical conditions.

Special Considerations

1. All endoscopic procedures may require urgent open operation should complications arise; always be prepared for an emergency laparotomy or thoracotomy.
2. Bleeding may be difficult to rapidly control without open surgical exposure; reliable large-bore intravenous access is recommended.
3. Access to the child may be limited by the equipment required for robotic surgery, which may impede access to the child and in some cases interfere with observation of monitors. Pad/protect the child's face from the articulating arms of the robot.
   (a) Laparoscopic procedures.
   - Physiologic changes secondary to a CO_2 pneumoperitoneum.
     - The diaphragm is splinted with a consequent decrease in chest wall compliance; this effect is increased in the Trendelenburg position. Elevation of the diaphragm is followed by decreasing lung volumes, increasing the potential for airway closure during tidal breathing, $\dot{V}/\dot{Q}$ mismatch, and resultant desaturation.
     - Increased intra-abdominal pressure (IAP) decreases venous return and cardiac output, and increases systemic vascular resistance. The magnitude of these effects depends on the IAP; they are increased in reverse Trendelenburg. These hemodynamic effects are magnified in the hypovolemic child.
     - Carbon dioxide is readily absorbed into the circulation increasing the $PaCO_2$ and thus ventilation requirements. Positioning, pneumoperitoneum, and the requirement for increased ventilation may increase the peak inspiratory pressure (PIP), which can be corrected by increasing the respiratory rate and reducing tidal volumes. Absorption of CO_2 during laparoscopic surgery in children is greater than in adults.

  - IAPs up to 5 mmHg cause little effect on hemodynamics and ventilation; 5–12 mmHg IAPs are generally well tolerated by healthy children in the horizontal position. Positions other than horizontal or IAPs exceeding 12 mmHg may compromise the cardiorespiratory systems necessitating interventions. Limiting the IAP and careful positioning may permit some children with cardiorespiratory disease to tolerate pneumoperitoneum but some may not be ideal candidates for this surgery, e.g., children with Fontan physiology and passive venous return to the lungs.
- Anesthesia management.
  - Careful preoperative assessment of cardiorespiratory status, state of hydration, and volume replacement is necessary. Respiratory or cardiac disease and/or volume depletion could cause adverse responses to induced pneumoperitoneum. Volume status should be optimized, e.g., infants with pyloric stenosis, and potential cardiorespiratory limitations considered preoperatively.
  - Controlled ventilation in pressure control, volume-guarantee mode is preferred. Oxygenation and $PetCO_2$ should be closely monitored although the latter may be unreliable and give falsely low readings in infants. Increases in FIO_2, PEEP (usually 5 cmH_2O), and minute ventilation (MV) may be required.
  - Nitrous oxide may be contraindicated (see item 7 under General Principles above).
  - For lower abdominal surgery, the bladder should be emptied either by the child preoperatively or by passing a urinary catheter after induction. A gastric tube may be indicated to empty the stomach and improve exposure. For pyloromyotomy, the gastric tube may be left in situ during surgery to later inject air and assess the integrity of the duodenal mucosa.

- In small infants, the cephalad movement of the diaphragm and lungs may cause the tip of the endotracheal tube to migrate into a bronchus; frequently assess bilateral ventilation. Pneumothorax occurs rarely but should be anticipated; PEEP may offset the atelectasis from high IAPs and reduce the potential effects of a pneumothorax.
- Intra-abdominal manipulations may induce a Bezold-Jarisch reflex especially with initial insufflation; brisk vagal reflexes may also require immediate cessation of surgical manipulations and treatment with atropine.
- Monitor for sudden decreases in $PetCO_2$ as carbon dioxide embolism may rarely cause unexplained cardiovascular collapse and the development of a water-wheel murmur. Treatment includes Trendelenburg position, left lateral decubitus (Durant maneuver) and aspiration from the right atrium if a central line is present.

(b) Visually assisted thoracic surgery (VATS).

- Physiologic considerations.
  - Infants have a high metabolic rate for oxygen and V_A/FRC ratio. Any compromise in ventilation rapidly leads to hypoxemia.
  - In older patients in the lateral decubitus position for intrathoracic procedures, ventilation of the uppermost lung exceeds that of the dependent lung, although perfusion favors the dependent lung increasing $\dot{V}/\dot{Q}$ mismatch. In infants, the distribution of blood to the dependent lung and $\dot{V}/\dot{Q}$ mismatch are less than in older children because of their small size and highly compliant ribs.
  - In order to visualize the intrathoracic structures, some degree of lung collapse must occur, resulting in further $\dot{V}/\dot{Q}$ mismatch. This may be obtained by selective one-lung ventilation (OLV) or as a result of gas insufflation into one hemithorax.

  - OLV tends to direct perfusion away from the unventilated lung because of hypoxic pulmonary vasoconstriction (attenuated in part by inhalational anesthetics) and mechanical effects within the collapsed lung, thus restoring in part, $\dot{V}/\dot{Q}$ relationships.
  - Absorption of insufflated CO_2 from the pleural cavity requires increased pulmonary ventilation.
  - PEEP preserves ventilation of the dependent lung.
  - In summary, oxygenation and ventilation during VATS are unpredictable thus requiring careful monitoring, and an increase in FIO_2, especially in small infants.
- Anesthesia management for VATS.
  - Carefully evaluate the cardiorespiratory system and volume status preoperatively.
  - Plan an approach for OLV if requested:
    - A *tracheal tube* (*no* Murphy eye) guided into the contralateral main bronchus is the usual option for small infants. An uncuffed tube 0.5 mm ID smaller or a cuffed tube 1 mm ID smaller than predicted for normal use is recommended. The tube can usually be inserted blindly into the (R) main bronchus, although right upper lobe atelectasis may result. A fiberoptic bronchoscope or stylet is usually necessary to enter the (L) main bronchus. When using this technique, it is not possible to suction or inflate the operated side without withdrawing the tube.
    - A *bronchial blocker* may be placed on the operated side. A Fogarty catheter has been used in small infants although there is no central channel for suction or to allow the lung to deflate completely; in addition, it has a high pressure cuff, which might cause damage to the bronchial mucosa. Low pressure cuffs are found on biliary catheters, which may also be used as a bronchial

blocker. Bronchial blockers in small infants may be difficult to accurately position and become displaced leading to airway obstruction. In children greater than 2 years of age, the Arndt 5 Fr pediatric bronchial blocker may be used, which has a high volume low pressure cuff. With the guide wire removed, this channel may also be used to suction or deflate the operated lung.
This blocker is inserted via a special adaptor into the tracheal tube and guided into position using a FOB. The use of the Arndt 5 Fr blocker passed through the trachea external to the tracheal tube has also been described. The blocker is passed into the trachea before intubation and positioned either by fluoroscopy or with the aid of the FOB.
- The *Univent tube* is a tracheal tube with a bronchial blocker within a separate lumen for children ~6–18 years. This coaxial arrangement requires a smaller diameter tracheal tube to maintain a nominal outer diameter. The 3.5 mm and 4.5 mm ID Univent tubes are suited for children between 6 and 8 years. FOB is required to position the blocker. The 4.5 mm ID tube has a separate channel to suction or administer CPAP. Since these tubes have a limited useful age range, they are infrequently used.
- *Double lumen tracheal tubes* (>26 Fr) may be placed in children 8 years of age (~25 kg) and older. Correct positioning should always be confirmed with the FOB.

– Anesthetic agents that interfere with normal hypoxic pulmonary vasoconstriction, e.g., inhaled anesthetics, should be used in limited concentrations to ensure that pulmonary blood flow is optimally distributed away from the collapsed lung. Low concentrations of sevoflurane or intravenous agents, e.g., propofol, fentanyl, are preferred.

- During OLV, the child must be closely monitored to detect displacement of the isolation device. If obstruction to ventilation occurs, the cuff of a blocker should be immediately deflated.
- After OLV, the lung on the operated side should be reinflated using a recruitment maneuver before closing the incision; a postoperative chest X-ray is recommended to exclude persistent atelectasis or residual pneumothorax.

Congenital Defects That May Necessitate Surgery During the Neonatal Period

Congenital Lobar Emphysema

Abnormal distention of a lobe (usually the upper or middle lobe) compresses the remaining normal lung tissue and displaces the mediastinum; respiratory distress and cyanosis result. When severe, this condition manifests as an extreme emergency during the early neonatal period. Obstruction of the bronchus supplying the distended lobe may be extrinsic, e.g., abnormal blood vessels, intraluminal, e.g., bronchial papilloma, or it may be caused by a defect of the bronchial wall, e.g., bronchomalacia. More than one lobe may be involved, and sometimes the disease may be bilateral. The chest radiograph demonstrates a hyperlucent area with sparse lung markings (differentiating it from pneumothorax) and a mediastinal shift. The lesion must be differentiated from congenital diaphragmatic hernia (CDH) or cystic adenomatoid malformation, which can have a similar radiologic appearance. Less severe forms may be unnoticed for months or even years; conservative management may be appropriate in some cases.

Associated Condition

1. Congenital heart disease (~40%)

Surgical Procedure

1. Lobectomy, if no intraluminal or extrinsic cause can be found and corrected; this may be performed using VATS in children other than those in extremis.

Special Anesthesia Problems

1. Severe respiratory failure may occur because normal lung tissue has been compressed.
2. There is the possibility of a "ball-valve" effect, which further increases the size of the affected lobe during positive-pressure ventilation.
3. N_2O may cause further distention of the lobe and is contraindicated.
4. Considerations for the use of VATS.

Anesthesia Management

1. Observe the usual special considerations for neonates.

Preoperative

1. These infants are usually cared for in the semi-upright position.
2. Check that blood is available.
3. Spontaneous ventilation after induction is recommended because the potential for "ball-valve" obstruction would greatly enlarge the obstructed lobe leading to catastrophic mediastinal shift.
4. Placing a gastric tube and suctioning gastric contents may prevent gastric distention which would further compromise ventilation.

5. Sudden cardiovascular collapse demands immediate thoracostomy to exteriorize the affected lobe, correct the mediatinal shift, and allow ventilation of normal lung tissue.

Perioperative

1. Bronchoscopy may be performed before thoracotomy or VATS to exclude intraluminal obstruction. If a bronchoscopy is planned, anesthesia is induced with either sevoflurane in O_2 or incremental doses of ketamine or propofol to prevent apnea. After the vocal cords are sprayed with 1% lidocaine, either a flexible fiberoptic bronchoscope is passed through a tracheal tube or a rigid bronchoscope is passed, while maintaining spontaneous ventilation. After the bronchoscopy, the trachea is intubated and anesthesia is maintained with either sevoflurane or propofol and spontaneous ventilation. If assisted ventilation is required, this should be applied very gently.
2. VATS is usually managed with a tracheal tube and gentle positive-pressure ventilation while the thorax is insufflated with CO_2. Rarely is there a need to isolate the lung. In such instances consider the following:
   (a) Selective endobronchial intubation by advancing the tracheal tube into the bronchus of the contralateral lung. FOB should be used to verify the location of the tip of the tube while the neonate is supine. Intubation of the right bronchus may occlude the right upper lobe bronchus causing desaturation. Advancing the tube into the left bronchus may be accomplished by rotating the tube 180° before advancing it. Correct tube position should be verified after repositioning in the decubitus position.
   (b) In older children, bronchial blockers may be inserted into the affected bronchus either endoscopically or radiographically. The blocker should be small, highly compliant, and its position verified. Blockers are inserted outside the tracheal tube lumen and positioned by passing a FOB through the tracheal tube and verifying its location after inflation. These blockers may dislodge easily during surgery and suddenly obstruct the tracheal tube. Be prepared to deflate them should this occur.

3. Continue spontaneous or gently assisted ventilation with 100% O_2 until the thorax is open or accessed. In children in extremis, the affected lobe balloons out of the chest on thoracostomy and ventilation must be controlled. If VATS is used, CO_2 may be insufflated into the affected hemithorax and permissive hypercapnia tolerated during this period.
4. A non-depolarizing neuromuscular blocking drug may facilitate controlled ventilation and minimize the need for high concentrations of inhaled anesthetic once the lobe has been isolated.
5. After the affected lobe has been excised, the remaining lung expands to fill the residual space, although a pneumothorax may remain.

Postoperative

1. Discontinue all anesthetic drugs, administer 100% O_2 and antagonize the paralysis.
2. Suction and remove the tracheal tube when the infant is awake.
3. Administer supplemental O_2 as required.
4. A chest drain, connected to underwater drainage and suction, will be required.

Anesthesia Management: Older Children

In approximately 10% of cases, a congenital emphysematous lobe is discovered at an older age. If surgery is planned, the child should be managed as outlined for infants. A double lumen endotracheal tube may be used to facilitate surgery or VATS.

Congenital Diaphragmatic Hernia

The incidence of CDH is 1 in 4000 live births. There are three common types: anterior through the foramen of Morgagni, posterolateral via the foramen of Bochdalek (80% of cases on the left), and at the esophageal hiatus. Herniation of abdominal contents into the thorax causes respiratory distress, mediastinal displacement ("dextrocardia"), and a scaphoid abdomen. Breath sounds are absent over the affected side; bowel sounds may be heard over the thorax. The radiographic appearance is usually diagnostic.

In many children with CDH, both lungs may be severely hypoplastic. Currently, CDH is thought to be a primary failure of lung and associated diaphragm development. These infants usually present with severe respiratory distress at or soon after birth; often the diagnosis has been made antenatally by fetal ultrasound.

Associated Conditions

1. Malrotation of the gut (~40%)
2. Congenital heart disease (~15%)
3. Renal abnormalities (less common)
4. Neurologic abnormalities
5. Cantrell's pentalogy, defined as CDH, omphalocele, sternal cleft, ectopia cordis, and intracardiac defect (VSD or diverticulum of left ventricle)

Surgical Procedure

1. Surgery involves reduction of the hernia and repair of the diaphragmatic defect; usually, a trans-abdominal laparoscopic approach is used.

Special Anesthesia Problems

1. *This is not a surgical emergency!* Reducing the herniated abdominal viscera to relieve lung compression does not improve either oxygenation or ventilation. The preferred approach is to treat the respiratory insufficiency using a combinaton of muscle paralysis, controlled gentle ventilation, and therapy to reduce pulmonary vasoconstriction: surfactant, hyperventilation, oxygenation, correction of metabolic acidosis, deep sedation with an opioid with paralysis, and nitric oxide. If these measures fail, ECMO may be instituted. Surgical correction is performed as an elective procedure, once the infant has stabilized and is improving, and can be weaned from respiratory support.

Anesthesia Management

Preoperative

The infant is usually nursed in a semi-upright, semilateral position, facing toward the involved side. A gastric tube is passed and maintained on low suction to prevent further distention of intrathoracic abdominal viscera. However, most infants require intubation; this is accomplished using incremental doses of midazolam and fentanyl or other sedatives followed by topicalizing the airway and tracheal intubation, while avoiding bag-mask ventilation to prevent further distending the stomach and compromising respiration.

1. Muscle paralysis after intubation facilitates controlled ventilation with low peak inflation pressures, minimizing the risk of barotrauma, pneumothorax, and increased pulmonary vascular resistance. Pneumothorax is a constant danger that must be anticipated and immediately treated.
2. Ventilate with low peak inflation pressures, allowing permissive hypercapnia to minimize additional lung damage.
3. High-frequency oscillating ventilation (HFOV) is another effective means to reduce lung injury and the risk of pneumothorax; surfactant therapy may be indicated for preterm infants.
4. Pulmonary vascular resistance may be reduced by sedating with a fentanyl infusion or other sedatives and minimizing handling of the child. Inhaled nitric oxide may further reduce pulmonary vascular resistance in some children.
5. If hypoxia, hypercapnia and acidosis persist despite the above measures, ECMO may be required until the pulmonary status improves.

Aggressive invasive monitoring and ECHO-derived pulmonary artery pressures ensure optimal treatment. The best predictors of the severity of pulmonary hypoplasia, and hence survival, are the oxygenation index (mean airway pressure x FIO_2/PaO_2, <0.08 which predicts >90% chance for survival) and the modified ventilation index (peak inflation pressure x respiratory rate x $PaCO_2/1000$, <40, which predicts ~90% chance for survival). Those children who are easy to ventilate and not severely hypercarbic have a better prognosis. Those who are chronically hypoxic, hypercarbic, and acidotic, with associated high mean airway pressures, are less likely to survive.

Perioperative

Infants who require ECMO and HFOV, and who are hemodynamically unstable undergo surgical repair of the hernia in the NICU; stable infants may undergo surgery in the OR.

1. Anesthesia is most commonly maintained with high-dose fentanyl; in some, low-dose inhalation agent may be added using an O_2/air blend to maintain SaO_2 in the OR; N_2O is contraindicated.
2. Peak airway pressures should *not* exceed 20 cm H_2O (greater pressures may cause further lung damage or contralateral pneumothorax).
3. Lung recruitment maneuvers after reduction of the hernia are generally avoided to prevent additional lung damage.
4. Frequent blood gases and acid-base status assessments allow appropriate corrective interventions.

For children having surgery while requiring ECMO:

1. A common approach is to administer additional doses of relaxant and opioids. However, infants on ECMO often develop tolerance to fentanyl and require very large doses to blunt cardiovascular responses to surgery. Instead, low concentrations of sevoflurane or isoflurane may be titrated to blunt the responses by adding it to the oxygenator gas supply.
2. Ensure ECMO cannulas do not become kinked during positioning for surgery.
3. Despite being anticoagulated, excessive bleeding is usually not a problem.

Postoperative

1. Some infants who have been salvaged by heroic intensive care measures may remain oxygen dependent for years.

Tracheoesophageal Fistula and Esophageal Atresia

Tracheoesophageal fistula (TEF) and interrelated esophageal atresia (EA) may occur in several combinations. The overall incidence is 1 in 3000 live births. Both maternal polyhydramnios and premature birth are common. EA may also be associated with duodenal atresia.

The most common form (approximately 90% of cases) is EA with a fistula between the trachea and the distal segment of the esophagus (Fig. 14.1, Type A). The fistula typically arises on the posterior tracheal wall. This condition might be detected when the neonate chokes/aspirates at the first feeding, but ideally it should be diagnosed antenatally by ultrasound or at birth by the inability to pass a soft catheter into the stomach. Plain radiography confirms the diagnosis, showing the catheter curled in the upper esophageal pouch and an air bubble in the stomach, indicating a fistula. Contrast medium should not be used because it may be aspirated and further damage the lungs.

EA without a fistula is the second most common form of the anomaly (Fig. 14.1, Type B); there may be a large gap between the upper and lower segments of the esophagus. In these defects, it is not possible to pass a catheter into the stomach, and there is no gastric air bubble. Pulmonary aspiration from the upper pouch is an immediate danger. Constant suctioning of the upper pouch until surgical repair should be instituted.

The third most common form is the H-type fistula without atresia (Fig. 14.1, Type C); diagnosis may be more difficult and is often delayed. In such cases, there is usually a history of repeated respiratory infections. The fistula may be difficult to locate even when contrast studies and endoscopy are used. Once the fistula is identified, surgical ligation is commonly performed via a neck dissection. Other, rarer anatomic variants of this disease have been reported including double H-fistulae and tracheal stenosis.

Associated Conditions

1. Prematurity (~30–40%).
2. Congenital heart disease (~22%).

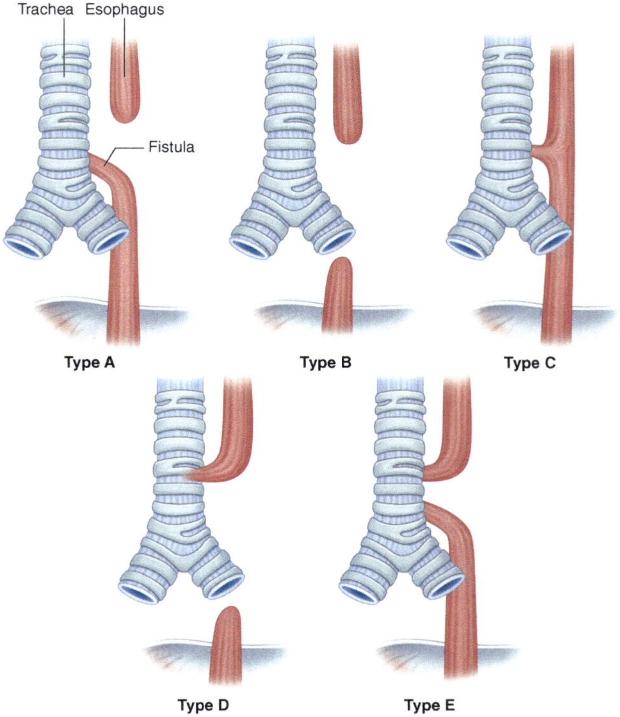

Fig. 14.1 Esophageal atresia fistula (see text for details)

3. Additional gastrointestinal abnormalities, e.g., pyloric stenosis.
4. Renal and genitourinary abnormalities.
5. The **VATER** and **VACTERL** associations: **VATER** association (***V***ertebral defects, ***A***nal atresia, ***T***racheoesophageal fistula, ***E***sophageal atresia, ***R***adial and ***R***enal dysplasia); **VACTERL** is VATER with ***C***ardiac and ***L***imb defects.
6. Tracheomalacia and other abnormalities of the trachea, e.g., subglottic stenosis.

Surgical Procedures

The infant's general condition and the anatomy of the defect govern the choice of surgical management:

1. Primary complete repair (ligation of fistula and esophageal anastomosis) is preferred.
2. Staged repair (gastrostomy followed by division of the fistula and later repair of the esophagus) is less optimal, but occasionally necessary.

The current trend is to perform an early primary repair with prior bronchoscopy to define the site of the fistula and exclude other tracheal defects.

Special Anesthesia Problems

1. Prematurity and other associated diseases, e.g., congenital heart disease.
2. Aspiration and pulmonary complications.
3. The possibility of intubating the fistula.
4. Positive-pressure ventilation may inflate the stomach via the fistula.
5. Surgical retraction during repair may obstruct ventilation.
6. Subglottic or tracheal stenosis may be present.
7. Children with repaired TEF may have an esophageal stricture and are prone to develop tracheal compression between the aorta and esophagus during feeding. The onset of symptoms of dyspnea and so-called "dying spells" during feeding, i.e., parents report an unresponsive infant 2–4 months of age who is pale and apneic. This condition arises when an abnormally soft trachea is compressed against the aorta by a dilated esophagus. Aortopexy usually relieves the symptoms, but some require an external stent to reinforce the trachea.

Anesthesia Management: Primary Repair

(a) Observe the usual special considerations for neonates.

Preoperative

1. The infant is nursed in a semi-upright position.
2. The proximal esophageal pouch is suctioned continuously to prevent aspiration of secretions.
3. Intensive respiratory care is initiated although their pulmonary status seldom improves until after the fistula is ligated. Thus, surgery should not be delayed in the hope that the infant's pulmonary status will improve.
4. Evaluate the infant for associated lesions, e.g., echocardiography to rule out a congenital heart defect.
5. Ensure that blood is available.
6. Continue maintenance IV fluids but recognize that neonatal fluid requirements during the first 24 h are small, and fluid and electrolyte depletion does not occur with esophageal obstruction.
7. In the preterm infant with respiratory distress syndrome and poor lung compliance, there is great danger of massive distention of the stomach (or massive leak from a gastrostomy if present) and consequent failure to ventilate. Rupture of the stomach and pneumoperitoneum may occur. It has been suggested that a gas leak through the fistula may be controlled by:

   (a) A balloon catheter passed via a gastrostomy retrograde into the lower esophagus.
   (b) A balloon catheter inserted into the fistula under bronchoscopic guidance.
   (c) Most commonly by early simple ligation of the fistula in infants with respiratory distress syndrome who might require high airway pressures. The operation is brief and can be followed by esophageal reconstruction after the child's respiratory function has improved.
8. Beware of the possibility of subglottic stenosis; have small tube sizes available.
9. TEF may be repaired using VATS in which case the considerations of one-lung surgery must be observed (see previous discussion).

Perioperative

1. Suction the upper pouch.
2. Apply the usual monitors and monitor ventilation using a precordial stethoscope taped in the left midaxillary line.
3. One of two approaches may be taken to secure the airway:
   (a) Induce anesthesia with sevoflurane (or halothane) in O_2, maintaining spontaneous ventilation. Perform laryngoscopy and topicalize the larynx with lidocaine (1%, maximum dose, 5 mg/kg). Continue inhalation anesthesia for several minutes before performing laryngoscopy and intubation.
   (b) Alternatively, and if a bronchoscopy is *not* planned, sedate with incremental doses of fentanyl and midazolam or other sedatives, and topicalize the larynx with lidocaine.
   Then:
   (a) Intubate the trachea with the bevel of the tube facing posteriorly (to avoid intubating the fistula).
   (b) Alternatively, if a rigid bronchoscopy is planned, once the surgeon passes the bronchoscope, attach the anesthesia circuit to the side arm of the bronchoscope and continue with spontaneous or gently assisted ventilation. When the bronchoscopy is completed, insert a tracheal tube with the bevel facing posteriorly, or
   (c) If a fiberoptic bronchoscopy is planned, insert the tracheal tube with the bevel posterior and attach a bronchoscopic adapter to accommodate the fiberoptic bronchoscope through the tracheal tube. Gently assist ventilation while the endoscopy proceeds.
4. Immediately after intubation, advance the tracheal tube into the right bronchus, rotate the tube so the bevel is anterior (to block the fistula on the posterior tracheal wall), and then slowly withdraw until breath sounds are heard over the left lung and bilaterally. *If ventilation proves to be unsatisfactory*, then readvance the tube into the right bronchus and repeat the above measures. This will place the tube with its tip just above the carina but beyond the fistula in most cases. If the fistula is at the level of the carina, it is imperative that the tube

is rotated so that the bevel faces anteriorly (to prevent inflating the fistula). More complicated methods to position the tube have been described but are unnecessary in our experience. Always check ventilation after taping the tube and positioning the child. It is preferable to use a tube without a "Murphy eye," to minimize the possibility of ventilating the fistula.

5. Once the tracheal tube has been properly positioned, perform tracheobronchial suction to remove any accumulated secretions.
6. Maintain anesthesia with air, O_2, and sevoflurane (or isoflurane) with spontaneous or gently assisted ventilation. If the inhalational anesthetic is not tolerated, small doses of fentanyl may be substituted.
7. If spontaneous ventilation is inadequate: assist respirations gently to minimize the risk of gastric inflation, while observing and auscultating over the stomach.
8. Continuously monitor ventilation during surgical manipulations since large airways may be kinked by retraction, especially as the fistula is ligated.
9. Once the fistula is ligated, give a muscle relaxant and control ventilation in the usual manner.
10. VATS has been used to repair TEFs since the view on the video-screen allows very precise repair of the esophagus. With this approach, it may not be necessary to advance the endotracheal tube into the bronchus and isolate one lung because with CO_2 insufflation the "up" lung is compressed, in effect, creating one-lung anesthesia by increasing intrathoracic pressure. The downside is that during this period, ventilation may become difficult requiring a high FIO_2. The upside is that by avoiding bronchial intubation, persistent right upper lobe atelectasis may be avoided.

Postoperative

1. The child with a clear chest who is awake and moving vigorously may be extubated in the OR. Some surgeons, however, prefer to keep the trachea intubated and a gastroesophageal

tube in place for several days to avoid reintubation and damage to the tracheal repair.
2. If there are pulmonary complications or any doubts about the adequacy of ventilation, continue controlled ventilation.
3. The pharynx is suctioned with a soft catheter that has a suitable maximum length of insertion clearly marked; it must not reach (and damage) the anastomotic site.
4. Prolonged intensive respiratory care may be required; swallowing is not normal postoperatively, and aspiration may occur.
5. Prognosis after the repair depends on the maturity of the infant, the presence of other congenital anomalies, and whether pulmonary complications develop. In the absence of these conditions, the prognosis is excellent.
6. Postoperative analgesia may be provided by a caudal epidural catheter inserted intraoperatively and threaded to the thoracic level; careful management of local anesthetic doses is required (see Chap. 7).

Anesthesia Management-Staged Repair

If staged repair is planned, a preliminary gastrostomy is performed under local or general anesthesia. Management of the second stage (to repair the atresia) should follow the sequence outlined for primary repair when the child's condition is optimal.

Late Complications

1. Diverticulum of the trachea at the site of the fistula is common. Be aware of this possibility and the danger of intubating the diverticulum during anesthesia in later life.
2. The tracheal cartilage is abnormal, and tracheomalacia may cause symptoms during infancy even after repair; episodes of stridor, dyspnea, and cyanosis ("dying spells") (see above) characteristically occur during feeding. Severe symptoms require surgical treatment by aortopexy or tracheoplasty with an external splint. These children often have a deep barking cough like children with croup.
3. Stricture may develop at the site of the esophageal anastomosis with episodes of esophageal obstruction, the classic "hot-

dog" in the esophagus; it may require repeated dilations and possibly resection with replacement using a colon graft. In some, a permanent gastric tube is required.

Congenital Laryngotracheoesophageal Cleft

This very rare anomaly is defined by the presence of a cleft in the posterior wall of the larynx that communicates with the esophagus. Four types are described, depending on the caudal extension of the cleft: Type 1 is confined to the larynx, type 2 extends to the trachea, type 3 extends to the carina, and type 4 extends into the bronchi.

Mild type 1 forms may be missed initially, and the child may later have a hoarse cry, cyanotic spells during feeding, and repeated episodes of aspiration pneumonia. Type 1 and type 2 clefts may be repaired endoscopically with the child breathing spontaneously and without a tracheal tube, thus ensuring excellent surgical access.

Cleft types 3 & 4 manifest early in life with severe respiratory distress, which may be relieved by passage of a gastric tube. Pulmonary damage from aspiration may be severe. Early tracheostomy and gastrostomy may be lifesaving.

Anesthesia Management for Type 1 and 2 Clefts

1. Exclude other significant congenital lesions.
2. All the usual considerations for neonatal anesthesia are observed.
3. An inhalational induction using sevoflurane or halothane is preferred.
4. After IV access has been established, administer an antisialogogue to limit secretions.
5. The larynx and trachea are topicalized with lidocaine (1%, 5 mg/kg maximum).
6. The suspension laryngoscope is positioned by the surgeon.
7. Anesthesia is maintained by insufflation of sevoflurane (or halothane) via a nasopharyngeal tube or alternatively by a propofol/remifentanil infusion.

8. An oxygen/air carrier gas (no nitrous oxide) with a low FIO_2 is preferred to reduce the fire risk.
9. Postoperatively biphasic positive airway pressure (BIPAP) may be applied to ensure unobstructed respirations; a feeding tube is left in the stomach.

   Note: This method of anesthesia (spontaneous ventilation, no tracheal tube, inhaled anesthetic, and meticulous topical anesthesia to the airway) is extremely useful for endoscopic surgery of the larynx and upper trachea. However, obsessive attention is required—the child must be maintained at a constant level of anesthesia and not allowed to awaken or move. The topical anesthesia must be thoroughly applied, and for long cases, it may need to be repeated. Halothane is a better anesthetic than sevoflurane for this purpose, as awakening is slower with the former if the concentration decreases. Otherwise, sevoflurane may be used—but maintain deep anesthesia (8% inspired sevoflurane). This is often difficult with sevoflurane alone; supplementation with propofol either intermittently or by infusion is advised. Alternatively, a TIVA technique with a propofol/remifentanil infusion may be utilized.

Anesthesia Management for Types 3 and 4 Clefts

These defects require open surgery; definitive repair may involve a combined cervical and thoracic approach. Secure control of the airway is vital and demands close cooperation between the anesthesiologist and surgeon. A cuffed tube may be inserted into the esophagus to prevent ventilation of the stomach. Cardiopulmonary bypass may be required for repair of lesions extending to the carina.

Congenital Hypertrophic Pyloric Stenosis

Congenital hypertrophic pyloric stenosis occurs in ~1 per 300 live births. First-born male infants are more commonly affected. Muscular hypertrophy of the pyloric sphincter causes gastric outlet obstruction, leading to persistent vomiting. Dehydration with hypochloremic, hypokalemic metabolic alkalosis develops after protracted vomiting. Currently the diagnosis is usually made promptly, resulting in less extreme electrolyte derangements and dehydration. Diagnosis is made based on the history, palpation of an olive-sized mass in the region of the pylorus, and confirmation by ultrasound.

Associated Conditions

1. Jaundice (~2%) is caused by glucuronyl transferase deficiency: no special therapy is required, and the jaundice clears after pyloromyotomy.

Surgical Procedure

1. Pyloromyotomy—open or by laparoscopy (see Special Considerations).

Special Anesthesia Problems

1. *Pyloromyotomy is never a surgical emergency* so dehydration and electrolyte imbalances should be fully corrected before surgery.
2. There is a risk of vomiting and aspiration.
3. If an endoscopic approach is intended, observe considerations for laparoscopic surgery (see above: "Minimally Invasive/ Endoscopic Surgery").

Anesthetic Management

1. Observe the usual anesthetic considerations for neonates.

Preoperative

1. A gastric tube is placed and continuous suction applied.
2. Rehydrate and correct the electrolyte imbalances. This may require 24–48 h.
3. Immediately before surgery, reassess the child to ensure that the fluid status (see Chap 6 for adequacy of hydration) and electrolyte concentrations are normal.

Perioperative

1. Replace the nasogastric tube with a vented orogastric suction catheter and suction the stomach in the supine, right and left lateral decubitus positions (even if the stomach has been on continuous gastric suction). This maneuver removes ~95% of gastric contents.
2. Perform an RSI (without cricoid pressure to facilitate tracheal intubation) with IV propofol (4–5 mg/kg) ± succinylcholine (2 mg/kg) or rocuronium 1.2 mg/kg. Maintain anesthesia with N_2O and a potent inhaled anesthetic.
3. The need for additional muscle relaxant is dictated by the duration of surgery, i.e., the speed of the surgeon. Low-dose rocuronium (≤0.3 mg/kg) or cisatracurium (0.1 mg/kg) may be used for brief procedures. No relaxant may be needed in some cases.
4. After the pylorus has been incised, the surgeon may request that a small amount of air be insufflated into the stomach to check the integrity of the mucosa.
5. Acetaminophen (30–40 mg/kg PR or 7.5 mg/kg iv perioperatively) may be administered. Do not give oral medications. The surgeons should infiltrate the wound with a long-acting local anesthetic to limit perioperative pain. Administering opioids during surgery, especially during laparoscopic pyloromyotomy, will delay emergence.
6. Extubate the airway when the infant is wide awake and in the lateral decubitus position.

Postoperative

1. If analgesia is insufficient, administer very small doses of IV morphine (0.02–0.03 mg/kg) after tracheal extubation.
2. Intravenous infusions are maintained until oral intake is adequate (usually 24 h). Hypoglycemia may occur if glucose-containing intravenous fluids are discontinued before oral intake is adequate.
3. Postoperative apnea may occur, possibly as a result of the effect of preoperative alkalosis on the pH of the cerebrospinal fluid; infants should be monitored for apnea for 24 h postoperatively.

Omphalocele and Gastroschisis

In omphalocele and gastroschisis, abdominal contents are herniated through the anterior abdominal wall. The incidence of these conditions ranges from 0.4 to 3 in 10,000 live births for gastroschisis and 1.5–3 in 10,000 for omphalocele.

The defect with gastroschisis is lateral to the umbilicus (usually on the right side), and the umbilical cord remains midline. Other congenital defects are rare, but the bowel is exposed to the damaging effects of amniotic fluid in utero. The incidence of associated extra-intestinal defects is greater with left-sided gastroschisis. In omphalocele, the umbilical cord is continuous with the apex of the sac, which is covered by peritoneum and amnion, and associated congenital defects are common (~75%). Preterm delivery is associated with a greater incidence of adverse outcomes.

The surgical objective is to close the abdominal defect without exposing the contained viscera to excessive intra-abdominal pressure (IAP).

Associated Conditions (Omphalocele)

1. Prematurity: ~30%.
2. Other gastrointestinal malformations, e.g., malrotation, diaphragmatic hernia: ~25%.
3. Genitourinary anomalies: ~25%.
4. Congenital heart disease: ~10%.
5. Beckwith-Wiedemann syndrome (omphalocele, macroglossia, hyperviscosity, and severe hypoglycemia). These infants are usually large and have visceromegaly of the liver, kidney, and pancreas.

Surgical Procedures

The size of the abdomen in relation to the lesion determines the surgical procedure.

1. Primary closure is preferred because there is less risk of infection and other gastrointestinal complications. However, primary closure usually increases IAP, which, if excessive, may lead to impaired ventilation, reduced cardiac output, hypotension, and splanchnic ischemia, with impaired hepatic, renal, and bowel function. It has been recommended that the intragastric or bladder pressure be used as a guide to the safety of primary closure: pressures greater than 20 mmHg are poorly tolerated (impaired renal perfusion and/or venous return).
2. Skin closure only may be indicated in some infants.
3. In others, the procedure is staged; this approach involves initial closure using a preformed silo and the defect progressively reduced over time without anesthesia.
4. Very large omphaloceles may simply be painted with silver sulfadiazine and allowed to epithelialize over a period of weeks or months with delayed surgical closure.

Special Anesthesia Problems

1. Heat and fluid loss from exposed viscera (greater with gastroschisis).
2. Severe fluid and electrolyte disturbance and hypovolemic shock from transudation of fluid into the bowel and from exposure of viscera to air (hypoproteinemia may occur and is more likely with gastroschisis).
3. Increased IAP after closure may lead to compromised ventilation, decreased cardiac output, renal failure, and impaired hepatic function (including delayed clearance of drugs, notably fentanyl).
4. Possible hypoglycemia in infants with Beckwith-Wiedemann syndrome.

Anesthesia Management

1. Observe the usual special considerations for neonates.

Preoperative

1. The child is usually nursed in a semi-upright position with exposed viscera wrapped in sterile plastic film and covered by towels; this is done to prevent infection and minimize heat and fluid losses.
2. A gastric tube is usually inserted to decompress the bowel.
3. Blood glucose is closely monitored. If the infant develops hypoglycemia (less than 40 mg/dl), a glucose infusion is initiated.

   N.B. Children with Beckwith-Wiedemann syndrome have increased insulin production; severe rebound hypoglycemia may occur if bolus doses of glucose are given.
4. Hypovolemia, electrolyte abnormalities, and oncotic status should be corrected preoperatively due to their very high fluid requirements (up to 140 mL/kg/24 h).
5. A type and cross should be sent for possible transfusion.

Perioperative

1. Warm the OR to 28 °C; a forced air warming device and heating lamp should be available. Aspirate the gastric tube.
2. Perform an RSI (with cricoid pressure). Note: children with Beckwith-Wiedemann syndrome may have a large trachea and require a larger or cuffed tracheal tube; their large tongue may interfere with normal laryngoscopy. In these children, a sedated awake intubation may be indicated. Have a videolaryngoscope immediately available.
3. Maintain anesthesia with sevoflurane (or halothane) in O_2 and air.
   (a) N_2O is contraindicated because it distends the bowel.
   (b) Opioids, e.g., fentanyl, may not be metabolized as rapidly as expected because increased IAP shunts blood past the liver.
4. Muscle relaxants (cisatracurium is preferred) may be required to facilitate ventilation and abdominal closure.
5. It is recommended that intragastric pressure be measured during abdominal closure to determine whether a primary closure will be tolerated (<20 mmHg, see above). Monitoring SaO_2 at post-ductal sites above and below the

abdomen, i.e., left hand and foot, may predict increased IAP; if the reading from the foot is less than the hand, or if the quality of the waveform is markedly less in the foot compared with the hand, then IAP may be excessive.

Postoperative

1. Assess the adequacy of spontaneous respirations; if in doubt leave the endotracheal tube in place and transfer to the NICU sedated and ventilated.

Biliary Atresia

Severe neonatal conjugated hyperbilirubinemia and subsequent jaundice are most commonly caused by neonatal hepatitis or biliary atresia. Atresia of the extrahepatic bile ducts may be a result of an intrauterine inflammatory process. Neonatal viral infections and tests for inborn errors of metabolism help to differentiate biliary atresia from biliary obstruction which is usually accompanied by elevated alkaline phosphatase and gamma-glutamyl transferase levels. Biliary obstruction leads to hepatocellular damage and ultimately to cirrhosis. The incidence of biliary atresia is 0.5–1 in 10,000 live births. The diagnosis of bile duct atresia is confirmed by percutaneous liver biopsy, scintography, and endoscopic retrograde cholangiography.

Associated Anomalies

1. Polysplenia syndrome with associated intestinal malrotation, preduodenal portal vein, situs inversus, absent IVC, cardiac defects, and anomalous hepatic artery supply.

Surgical Procedure

1. Hepatic portoenterostomy (Kasai procedure). The extrahepatic bile ducts are resected, and the porta hepatis is dissected to a depth of 2–3 mm; then a Roux-en-Y jejunal anastomosis is performed. The major preoperative determinant of survival seems to be the age at which the operation is performed; success is less likely in infants >12 weeks of age.

Anesthesia Problems

1. Hepatic function is impaired, especially in the older child, potentially altering drug metabolism.
2. Hypoprothrombinemia may lead to coagulopathy.
3. Blood loss may be extensive.
4. The procedure may be performed using robotic surgery via a laparoscope (See above for Special Considerations for Minimally Invasive Surgery).
5. Some infants with hypersplenism have associated thrombocytopenia.
6. Reoperation may be required if bile drainage is inadequate.

Anesthesia Management

Preoperative

1. Observe the usual anesthetic considerations for neonates.
2. Check the coagulation profile and verify that the child has received vitamin K_1.
3. Check that adequate blood, fresh frozen plasma, and platelets are available.

Perioperative

1. Induce anesthesia intravenously or by inhalation.
2. Administer a muscle relaxant and intubate; cisatracurium is preferred because of possible impaired hepatic function.
3. Maintain anesthesia with low concentrations of sevoflurane or isoflurane in an O_2/air mixture. Fentanyl or remifentanil may be used for analgesia.
4. Insert large-bore intravenous lines into the upper extremities or neck. Insert a gastric tube.
5. Sudden hypotension may occur because the IVC becomes obstructed when the liver is manipulated. Placing the infant in a slight head-down position may minimize decreases in BP during manipulation of the liver.
6. Infuse glucose-containing solutions at maintenance rates and monitor blood glucose concentrations.

7. Use a forced air warming device or radiant overhead heater (or both) in addition to warming the OR to maintain normothermia.
8. Consider a continuous caudal or epidural catheter for postoperative analgesia provided the child is not coagulopathic; reduced doses of long-acting local anesthetics are required in this age group.

Postoperative

1. Prolonged IV alimentation may be required.
2. Ascending cholangitis is common, and portal hypertension may develop.
3. Many children develop esophageal varices in later years with repeated bleeding episodes.
4. If the trachea is intubated postoperatively, titrate fentanyl or morphine to provide analgesia.

Intestinal Obstruction in the Neonate

Intestinal obstruction in the neonate may result from various lesions, e.g., duodenal atresia, duplication, midgut volvulus, malrotation, or accumulation of viscid meconium ("meconium ileus"). Laparoscopic rather than open procedures are common.

Associated Conditions

1. Prematurity.
2. Down syndrome with associated congenital heart disease (~40–50%).
3. Cystic fibrosis (invariably accompanies meconium ileus).
4. Subglottic stenosis with duodenal atresia.

Special Anesthesia Problems

1. Hypovolemia; acid-base and electrolyte imbalance.
2. Gross abdominal distention in some cases.
3. Risk of regurgitation and aspiration.

Anesthesia Management

1. Observe special considerations for neonates.

Preoperative

1. Ensure adequate fluid volume replacement.
2. Check acid-base and electrolyte status and correct imbalances.
3. Ensure that the gastrointestinal tract has been decompressed via a gastric tube.
4. Ensure the availability of blood and blood products.

Perioperative

1. Aspirate the stomach contents via a vented gastric tube in the supine, right and left lateral decubitus.
2. Intubate the trachea with the child sedated or after an RSI; subglottic stenosis may be present.
3. Maintain anesthesia with isoflurane or sevoflurane in an air/O_2 mixture. Avoid N_2O to prevent further bowel distention.
4. Use incremental doses of muscle relaxants (cisatracurium is preferred because it is metabolized by nonspecific plasma esterases).
5. Despite apparently adequate preoperative fluid resuscitation, some infants become hypotensive upon opening the abdomen, especially those with small bowel atresia or midgut volvulus. They may need surprisingly large volumes of intravenous fluid (albumen and even blood or plasma) to restore the BP.
6. Some children will benefit from placement of a caudal catheter for postoperative pain management; recall that reduced total doses of long-acting local anesthetics are required in this age group.

Postoperative

1. Extubate the trachea when the infant is fully awake and vigorous and turn the infant to the lateral position.
2. Prolonged intravenous or gastrostomy feeding may be required.
3. After meconium ileus, problems including prolonged bowel dysfunction, sepsis, and pneumonia must be anticipated.

Neonatal Necrotizing Enterocolitis

Neonatal necrotizing enterocolitis (NEC), a disease of low-birth-weight infants (usually less than 34 weeks gestation), is characterized by inflammation of the intestinal mucosa, which may be due to a variety of factors leading to localized areas of bowel ischemia that often results in perforation and peritonitis. Severe fluid and electrolyte disturbances, especially life-threatening hyperkalemia, endotoxic shock, renal failure, and coagulopathy, including thrombocytopenia, may ensue. As the disease progresses, multisystem organ failure occurs. The cause of NEC is uncertain, but the disease usually affects infants with a history of birth asphyxia, respiratory distress syndrome, and those fed formula rather than breast milk. Other associated factors include early enteral feeding, liberal intravenous fluid administration, restrictive target oxygen therapy (SpO_2 90–95%), infection, and umbilical artery catheterization. The administration of probiotics may reduce the incidence and severity of NEC.

The clinical picture is one of abdominal distention, bloody diarrhea, temperature instability, lethargy, and apnea. Abdominal radiography may reveal intramural bowel gas (pneumotosis intestinalis) or portal venous gas.

The medical management of NEC includes cessation of feeding, institution of continuous gastric suction, liberal administration of intravenous fluids and alimentation, IV antibiotics, correction of anemia, hyperkalemia, and/or coagulopathy. Steroids and inotropes may be needed to treat shock; bowel perforation is the usual indication for surgery.

Special Anesthesia Problems

1. Prematurity and respiratory distress.
2. Shock, hypovolemia, electrolyte disturbance, especially life-threatening hyperkalemia, and coagulopathy.
3. Sepsis, acidosis, and congestive cardiac failure.
4. Interstitial gas in the bowel wall.

Anesthesia Management

Preoperative

1. Restore blood and fluid volumes: blood, fresh frozen plasma, platelets, and crystalloid solutions are indicated; third-space losses are considerable. If volume replacement does not improve the BP, inotropic support is required.
2. Check coagulation: thrombocytopenia must be corrected with platelet infusions.
3. Check potassium values and correct hyperkalemia if time permits; otherwise be prepared for cardiac dysrhythmias and possible electromechanical dissociation.
4. Exchange transfusion may be required for severe sepsis. Correct the acid-base status.
5. Emergency medications including epinephrine for hypotension and cardiac arrest, calcium gluconate or calcium chloride for hypocalcemia during massive blood transfusions or hyperkalemia, and infusions of dopamine and epinephrine for intraoperative hemodynamic support should be prepared.

Perioperative

1. Observe all special considerations for the preterm infant. Reliable intravenous routes and an arterial line are essential.
2. Avoid inhalation agents and titrate fentanyl as tolerated; avoid N_2O to prevent expanding intramural bowel gas.
3. Administer rocuronium or cisatracurium.
4. Continue warmed fluid resuscitation with 5% albumen and balanced salt solutions as dictated by clinical status.
5. Anticipate that major fluid infusions including a massive transfusion may be required to maintain cardiovascular homeostasis when the abdomen is opened. Up to one blood volume or more of 5% albumen may be required to maintain intravascular volume due to massive third-space losses.

Postoperative

1. Return the infant to the NICU for continued management of possible multisystem dysfunction (cardiac, pulmonary, renal, etc.).

Other Major Thoraco-Abdominal Lesions and Procedures

Neuroblastoma and Ganglioneuroma

Neuroblastoma is the most common solid malignant tumor of infancy. More than 50% of such tumors appear in the retroperitoneal space, but they may occur anywhere along the sympathetic chain. Four stages of the disease are described: Stage 1, limited to the primary site; stage 2, extension from primary but not across the midline; stage 3, beyond the midline; and stage 4, beyond the midline with metastases. Metastases are present at diagnosis in more than 50% of cases.

The diagnosis is occasionally based on fetal ultrasound but in neonates and young infants, it is usually made by palpation of an abdominal mass. The older child frequently has evidence of chronic disease, including fever, weight loss, and anemia. The tumor may also cause symptoms because of its extension to involve other tissues, e.g., the extradural space with accompanying neurologic signs. The tumor may also wrap around or compress major vessels such as the vena cava or aorta. These tumors secrete catecholamines, which may cause hypertension, and vasoactive intestinal peptides, which may cause watery diarrhea, dehydration, and electrolyte disturbances; most have increased levels of catecholamines and metabolites in the urine (positive vanillylmandelic acid). Computed tomography (CT) and magnetic resonance imaging (MRI) permit localization of the tumor and identification of metastases.

Treatment of stage 1 or 2 disease is by surgical excision. Stage 3 or 4 disease is treated by initial chemotherapy or radiotherapy, or both, and may later be followed with surgical resection.

Special Anesthesia Problems

1. Massive blood loss may occur during surgery, especially in those who had preoperative radiotherapy. Major vessels, e.g.,

the IVC, may be invaded by tumor and may be a source of rapid blood loss or clot/tumor emboli.
2. Increased circulating catecholamine levels may cause hypertension, but cardiac arrhythmias are unusual. Those with severe hypertension will have a contracted blood volume and may benefit from preoperative preparation as outlined for pheochromocytoma.
3. Thoracic tumors may compress the lungs causing airway obstruction and compromised ventilation. Cervical tumors may displace the trachea and compress the airway.
4. Children with extension to the extradural space (dumb-bell tumor) may need a combined abdominal and neurosurgical approach with laminectomy.
5. Hyperthermia (*not* MH) has been reported during surgery for neuroblastoma.

Anesthesia Management

Preoperative

1. Assess for systemic disease manifestations (hemoglobin, electrolytes, indices of coagulation, and a baseline platelet count). Review the CT or MRI for evidence of major blood vessel or neurologic involvement.
2. Assess the severity of hypertension and its control.
3. Assure the availability of adequate supplies of blood for potential massive transfusion; a rapid infusion device is recommended.
4. Anticipate the need for resuscitation with vasopressors and IV calcium.
5. Review the case with the surgeon to anticipate problems and plan appropriately.

Perioperative

1. Observe all special considerations for infants.
2. Place monitors and induce anesthesia.
3. Maintain anesthesia with an inhalation agent, which can be titrated to control BP and avoid N_2O.

4. Rocuronium or vecuronium is preferred for relaxation; both provide cardiovascular stability and cause minimal histamine release.
5. Establish reliable large-bore intravenous routes (preferably rapid infusion catheters) in the upper limbs or neck.
6. Routine monitors should be supplemented with an arterial line and a urinary catheter. A double lumen central line provides a route for infusions and monitoring of central venous pressure (CVP).
7. Anticipate fluctuations in BP during surgical manipulation of the tumor, most often caused by venacaval compression. Hypotensive events can usually be resolved by asking the surgeon to readjust her/his retractors or cease tumor manipulations. Hypertensive events usually resolve by asking the surgeon to stop manipulating the tumor but occasionally may require small doses of phentolamine (0.2 mg/kg) or a brief infusion of sodium nitroprusside.
8. Be prepared to provide rapid infusions of warmed blood or IV fluids, especially as the tumor is removed.
9. If blood loss exceeds one blood volume, anticipate the need for FFP (usually 1/3 of each successive blood volume loss). If the child had a normal platelet count before surgery, anticipate the need for additional platelets after 2–3 blood volumes have been lost and replaced.
10. Hypocalcemia during the rapid infusion of FFP or platelets (>1 mL/kg/min) should be anticipated and treated with IV calcium.
11. Some children benefit from a continuous caudal or epidural catheter for postoperative pain management; the doses of long-acting local anesthetics are reduced in infants <6 months of age.

Postoperative

1. Most children can be extubated at the end of surgery; if the child is unstable, do not extubate.
2. Continue to monitor volume status and urine output to ensure adequate fluid replacement.

N.B. Ganglioneuromas are benign tumors arising from sympathetic ganglia. They do not invade other tissues but gradually enlarge and may produce symptoms because of their size and pressure on adjacent structures. They do not generally secrete significant amounts of catecholamines or other active peptides; however, in atypical forms this may occur. In such a case, despite normal preoperative catecholamine levels, intraoperative hypertension may occur when the tumor is manipulated. Surgical excision is usually simpler than for neuroblastomas and suitable for endoscopic removal, but others may be complicated by the tumor's location and size.

Lung Surgery

Lung surgery may be indicated for the following conditions:

1. Lung abscess
2. Bronchiectasis
3. Lung cysts
4. Bronchogenic cysts
5. Diagnostic biopsy (in children, usually to confirm or exclude infection by a virus or other pathogen)
6. Pulmonary arteriovenous malformation
7. Sequestrated pulmonary lobe
8. Pulmonary neoplasm
9. Chronic pulmonary infection

Special Anesthesia Problems

1. For open thoracic surgeries, major $\dot{V}/\dot{Q}$ inequalities should be anticipated; increase the FIO_2 and monitor SaO_2. Blood and secretions within the bronchial tree may require frequent tracheal suction.
2. Major hemorrhage may suddenly occur if a large vessel is accidentally cut or torn. Reliable large-bore infusion routes are

essential, and blood for transfusion must be immediately available; have a rapid transfusion device nearby.

3. Postoperative pain limits coughing and deep breathing, especially in older children, predisposing to atelectasis. Plan for optimal analgesia, e.g., thoracic epidural catheter.
4. Pulmonary function may be impaired, resulting in respiratory failure. In such children, even minor fluid overload can precipitate serious deterioration in postoperative lung function; avoid excessive fluid therapy.
5. Pus from purulent lesions, e.g., lung abscess, bronchiectasis, may become dispersed during surgery unless a lobe or lung can be isolated. Preoperative bronchoscopy to remove accumulated secretions is useful for some children.
6. Methods for VATS and OLV are described at the beginning of this chapter.

Anesthesia Management

Preoperative

1. Assess the child's pulmonary function (only limited data may be obtainable for children too young or unable to cooperate in the full range of tests). Check the blood gases and other available studies. Ensure that the child is in the best possible condition for the planned surgery.
2. Ensure that adequate blood products are available.

Perioperative

1. Apply monitors.
2. Induce anesthesia by inhalation of either sevoflurane or halothane; if an IV is in place then propofol (or thiopental) followed by rocuronium to facilitate bronchoscopy and tracheal intubation.
3. If lung isolation is required, use one of the techniques described above.
4. Establish large-bore venous access.
5. Place an arterial line (except for "minor" procedures in healthy children).

6. Maintain anesthesia with sevoflurane (or isoflurane) in oxygen/air with opioid, adding sufficient O_2 to maintain the saturation at 95–100%. Nitrous oxide may be used if a gas-filled cavity is not present.
7. Control ventilation aiming for a $PaCO_2$ of 35–40 mmHg.
8. After positioning, recheck bilateral lung ventilation.
9. Suction the tracheal tube as needed.
10. Periodically inflate the lungs; as the chest is being closed, give several large breaths with high peak pressures while observing re-expansion of the lung. The surgeon may also fill the chest with saline and ask for large breaths to check for possible air leaks.
11. Ensure that chest drains are appropriately functioning.
12. Ensure that the child is awake, responding appropriately, and has adequate spontaneous respirations before extubation. If in doubt, leave the tracheal tube in place and transport to the ICU.

Postoperative

1. Analgesia may be provided with a thoracic epidural (bupivacaine or ropivacaine with fentanyl is ideal) which may be left in situ for up to 72 h postoperatively. Alternatively, intercostal nerve blocks plus an opioid infusion, a continuous paravertebral block or patient-controlled analgesia may be used.

Anterior Mediastinal Masses

Anterior mediastinal masses (AMM, bordered by the retrosternum, pericardium, xiphoid, and angle of Louis) may press on middle mediastinal structures (trachea/bronchi or heart [pulmonary artery, right atrium]) resulting in impaired or life-threatening reduced cardiac output. Four tumors that are common in the anterior mediastinum in children are:

1. Lymphoma, Hodgkin disease, etc.
2. Teratoma
3. Thyroid
4. Thymoma (less common)

Tumors also arise in the middle and posterior mediastinum, e.g., neuroblastoma, ganglioneuroma, and dermoid cysts, although they do not usually present substantive anesthetic challenges.

Children with AMM may need general anesthesia for cervical node biopsy, placement of a venous port, radiologic investigations, or excision of the tumor. A biopsy in a child with significant airway compression is most safely managed using local anesthesia and mild sedation.

Special Anesthesia Problems

1. Acute airway obstruction may occur after induction, even in children with no history of dyspnea. Tracheal intubation may fail to relieve the obstruction and require advancing the tube into a bronchus to reestablish an airway and successful ventilation. This is especially likely in children with massively enlarged hilar nodes or those with tumor compression causing obstruction or tracheomalacia; anesthesia even for a minor procedure may be extremely dangerous.
2. An AMM mass may also compress the heart (right atrium and/or pulmonary artery), compromising ventricular filling, resulting in acute hypotension and sudden disappearance of the capnogram if supine.
3. Major blood loss should be anticipated.
4. Myasthenic children require special consideration.

Anesthesia Management

Preoperative

1. A focused airway examination is essential for assessing the potential for airway and cardiovascular problems. A night cough and several pillows for orthopnea are classic signs of airway compromise and the potential for disaster. Inquire about any postural dyspnea and which position provides the easiest breathing as this position may be most appropriate to use during induction. Additionally, look for signs of superior

vena cava obstruction or upper body edema. In severe airway compromise it is best to delay surgery until the size of the tumor can be reduced by steroids or radiation after a measured discussion with the surgeon and oncologist (See below).

2. Examine radiologic studies and pulmonary function tests:
   (a) The chest X-ray in anterior/posterior view provides information regarding a compressed, deviated, or scabbard trachea (suggesting tracheomalacia).
   (b) The CT scan will define the extent of airway compromise; if the area of the airway is decreased by more than 50%, extreme caution is recommended, i.e., consider preoperative steroids, radiation or local anesthesia only. Evidence of main stem bronchial compression is ominous. Cardiac and great vessel compression by the tumor should also be assessed.
   (c) An echocardiogram provides guidance regarding structural compression of the right atrium and/or pulmonary artery and determines the presence of a pericardial effusion or constrictive pericarditis.
   (d) Pulmonary function testing flow-volume loops in older children able to cooperate also help to determine the severity of airway obstruction; a reduction of the expiratory flow rate of 50% is very worrisome (see previous discussion).
3. Anticipate the possibility of rapid massive blood loss; ensure that adequate blood is immediately available and that a rapid infusion device is nearby.
4. Avoid premedication if there is any danger of airway obstruction.
5. A full range of endotracheal tubes, stylet, and laryngoscope blades should be prepared; an armored tube on a rigid stylet may be required. Ensure that a skilled surgeon with a rigid bronchoscope is present during induction.

Perioperative

N.B. Cervical lymph node biopsy in the child with a very large AMM that prevents the child from lying flat requires special consideration. Preoperative steroids or radiation for 12 h should be considered. However, some oncologists prefer to avoid preoperative steroids because steroids may cause necrosis of the tissue rendering diagnosis more difficult and, if the tumor is a lymphoma, tumor lysis syndrome may ensue. Even after a single dose of steroids life-threatening hyperkalemia with a fatal outcome is possible. In such cases lymph node biopsy may be most safely accomplished with the child in the sitting position using local anesthetic and very mild sedation. If that is not possible or if more extensive surgery is planned, general anesthesia may be induced using inhalational anesthesia with the child in the position previously assessed to provide the maximum airway dimensions, most often the left lateral decubitus position.

For general anesthesia:

1. Establish IV access before induction.
2. Confirm with the awake child that they can tolerate the position chosen for surgery. An inhalation induction while maintaining spontaneous respirations is preferred.
3. Breath sounds, the shape of the capnogram, and SaO_2 should be assessed after induction and reassessed after any changes in the child's position.
4. If the airway obstructs or the capnogram suddenly becomes flat before tracheal intubation:
   (a) Intubate the trachea and turn the child to the left lateral decubitus position. If vital signs are not restored, turn the child prone. In this position, gravity pulls the tumor off the mediastinal structures. An alternative to turning the child prone is to apply towel clips to the xiphoid and suprasternal notch and lift the sternum to pull the retrosternal mass off the mediastinal structures.
   (b) Advance the tube with a rigid stylet past the obstruction, even endobronchial if necessary.
   (c) If this fails, perform rigid bronchoscopy.
   (d) In extreme cases, an emergency thoracotomy may be required.
5. Maintain anesthesia with sevoflurane or isoflurane in 100% O_2; spontaneous ventilation is preferable.
6. Expect cardiac arrhythmias during surgical manipulations.
7. Intercostal nerve blocks with long-acting local anesthetics or a thoracic epidural may provide postoperative analgesia.

8. At the completion of surgery, confirm the adequacy of respirations before extubation. If inadequate, leave the trachea intubated and transfer the child to the PICU.

Postoperative

1. Inform the PACU team that airway obstruction or cardiac compromise might occur in certain positions and describe the maneuvers to restore cardiorespiratory homeostasis.
2. Review the postoperative chest radiograph for residual pneumothorax.

Myasthenia Gravis

Myasthenia in infants and children presents in three forms:

1. Neonates of myasthenic mothers develop *transient neonatal myasthenia* that presents with hypotonia and feeding difficulty within a few hours of birth. Improvement usually occurs within a few weeks, and anticholinesterases are needed until recovery.
2. *Juvenile myasthenia gravis* (autoimmune myasthenia) usually manifests in childhood or adolescence. The disease may be generalized or limited to the ocular muscles. Abnormal fatigability, limb weakness, and ptosis are the usual presenting clinical features. The diagnosis is confirmed by a decreased compound muscle action potential on repetitive nerve stimulation or by improved muscle power after an intravenous anticholinesterase drug (edrophonium).
3. *Congenital myasthenic syndromes* due to various defects of neuromuscular transmission may cause symptoms during infancy or childhood and are difficult to distinguish from autoimmune myasthenia without complex testing.

Associated Condition

1. Hyperthyroidism may be present.

Treatment

1. Anticholinesterase therapy produces symptomatic improvement, but secretions may become a problem.
2. Plasmapheresis or intravenous immunoglobulin may result in temporary improvement reducing the need for thymectomy.
3. Prednisone and azathioprine have been effective in some children.
4. Others may benefit from intravenous immunoglobulin, plasmapheresis, as well as immunosuppression with rituximab.
5. Thymectomy may increase the probability of remission, especially if performed early after symptoms appear.

Surgical Procedure

Thymectomy is performed in some children with severe generalized myasthenia gravis who fail to respond to other treatment, even if there is no thymoma; the best long-term outcomes occur in prepubescent children. Complete thymectomy can be accomplished via minimally invasive surgery. This is preferred for the myasthenic child because it significantly decreases postoperative problems with incisional pain.

Special Anesthesia Problems

1. Muscle weakness may lead to ventilatory failure.
2. Treatment with anticholinesterases increases respiratory tract secretions.
3. Potential sudden deterioration in muscle power may be caused by:
   (a) A myasthenic crisis or
   (b) A cholinergic crisis (sweating, salivation, bronchial secretions, miosis, and muscle paralysis with respiratory failure) induced by excessive anticholinesterase dosage.
4. Postoperative pain may limit ventilation; regional analgesia, e.g., a thoracic epidural or parasternal blocks, is ideal.
5. Extreme sensitivity to non-depolarizing relaxants may occur. Regional anesthesia, inhalational anesthesia, or TIVA alone have proved very successful.

Anesthesia Management

Preoperative

1. The child should be admitted to the hospital for a period of rest, and anticholinesterase drugs carefully reduced or withdrawn in consultation with the child's neurologist.
2. Ensure that blood is available.
3. Avoid heavy premedication, especially with opioids.
4. Preoperative plasmapheresis may be useful in children with severe symptoms.

Perioperative

1. Induce anesthesia with either inhalational or intravenous agents.
2. Avoid muscle relaxants; intubate the trachea after the airway has been topicalized and the child adequately anesthetized. These patients are very sensitive to the effects of non-depolarizing muscle relaxants but resistant to the relaxant effects of succinylcholine. Chronic anticholinesterase therapy may inhibit the metabolism of succinylcholine potentially prolonging its effect or causing a phase II block. For VATS surgery, a double lumen tube or bronchial blocker is required (see previous discussion).
3. Regional anesthesia is preferred to treat postoperative pain. If a thoracotomy is planned, a thoracic epidural will also reduce intraoperative inhalation agent requirements.
4. At the completion of surgery, allow the child to recover and resume spontaneous respirations with the tracheal tube in place. Check the vital capacity; if this is adequate (more than 20 mL/kg), proceed cautiously with extubation.

Postoperative

1. Close observation and respiratory care in the PICU are essential.
2. Reduce or discontinue anticholinesterase therapy (to lessen the likelihood of a cholinergic crisis).
3. Regional analgesia, e.g., continuous epidural or parasternal blocks, is preferable; minimize opioid use.

Splenectomy

See Idiopathic Thrombocytopenic Purpura (Appendix A).

Pheochromocytoma

Pheochromocytomas are rare in children (~5% of all tumors) and are usually located in the adrenal medulla; ~20% of cases occur bilaterally. Most are benign; only 5–10% are malignant. About 50% are inherited as autosomal dominant, e.g., neurofibromatosis 1 and multiple endocrine neoplasia; the remainder are spontaneous.

Patients commonly present with headache, nausea, vomiting, and abdominal pain, with sustained or, less commonly, episodic hypertension. The diagnosis is confirmed by measuring free plasma metanephrine and normetanephrine concentrations rather than urinary vanillylmandelic acid. The secretion from the tumor is predominantly norepinephrine resulting in sustained hypertension with vasoconstriction, contraction of the intravascular volume, and an increased hematocrit. Paraganglioneuromas may mimic pheochromocytoma since they also secrete vasoactive peptides. A laparoscopic rather than open approach is preferred, leaving some viable adrenal cortex, especially if the tumors are bilateral, to preserve adrenal function; ~20% will have a recurrence of the tumor.

Associated Conditions

1. Neurofibromatosis 1
2. Thyroid tumor
3. Multiple endocrine adenomatoses, e.g., Sipple syndrome

Special Anesthesia Problems

Note: Anesthesia is very dangerous in the unprepared child as extreme swings in BP may occur.

1. Management of the BP and volume status of the child can be difficult.
2. Anticipate significant blood loss from extensive dissection to locate and remove multiple tumors.
3. Avoid anesthetic medications that might increase the release of catecholamines, e.g., pancuronium or droperidol, or sensitize the heart to these substances, e.g., halothane. Drugs that release histamine, e.g., morphine and atracurium, are best avoided.
4. A heavy premedication and a smooth induction are essential to prevent release of catecholamines.

Anesthesia Management

Preoperative

1. These children are usually treated with α-blocking drugs, e.g., phenoxybenzamine HCl, for several days until:
   (a) BP is consistently normal, and postural hypotension is minimal.
   (b) The hematocrit has decreased indicating re-expansion of the intravascular volume. β-blockers, if they are needed, are only initiated after the child is α-blocked to prevent a hypertensive crisis. However, a brief infusion of a short-acting β blocker such as esmolol may be appropriate in some (500 μg/kg over 2 min then an infusion of 50–250 μg/kg/min) to treat tachycardia.
2. Ensure that adequate supplies of blood are available.
3. Check that drugs are available to treat anticipated swings in blood pressure or disturbances in cardiac rhythm including:
   (a) Phentolamine—to decrease BP (usually necessary).
   (b) Isoproterenol—to increase heart rate.
   (c) Norepinephrine or phenylephrine—to increase BP.
   (d) Magnesium sulphate (25–50 mg/kg over 20 min) to control hypertensive events.
   (e) Consider a remifentanil-based anesthetic to control heart rate and BP.

4. Administer an anxiolytic as needed.

Perioperative

1. If the child remains apprehensive after premedication, supplemental midazolam, remimazolam, clonidine, or dexmedetomidine may be administered.
2. An intravenous induction, titrating doses of either propofol or thiopental, is recommended.
3. Paralysis with relaxants that have minimal effects on heart rate is suggested, e.g., rocuronium or vecuronium.
4. Consider lidocaine (1.5 mg/kg) and fentanyl (2–5 μg/kg) before instrumenting the airway.
5. Maintain anesthesia with O_2, air, and either isoflurane or sevoflurane.
6. Establish arterial and CVP access. Epidural analgesia to provide perioperative analgesia and improve hemodynamic stability.
7. Anticipate the need for fluid boluses and/or initiate a phenylephrine or norepinephrine infusion as necessary to support the blood pressure as the block is established.
8. An initial bolus of fentanyl (5–10 μg/kg) before incision may be followed by an infusion of 2 μg/kg/h or remifentanil (0.05–0.15 μg/kg/min) piggybacked with a carrier infusion on a pump through a dedicated IV. The context-sensitive half-life of a fentanyl infusion increases dramatically after 1 h.
9. When manipulating and excising the tumor:
   (a) Multiple IV fluid boluses may be required to maintain arterial pressure.
   (b) A target CVP of 9–11 cm H_2O is optimal.
   (c) If hypertension persists or recurs after excision, suspect additional tumors.
10. After the tumor has been removed:
   (a) Discontinue the inhalation agent.
   (b) Continue anesthesia with O_2, fentanyl, or remifentanil infusions, and a muscle relaxant as indicated.

(c) Recall that the duration of phenoxybenzamine will last far into the recovery period and that blood pressure support may be needed.

Postoperative

1. Check blood glucose levels as hypoglycemia may result from the decrease in circulating catecholamines and secondary rebound hyperinsulinism.
2. Continue epidural analgesia or intravenous analgesics as required.

Wilms Tumor (Nephroblastoma)

Wilms tumors constitute 50% of the retroperitoneal masses in children but they usually present as abdominal masses. Stage 1 = one kidney only (~40%), Stage 2 = local spread outside of kidney but resectable (~23%), Stage 3 = spread outside of kidney but not resectable, e.g., to lymph nodes (~23%), Stage 4 = tumor spread to liver, brain, and bone (~10%), Stage 5 = tumors in both kidneys (~5%). Abdominal pain and fever are common presenting symptoms. Hypertension may develop from ischemia of renal tissue adjacent to the tumor, but the BP may remain increased after removal of the entire affected kidney. Laparoscopic techniques, a retroperitoneal approach (possibly less pain), and renal tissue sparing techniques are preferred.

Associated Conditions

Hemihypertrophy, absence of the iris (aniridia), Beckwith-Wiedemann syndrome, Sotos syndrome, Denys-Drash syndrome, Fanconi anemia, and others.

Special Anesthesia Problems

1. Massive blood loss may occur (arterial and CVP lines should be placed) (see Chap. 18).
2. Surgical manipulations may kink the IVC and cause an abrupt decrease in cardiac output resulting in severe hypotension.
3. A thoraco-abdominal approach may be required for large tumors.
4. The size of the tumor and previous whole-body radiation may impair pulmonary function.
5. Hypertension may be present (60% of cases) secondary to renin secretion. It may be severe in some children requiring perioperative treatment. Preoperative treatment with angiotensin-converting enzyme (ACE)-inhibiting drugs, e.g., captopril, and beta blockers has been suggested.
6. Rarely, the tumor may invade the IVC; in such cases, an intra-operative pulmonary tumor or thrombus embolism may develop and cause sudden catastrophic hypotension.
7. A coagulopathy, acquired von Willebrand disease, may develop in association with Wilms tumor. This may require desmopressin (DDAVP) or replacement of von Willebrand Factor (VWF) preoperatively but improves after resection of the tumor.
8. Anemia is common.
9. Large intra-abdominal tumors may delay gastric emptying, increasing the risk of regurgitation at induction of anesthesia.

Anesthesia Management

Preoperative

1. An adequate supply of blood products should be available.
2. Do not palpate the child's abdomen as this may release vaso-active compounds.
3. Consider giving antacids and metoclopramide to reduce the risk of acid aspiration.
4. Prepare for a possible massive and rapid blood loss.

5. Anticipate the need for vasopressors; have them ready for emergent use.
6. Prepare for severe hypocalcemia if blood products (FFP or platelets, > 1 mL/kg/min) are rapidly infused.
7. Anticipate the need to treat episodic hypertension.
8. Consider magnesium sulphate boluses (25–50 mg/kg over 20 min) to control hypertensive events.
9. Consider a remifentanil-based anesthetic to control heart rate and BP.
10. Consider an epidural for postoperative analgesia.

Perioperative

1. Apply monitors and induce anesthesia; an RSI is preferred.
2. Insert large-bore or rapid infusion catheters in the upper extremities and/or neck veins.
3. Maintain anesthesia with isoflurane or sevoflurane and a relaxant (rocuronium or vecuronium) or low-dose inhalation agent and remifentanil infusion through a separate dedicated IV piggy backed to a carrier infusion.
4. Insert an arterial line and a double lumen CVP to monitor volume status and provide a reliable route for vasopressors or vasodilators.
5. Be vigilant for abrupt decreases in BP (due to surgical compression of the IVC); communicate with the surgeon to desist surgical manipulations if this happens.
6. If hypertension occurs (unusual), ask the surgeon to cease manipulating the tumor and treat the hypertension with increased concentrations of inhalation agents and IV infusions of magnesium, esmolol, and/or increased infusions of remifentanil.

   N.B. Significant blood losses and hypotension may occur after the tumor has been excised and during wound closure: continue transfusions to match losses and administer vasopressors as needed.

Postoperative

1. Hypertension may continue and require treatment postoperatively.

2. Blood loss into the wound may continue, requiring ongoing transfusions.
3. Postoperative analgesia may be provided with an epidural catheter.

The Acute Abdomen

In children, an "acute abdomen" most commonly represents acute appendicitis, intussusception, or perforated Meckel diverticulum.

Appendicitis

Appendicitis is the most common cause of acute abdomen in childhood. The concerns for the anesthesiologist are possible fluid and electrolyte disturbance (secondary to emesis) and the presence of sepsis and high fever. Adequate fluid resuscitation should be ensured before proceeding to general anesthesia.

Intussusception

Intussusception is a common cause of obstruction in the first 5 years of life. A segment of small bowel passes into more distal bowel and may become ischemic and gangrenous. Enlarged Peyer patches, caused by viral infection, may precipitate this lesion by providing the lead point. The diagnosis is confirmed by contrast enema, which may also serve to reduce the intussusception. If this fails, a second attempt at hydrostatic reduction under general anesthesia may be successful; inhalation anesthetics may facilitate the process by relaxing abdominal muscles, decreasing smooth muscle activity, and reducing splanchnic blood flow. Pneumatic pressure with air or oxygen has also been used to reduce an intussusception but risks creating a gas embolism, so avoid N_2O. Laparotomy or a laparoscopic approach is usually indicated for peritonitis, failed reduction, and repeated episodes. It should be noted that significant hidden blood loss may occur within the intussusception; some children will require transfusion.

Meckel's Diverticulum

Meckel's diverticulum is partial persistence of the omphalomesenteric duct, which is present in ~2% of the population; it may provide a site for bleeding, perforation, or intestinal obstruction. Severe bleeding may occur from ectopic gastric mucosa within the diverticulum resulting in hypovolemic shock.

Special Anesthesia Problems

1. Assume that the child has a full stomach, even if the child has been NPO for several hours.
2. Fluid and electrolyte disturbances may occur secondary to vomiting.
3. The child may have a high temperature; this increases the metabolic rate for oxygen and compounds the risk should any interruption of ventilation occur. It also increases the maintenance fluid requirements by 10–12% per 1 °C increase in body temperature.

Anesthesia Management

Preoperative

1. Assess the child's general condition. Check the volume status, fluid intake, serum electrolytes, and urine output. Ensure that fluid resuscitation has been sufficient to correct deficits and urine output.
2. Ensure that blood has been cross-matched and sent to OR.
3. If the child's temperature is increased, avoid atropine or hyoscine.

Perioperative

1. Establish reliable intravenous access.
2. Apply standard monitors.
3. Preoxygenate as tolerated.
4. Perform an RSI and intubate the trachea.

5. Consider placement of an epidural catheter for postoperative pain relief.
6. Maintain anesthesia with N_2O, an inhalation agent, and a non-depolarizing muscle relaxant.
7. At the end of surgery, when the child is fully awake and muscle relaxants have been antagonized, extubate the trachea with the child in the lateral decubitus position.

Postoperative

1. Continue the epidural catheter for 48–72 h.
2. Advise the PACU team that hyperthermia may continue postoperatively and initiate appropriate treatment if indicated.

Testicular Torsion

Testicular torsion requires immediate surgery to save the testis. Therefore, in most cases, it is not possible to prepare the child; always assume that the patient has a full stomach.

Anesthesia Management

Preoperative

1. Prepare and check all equipment for an RSI (Chap. 4).

Perioperative and Postoperative

1. As for "Acute Abdomen" (see above).

Liver Transplantation

Major advances have increased the frequency of liver transplantation in infants and children; transplantation of a portion of a living-related donor organ or split liver from a cadaver donor has markedly improved organ availability. Common indications for pediatric liver transplantation include the following:

1. Biliary atresia
2. Metabolic disease, e.g., α_1-antitrypsin deficiency
3. Liver tumors
4. Ingestion of liver toxins
5. Cirrhosis

Special Anesthesia Problems

1. Anticipate massive blood losses.
2. Intraoperative circulatory instability may result from preexisting myocardial disease, plus mechanical factors (surgical manipulation), electrolyte disturbances (K^+, Ca^{++}), acidosis, hepatic encephalopathy, and release of vasoactive and cardiotoxic factors on reperfusion.
3. Coagulation defects may pre-exist secondary to impaired preoperative hepatic function and secondary hypersplenism and are compounded by massive blood losses.
4. Metabolic derangements include hypothermia, hypoglycemia (rare), hyperglycemia (more common), hypernatremia secondary to bicarbonate therapy, ionized hypocalcemia secondary to citrate, especially during the anhepatic phase when citrate cannot be metabolized, and hyperkalemia during reperfusion.
5. Pulmonary function may be severely impaired secondary to liver disease (hepatopulmonary syndrome). Portopulmonary hypertension (PPHTN) may be present in older children; it should be assessed by echocardiogram and if necessary by right heart catheterization. Mild PPHTN resolves after transplantation; severe PPHTN should be controlled preoperatively. Irreversible severe PPHTN is a contraindication to transplantation. Restrictive disease may be present secondary to ascites and pleural effusions.
6. Renal dysfunction may be present, as may hepatorenal syndrome, due to previous renal tubular damage.
7. Central nervous system dysfunction may be present as a result of hepatic coma with increased ICP.

Anesthesia Management

Preoperative

1. Preoperative angiography to assess the vascular connections of the liver may require general anesthesia. Urgent admission at the time a donor organ becomes available is the norm.
2. Transplant candidates should be evaluated by anesthesiology before the day of the transplant.
3. Children with PPHTN and those with possible cardiomyopathy will benefit from ECHO cardiogram assessment.
4. On the day of surgery, confirm that the child has not developed an acute disease that might affect the transplanted liver. Reassess the coagulation status (an increased INR is reliably predictive of massive blood loss), BUN, creatinine, electrolytes (especially potassium which could be elevated or low), glucose, albumen, ionized calcium, and magnesium, and correct as indicated and time permits. Obtain a chest X-ray to assess possible pleural effusions.
5. Preoperatively, a bowel preparation is performed, which may result in hypovolemia.
6. Immunosuppressive therapy with high-dose steroids and other medications is initiated.
7. Anticipate increased blood losses in children <2 years of age, those who have had previous abdominal surgery, those with increased prothrombin times, acute liver disease, bleeding varices, or encephalopathy. Ensure that adequate quantities of blood products are available and set up a rapid infusion device.
8. Avoid intramuscular injections in coagulopathic children; IV or oral premedication is preferred. If an IV is started preoperatively, use the feet to preserve IV access in the upper extremities for surgery.
9. Most children are at risk for pulmonary aspiration due to recent food intake, delayed gastric emptying, and abdominal distention; plan for an RSI.
10. Plan for frequent (~hourly) determinations of glucose, electrolytes, acid-base, hematocrit, and coagulation factors.

11. Prepare size appropriate infusions of dopamine and epinephrine.
12. Prepare infusions of fentanyl and muscle relaxant (cisatracurium).
13. Prepare resuscitation drugs (dilute epinephrine, calcium chloride, calcium gluconate, sodium bicarbonate).

Perioperative

First Stage

The first stage includes mobilization of the diseased liver before its removal.

1. Anesthesia may be induced with ketamine or etomidate and an RSI.
2. Maintain anesthesia using air/O_2/inhalation agent (usually sevoflurane) as tolerated, with a supplemental opioid infusion, e.g., fentanyl or remifentanil. Avoid N_2O to prevent bowel distention and exacerbate an intraoperative air embolization. Control ventilation with PEEP (usually 5 cm H_2O) and maintain normocarbia.
3. A cisatracurium infusion is recommended to maintain neuromuscular block since hepatic metabolism is not required; it is recommended that all infusions, especially vasoactive drugs, be infused with a carrier via a central vein.
4. Insert at least three large-bore intravenous lines into the upper limbs and neck; rapid infusion catheters are especially helpful. Place a large double/triple lumen CVP line; prime rapid blood transfusion and blood warming devices. Insert an arterial line, preferably in the radial artery (the abdominal aorta may have to be clamped). Place a urinary catheter, esophageal, and rectal temperature probes. Remember that a multi-lumen CVP is not adequate for rapid blood administration because of the luminal resistance and that large-bore IVs, rapid infusion catheters, or introducer sheaths are essential. The use of transesophageal echo to assess RV function is recommended if PPHTN is present.
5. The child should be carefully positioned, padded, and a forced air warmer placed over the upper body.

6. Monitor blood gases, electrolytes, glucose, ionized calcium, Hct, platelet count, prothrombin time, and partial thromboplastin times frequently (usually hourly). Point-of-care devices for these assessments are preferred. Other studies of coagulation, e.g., thromboelastogram, may be helpful to guide replacement therapy.
7. During mobilization of the liver, major bleeding may occur (especially if a Kasai procedure had been performed), depending on the extent of intra-abdominal adhesions from previous surgery. The intravascular volume should be replaced as necessary to maintain the CVP, BP, urine flow, and the Hct. Generally, surgeons prefer that the CVP be kept in a lower range so as to minimize venous pressure.
8. Hypotension may occur as a result of manipulation of the liver on its pedicle and compromise of IVC flow. Hypotension may also occur as a result of a sudden decrease in ionized calcium during the rapid administration of citrate containing blood products (FFP, platelets)(>1 mL/kg/min). Mannitol (0.5 g/kg) may be administered to establish a brisk diuresis before clamping of hepatic and portal veins and the hepatic artery.

Second (Anhepatic) Stage

1. When the IVC is clamped, venous return from the lower body becomes dependent on collateral anastomotic channels unless a veno-venous bypass system is used. In this case, venous return is maintained but the hazards of hypothermia, thromboembolism, and air embolism are introduced. Veno-venous bypass may, however, reduce blood loss and improve intraoperative splanchnic and renal blood flow, with associated reduced morbidity. Veno-venous bypass is not usually used in infants weighing less than 10–15 kg because it is difficult to maintain flow in small cannulas, and small infants seem to tolerate IVC clamping.
2. Hypoglycemia is a potential problem during the anhepatic stage, but it is uncommon because the dextrose content of infused blood products maintains normal to high blood glucose levels.

3. It is during this stage that patients are at greatest risk for ionized hypocalcemia, hypomagnesemia, and acidosis in association with transfusion of FFP because there is no liver to metabolize the citrate preservative.

Third Stage

1. When the donor liver is reperfused, severe hypotension, arrhythmias, heart block, and cardiac arrest from hyperkalemia are possible. These complications arise from the combined acute changes in acid-base and electrolyte levels and the effects of vasoactive and cardiotoxic factors released from reperfused, previously ischemic tissues.
2. To minimize these changes:
   (a) Before reperfusion, the ionized calcium and bicarbonate (pH) levels should be increased with exogenous calcium and bicarbonate. Be prepared to treat hyperkalemia: calcium chloride/calcium gluconate, bicarbonate, a β-agonist, and possibly glucose/insulin.
   (b) Volume expansion with crystalloid or colloid solutions to maintain a CVP greater than 10 mmHg.
   (c) Rapid evaluation and correction of adverse electrolyte changes must be performed.
   (d) Previously prepared vasopressors should be in line for instant infusion as required.
3. During the third stage, large blood losses may continue. Platelet transfusions are usually withheld until this stage to minimize the risk of vascular thrombosis in the transplanted liver.
4. The need to treat coagulopathy is based on both coagulation studies and observation of the surgical field. If oozing occurs, replacement therapy must be instituted after discussion with the surgeon because after transplantation some children become hypercoagulable due to decreases in antithrombin III and protein C.
5. Hypertension is common late in the operation and is often unresponsive to additional opioids and antihypertensive medications. It has been attributed to multiple factors: volume overload, impaired renal function, cyclosporine, and

steroid therapy. Postoperative treatment with salt restriction, diuretics, and ACE inhibitors may be indicated.

6. There may be difficulty in closing the abdomen because of the size of the implanted liver and distention of the bowel. Ventilation may be compromised, and in extreme cases the use of a Silastic pouch to close the abdomen temporarily (as in children with omphalocele) may be required.

Postoperative

1. Immediate extubation in the OR is preferred if the hemodynamics are stable and there are no other contraindications. A team discussion and decision as to the disposition of the child and airway management should occur. If surgery has been prolonged or the child is cold or unstable, he or she is returned to the ICU intubated for continued support. Pulmonary problems are common and require aggressive therapy.
2. In some cases, return to the OR is necessary to re-explore for continued bleeding, impaired liver perfusion due to vascular thromboses, biliary obstruction, or hematoma washout.
3. Renal function may be impaired, and hypertension may be a continuing problem. Acid-base and electrolyte disturbances must be anticipated and treated.
4. There is a high risk of infection, and careful aseptic precautions are essential.
5. Neurologic complications, manifesting as seizures, are common.

Common Minor Surgical Procedures

N.B. Some children who require minor elective surgery have conditions that may complicate anesthesia and require special attention:

1. Anemia or an upper respiratory infection (see Chap. 8).
2. A history of prematurity and respiratory distress syndrome. These infants must not be considered absolutely normal even if they are now older and apparently healthy. See Chap. 6 for a discussion of these medical conditions.

Division of "Tongue-Tie"

If the frenulum is so short that the child has difficulty passing the tongue around the buccal sulcus, surgical division of the "tongue-tie" is probably advised.

Special Anesthesia Problems

1. This is a very brief, minor procedure, but the surgeon must have good access to the oral cavity and a clear airway ensured.
2. The surgeon may use one of the several techniques to free the tongue: clamp the frenulum and then cut with scissors or cauterize the frenulum; sutures may be needed.

Anesthesia Management

Preoperative

1. Premedication: sedative premedication (oral midazolam) if required.

Perioperative

1. Induce anesthesia by inhaled sevoflurane or halothane or IV propofol.
2. If the surgeon does not cauterize the frenulum, maintain deep anesthesia with 8% sevoflurane in N_2O and O_2 and hold the elbow of the circuit (face mask removed) over the mouth while the surgeon clamps the frenulum. Alternatively, cut a tracheal tube to a length of 5 cm and insert it into the mouth to insufflate gases. Both techniques require ingenious scavenging to minimize OR pollution. Caution is advised with electrocautery and the potential for an airway fire; use an air/O_2 blend with the lowest FIO_2. Otherwise, a tracheal tube may be inserted. IV anesthesia is probably an ideal technique (it avoids the need to scavenge); administer intermittent propofol.
3. Suction the pharynx to remove blood. Apply lidocaine gel to the sublingual wound.

4. The child should be fully awake before transfer to the PACU.

Postoperative

1. Further analgesics are not usually required.

Inguinal Herniorrhaphy

Inguinal hernia is the most common elective general surgical procedure in children. Because they readily become incarcerated during the first year of life, their repair should not be unduly delayed. Once incarceration has occurred, conservative treatment is usually instituted. Virtually all hernias can be reduced, and then, after 24–48 h, herniorrhaphy is performed.

The former preterm infant may benefit from spinal analgesia for herniorrhaphy, especially if there is a history of prematurity or residual pulmonary disease and as a means for reducing the potential for post-anesthesia apnea (see Chap. 2).

Anesthesia Management

Preoperative

1. Assess the child's general condition.
2. Former preterm infants < ~65 post-menstrual age are at risk for post-anesthesia apnea and should be admitted for postoperative apnea monitoring regardless of anesthesia technique (see Chap. 2).

Perioperative

The choice of anesthesia technique for hernia repair depends on the surgeon. There are pediatric surgeons who can perform a unilateral inguinal herniotomy in 10 min—there are also those who can stretch this procedure out to last well over an hour. For the faster surgeon, general inhalational anesthesia delivered by face mask or LMA, or spinal or caudal anesthesia (for infants) is ideal; for more prolonged procedures, it is probably wise to use general anesthesia and place an LMA or intubate the trachea.

1. For general anesthesia, induce with an inhalational or intravenous technique. Anesthesia may be maintained by mask with spontaneous ventilation and sevoflurane (or halothane) in N_2O/O_2.
2. For prolonged procedures, place an LMA or tracheal tube. Maintain anesthesia with N_2O and sevoflurane or halothane with assisted or controlled ventilation. A laparoscopic approach is also commonly used but this approach requires endotracheal intubation.
3. Ilioinguinal and iliohypogastric nerve blocks or a caudal block are usually placed. Surgeons can perform these nerve blocks while the nerves are exposed. Acetaminophen, 10–15 mg/kg PO/IV (7.5 mg/kg IV in infants) or 30–40 mg/kg PR, is given before surgical incision to augment postoperative analgesia. Opioids are generally avoided because they increase the incidence of PONV.

Postoperative

1. Analgesia for children who have intraoperative nerve blocks or a caudal block is usually managed with postoperative oral acetaminophen.

Orchidopexy

Anesthesia management for orchidopexy is the same as for inguinal herniorrhaphy. A caudal block for postoperative analgesia is best placed before the surgery commences; ilioinguinal nerve blocks do not provide adequate analgesia.

Circumcision

Indications for circumcision vary in different communities and from time to time. It remains a common outpatient procedure in pediatric surgery.

Special Anesthesia Problems

1. Management of postoperative pain.

Anesthesia Management

Preoperative

1. Assess the child's general health.

Perioperative

1. Induction and maintenance of anesthesia as for herniorrhaphy. Face mask or LMA anesthesia is usually adequate.
2. Analgesia may be provided by:
   (a) A dorsal penile nerve block using 0.25% bupivacaine *without epinephrine* or 0.2% ropivacaine; maximum dose 2 mg/kg.
   (b) Performing a ring block around the base of the penis.
   (c) Applying lidocaine jelly to the wound.

Postoperative

1. If regional anesthesia is unsatisfactory, commence opioids during surgery and repeat as needed in the PACU until the child is comfortable.

Organ Transplantation: Care of the Donor

Transplantation of solid organs is common, although transplantation (apart from kidneys) tends to be limited to specialist centers; organ procurement may be performed in any hospital. The anesthesiologist has a major role to play in the care of the donor to ensure that the donated organs remain in optimal condition. Donation from living-related donors is also increasing; thus, anesthesia care will be needed for two patients, often in adjacent operating rooms.

Determination of Brain Death

Guidelines for determination of brain death are based on the Uniform Determination of Death Act (UDDA) and based on the following: irreversible cessation of all brain function including the brainstem and two examinations by qualified physicians assessing the absence of brainstem reflexes and ability to breathe (apnea test) 24 h apart for newborns and 12 h apart for older children. Additional tests include absence of cerebral blood flow and lack of EEG activity. Before brain death is declared, all local criteria for "brain death" in an infant or child must be satisfied. A new advance to increase organ donations is donation after withdrawal of life support known as Donation after Circulatory Death (DCD). In such situations, death is based upon cessation of cardiac and pulmonary function; it is common for the donor to be brought to the OR, where care is withdrawn under controlled conditions and the organs are harvested. Uncontrolled DCD involves organ harvest after an unexpected cardiac arrest with no attempts at resuscitation. A further strategy to improve organ donations is to institute extracorporeal support even in newborns after circulatory determination of death. Each institution has specific guidelines based on national and local norms in the care of such donors.

Care of the Donor

When cerebral death occurs, a sequence of physiologic changes occurs that may compromise the survival of organs destined for transplantation that may require intensive measures to preserve them. The anesthesiologist involved in caring for the donor during organ retrieval should discuss management strategies with the surgical harvest teams as the goals of one, e.g., liver, may differ from those of another, e.g., heart. These strategies are particularly essential for donors after withdrawal of care and those that suffer out of hospital cardiac arrest.

After "brain death," the following events occur:

1. Hemodynamic instability: There is widespread vasodilation resulting in hypotension which may be compounded by hypovolemia secondary to the use of diuretics for previous attempts at cerebral resuscitation. Myocardial function may also be depressed. As the brain stem fails or in the presence of raised intracranial pressure, hypertension may occur. In the gravest situations, wide swings from hypotension to hypertension occur.
2. Central diabetes insipidus leads to polyuria, dehydration, hyperosmolarity, and hypernatremia.
3. Arrhythmias, atrial or ventricular, are frequent owing to intracranial pressure changes, electrolyte disturbances, and myocardial injury.
4. Hypothermia is present owing to loss of central thermoregulation.
5. Coagulopathy occurs secondary to disseminated intravascular coagulation as a result of released necrotic brain substrates.

To counter these changes, the following management regimen is suggested:

1. The circulating volume should be restored with a balanced salt solution (20–40 mL/kg); avoid overhydration.
   (a) Lactated Ringer's solution or normal saline is recommended; D_5W is indicated if the Na concentration is greater than 150 mEq/L; however, it is important to avoid hyponatremia and hyperglycemia.
   (b) Volume expansion to maintain the CVP greater than 8 cm H_2O and an adequate urine output may be assisted with 5% albumen boluses.
   (c) Packed red blood cells are administered to maintain the Hct at ~30%.
   (d) Warm fluids to prevent hypothermia.
2. If hypotension persists despite adequate volume expansion commence vasopressors:
   (a) Dopamine 5–15 μg/kg/min first.
   (b) Epinephrine up to 0.1 μg/kg/min if dopamine fails to correct the hypotension.

Vasopressor infusion rates should be reduced or discontinued before organ harvest to minimize ischemic injury. The use of dopamine in cardiac donors should be limited to that required to stabilize hemodynamics; excessive doses (>20 μg/kg/min) may deplete energy stores and damage the myocardium.

3. Renal function should be maintained by fluid loading:
   (a) If urine output decreases to <1 mL/kg/h, give furosemide 1 mg/kg.
   (b) For diabetes insipidus, give *either* 1-deamino-8-D-arginine vasopressin (DDAVP), 1–4 μg IV, *or* pitressin infusion, 0.5–2 mU/kg/h titrated to maintain the desired output.
   (c) Suitable electrolyte solutions should be administered to correct hypernatremia and hypokalemia.
4. Hepatic function should be preserved by maintaining oxygenation and perfusion.
5. Other measures:
   (a) Measure esophageal and rectal temperatures and maintain normothermia.
   (b) Correct acid-base and electrolyte abnormalities.
   (c) Optimize ventilation and oxygenation.
   (d) Use aseptic techniques; prophylactic antibiotics may be requested.

Suggested Reading

Ahuja J, Strange CD, Agrawal R, et al. Approach to imaging of mediastinal masses. Diagnostics. 2023;13:3171.

Bhat V, Moront M, Bhandari V. Gastroschisis: a state-of-the-art review. Children. 2020;7:302.

Canchi-Murali N, Stendall C, Arul GS. Perioperative management of tracheo-oesophageal fistula and oesophageal atresia. BJA Educ. 2025;25:226–33.

Cassaro F, Impellizzeri P, Maiorana M, et al. Bedside vs. conventional operating room surgery in critically ill newborns: systematic review and meta-analysis. J Pediatr Surg. 2025;60:162419.

Cross K, Carachi P, Wilmhurst S. General and Thoracoabdominal surgery Including Management of Conjoined Twins. In: Lerman J, editor. Neonatal anesthesia. 2nd ed. Springer Nature; 2023. Chap 9

Dhar M, Prakash S, Pandey V, Pai VK. Intraoperative tumor lysis syndrome in a child with Wilms' tumor. Anesthseia; essays and Researches. 2016;10:145–7.

Francisco S, Muise E, D'Anna R, et al. Pulmonary and radiographic findings in pediatric type 1 laryngeal cleft. Laryngoscope. 2025;135:3404–11.

Hunt RW, Perkins EJ, King S. Peri-operative management of neonates with oesophageal atresia and trachea-oesophageal fistula. Paediatr Respir Rev. 2016;19:3–9.

Kamata M, Hakim M, Walia H, et al. Changes in cerebral and renal oxygenation during laparoscopic pyloromyotomy. J Clin Monit Comput. 2020;34:699–703.

Khater N, Swinney S, Fitz-Gerald J, et al. Robotic pediatric urologic surgery-clinical anesthetic considerations: a comprehensive review. Anesth Pain Med. 2024;14:e146438.

Marret J-B, Dupont-Lucas C, Petit T, et al. Safety of laparoscopic fundoplication in children under 5 kg: a comparative study. Surg Endo. 2018;32:4191–9.

McDonnell C, Barlow R, Campisi P, Grant R, Malkin D. Fatal peri-operative acute tumour lysis syndrome precipitated by dexamethasone. Anaesthesia. 2008;63:652–5.

Nichols JH, Nasr VG. Sternal malformations and anesthetic management. Pediatr Anesth. 2017;27:1084–90.

Syal K, Chandel A, Kanwar MS. Ultrasound guided pediatric caudal dose: a two-center randomized controlled trial. BMC Anesthesiol. 2024;24:401.

Tan A, Nolan JA. Anesthesia for children with anterior mediastinal masses. Paediatr Anaesth. 2022;32:4–9.

Taverner F, Krishan P, Baird R, von Ungern-Sternberg BS. Perioperative management of infant inguinal hernia surgery; a review of the recent literature. Pediatr Anesth. 2023;33:793–9.

Tognon C, Pulvirenti R, Fati F, et al. Anesthesia in children with neuroblastoma, perioperative and operative man agement. Children (Basel). 2021;8:395.

Way C, Wayne C, Grandpierre V, et al. Thoracoscopy vs. thoracotomy for the repair of esophageal atresia and tracheoesophageal fistula: a systematic review and meta-analysis. Pediatr Surg Int. 2019;35:1167–84.

Whyte SD, Ansermino M. Anesthetic considerations in the management of Wilms' tumor. Pediatr Anesth. 2006;16:504–13.

Cardiovascular Surgery and Cardiologic Procedures

15

Heart surgery in children is performed almost exclusively for congenital heart disease (CHD). The incidence of CHD is approximately 6 per 1000 live births. The lesions listed in Table 15.1 account for more than 90% of all congenital heart defects.

N.B. The reported incidence has increased since diagnostic methods have improved and access to infant healthcare extended. There may be geographic and racial variations.

Table 15.1 Approximate incidence of congenital heart defects (CHD) in children

	Per 1000 live births	% of Total CHD cases
Ventricular septal defect	2.62	34
Atrial septal defect	1.64	13
Patent ductus arteriosus	0.87	10
Pulmonary stenosis	0.5	8
Tetralogy of Fallot	0.34	5
Coarctation of aorta	0.34	5
Transposition great arteries	0.31	5
Aortic stenosis	0.22	4

From: Van der Linde D, Konings EEM, Slager MA et al. Birth Prevalence of Congenital Heart Disease Worldwide. J Am Coll Cardiol 58: 2241–7, 2011

J. Lerman, C. J. Coté, *Steward's Manual of Pediatric Anesthesia*,
https://doi.org/10.1007/978-3-032-24545-8_15

The Child with Congenital Heart Disease

Diagnosis of Congenital Heart Disease

Many infants and children with CHD are diagnosed in utero, although some may remain undiagnosed throughout the neonatal period or even until later in life. In neonates, the diagnosis of CHD can be quite difficult:

1. Heart murmurs are common in the perinatal period and may not be indicative of a structural heart defect.
2. Serious cardiac lesions may be present in the absence of a loud murmur.
3. The transitional circulation of the neonate may obscure a diagnosis: high pulmonary vascular resistance (PVR) limiting left-to-right shunts, and a patent ductus arteriosus (PDA) providing blood flow to the lower body, e.g., in children with coarctation or interrupted aortic arch.

Signs that suggest CHD in the neonate include cyanosis, tachypnea, prominent precordial pulsations, bounding peripheral pulses, hepatomegaly, poor feeding, cyanotic spells, and a large heart on chest X-ray. An echocardiogram (ECHO) is essential to diagnose the defect and should be requested whenever CHD is suspected. Depending on the malformation, further workup may require additional imaging studies (cardiac catheterization, cardiac MRI, CT, or nuclear scan).

In older infants and children, a murmur may be discovered during a routine medical examination, or children may present with decreased exercise tolerance, recurrent respiratory infections, shortness of breath, chest pain, or syncope.

General Systemic Effects

- Poor weight gain and development delay.

  Usually, the child's height and weight are below average. Children with CHD, and especially those with cyanotic CHD, may also demonstrate some developmental delay. Children in cardiac failure, with increased work of breathing and cardiac volume or pressure load, are unable to meet the additional metabolic demands for age-appropriate growth and development. Any further metabolic stress (infection, fever, or hypothermia) can lead to further decompensation.

Effects on the Respiratory System

- **Increased pulmonary blood flow**:
  Increased pulmonary blood flow results in small airway obstruction, decreased compliance, increased resistance, and ventilation-perfusion ($\dot{V}/\dot{Q}$) imbalance. Accumulation of interstitial lung water and pulmonary edema lead to increased work of breathing. Chronic exposure to excessive pulmonary blood flow causes structural changes in the pulmonary vasculature (medial muscle hypertrophy and peripheral extension of the muscular layer into normally non-muscular arterioles) and may lead to irreversible pulmonary hypertension (PAH). Early repair or temporary banding of the pulmonary artery can protect against these changes.
- **Decreased pulmonary blood flow:**
  Children with decreased pulmonary blood flow compensate with increased minute ventilation to eliminate carbon dioxide. The gradient between end-tidal and arterial carbon dioxide levels may be increased. The uptake of inhaled anesthetics is delayed (due to shunting blood which slows induction of anaesthesia); however, the alveolar (and hence end-tidal) levels may increase rapidly. Cyanosis is associated with a reduced ventilatory response to hypoxemia.

Effects on the Heart

In addition to the special characteristics of the child's heart (see Chap. 2), CHD may cause other changes:

1. **Obstructive lesions** impose a pressure load on the affected ventricle. This ventricle then hypertrophies (becomes less compliant and less able to increase stroke volume) and becomes subject to subendocardial ischemia and consequent arrhythmias.
2. **Large shunts or valvular incompetence** are associated with a significant ventricular volume load; initially the ventricle compensates by increasing the stroke volume but later the ventricle dilates and fails. The dilated ventricle requires an increased wall tension to mount the pressure within the chamber (Laplace's law) rendering it vulnerable to myocardial depressants and preventing it from coping with additional loads.
3. **Myocardial ischemia** may result from reduced aortic diastolic pressures and rapid heart rates in some children, e.g., those with a PDA.

Effects on the Blood

- **Polycythemia and coagulopathy** in cyanotic children.

  Cyanosis is compensated by polycythemia and an increased blood volume. The increased hematocrit (Hct) may lead to poor microcirculation with thrombosis (subendocardial, cerebral) and abscess formation. Cyanotic CHD is also commonly accompanied by coagulopathy secondary to thrombocytopenia, impaired platelet function, and decreased clotting factors.

Effects on Hepatic and Renal Function

- **Impaired organ perfusion and reduced drug clearance**.

  Hepatic and renal functions are impaired in cyanotic CHD and especially in those with CHF; splanchnic blood flow is reduced and clearance of drugs via the liver or kidneys is delayed, e.g., morphine clearance may be greatly reduced in children with CHD.

Principles of Anesthetic Management

Pathophysiologic Implications

1. **Right-to-left shunts result in**:
   (a) Reduced PaO_2, which is only minimally improved by increasing the FIO_2.
   (b) Delayed uptake of inhaled anesthetics.
   (c) Extreme danger of systemic emboli from venous air embolism; all IV solutions and syringes must be bubble free.
   (d) A brief arm to brain circulation time, with no pulmonary transit creating the possibility of an extremely rapid onset and relative overdose of intravenous drugs.
   (e) Less efficient ventilation and gas exchange that requires a compensatory increase in ventilation to maintain normocapnia, whether the child is awake or anesthetized.
   (f) An increased arterial to $PetCO_2$ gradient because the $PetCO_2$ levels underestimate the arterial levels.
   (g) Hemoconcentration
      - Polycythemia. (Hct > 55% in cyanotic lesions) is associated with poor rheology, increased cardiac work, greater risk for thrombosis (especially with dehydration or venous stasis), and possible formation of cerebral abscesses. Acute hemodilution to Hct < 40% may cause myocardial ischemia leading to cardiovascular collapse; hence maintain the child's usual Hct.
      - Iron-deficiency anemia that responds to exogenous iron therapy.

   (h) Coagulopathy may be present.
2. **Left-to-right shunts result in**:
   (a) Pulmonary vascular overperfusion is initially associated with good ventilatory efficiency and gas exchange.
   (b) Later, PAH develops and progresses to irreversible increased PVR, which may limit surgical correction.
   (c) CHF.
   (d) Some infants with large left-to-right shunts are at extreme risk of pulmonary hypertensive crises during and after surgery, e.g., truncus arteriosus, arteriovenous (AV) canal. A

sudden increase in PVR can be triggered by hypoxia, hypercapnia, or a sudden catecholamine surge during stimulation and lead to RV failure, ischemia, and cardiac arrest. Management may require deep sedation/anesthesia, minimal handling postoperatively, controlled moderate hyperventilation ($PaCO_2$ 25–30 mmHg), and analgesia with opioid, a vasodilator such as sodium nitroprusside, and/or inhaled nitric oxide (NO). Prophylactic IV fentanyl or lidocaine and 100% oxygen should be considered before undertaking a stimulating procedure (such as suctioning the airway).

3. **Obstructive lesions may result in**:
   (a) Fixed cardiac output, and very limited ability to compensate for changes in metabolic demand or a decrease in SVR.
   (b) Myocardial hypertrophy, with possible inadequacy of myocardial perfusion, especially to the subendocardium. Reduced ventricular compliance results in dependence on a high cardiac filling pressures.
   (c) CHF.
   (d) Sudden serious arrhythmias.
4. **Complex “mixing” lesions**:
   (a) Venous and arterial blood are mixed at various levels before reaching the systemic circulation; often additional intra- or extracardiac flow obstructions are present.
   (b) Arterial oxygen saturation and adequate tissue perfusion depend to a large extent on a well-balanced ratio of pulmonary and systemic blood flow.
   (c) Pulmonary overcirculation will maintain oxygenation, but result in inadequate cardiac output and metabolic acidosis. Poor pulmonary perfusion will maintain systemic circulation, but lead to significant hypoxemia and cyanosis.
5. **Ductal-dependent defects**:
   (a) Some infants depend on a PDA and the shunting of blood for adequate pulmonary or systemic blood flow, e.g., pulmonary atresia, TGA with intact septum, interrupted aortic arch, hypoplastic left heart syndrome (HLHS). If a prosta-

glandin E_1 (PGE_1) infusion is required to keep the ductus open, it should be continued until the surgical procedure is completed.

6. **Congestive heart failure (CHF)**:
   (a) Depressed myocardial function with poor tolerance for increases in afterload or cardio-depressing effects of drugs prolongs the circulation time.
   (b) Pulmonary edema and poor lung compliance result in rapid desaturation with apnea.
   (c) Hepatic and renal dysfunction may result in electrolyte disturbances and altered drug metabolism/excretion.

General Principles

1. Minimize the demands on the cardiovascular system:
   (a) Give adequate premedication to reduce anxiety, agitation, and O_2 requirements.
   (b) A smooth induction of anesthesia, with minimal crying or struggling, is most desirable.
   (c) High-dose opioid anesthesia, combined with appropriate postoperative analgesia, may favorably influence the neuroendocrine and metabolic responses to surgery and improve survival as well as preventing hypertension and tachycardia by ensuring adequate analgesia.
   (d) PAH must be controlled (See above).
2. Maintain myocardial function and cardiac output by:
   (a) Avoiding agents that depress the myocardium excessively.
   (b) Optimizing cardiac filling pressures.
   (c) Ensure adequate myocardial perfusion and oxygen supply by allowing adequate filling times:
      - The duration of diastole and the diastolic pressure are important factors in maintaining myocardial perfusion, which is especially vulnerable if left-to-right shunting (causing low aortic root diastolic pressure) and ventricular hypertrophy are present. Avoid tachycardia, hypotension, anemia, and hypertension, which may impair subendocardial perfusion.

- Maintain an adequate hematocrit for sufficient oxygen delivery. Cyanotic children depend on a greater hematocrit (Hct > 40–45%); anemia may cause subendocardial ischemia.

3. Optimize ventilation to maintain normocapnia while avoiding hyperventilation, unless indicated to manage pulmonary HTN. Hypocapnia:
   (a) Reduces cardiac output.
   (b) Vasoconstricts and increases SVR.
   (c) Decreases PVR and increases left-to-right shunts.
   (d) Shifts the hemoglobin/oxygen (Hb/O_2) dissociation curve to the left and limits O_2 transfer.
   (e) Decreases myocardial blood flow.
   (f) Decreases the serum potassium level, possibly resulting in arrhythmias.
   (g) Decreases cerebral blood flow.
4. Prevent detrimental changes in cardiac shunts:
   (a) Administer anesthesia with medications that have minimal effects on SVR.
   (b) Be aware of the ventilatory effects on shunts; avoid high intrathoracic pressures, but maintain the lung volumes with optimal positive end-expiratory pressure (PEEP). PVR is minimally affected at optimal lung volumes, but increases at greater or lesser degrees of lung inflation.
   (c) Drugs that produce a controllable degree of myocardial depression, e.g., inhalational agents, may be indicated when hyperdynamic ventricular muscle causes obstruction to blood flow and increased shunting, e.g., TOF, idiopathic hypertrophic subaortic stenosis (IHSS).
   (d) Children who depend on systemic-to-pulmonary shunts will desaturate if the systemic arterial pressure decreases.
   (e) Anemia may increase left-to-right shunts; conversely left-to-right shunting may be reduced by increasing the Hct. Changes in blood viscosity have a greater effect on PVR than on SVR.
   (f) Be prepared to use drugs or other methods to manipulate PVR or SVR.

5. The time to maximum effect of non-depolarizing agents in children with CHD is greater than in those without CHD; a more prolonged period of mask ventilation may be needed before intubation. Provide adequate additional neuromuscular blockade to prevent ventilatory efforts especially when the heart is open (air emboli).
6. Maintain normothermia and prevent cold stress unless induced hypothermia is indicated. Temperature control may be especially poor in neonates with cyanotic CHD; body temperature decreases rapidly if they are exposed to a cool environment.
7. Heparin has a larger volume of distribution and a more rapid plasma clearance in infants than in adults. Therefore, larger doses/kg may be required initially; an activated clotting time (ACT) ≥480 s is required before initiation of cardiopulmonary bypass (CPB). It is then recommended that the ACT be reassessed at ~30 min intervals. Some advocate a greater ACT, i.e., 600 s, in hemodiluted hypothermic infants. Some centers determine blood heparin levels.
8. During CPB the myocardium may be protected by:
   (a) Cardioplegic solutions that are infused into the coronary circulation after aortic clamping. Most solutions contain increased concentrations of potassium with added dextrose and pH buffers. The addition of free radical scavenger agents and calcium ion channel blockers has been advocated by some. The ideal cardioplegic solution:
      - Produces immediate arrest and prevents energy depletion.
      - Provides substrate for anaerobic metabolism.
      - Buffers tissue metabolic acidosis.
      - Minimizes tissue edema by its osmolar effects.
      - Stabilizes cell membranes.
      - Minimizes reperfusion injury.
      - Blood cardioplegia is preferred by many institutions; cardioplegia is redosed every 15–20 min.

   (b) The heart temperature readily increases because of surgical manipulation and heat from operating room lights. Therefore, during prolonged surgery, cold cardioplegic solutions are usually repeatedly applied; a pericardial cooling bath may also be indicated.

(c) Some centers administer pre-CPB systemic corticosteroids to reduce myocardial ischemic injury during periods of cardiac arrest.

(d) An optimal reperfusate solution to flush out metabolites and prevent reperfusion injury may be used after a period of ischemic arrest; a repeat dose of warmed cardioplegic solution is often given just before reperfusion.

Preoperative Assessment and Preparation

1. Review the child's current and past medical history and previous anesthetic records to identify any difficulties.
2. Identify syndromes that may require special considerations.
3. The physical examination should focus on the cardiovascular and respiratory systems, as well as the child's airway and state of dentition. Signs of cardiac failure (tachypnea, sweating, and hepatomegaly in infants), and a stable respiratory status to exclude acute disease that might compromise the child perioperatively, should be sought. If the child had a recent lower respiratory tract infection, a discussion of the additional perioperative risks this introduces is warranted with the parents and surgeon.
4. Review the cardiology notes, most recent ECHO, cardiac catheterization, and angiographic data to fully understand the current cardiac pathophysiology; think about the course an RBC must take so as to clearly understand the clinical implications of shunts, obstructions, and past surgical procedures.
5. Review current medications and laboratory tests. Long-acting ACE inhibitors, digitalis, and diuretics are usually withheld on the day of surgery, whereas antiarrhythmic drugs and β-blockers are continued (to avoid rebound effects). Many cardiac drugs have significant anesthetic implications:
   (a) Diuretics can cause hypovolemia, electrolyte disturbances (hypokalemia, hypocalcemia, and hypomagnesemia), and potentiate perioperative arrhythmias especially in association with hypothermia or digitalis.

   (b) Digitalis is rarely used because the therapeutic index is low, and toxicity is a hazard, especially in young children. If digitalis is prescribed, check for therapeutic values.
   (c) ACE inhibitors (particularly if taken on the day of surgery) can cause refractory hypotension after induction of general anesthesia; long-acting ACE inhibitors are generally withheld.
   (d) β-adrenergic blocking agents may impair cardiac contractility, but are often indicated as antiarrhythmics or to prevent "hypercyanotic spells" in those with TOF; they should not be stopped abruptly.
   (e) Calcium channel-blocking agents are only occasionally used in children and adolescents mainly to treat PAH. The combination of β-adrenergic blocking agents with calcium channel blockers is best avoided.
   (f) Anticoagulants can increase the risk of bleeding but are often essential for thrombosis prophylaxis; occasionally bridging with heparin is indicated.
6. Plan postoperative pain management and discuss this with the parents. In those whose tracheas may be extubated early, spinal or epidural opioids may be useful; in others an opioid infusion ± PCA is indicated.

Premedication

1. Children with CHD require adequate preoperative sedation to reduce excitement, anxiety, and crying (and thus reduce O_2 consumption).
2. Oral premedication is preferred:
   (a) Midazolam 0.5–1 mg/kg PO (maximum 20 mg) is very effective (10–30 min for the peak effect).
   (b) Ketamine (5 mg/kg PO) or
   (c) A combination of midazolam (0.25–1 mg/kg) and ketamine (3–5 mg/kg) is also effective.
   (d) Lorazepam 1–2 mg PO is effective for adolescents
3. Children should be constantly observed, and SpO_2 monitored. Suction and airway equipment should be nearby. Topical local anesthetic cream will facilitate pain-free IV placement.

4. For cyanotic children with a high Hct, ensure that oral fluids are offered up to 2 h before the anesthesia to prevent dehydration; alternatively, preoperative maintenance IV fluids may be initiated.

Blood Supplies

An adequate supply of blood and blood products should be in the OR by the time surgery begins.

Special Blood Requirements

1. For cyanotic children with an Hb >16 g/dL, plasma should be available.
2. For infants, the blood should preferably be <3 days old and negative for cytomegalovirus; washed cells reduce the danger of hyperkalemia. Radiated RBCs or leucocyte poor blood is indicated for some children (immune deficient, Di George Syndrome or transplant children); these RBCs may have very high levels of potassium.
3. Ensure that appropriate quantities of packed cells, FFP, and platelets (1 unit/5 kg) and cryoprecipitate are available. Fresh whole blood is considered advantageous to reduce bleeding after CPB. Alternatively, "reconstituted blood," (packed cells and FFP) is used to prime the CPB circuit.
4. Where "relatively minor" cardiac surgery is planned for older children and those with an initially high Hct, hemodilution with a clear fluid prime in the pump oxygenator may avert the need for blood transfusion. At the end of CPB, modified ultrafiltration may be used to remove the fluid prime and restore the Hct. Alternatively, the contents of the pump circuit may be washed and hemoconcentrated via a cell-saver for use in the postoperative period.

Anesthesia Management

Routine Anesthesia Management

Preoperative

1. Complete a standard anesthesia and monitoring check.
2. Emergency drugs should be prepared:
   (a) Sodium bicarbonate
   (b) Atropine
   (c) Calcium chloride or calcium gluconate
   (d) Epinephrine
   (e) Phenylephrine

   Solutions of inotropic drugs in concentrations that permit their infusion at a therapeutic rate with limited fluids should be prepared with a carrier infusion of balanced salt solution (see Appendix C).
3. Establish IV access after applying a topical local anesthetic cream. IM Ketamine may be used for sedation in the absence of IV access, but an IM injection will briefly upset the child. Ketamine increases $CMRO_2$ and may cause systemic hypertension and is best avoided in those with aortic stenosis (e.g., Williams syndrome) or cardiomyopathy.
4. On arrival in the OR, apply standard ASA monitors. Do not prolong this process, especially if the child is apprehensive.

Perioperative

1. Administer high-flow O_2 by a face mask as tolerated.
2. Induction of anesthesia.

   Any induction technique may be used; if well conducted, the SaO_2 increases with all of them, even in cyanotic children. An intravenous induction using an opioid, a “sleep” dose of propofol (or etomidate), and a non-depolarizing relaxant is preferred in children with right-to-left shunts over inhalation inductions, as the latter induces anesthesia slowly in cyanotic children. This approach enables manual ventilation, rapid airway control, and stable hemodynamics. A common prescription is fentanyl (2–5 μg/kg) followed by propofol (3–5 mg/kg) and a non-depolarizing muscle relaxant. In small infants, a small dose of atropine (0.01 mg/kg) or an appropriate dose of pancuronium prevents bradycardia. Alternatively, rocuronium (0.5–1 mg/kg) or vecuronium (0.1 mg/kg) produce good or excellent intubating conditions within 3 min. For the unstable child, administer larger doses of fentanyl (5–10 μg/kg) slowly and IV midazolam (up to 0.2 mg/kg) or etomidate (0.2–0.3 mg/kg) for induction but be vigilant, large doses of fentanyl rapidly administered before paralysis can cause chest wall rigidity.

3. If a right-to-left shunt is present, all intravenous drugs should be administered in small doses and *slowly* as their onset will be much more rapid due to the shunt. Conversely, if the circulation time is slow, the onset may be slow.

   NB: Subglottic stenosis in children with CHD is common, be prepared with a smaller diameter tracheal tube.
4. Use a cuffed tracheal tube to ensure adequate ventilation. The tube should pass easily through the glottis and subglottic space; otherwise, use a smaller diameter tube. Confirm bilateral ventilation; the cuff may not need to be inflated in infants to prevent leaks at normal inflation pressures.
5. Ventilate with a suitable mixture of air/O_2; >50% O_2 is rarely required. If a large right-to-left shunt is present, an increase in the FIO_2 has very little effect on the PaO_2. Avoid N_2O, which can increase the size of air bubbles in the circulation.
6. If myocardial function is good, low concentrations of inhaled agents may be used. Otherwise, for all complex lesions, supplement with opioids as indicated.
7. Control ventilation to produce the desired carbon dioxide tension. Note that $PetCO_2$ is a satisfactory means to monitor $PaCO_2$ in acyanotic children but may underestimate the $PaCO_2$ in those with cyanotic CHD. Always compare the $PetCO_2$ with the $PaCO_2$; the $PetCO_2$ can then be used to follow trends.
8. Steroidal muscle relaxants have very little effect on cardiovascular parameters, have an intermediate duration of action,

and may be antagonized for early extubation with sugammadex.

9. Monitor temperature from multiple sites (nasopharyngeal, rectal, or bladder); an esophageal stethoscope should not be inserted if a transesophageal echocardiography (TEE) probe will be used.
10. Insert adequate-bore intravenous routes, an arterial line (in the non-dominant hand), a double lumen central venous line (see Chap. 5), and a urinary catheter. In older children who may be extubated early.
11. Give maintenance fluids as outlined in Chap. 6. All fluid administration should be regulated by infusion pumps. Depending on NPO time and cardiac function, the cyanotic child with an increased hematocrit might benefit from a small fluid bolus of a balanced salt solution to improve the rheology and microcirculation. For CPB cases, slow cooling is preferred so a fluid warmer is not needed pre-bypass.
12. For those whose trachea may be extubated early after surgery, consider using epidural or spinal opioids (see Chap. 7).

Open-Heart Surgery

1. Follow routine management (see above). Cerebral oximetry via near infrared spectroscopy (NIRS) and/or transcranial Doppler (TCD) can be used to monitor cerebral perfusion. For older children and adolescents, processed EEG monitoring can be helpful to minimize the risk of awareness, especially during the rewarming phase of CPB.
2. Intraoperative TEE is usually used to define the anatomy and assess the success of the repair (including flow characteristics in conduits and shunts) immediately after bypass. TEE also diagnoses residual shunts, air bubbles, valve function, ventricular filling, and myocardial contractility. Because the probe may trigger autonomic reflexes, compromise ventilation, displace the tracheal tube, and/or compress the major vessels in small infants, monitor ventilation, SaO_2, the $PetCO_2$ waveform, and systemic BP.

3. Maintain anesthesia with:
   (a) Use an air/O_2 mixture to achieve an acceptable SaO_2. For lesions with significant pulmonary overcirculation, it may be necessary to reduce the FIO_2 to 18–21% oxygen and increase the $PetCO_2$.
   (b) Isoflurane or sevoflurane may be used to supplement larger doses of fentanyl.
   (c) Children with a history of CHF who may benefit from afterload reduction will probably do well with low-dose or no inhalation agent, e.g., VSD with left-to-right shunt. Children with dynamic ventricular outflow obstruction may benefit from a degree of myocardial depression and usually do well with low-dose isoflurane or even better low-dose halothane, e.g., TOF with dynamic RV outflow obstruction, hypertrophic obstructive cardiomyopathy.
4. Give incremental doses of muscle relaxants as needed; administer an additional bolus before initiation of bypass to ensure complete immobility.
5. Give appropriate volumes of balanced salt solution to restore euvolemia and maintain urine output greater than 1 mL/kg/hr; fluid loading before CPB is not advantageous. Avoid dextrose-containing fluids; hyperglycemia may exacerbate a neurologic injury in case of cerebral hypoxia/ischemia. Monitor blood glucose concentrations in small infants.
6. Blood loss from sponges, suction, drapes, and blood specimens, i.e., blood withdrawn for analysis, should be measured and replaced. It is seldom necessary to transfuse blood before CPB unless major blood loss occurs during opening of the chest or dissection around the heart, e.g., during repeat operations. For repeat operations, warmed lactated Ringer's solution or blood should be ready for urgent infusion at the time of sternotomy.
   (a) Aim to maintain the Hct near the preoperative level and the intravascular volume at a level to maintain CVP.
   (b) If the Hct was markedly increased preoperatively, replace initial losses with albumin, but refrain from significant hemodilution before CPB. Excess hemodilution may compromise oxygen delivery in cyanotic CHD.

(c) During venous cannulation in small infants, a significant volume of blood may be sequestered into the cannulae. Ensure that this volume is replaced, usually by transfusion from the CPB circuit via the aortic cannula.

7. Children with cyanotic CHD or those scheduled for repeat procedures may benefit from an antifibrinolytic agents, e.g., tranexamic acid, to reduce bleeding.
8. Arrhythmias are common during dissection around the heart; most are innocuous. If hypotension or arrhythmia persists, notify the surgeon until the condition corrects itself; continued hypotension suggests hypovolemia, poor contractility, or ischemia. Depending on the most likely cause, it should be treated with fluids, inotropic support, or surgical maneuvers to improve coronary perfusion.
9. Although we do not recommend the use of N_2O, if used, discontinue it before cannulation to prevent expanding air embolism.
10. Obtain a baseline ACT. Before the heart is cannulated, give the initial dose of heparin (300–400 units/kg), and recheck the ACT after 2–3 min; the ACT should be at least 480 s before initiation of CPB. Small infants may require more heparin and demonstrate more variation in dose requirements than older children.
11. Once CPB is established, the pump flow will be adjusted to establish satisfactory perfusion. Indicators of adequate perfusion are cerebral oximetry (NIRS), urine output, and the absence of metabolic acidosis. In children with cyanotic CHD, early bypass perfusion pressures may be low because of the child's decreased vascular resistance (children with cyanotic CHD have larger vessels) and the use of a low-viscosity perfusate. Those with TOF may have extensive collateral flow into the lungs requiring high flows initially; the systemic pressure will then increase as cooling progresses. The use of vasoconstrictors is not usually necessary but should be considered if hypotension persists. When the perfusion pressure is low, it is vital that the superior vena cava (SVC) pressure should also be at or near zero. Under these circumstances, any increase in jugular venous pressure, often

caused by a malpositioned obstructing SVC cannula, may have a serious effect on cerebral blood flow. Monitor CVP and NIRS to detect compromised SVC venous return and alert the surgeon immediately.

12. During partial bypass, ventilate the lungs with 100% O_2. Never use N_2O because of the possible presence of an air embolism in the circulation.
13. During total bypass:
    (a) Keep the lungs inflated at a low pressure.
    (b) Add 0.5% isoflurane to the oxygenator or give additional doses of fentanyl to continue anesthesia, analgesia, and improve perfusion during bypass. They are usually discontinued during rewarming. Fentanyl may bind to the plastic components of the CPB circuit, so blood levels decrease precipitously on bypass. Note that the tissue solubilities of inhalational agents are increased at low body temperatures and they may cause residual cardiac depression effects after rewarming and during weaning from CPB or delayed emergence. Discontinue inhalational agents during rewarming and supplement with IV anesthetics.
14. Treat hypertension with phentolamine (0.2 mg/kg). During hypothermic CPB, children respond to the cold-induced stress with increased levels of vasoconstricting catecholamines. Phentolamine improves perfusion and delays the development of metabolic acidosis through its α-adrenergic blocking action.
15. During bypass (partial and total), repeat the ACT every 30 min and administer additional heparin to maintain the ACT above 480 s.
16. Assess acid-base, electrolyte, Hct (and glucose in small infants) frequently and just before CPB is discontinued.
17. Before discontinuing CPB:
    (a) Inflate the lungs, suction the trachea/bronchi, and check ventilation by observing the movement and full re-expansion of both lungs.
    (b) Commence pacing if the heart rate is slow or if sinus rhythm is absent; infants and children need an atrial con-

traction to maintain a good cardiac output at this stage. Atrial pacing can be used for slow heart rates with normal conduction. AV sequential pacing is required if conduction is abnormal. If AV block is present, it is usually possible to sense the atrial contraction and use it to pace the ventricle (AV sequential pacing).

(c) If cardiac function is impaired, inotropic agents should be commenced before weaning; combinations of dopamine, milrinone, dobutamine, and/or low-dose epinephrine are commonly used.

(d) If myocardial contractility is severely depressed, an infusion of epinephrine (0.01–0.1 μg/kg/min) may be indicated.

(e) Be aware of the impaired calcium regulation in neonates and infants, especially when administering FFP or platelets. Hypotension during transfusions should be immediately treated with exogenous calcium. A calcium infusion may be required for small infants.

18. For children with PAH, consider the following before weaning:
    (a) A pulmonary artery line to monitor pressure and assess treatment.
    (b) Mild hyperventilation with 100% oxygen.
    (c) Maintain adequate levels of anesthesia and analgesia.
    (d) Correct preexisting metabolic acidosis.
    (e) In children with a mild increase of pulmonary artery pressure, a bolus of milrinone (50 μg/kg) followed by an infusion of 0.5 μg/kg/min may be useful before weaning from CPB.
    (f) If the PVR is high, consider adding nitric oxide (NO) to the inspired gases.
19. As CPB is discontinued:
    (a) Administer calcium chloride or calcium gluconate to improve cardiac function if necessary (calcium should not be given until the heart has resumed a steady regular rhythm).
    (b) Blood from the pump may be infused until the heart appears adequately filled. Monitor CVP and/or left atrial

pressure. Depending on the heart defect and the repair, the initial post-bypass ventricular compliance can be quite poor or rapidly changing; the pre-bypass levels may no longer apply. The Hct during bypass is usually reduced; age, type of repair, cardiac function and the presence of bleeding will determine the need for additional transfusion of packed cells. After complex repairs in neonates and small infants, a Hct of 35–40% should be the goal. Older children, especially those having more minor procedures, may be weaned at a lower Hct, given a diuretic, and have the pump contents re-infused over the ensuing period; this approach may prevent the need for exogenous blood.

20. If the child remains hypotensive despite a good rate and rhythm:
    (a) Adjust the dopamine infusion (5–10 μg/kg/min). Larger dopamine doses are often required in infants compared with older children and adults.
    (b) Dobutamine (5–10 μg/kg/min) may be added since it increases inotropy and heart rate, and decreases SVR.
    (c) A calcium infusion may improve cardiac function in some children, especially small infants and those with DiGeorge syndrome.
    (d) If these measures fail, an epinephrine infusion (0.1–0.5 μg/kg/min) may be indicated.
21. Modified ultrafiltration (MUF) may be employed after CPB to remove excess intravascular fluid and increase the Hct. The bypass circuit is used to withdraw blood from the aortic cannula, pass it through an ultrafiltration unit, and return it to the right atrium. In addition, it may clear some inflammatory mediators released during CPB, reduce bleeding, and enhance postoperative cardiopulmonary function.
22. When the child's condition is stable, give protamine slowly (preferably diluted for small infants). A common practice is to give a dose of protamine at least equal to that of the heparin (mg per 100 U/kg), which was administered before bypass. After 50% of the protamine is given, the surgeons stop using the pump suction to protect the CPB circuit and switch to the

wall suction. If hypotension occurs after protamine, it can be reversed by calcium and/or a fluid bolus. After the heparin has been reversed and cardiac function and filling pressures reassessed, the cannulae are removed.

23. Measure the ACT, electrolytes, and blood gases 2–3 min after the administration of protamine. Give more protamine and repeat the ACT as needed.
24. If bleeding persists, check coagulation indices; give platelets (1 Unit/5 kg), cryoprecipitate, and/or other coagulation factors, e.g., recombinant factor VII, as indicated by the ACT.

    N.B. Anticipate continued bleeding because of platelet dysfunction and other factor deficiencies:

    (a) After a long pump run
    (b) In children with cyanotic CHD
    (c) In small infants, in whom the pump-priming volume is very large in relation to blood volume
    (d) After a complex re-do sternotomy

    All bleeding must be well controlled before the chest is closed.

25. After some complex intracardiac repairs, sternal closure may be delayed, and a plastic membrane sewn in place to cover the heart in the interim. When myocardial edema is present, leaving the chest open prevents compression of the heart and may increase BP and urine output while decreasing CVP. It also allows for easy access to the heart in case of tamponade or the need for emergency cannulation for ECMO. The sternum is closed when myocardial function has improved and the child is able to tolerate this maneuver.
26. At the end of surgery, the decision must be made whether to extubate the trachea immediately or to continue with ventilatory support. The decision depends on the disease that was present and the intraoperative course.
27. The trend toward “fast-tracking” some children after cardiac surgery is well established; it may be very appropriate with minimally invasive surgical procedures. After simple operations, e.g., closure of ASD, the trachea may be extubated in the OR and the child may be expected to have a very short stay in the ICU. In such cases:

(a) Employ an anesthesia technique that permits early brisk recovery; avoid large doses of opioids or muscle relaxants that cannot be easily antagonized.
(b) Plan for good postoperative analgesia; a single-shot caudal morphine injection is safe and effective (see Chap. 7).
(c) Ensure that excess pump-priming fluid is removed by means of modified ultrafiltration after CPB is discontinued.

It may be more appropriate for some children to be transferred to the ICU for extubation depending on local circumstances.

- Some infants with large left-to-right shunts are at extreme risk of pulmonary hypertensive crises during and after surgery (see Principles of Anesthetic Management, Chap. 15)

(d) A milrinone infusion (0.5–0.75 μg/kg/min) may be infused to maintain adequate coronary perfusion pressures for the "pressure loaded" right ventricle.
(e) NO has specific pulmonary vasodilating properties and is extremely useful to control PVR. It is usually added to the inspired gas (as close to the tracheal tube as possible) in a concentration of 20–80 ppm, but its use requires special equipment and monitoring. When mixed with oxygen, nitrogen dioxide (NO_2) is formed, which is damaging to the lungs. Hence NO is added to the breathing circuit as close to the child as possible, and the FIO_2 should be limited to that needed to ensure an acceptable saturation level. Large doses of NO can also lead to methemoglobinemia. A sudden withdrawal of NO can cause severe rebound PAH; therefore, the child has to be weaned slowly.

28. Many children require post-bypass ventilatory support.
    (a) Including:
        - Those with hypoxemia despite a high FIO_2
        - Low cardiac output
        - Pulmonary hypertension
        - Diminished lung compliance
        - Persistent arrhythmias

- Hypothermia (<34 °C)
- Ongoing bleeding

(b) In such children:

- Plan for continuing ventilatory support. Controlled ventilation and CPAP are particularly beneficial during the immediate postoperative period because these patients have reduced lung volumes and increased lung water (especially the infant).
- Do not antagonize the muscle relaxants.
- The choice of a nasal versus an oral tracheal tube depends on institutional preference and the age of the child; for infants we insert nasal tubes at induction of anesthesia, especially if the child may require postoperative ventilation. Infants tolerate nasal tubes extremely well; these tubes are less likely to kink, cannot be occluded by the teeth, are easier to secure at a specific depth, and less likely to be pulled out during removal of the TEE probe. Nasal tubes do not predispose to middle ear or sinus disease. We avoid changing tracheal tubes from oral to nasal at the end of the surgery to preclude bleeding from the nasopharynx or if the infant's condition is unstable. Older children are readily managed with oral endotracheal tubes.

29. During transport to the ICU (all children):

(a) Attach a full bag of blood (or other appropriate fluid) to the IV line to ensure immediate replacement volume availability in case of sudden hemorrhage.

(b) Cover the child with warm blankets.

(c) Administer O_2 by mask or, if the trachea is still intubated, continue controlled ventilation with O_2. Make sure that the tank has an adequate supply of O_2 for the transfer to ICU.

(d) A portable monitor should provide:

- Pulse oximetry
- ECG
- Intravascular pressures
- $EtCO_2$ monitoring is desirable.

(e) Continue the infusions of inotropic drugs and/or vasodilators with battery-powered pumps. If NO is used, this must be continued during transport and in the ICU. Beware of interruptions or changes to the flow of any of these drugs during transport to the ICU. Kinking of infusion lines may interrupt flow and result in a bolus dose as the kink is relieved.

Deep Hypothermia with Circulatory Arrest

Deep hypothermia with circulatory arrest (DHCA) is used for some neonates and infants undergoing cardiac surgery, particularly when surgery involves the aortic root.

Hypothermia is achieved by means of bloodstream cooling on CPB. The debate concerning the safety of profoundly hypothermic circulatory arrest versus continued perfusion is ongoing; many infants have been successfully managed by DHCA and have shown little evidence of cerebral impairment as they grow to adulthood. However, with the extension of cardiac surgery to more complex repairs in smaller infants many centers prefer to limit the duration of DHCA and possibly use antegrade cerebral perfusion (ACP) during aortic arch reconstruction procedures.

Anesthesia Management

Anesthesia management is as described previously, with the following modifications:

1. Dextrose-containing solutions are avoided because hyperglycemia may increase the risk of cerebral damage during total circulatory arrest. The blood glucose concentration should be monitored and hypoglycemia treated. Large doses of fentanyl (more than 50 μg/kg) may limit the increase in blood glucose concentration that often occurs during hypothermic CPB.
2. Give methylprednisolone (Solu-Medrol) (15–30 mg/kg) IV slowly to prevent hypotension due to a systemic inflamatory

response or which may also induce arrhythmias, before cooling on CPB. Ensure that adequate doses of relaxants have been given since once circulatory arrest has occurred, no additional drugs can be given.

3. Phenytoin (Dilantin) 5 mg/kg may be added to the CPB prime solution for neuroprotection.
4. After CPB is begun, ensure that the difference between the esophageal temperature and the temperature of the pump's output does not exceed 10 °C. Set the cooling mattress to 10 °C, turn down the room temperature, and pack the head in ice bags.
5. Two approaches are used to manage blood gas tensions and acid-base balance during profound hypothermia; which approach is optimal remains a subject of debate:
   (a) The "pH stat" approach, which corrects the blood gases to the child's body temperature, requires that CO_2 be added to the oxygenator during cooling. This has the advantage of increasing CBF, allowing for more even cooling and better oxygen delivery, and thereby improved neurologic outcomes in infants. pH stat is the recommended strategy for pediatric patients.
   (b) The "alpha stat" approach, which corrects measurements of blood gases to 37 °C irrespective of the child's body temperature, i.e., pH alkalotic when corrected for the actual body temperature, is used in adults. Blood gas analysis shows a normal or low $PaCO_2$ during cooling.
6. Some practitioners administer phentolamine (0.2 mg/kg) to improve tissue perfusion, ensure rapid even cooling, and minimize acidosis on rewarming.
7. When the esophageal temperature is 16 °C and the rectal temperature is <20 °C, CPB is discontinued, blood is drained to the oxygenator, and the venous cannulas are removed.
8. Record the duration of circulatory arrest. The duration of safe circulatory arrest at a given temperature is unknown, but the current limit is 20–30 min at a 15–18 °C core temperature.
9. Keep the lungs slightly inflated at 5 cm H_2O with an air/O_2 mixture and the ventilator turned off.
10. When the repair is complete, the venous cannulas are reinserted and the child rewarmed until the esophageal tempera-

ture reaches 37 °C. The temperature of the blood from the pump should never exceed 39 °C, and the child's temperature should not exceed 37 °C.

11. Do not correct the metabolic acidosis often seen during rewarming as it will spontaneously correct as the child's metabolism resumes. Administering sodium bicarbonate usually results in postoperative metabolic alkalosis.
12. Maintain Hct levels at 30% during CPB cooling and rewarming as it may lead to superior postoperative neurologic function.

Principles of Postoperative Care

Respiratory System

The status of the respiratory system after cardiac surgery in infants and children may be determined by the factors listed in Table 15.2:

Many children benefit from a period of controlled ventilation and/or PEEP or CPAP. This assists in restoring the lung volumes to normal and improves gas exchange. Levels of added O_2 and PEEP or CPAP can be reduced as the pulmonary status improves. Diuretic therapy may be indicated to reduce

Table 15.2 Factors affecting the respiratory system

1. Preexisting status
(a) Immaturity of respiratory system in young children (especially infants).
(b) Effects of the cardiac disease on the lungs.
2. Effects of anesthesia, operation, and CPB on the respiratory system:
(a) Decreased lung volume.
(b) Increased lung water.
3. Intraoperative events:
(a) Atelectasis, especially the right upper lobe.
(b) Phrenic nerve injury.
(c) Pleural effusions.

lung water. Special measures to control PVR may be required in children with PAH.

Cardiovascular System

After cardiac surgery, the cardiovascular status is determined by the following factors, Table 15.3.

After all but the most minor cardiac operations, cardiac function may deteriorate postoperatively. This deterioration progresses for the first few hours after surgery, probably associated with edema of the myocardium and other changes that decrease the compliance of the ventricles and reduce contractility. Treatment at this time must be directed toward:

1. Ensuring optimal filling pressures. Because the compliance of the ventricles is reduced in infancy and reduced in all children after cardiac surgery, increased filling pressures, i.e., 8–12 mmHg, may be required.
2. Producing an optimal cardiac rate and rhythm. This is most effectively achieved by the use of sequential pacing when necessary. Sinus rhythm, i.e., atrial contraction, significantly augments cardiac output.
3. Reducing afterload. The use of vasodilators in children with ventricular dysfunction increases cardiac output with little change in cardiac work or arterial BP. When vasodilators are used, the preload must be maintained by infusion of appropri-

Table 15.3 Factors affecting the cardiovascular system

1. Preexisting status:
   (a) Immature heart and circulatory system in infants.
   (b) Effects of the cardiac disease on the cardiovascular system.
2. Effects of anesthesia, surgery, and CPB, which are dictated by:
   (a) Duration of anesthesia and surgery.
   (b) Duration of CPB.
   (c) Duration of induced cardiac arrest.
   (d) The success of myocardial protection measures.

ate fluids; a SNP infusion is commonly used to produce vasodilation. Alternatively, milrinone or phenoxybenzamine may be used to provide afterload reduction, the latter yielding a long-lasting adrenergic blockade. Caution: some children do not tolerate LV afterload reduction, e.g., those with impaired RV function (TOF, etc.).

4. Inotropic support: If a low cardiac output persists despite these measures, administer an inotropic agent:
   (a) Dopamine (5–10 μg/kg/min) has been shown to be effective in increasing cardiac output in infants and children, *but*:
      - The doses required in children are greater than those in adults.
      - The vasodilating effect is less than in adults. Hence the concurrent infusion of a vasodilator (SNP or milrinone) is usually warranted. The combination of dopamine and SNP may also be effective in reducing PVR in children with PAH, but must be given as soon as the child is weaned from bypass.

   (b) Calcium should be administered to maintain the serum Ca^{++} at a high-normal level (1–1.2 mmol/dL).
   (c) If low cardiac output persists despite these measures, an epinephrine infusion (0.05–0.1 μg/kg/min) may be needed.

Fluid and Electrolyte Therapy

1. Blood should be administered to maintain the hemoglobin level at near-normal levels (14–15 g/dL), especially when cardiac dysfunction is present.
2. Acid-base status should be monitored and acidosis corrected.
3. Balanced salt solutions, e.g., lactated Ringer's solution, should be infused at rates sufficient to maintain urine output and CVP indices.
4. KCl, 2 mEq/kg/day, may be added, *provided* there is a urine output greater than 1 mL/kg/h.
5. Hypomagnesemia may occur perioperatively, especially with aggressive diuretic therapy. Magnesium sulfate may be administered if necessary.

6. If urine output is <1 mL/kg/h in the absence of hypotension, a "fluid challenge" may be administered. If the urine output does not respond, a diuretic may be indicated.

Special Considerations for Specific Operations

PDA Ligation

A PDA should be suspected in preterm infants who cannot be weaned off the ventilator, have refractory CHF, or develop NEC. Older infants or children are relatively asymptomatic and present with a continuous "machinery-like" murmur.

Preterm Infants

A PDA may occur in preterm infants, especially those weighing less than 1500 g. In addition to prematurity, respiratory distress syndrome, excessive fluid therapy, neonatal asphyxia, hypoxia, and acidosis predispose to this condition. A PDA results in a large left-to-right shunt, with pulmonary vascular engorgement and CHF. Clinical signs include tachypnea, hepatosplenomegaly, and bounding pulses.

Diagnosis is confirmed by auscultation of the typical murmur, radiographic evidence of increased vascularity, and ECHO findings of a large left atrium:aorta ratio. A PDA may prevent weaning from ventilatory support of infants with RDS.

Treatment for PDA

1. *Medical treatment.* Administration of indomethacin, a prostaglandin inhibitor, daily for several days may induce closure. Indomethacin may also cause renal damage and suppress bone marrow. Therefore, it is contraindicated in children with renal failure or coagulopathy. Very small infants (those weighing

less than 1000 g) do not respond as well with closure of the PDA after indomethacin.

2. *Surgical treatment (Clipping) and Interventional Cardiology.* These approaches may be necessary if indomethacin therapy fails or is contraindicated. Currently, the majority have their PDAs closed by interventional cardiologists with either an occluder device (those >700 g) or vascular plug (those <700 g). An ECHO determines which infants cannot be managed with an occluder or vascular plug (age <3 days, left PA stenosis, duct dependent cardiac output, PDA length <3 mm, PDA diameter >4 mm at narrowest point) and require a surgical approach.

Special Anesthesia Problems

1. Observe all special precautions for the preterm infant.
2. Be prepared for sudden blood loss; the ductus is very thin and tears easily.
3. If a surgical approach is chosen, it may be preferable to operate in the NICU to avoid transport problems, allowing the infant to remain on the NICU ventilator (including HFOV). However, this limits the anesthetic prescription to TIVA, results in electrocautery interference of the pulse oximeter, and ECG, and no capnography. Currently the majority of these infants are transported to the interventional cardiology suite (with the NICU ventilator), where standard operating room monitors are available and anesthesia is provided by TIVA.
4. Preoperative management:
    (a) Assess the infant for anemia, which may predispose to CHF and consider transfusing with packed red blood cells. The increased Hct may improve myocardial oxygenation and reduce the extent of left-to-right shunting.
    (b) For those infants who are transferred to the OR or interventional cardiology suite, use a heated transport incubator.
    (c) Premedication is unnecessary.

5. Perioperative Management
   (a) Heat the OR or cardiology suite (>80 °F) and prepare a forced air heating device before transferring the infant to the table.
   (b) Monitor SaO_2 in a preductal site (right hand) and in the foot; measure the BP in the right arm (see previous discussion).
   (c) Tracheal intubation:
      - If the trachea is already intubated, ensure that the tube is firmly fixed, patent, and optimally positioned; otherwise, reintubate.
      - If the trachea is not intubated, then intubate the trachea and ventilate the lungs with an air/O_2 mixture and the minimal FIO_2 necessary.
   (d) Our preference is to induce and maintain anesthesia with high-dose fentanyl and rocuronium.
   (e) Establish at least one large IV line; blood loss is usually minimal but can be catastrophic if a vessel is torn.
   (f) Have a dopamine infusion prepared if there is LV dysfunction.
   (g) Administer prophylactic antibiotics.
   (h) These infants are often diuresed in the NICU in an attempt to either close the PDA or reduce the severity of RDS. Be prepared to give balanced salt solution to offset hypotension.
   (i) Manual ventilation is often useful as the ductus is approached as many of these infants have congested lungs and poor compliance. To ensure adequate surgical exposure and dissection, a large part of the lung will be compressed, which often necessitates increasing the FIO_2. Watch for surgical retraction compromising cardiac output and oxygenation; if the infant becomes hypotensive or suddenly desaturates despite the above maneuvers, ask the surgeons to remove the retractors. If a transthoracic ECHO probe is used, anticipate the probe possibly causing airway obstruction and impaired ventilation.
      - Either local or cryo intercostal nerve blocks should be considered.

6. Postoperative
   (a) Continued ventilation is necessary for the majority of infants.

Post PDA ligation, the degree to which the infant's the respiratory status improves will be determined by how much the pulmonary vascular congestion decreases and the severity of the pulmonary disease (RDS or bronchopulmonary dysplasia).

Older Infants and Children

In older infants and children, a persistent PDA is treated either by insertion of an occluding device in the catheterization lab (see Interventional Cardiology below) or by ligation during a video assisted thoracotomy (VATS—see Chap. 14). Exceptions may be made for the very large ductus in a small infant.

1. PDA as the sole lesion in older infants and children usually presents few problems. Ligation or device occlusion is necessary to prevent later complications including PAH and cardiac failure, SBE, or aneurysm formation.
2. If VATS is planned, establish a reliable large-bore-IV route to manage possible bleeding, administer prophylactic antibiotics, and prepare for a thoracotomy.
3. An arterial line is not essential. The BP must be monitored in the right arm; in the unlikely event of a torn ductus, it may be necessary to clamp the left subclavian artery. Monitor SaO_2 in the right hand (preductal) and a foot (post-ductal).
4. Post-VATS, pain may be controlled by infiltrating the incision sites with local anesthetic. Post-thoracotomy, use intercostal or cryo nerve blocks, or an ultrasound-guided paravertebral block for pain control; these children may go to the ward after PACU. In infants and small children, a single dose of caudal morphine is another option, but the analgesia may have delayed onset. These children should be admitted to the PICU.

5. During the procedure, monitor:
   (a) For bradycardia during dissection near the vagus nerve.
   (b) Post-ligation, the continuous murmur ceases and a soft systolic murmur remains. The BP (especially diastolic) may increase slightly at this time, but large changes are unusual.

       Major changes in BP might suggest that the wrong vessel has been ligated or occluded. If the aorta has accidentally been occluded, hypertension and loss of the oximeter signal from the foot will occur. If a PA has accidentally been ligated, the continuous murmur of the ductus will remain. If a bronchus has been ligated, airway pressures will increase and the murmur will persist unchanged.
6. Blood loss is usually minimal, seldom necessitating transfusion, but it may be sudden and massive if a major vessel is torn: check that blood is immediately available.

Postoperative Care

(a) Routine post-thoracotomy care should be applied.
(b) Rarely, the thoracic duct may be injured during PDA ligation. The resulting chylothorax may require drainage, and continued losses of chyle may impose a severe nutritional challenge.
(c) Damage to the left recurrent laryngeal nerve in the region of the ductus is also a rare complication.

Division of Vascular Rings and Suspension of Anomalous Innominate Artery

Abnormalities of the great vessels may encircle or compress the trachea, bronchi, and esophagus. Typical examples are a *double aortic arch*, a vascular ring that is completed by a PDA or ligamentum arteriosum, or an *abnormal course of the subclavian artery*. Severe compression by vascular rings can lead to stridor and/or difficulty with feeding during early infancy.

The infant with a vascular ring often assumes a characteristic opisthotonic position. A chest radiograph with barium swallow can be a helpful diagnostic tool. Anomalous vessels may compress the bronchi and cause gas trapping in an individual lobe of the lung, compressing the adjacent lung by the emphysematous lobe. In addition, dynamic CT and cardiac MRI are frequently used to delineate the anatomy and plan the surgical repair (aortopexy, simple ligation, or complex reconstruction). Infants with vascular compression are prone to sudden cardiorespiratory arrest (see also Chap. 14, Tracheaesophageal fistula).

Special Anesthesia Problems

1. Respiratory failure may exist.
   (a) Chronic or recurrent respiratory infection may cause impaired pulmonary function.
   (b) Vascular compression may cause emphysema of one or more lobes, compressing other lung tissue.
2. Airway compression may occur at the level of the carina or main bronchi, which will not be relieved by a normally positioned tracheal tube.
3. Tracheal intubation may be required preoperatively to relieve serious symptoms. Air trapping in a lobe that results from vascular compression may be alleviated by PEEP.
4. An esophageal stethoscope in infants with vascular rings has been reported to cause acute airway obstruction.
5. VATS may be used for the procedure (see Chap. 14). Be prepared for thoracotomy if problems arise.

Anesthesia Management

Preoperative

1. The infant should be positioned for optimal ventilation.
2. Bronchoscopy may be required to evaluate the site of airway compression and for endobronchial suction.

Perioperative

1. For intubation, use a method that ensures a patent airway past the obstruction. If the obstruction is mid-trachea, this is relatively simple. If the obstruction is low or at the carina, do one of the following:
2. Pass a long tracheal tube past the obstruction into a main bronchus; use a tracheal tube with a side hole, e.g. Murphy eye, to allow ventilation the other bronchus. Alternatively:
3. Ventilate the lungs via a rigid bronchoscope (placed under direct vision and adjusted intraoperatively if necessary).
4. Monitor the BP via an arterial line in the right radial artery. Operations on the great vessels can cause serious bleeding; secure a reliable, large-bore IV access.
5. For aortopexy, a post-repair bronchoscopy is performed to ensure that compression of the trachea has been relieved; always assess the tracheal compression during spontaneous ventilation and coughing.
6. If the bronchoscope is used instead of a tracheal tube, topicalize the airway with lidocaine and use general anesthesia with spontaneous respirations. During the remainder of the operation, ventilation may be assisted; try to avoid muscle relaxants.
7. Complex tracheobronchial reconstructions are occasionally performed on CPB.

Postoperative

1. If residual obstruction persists, continue with tracheal intubation for 24 h, then reassess.
2. Partial obstruction may be improved by placing a small bolster, 1–2 in. thick, below the shoulders.
3. Racemic epinephrine and/or dexamethasone may be required for post-instrumentation croup.
4. After complex tracheobronchial reconstructions the children are usually immobilized for several days in a specific head-neck position to avoid tension on the sutures.

Resection of Aortic Coarctation

All coarctations are classified as juxtaductal. There are two distinct presentations: in infancy with CHF or in later life with systemic hypertension. The infantile type is frequently accompanied by other anomalies, e.g., VSD, PDA, and usually manifests as cardiac failure in infants <6 months of age. The later life type is usually diagnosed during investigation of hypertension in preschoolers.

CoA can be treated medically by balloon angioplasty or surgically by resection. Re-coarctation is optimally treated by angioplasty and that long segment coarctation is best treated surgically, both under general anesthesia (see Interventional Cardiology below).

Coarctation of the aorta is recognized as a lifelong disorder; later in life many children will have continuing problems with hypertension and its complications possibly attributed to an altered renin angiotensin system or baroreceptors.

Infantile Coarctation

Special Problems

1. Most infants have severe cardiac failure requiring inotropic support, diuretics, and assisted ventilation.
2. Severe cardiovascular anomalies are commonly associated.
3. Blood flow to the lower portion of the body depends on the ductus arteriosus. Prostaglandin (0.05–0.15 μg/kg/min) is infused to maintain patency until surgical repair.
4. Hypoplasia of the aortic arch may be present and, if significant, may require repair with CPB (see later discussion).

Anesthesia Management

Preoperative

1. Review recent blood gases.
2. Continue the prostaglandin infusion.

3. Ensure that supportive drugs are immediately available, e.g., epinephrine, dopamine.
4. Ensure that blood is available in the OR and checked before incision.

Perioperative

1. Passive cooling to 34 °C for neuroprotection.
2. While the aorta is clamped, maintain the systolic pressure < 100 mmHg with small concentrations of isoflurane. A small dose of heparin (1 mg/kg) is usually given before clamping or balloon angioplasty, check that the ACT is ≥ ~250 s.
3. Be prepared to support the circulation when the aortic obstruction has been removed; an infusion of fluid and/or cardiotonic drugs may be required.
4. Prostaglandin is discontinued once the ductus is ligated and the CoA relieved.

Postoperative

The course is sometimes stormy. Therefore:

1. Transfer the child to the ICU with a tracheal tube in place.
2. Controlled ventilation is usually necessary for at least 48–72 h.

Adult Type

Special Considerations for Surgical Repair

1. Clamping the aorta could compromise the blood supply to the spinal cord; maintain mean BP in the distal aorta of ~45 mmHg.
2. While the aorta is clamped, severe proximal hypertension may occur and require treatment.
3. Hypertension can be troublesome postoperatively; this may be controlled with short-acting β-blockers, but may also require SNP.
4. Although blood must be available for transfusion, it is rarely required.

5. In the very rare event that severe proximal hypertension cannot be controlled after aortic clamping or if the distal pressure is very low, a temporary shunt must be placed to bypass the site of anastomosis, or left heart bypass must be used.

Anesthesia Management

Preoperative

1. Monitor BP and SaO_2 in the right arm. Place a second oximeter probe on a foot.
2. Establish reliable intravenous infusions at sites other than in the left arm.
3. An epidural/caudal catheter may be placed to administer morphine and/or bupivacaine for postoperative pain management, although this may raise medicolegal concerns if paraplegia occurs.

Perioperative

1. Maintain anesthesia with N_2O, an inhalation agent, and a non-depolarizing agent.
2. Place an arterial line in the right radial artery, and a central venous line; the latter to infuse vasodilators.
3. During aortic clamping, control the BP (< 140 mmHg) by increasing the concentration of inhalation agent; do not reduce the BP if it remains <140 mmHg. Distal aortic pressure during clamp-off varies directly with the proximal pressure; distal pressure should be maintained at or above a mean of 45 mmHg to ensure perfusion of the spinal cord.
4. The surgeon first removes the distal clamp and then slowly removes the proximal clamp. Monitor the BP; if hypotension develops, first infuse fluids and second ask the surgeon to partially reapply the proximal clamp. The BP may remain slightly reduced for a brief period of time but usually returns to above-

normal levels by the end of the operation. Anticipate the need to treat postoperative hypertension with:
   (a) SNP(1–10 μg/kg/min) or
   (b) Esmolol, (loading dose 100–500 μg/kg over 1 min), followed by an infusion (50–100 μg/kg/min) to control hypertension.
5. Blood loss is usually minimal and transfusion exceedingly rare.
6. In most cases the trachea is extubated at the end of surgery.

Postoperative

1. Postoperative hypertension usually persists for several days and may necessitate therapy with SNP and/or esmolol. Prevention of hypertension is essential to prevent arteritis (see later discussion).
2. Very rarely, the postoperative course is complicated by post-coarctectomy syndrome which consists of intestinal ileus caused by mesenteric arteritis secondary to increased pulsatile flow in the mesenteric artery. In extreme cases, bowel resection may be required.
3. Other serious postoperative complications include recurrent laryngeal nerve palsy, phrenic nerve palsy, chylothorax, and paraplegia because of spinal cord ischemia during repair (very rare).
4. Re-coarctation may occur in later years, particularly after repair in infancy. Repeat operation may be technically much more difficult and may involve major blood loss. Hence balloon angioplasty is preferred.

Interrupted Aortic Arch

This lesion is frequently associated with a VSD and DiGeorge syndrome and requires repair using CPB with profound hypothermic circulatory arrest. The PDA must be maintained with a prostaglandin infusion until surgery.

Palliative Surgery to Increase Pulmonary Blood Flow

Palliative surgeries may include:

1. Blalock-Taussig procedure (systemic artery anastomosed to the PA). A modified Blalock procedure using a synthetic graft between the aorta or innominate artery and the central portion of the PA is the most commonly performed procedure.
2. The Potts operation (PA anastomosed to descending aorta) and the Waterston procedure (PA anastomosed to ascending aorta) are rarely performed because they become too large and may cause unilateral pulmonary edema.

These surgeries are indicated for infants and children with right-sided cardiac lesions such as TOF, tricuspid atresia, and other conditions with decreased pulmonary blood flow. The surgeries, which increase pulmonary blood flow and stimulate growth of the PAs until complete correction, are usually performed during infancy. Complete correction of the defect is usually performed at an older age. Total correction of CHD in infancy has resulted in many fewer palliative procedures.

Special Anesthesia Problems

1. Many of these children are severely hypoxemic and polycythemic.
2. During surgery, the PA is partly occluded so that the anastomosis can be completed; this causes a further temporary decrease in pulmonary blood flow.
3. Children with polycythemia may have a coagulation defect, although this is rarely a problem.
4. In small infants, the narrow lumen of the new shunt is prone to thrombose. This may be prevented by using a small dose of heparin and appropriate fluid therapy.

Anesthesia Management

Preoperative

1. These are often urgent or semi-urgent surgeries to increase pulmonary blood flow after failure to stent the PDA or dilate a stenotic or atretic pulmonary valve in the cardiac catheterization laboratory.
2. Continue β-blocking drugs.
3. Allow liberal oral fluids up to 2 h before surgery and administer an IV infusion if the preoperative fasting period is prolonged for any child with a Hb >16 g/dL.

Perioperative

1. Follow Routine Anesthesia Management, under "Anesthesia Management" above.
2. Induce anesthesia with IV ketamine or propofol followed by fentanyl and rocuronium.
3. An arterial line should be placed either in the radial artery—*in the rare event that the subclavian artery will be used, place the line in the contralateral side*—or in the femoral artery.
4. Maintain anesthesia with an inhaled agent in at least 50% O_2 in air.
   (a) If halothane is available, use it in children with TOF because it decreases the RV contractility and outflow obstruction; alternatively, sevoflurane may be used.
   (b) If the child with TOF desaturates, give esmolol (500 μg/kg IV slowly) and/or IV phenylephrine (1–10 μg/kg).
   (c) If excessive hypotension occurs, discontinue the inhaled agent and administer fentanyl.
5. Immediately before the PA is clamped, switch to 100% O_2, inflate the lungs, and give a further dose of relaxant.
6. Once the clamps are in place and if the SaO_2 is stable, the surgeon should proceed. *Once this is commenced, the PA will be open and the clamps cannot come off until the anastomosis is completed.*
7. While the anastomosis is being created, administer cardiotonic drugs, e.g., epinephrine (1–5 μg/kg), if the systemic BP decreases profoundly or bradycardia occurs.

8. A "modified" Blalock anastomosis usually involves a synthetic graft. In small infants, administer a small dose of heparin (100 U/kg) to prevent thrombosis of the shunt. An IV bolus of a balanced salt solution after the clamps are released may enhance flow through the shunt.
9. Give 5% albumin to replace blood loss and decrease the Hct.

Postoperative

1. Auscultate the chest to confirm the presence of a new murmur indicating that the shunt is functioning.
2. If the anastomosis is small and likely to be blocked by thrombosis, heparin and/or an anti-platelet function medication may be indicated for several days postoperatively.

Palliative Surgery to Decrease Pulmonary Blood Flow

PA banding is performed to diminish blood flow to the lungs in infants who have a large left-to-right shunt, thereby improving systemic perfusion, decreasing pulmonary vascular congestion, and preventing the development of irreversible PAH. This is usually performed as an emergency procedure in the neonate who has other significant congenital abnormalities. Many children present with CHF.

Anesthesia Management

Preoperative

1. Follow Routine Anesthesia Management under "Anesthesia Management" above.
2. Optimize the infants' general status before surgery including treating CHF.

Perioperative

1. Avoid myocardial depressants.
2. Monitor the infant closely as the band is applied. With an optimal band tightness:

(a) The systemic BP should increase, and the saturation may decrease slightly.
(b) The distal PA pressure should decrease to ~30–50% of systemic pressure.
(c) The change in $PetCO_2$ is a reliable guide to optimal PA banding. The $PetCO_2$ value may decrease very slightly after the band is applied, but a large decrease indicates that the band is too tight.

Postoperative

1. Controlled ventilation may be required for several days.

Specific Open-Heart Procedures

The considerations discussed here are a supplement to all the other important general principles outlined previously.

Atrial Septal Defect (ASD) (Secundum Type)

The secundum-type ASD is the most common form of an ASD and located in the fossa ovalis. Simple small ASDs are commonly closed by interventional cardiology using an "Umbrella" device (see Interventional Cardiology, page 507). A large ASD may require surgical closure, although this may be performed using minimally invasive techniques. Other forms of ASD may be associated with a cleft in the mitral valve (primum ASD) or with partial anomalous pulmonary venous drainage (sinus venosus type, most often located at the junction of the right atrium with the SVC), in which case a baffle is required to redirect this flow to the left atrium. This may complicate and prolong the simple ASD closure procedure slightly.

1. For simple secundum ASDs in healthy children, plan to extubate the trachea at the end of the procedure. Many different "fast-track" techniques have been described, depending on the child's age and general condition. A single dose of caudal morphine (33 μg/kg of Duramorph) given after induction of anes-

thesia can provide early postoperative analgesia for up to 24 h, but may require admission to PICU overnight.

2. Surgical closure of the ASD is performed either with cardioplegia or with induced ventricular fibrillation to prevent the possibility that air may enter the LV and be pumped into the circulation. Ensure that the child is completely paralyzed during CPB to prevent the child from taking a breath while the atrium is open, which could draw air into the left side of the heart; give an additional dose of relaxant as the heart is being cannulated.
3. As the last suture is being tightened to close the defect, the surgeon may request sustained lung inflation to promote flow of blood via the pulmonary veins into the left atrium to remove any residual air from the left side of the heart.
4. Bypass is brief and post-CPB inotropic therapy is unlikely to be needed.

Total Anomalous Pulmonary Venous Drainage (TAPVD)

The pulmonary veins typically drain into the right atrium or its venous connections. There are three common types of anomalous venous drainage:

1. *Supracardiac (50% of cases):* Pulmonary veins drain into the left SVC.
2. *Cardiac (30% of cases):* Pulmonary veins drain into the coronary sinus or right atrium.
3. *Infracardiac (10% of cases):* Pulmonary veins drain into the inferior vena cava via a common trunk below the diaphragm.

TAPVD manifests in early neonatal life with severe cyanosis and acidosis. Obstruction of the pulmonary veins may be present causing pulmonary edema and cardiac failure. Survival depends on a right-to-left shunt, usually via an ASD or patent foramen ovale (PFO), which may need enlarging by balloon dilation in the catheterization suite. The presence of obstruction to the pulmonary veins exacerbates the symptoms and if severe, may dictate emergency surgery.

Special Considerations

1. If the pulmonary veins are obstructed, pulmonary edema, PAH, and cardiac failure may be present.
2. Preoperative ventilation may be required to treat pulmonary edema and improve oxygenation.
3. The left atrium and LV may be small, and the LV compliance reduced; aggressive inotropic therapy may be required after bypass.
4. The pulmonary vasculature may have a thick medial layer, and PVR may remain increased after repair.

Anesthesia Plan

1. Maintain controlled ventilation and PEEP; monitor acid-base status frequently.
2. A high-dose opioid technique is preferred.
3. After repair, the LV may require inotropic support and afterload reduction to maintain cardiac output. A high left atrial pressure should be avoided as this may lead to fluid overload.
4. Active measures to reduce PVR and prevent pulmonary hypertensive crisis must be instituted. The PA pressure should be monitored; prepare to administer NO.
5. TEE may be contraindicated as it may further obstruct the venous drainage and induce a pulmonary hypertensive crisis.

Ventricular Septal Defect (VSD)

VSD is the most common single cardiac defect (20% of CHD cases). The position of the VSD is used to classify the disease and predict complications:

1. *Type I (supracristal, ~5%):* under the annulus of the aorta, which may affect the adjacent cusp and cause aortic valve incompetence; also associated with a narrow aortic isthmus.
2. *Type II (infracristal, most common, ~80%):* in the membranous septum—often large with a big shunt.
3. *Type III (AV canal type, ~1%):* beneath the tricuspid valve
4. *Type IV (muscular ~ 4%):* may be multiple ("Swiss cheese" defect)

The physiologic effects of the VSD depend on size. If it is large (non-restrictive), the left-to-right shunt is similarly large, resulting in early CHF and subsequent pulmonary vascular obstructive disease (PVOD). Small defects (restrictive) allow only a limited left-to-right shunting, which may be physiologically insignificant. Early operation is performed for large defects to prevent the onset of PVOD. Hybrid techniques (combined surgical and interventional cardiology) may be used to close small defects.

Special Considerations

1. Infants with severe CHF may benefit from sedation, intubation and ventilation preoperatively.
2. Infants with CHF may only tolerate a high-dose fentanyl anesthetic.
3. Anticipate postoperative conduction disturbances, which may be temporary (possibly due to edema around a suture).
4. Pulmonary vascular crisis may occur postoperatively in small infants with previously large left-right shunts.

Anesthesia Plan

1. High-dose opioids are preferred; caution with myocardial depressants.
2. Bidirectional shunts are common; avoid air bubbles in the IV lines.

3. Maintain PVR (avoid hyperventilation) to prevent increasing left-to-right shunting. A limited reduction in SVR (low-dose inhalation agent) may be beneficial.
4. If a conduction defect is detected after repair, consider pacing.
5. In the case of large defects, post-bypass therapy to reduce PVR and prevent pulmonary vascular crisis may be required.

Atrioventricular Canal

Atrioventricular (AV) canal is frequently associated with Down syndrome and may be complete (ASD, VSD, and cleft AV valve) or partial (ostium primum ASD plus cleft mitral valve). The most significant hemodynamic changes are a large left-to-right shunt, leading to PAH, and mitral incompetence. Early surgical repair in infancy is preferred.

Special Considerations

1. Down syndrome is often present (see Chap. 8).
2. PAH may require treatment postoperatively; aggressive inotropic therapy may also be indicated.
3. Conduction disturbances are relatively common after repair and may persist; a pacemaker may be required.
4. Mitral valve malfunction may occur in the early or late postoperative period, and reoperation to repair the valve may be required.

Tetralogy of Fallot

The combination of a large VSD and RV outflow obstruction produce a large right-to-left shunt, which gives the clinical presentation of cyanosis and exercise intolerance. Additional features of TOF include an overriding of the aorta and RV hypertrophy. RV obstruction may be infundibular (~50%), valvular (~10%), PA (~10%), or combined (~30%). Acute dynamic increases in infundibular obstruction may lead to severe desaturation episodes ("tet" spells). Most children are treated by complete repair in infancy, except those with small PAs, who are treated initially with a systemic-to-pulmonary shunt.

Special Considerations

1. Adequate preoperative sedation and sufficient anesthesia and analgesia to suppress responses to surgical stimulation are important to prevent "tet" spells. Avoid drugs that reduce SVR, e.g., isoflurane; a high-dose opioid technique is preferred.
2. Halothane may be administered, if available, in low concentrations to depress the muscle of the RV infundibulum and prevent desaturation due to increased shunting.
3. Treat a sudden desaturation with oxygen, fluid infusion, esmolol (0.5 mg/kg slowly) and/or phenylephrine (1–10 μg/kg).
4. After CPB, a high filling pressure may be required owing to the thickened, poorly compliant right ventricle. Rarely, conduction defects require AV pacing. Junctional ectopic tachycardiac (JET) may occur in the postoperative period and is usually treated with cooling, sedation, reduction of inotropic support and antiarrhythmics, e.g., procainamide or amiodarone.
5. Afterload reduction of the LV may be poorly tolerated because the overall cardiac output is limited by the RV output. In neonates, a small intra-atrial communication (PFO or ASD) is often left open or created to decompress the RV and maintain LV filling.

Transposition of the Great Arteries (TGA)

The most common cause of cyanotic CHD in the neonate is TGA in which the aorta arises from the RV and the PA arises from the LV. Here, the pulmonary and systemic circulations are separate and in parallel; survival depends on adequate mixing of blood via a PFO, ASD, VSD, and/or PDA. Without treatment, 90% of infants die within 12 months. Current surgical treatment is the arterial switch procedure performed in neonates with an intact septum; it may be performed later in those with a large VSD and subpulmonary obstruction.

Special Considerations

1. The neonate with an intact septum depends on mixing via the PFO and PDA. When the PDA closes, the neonate becomes desperately hypoxic. Balloon atrial septostomy (BAS) creates a shunt to improve mixing, or, if the neonate is having early surgery, PGE_1 may be used to maintain the PDA.
2. The effective pulmonary or systemic blood flow is limited to that volume of blood that shunts between the circulations.

Anesthesia Plan

1. A technique that maintains myocardial function and cardiac output should be used; a high-dose opioid technique is preferred.
2. Moderate hyperventilation with a high FIO_2 may reduce PVR thereby increasing pulmonary blood flow, mixing, and arterial saturation.
3. The PGE_1 infusion must be continued until bypass, although the PDA is usually ligated once on bypass to prevent run-off during surgery.
4. Post-CPB measures to optimize blood flow in the re-implanted coronary arteries are required. An infusion of nitroglycerin (1 μg/kg/min) is usually started before weaning from CPB.
5. Maintain an optimal preload; there must be an adequate balance between coronary perfusion and afterload reduction for the deconditioned LV that was previously exposed only to the lower PVR. Monitoring the EKG for ST changes is not very reliable.

6. Bleeding from multiple suture lines should be anticipated; coagulopathy is common after CPB and platelets, FFP, and cryoprecipitate may be required.

Aortic Stenosis

Critical aortic stenosis can cause severe CHF in the neonate. Older children with aortic stenosis may be asymptomatic, but are predisposed to angina, syncope, and sudden death. Aortic stenosis may be subvalvular; valvular (~80% of cases), usually with a bicuspid valve; or supravalvular (often associated with Williams syndrome [see Appendix A]). Critical aortic stenosis in the neonate is usually treated by balloon dilation. On occasion an infant with a small aortic annulus or with associated cardiac lesions may require surgery. The principles outlined below apply equally to those children who require anesthesia in the cardiac catheterization lab.

Special Considerations

1. Infants with critical aortic stenosis are hypotensive, poorly perfused, and acidotic, with respiratory distress and hepatomegaly. The disease often becomes apparent as the ductus arteriosus closes. The thickened LV is prone to ischemia and arrhythmias. Subendocardial fibroelastosis may also be present. These infants require aggressive resuscitation, early operation, and have a high mortality rate.
2. Older children with valvular aortic stenosis usually have good cardiac function despite a high gradient across the stenosed valve.

Anesthesia Plan: Infants

1. Continue infusing prostaglandin to maintain the ductus arteriosus.
2. A high-dose opioid and relaxant technique is preferred.
3. Maintain body temperature.

4. Serious arrhythmias, including ventricular fibrillation, may occur as the heart is manipulated, especially if any cooling has occurred.

Anesthesia Plan: Older Children

1. Maintain the heart rate and avoid tachycardia or bradycardia; prevent a major decrease in SVR and aortic root pressure. A high-dose opioid plus muscle relaxant technique is usually satisfactory.
2. Halothane or other potent inhalation agent may be useful to reduce dynamic LV outflow tract obstruction in those with subvalvular aortic stenosis.
3. Children with supravalvular aortic stenosis and Williams syndrome may have a difficult airway. These children require meticulous management due to their high (~1%) cardiac arrest risk (See Appendix A)
4. Postoperative hypertension is common after aortic valvotomy requiring treatment with esmolol and/or SNP.

Hypoplastic Left Heart Syndrome

In HLHS, the LV and ascending aorta are hypoplastic and the LV is nonfunctional. Immediate survival depends on the pumping action of the RV and systemic flow via the PDA with retrograde flow in the aortic arch. Blood mixes in the right atrium (via an ASD or PFO), and pulmonary-to-systemic flow ratio depends on the size of the intra-atrial communication, the PVR, and the SVR. Treatment of this condition involves conversion to a univentricular series type of circulation by means of a staged repair. Alternatively, a heart transplant may be considered.

1. *Stage 1:* Norwood procedure. Division of the PA, connection of the RV to a reconstructed aortic arch (neoaorta created from the PA and AO), atrial septectomy, and a modified Blalock-Taussig shunt (innominate or subclavian artery to PA). The Sano modification of the Stage 1 Norwood procedure is to place the shunt from RV to PA.

2. *Stage 2:* Bidirectional Glenn (SVC-RPA) anastomosis or hemi-Fontan procedure (and take down of the B-T shunt). This procedure is designed to direct some of the blood flow directly to the lungs and so reduce the load on the RV.
3. *Stage 3:* Completion of the Fontan procedure, which connects the IVC to the PA by means of an intra-atrial lateral tunnel or extracardiac Gortex conduit, which then places the systemic and pulmonary circulations in series. There is no subpulmonary pumping chamber; the conduit/tunnel is fenestrated to decompress high right-sided pressures.

Special Considerations

1. Preoperative management is aimed at maintaining the ratio of pulmonary-to-systemic blood flow (Qp:Qs) close to 1. The ease with which this can be achieved depends on the child's anatomy, i.e., the size of the interatrial communication.
   (a) If it is large and unrestrictive, pulmonary blood flow is excessive, and systemic hypoperfusion with metabolic acidosis occurs.
   (b) Children with relative restriction (a high percentage) may achieve Qp:Qs near 1 when breathing room air. These infants must be managed to maintain the status quo, i.e., to prevent changes in ventilation or oxygenation.
   (c) Children with a very small or absent ASD have left atrial and PAH, decreased pulmonary blood flow, and are profoundly hypoxic at birth. These infants require an immediate balloon atrial septostomy and early surgery.
2. All infants require a continuous infusion of PGE_1 to maintain patency of the ductus arteriosus.
3. Some infants require inotropic support to increase cardiac output and systemic perfusion but also prevent adverse changes in SVR.

Anesthesia Plan-Norwood Stage 1

1. Maintain the FIO_2 (an oxygen blender) and ventilation (self-inflating bag) unchanged during transport to and from the OR. It is very easy to hyperventilate the lungs causing a disastrous decrease in PVR and thus in systemic blood flow.
2. Care during the pre-bypass stage is similar for those undergoing either the Norwood procedure or transplantation; maintain the level of ventilation and oxygenation to balance the PVR:SVR ratio. The arterial saturation should be ±80%.
3. High-dose opioid anesthesia is preferred, but fentanyl (50–75 μg/kg) must be titrated to prevent hypotension.
4. Post-CPB after a Norwood procedure, measures to maintain the PVR and limit pulmonary blood flow may still be required, depending on the size of the shunt. Expect the saturation to be 70–80%.
5. If pulmonary blood flow is inadequate and the infant is severely hypoxic, a larger shunt will be needed.

Fontan Procedure

In addition to the HLHS, the Fontan procedure and its modifications are used to treat other forms of CHD with a single functional ventricle: the SVC is connected directly to the PA (Glenn procedure), and the venous return from the IVC is redirected to the PA via an intra-atrial lateral tunnel or an extracardiac conduit. This creates a serial circulation in which the all the kinetic energy for blood flow through the pulmonary and systemic vascular beds is provided by the single ventricle.

Special Considerations

1. After the operation, the total cardiac output is directed to the systemic circulation, resulting in the pulmonary circulation being driven by the systemic venous return; hence, a low PVR

is vital. There is no shunting, so SaO_2 is improved and the load on the ventricle is reduced.

2. For a successful operation, a PVR < 4 Wood units/m^2 is desirable and PVR must not be allowed to increase. However, in some children with mildly increased PVR, a Fontan operation is performed but a fenestration is left in the vena cava-to-PA baffle. This allows for some right-to-left shunting and relieves the right atrial pressure; cyanosis may occur, but ventricular filling and cardiac output are maintained.
3. Pleural and pericardial effusions are common and may require drainage.
4. Plastic bronchitis leading to acute airway obstruction and requiring bronchoscopic removal may occur post-Fontan, the result of the high venous pressures.

Anesthesia Plan

1. Establish reliable IV access; postoperatively, edema may make later venous access difficult.
2. A reliable CVP line is essential for postoperative monitoring. The surgeons will place a direct atrial line to monitor the transpulmonary gradient (SVC pressure—atrial pressure)
3. Before coming off bypass, ensure that sinus rhythm is present or institute sequential pacing; sinus rhythm is essential. Hyperventilate using a short inspiratory phase, minimal peak inspiratory pressure, and PEEP just adequate to maintain optimal lung volumes.
4. After bypass, maintain the CVP at 14–16 mmHg and atrial pressures of 4–8 mmHg to maintain pulmonary blood flow. The gradient across the pulmonary vascular bed should be less than 10 mmHg.
5. Early return to spontaneous ventilation and extubation augment pulmonary blood flow.
6. Fluid retention with peripheral edema, pleural and pericardial effusions, and ascites is common. Protein-losing enteropathy may occur in some children.

Tricuspid Atresia

Tricuspid atresia is a condition in which there is no communication between the right atrium and the RV, which is usually hypoplastic. Survival depends on the presence of an adequate atrial communication (PFO or ASD) and a systemic-to-pulmonary shunt (VSD or PDA). Palliation in the neonate is required, and the ASD may have to be enlarged by balloon septostomy. For those children with diminished pulmonary blood flow, a systemic-to-PA shunt, e.g., modified Blalock operation, is performed. Those with increased pulmonary blood flow, CHF, and systemic hypoperfusion need a PA band. Later in life, when the pulmonary vasculature is more developed, palliative procedures toward the single ventricle circulation (bidirectional Glenn and Fontan) are possible.

Truncus Arteriosus

Truncus arteriosus occurs when the pulmonary artery fails to completely separate from the aorta resulting in a communication between the two vessels. Several types have been described:

1. *Type I:* PA arises from the truncus and then divides.
2. *Type II:* separate PAs arise from the posterior truncus.
3. *Type III:* separate PAs arise from the sides of the truncus.

The different types are further classified according to the presence (type A) or absence of a VSD (type B).

Special Considerations

1. DiGeorge syndrome is present in 25% of cases (see Appendix A). In such cases monitor the Ca^{++} level. Immune deficiency is present: use irradiated red blood cells.

2. Increased pulmonary blood flow predisposes to pulmonary vascular hypertensive crises.
3. Low aortic diastolic pressure may result in inadequate coronary flow and myocardial ischemia.
4. The truncal valve is semilunar and usually incompetent.

Anesthesia Plan

1. Children may require preoperative ventilation and inotropic support.
2. SVR and PVR should be maintained to support aortic diastolic pressure and coronary flow. Therefore, avoid hyperventilation, excess O_2, and vasodilating drugs.
3. A high-dose opioid technique is preferred.
4. After CPB and postoperatively, institute measures to protect against pulmonary vascular crisis.

Heart Transplantation

Indications

1. Severe congenital malformations, e.g., HLHS, or failed previous surgical corrections of CHD not amenable to further surgery.
2. Cardiomyopathy—progressive with no chance of timely remission.
3. Myocardial tumors not amenable to resection (rare).

General Principles

1. The preoperative PVR is the most important determinant of the suitability of the infant or child for transplantation. Neonates have a high PVR, but a neonatal donor heart should be able to cope with this as PVR decreases over the first weeks of life. Otherwise, for older children, strategies must be used

to reduce PVR or, failing this, heart-lung transplantation must be considered.

2. Other contraindications to transplantation include serious hepatic, renal, or central nervous system disease and chronic infections, e.g., hepatitis, cytomegalovirus, and human immunodeficiency virus.
3. A stable family and social environment is most desirable to ensure the continued care that will be required after transplantation.

Care of the Donor

Care of the donor child during the organ harvesting is discussed in Chap. 14.

Anesthesia Management of the Recipient: Special Considerations

1. The basic management is similar to that for other open-heart procedures. However, the child may have been urgently admitted and may not have been fasted. Precautions for dealing with the full stomach may be necessary. If a rapid sequence induction is planned, the selected drugs and doses should aim to minimize adverse cardiovascular effects. Ketamine or etomidate may be optimal induction agents for the child with minimal reserve, but exercise caution in children with chronic cardiomyopathy or depleted catecholamine stores.
2. Do not aspirate the stomach after induction if oral cyclosporin was recently given pre-transplant as a component of the antirejection therapy.
3. Most children have very poor cardiac function and a dilated heart; therefore take care to prevent inducing tachycardia, bradycardia, or any additional myocardial depression. A fentanyl-O_2 midazolam, muscle relaxant anesthetic is usually preferred; do not interrupt inotropic agents and/or PGE_1

infusions. Some require additional inotropic support as surgery commences.

4. In children who have had previous cardiac surgery, consider tranexamic acid to reduce perioperative bleeding.
5. PVR should be managed to prevent any further pulmonary vasoconstriction.
6. Neonates with HLHS should be treated for the Norwood procedure before CPB.
7. Infusions of dopamine and dobutamine, isoproterenol, and SNP should be primed for immediate use during weaning from bypass.
8. On weaning from CPB or as the clamps are removed and reperfusion starts, give antirejection drugs as indicated. Sinus tachycardia is often present at this stage, and the action of two atrial pacemakers may be observed (one from the remains of the child's native atrium and one from the implanted atrium). In the absence of sinus rhythm, AV pacing should be commenced. A slow sinus rhythm usually responds to an isoproterenol infusion. Infuse other inotropic solutions, e.g., dopamine, as indicated (see later discussion).
9. Continue measures to minimize PVR.
10. Remember the special properties of the newly implanted but denervated heart:
    (a) Cardiac drugs exert *only their direct effects*; atropine will have no chronotropic effect; anticholinesterases will not affect heart rate. Epinephrine, isoproterenol, and norepinephrine will all increase the heart rate; dopamine and dobutamine remain effective inotropic agents.
    (b) Increased filling pressure will, through the Frank-Starling mechanism, result in increased stroke volume. A CVP of 10–12 mmHg is usually optimal; hypovolemia is poorly tolerated.
    (c) There is no change in heart rate with the respiratory cycle or with a Valsalva maneuver.
    (d) Arrhythmias are uncommon in children, but the response to those antiarrhythmic drugs that have both direct and indirect effects on the heart will be altered:

Digoxin and procainamide normally exert a mixture of direct and indirect effects on the heart and will have a less predictable effect on the denervated heart.

(e) The effects of lidocaine, phenytoin, β-adrenergic blocking drugs, and calcium channel-blocking drugs are direct and similar to those in the intact heart.

Heart-Lung or Lung Transplantation

Lung transplantation is usually performed with the aid of CPB; the considerations are similar to those for heart-lung transplantation.

Indications

1. The indications for heart-lung transplantation are:
   (a) Eisenmenger syndrome.
   (b) Other congenital defects with pulmonary vascular disease.
   (c) Complex CHD, inadequate pulmonary vessels not amenable to further repair.
2. The indications for lung transplantation are:
   (a) Primary PAH.
   (b) Pulmonary fibrosis.
   (c) Cystic fibrosis.

Anesthesia Management of the Donor

The general principles are outlined in Chap. 14. Selection of a donor for lung transplantation is difficult:

1. The lungs must be of appropriate size to fit the thorax of the recipient; if they are too large, atelectasis will result. Perfect match or slightly smaller donor lungs are accepted; otherwise, lobar transplantation or tailoring of the donor lung is required.

2. Before harvesting the lungs, the donor is usually given methylprednisolone and an infusion of PGE_1, which is increased until the systemic arterial pressure decreases by ~10–20%. This produces maximal pulmonary vasodilation before infusion of the pulmoplegic solution.
3. Cardioplegia and pulmoplegia are induced, and the lungs are held inflated before tracheal clamping.
4. In selected cases, donor lung tissue may be obtained from living-related donors, e.g., one lobe from each parent may be transplanted.

Anesthesia Management of the Recipient

1. Older children with critical respiratory disease may be very apprehensive and require sedation with constant measurement of their SaO_2.
2. Before induction, verify administration of immunosuppressants and antibiotics.
3. Induction and maintenance of anesthesia should be planned as for CPB, bearing in mind the advanced respiratory disease.
4. Use a cuffed tube with the cuff positioned just below the vocal cords. Children with cystic fibrosis will require frequent suctioning of the tube during dissection of the native lungs.
5. Maintain meticulous aseptic technique for all procedures; remove all existing intravenous lines and replace them with new lines using strict asepsis. A pulmonary artery catheter may be indicated.
6. Fluid therapy should be limited to basal rates.
7. Antifibrinolytic therapy (ε-aminocaproic acid or tranexamic acid) is recommended to decrease postoperative bleeding.
8. During bypass, be prepared to aseptically reintubate with a new sterile tracheal tube. For children with pulmonary infections, e.g., those with cystic fibrosis, it is reasonable to change the entire breathing circuit. In addition, once the native lungs are removed, the surgeon may request that the proximal trachea and bronchi be lavaged with a tobramycin solution.

After transplant anastomoses are completed fiberoptic bronchoscopy will assess their integrity.

9. Before surgery, dopamine, dobutamine, and PGE_1 infusions should be set up and primed with a carrier solution; those with pulmonary infections may require a phenylephrine infusion (see later discussion). Nitric oxide should be available.
10. Immediately on weaning from CPB or once reperfusion has started, the surgeon may request methylprednisolone and furosemide. Institute inotropic agents as required. Pulmonary function may be improved by albuterol inhalations and aggressive diuretic therapy.
11. Adjust the FIO_2 to maintain oxygen saturation at ±93% to prevent hyperoxic lung damage. Moderate, low peak inflation pressure, and hyperventilation are indicated to maintain pulmonary blood flow; usually PEEP (6–10 cm H_2O) is added to maintain optimal lung volumes, minimize PVR, and prevent pulmonary edema.
12. Children with a history of severe lung infections, e.g., cystic fibrosis, may demonstrate signs of sepsis, i.e., a low BP despite good cardiac function. In such cases, a norepinephrine infusion or low-dose vasopressin may be required.
13. Persistent high PA pressures after transplantation should be treated by the addition of NO to the inhaled gases.
14. Extensive bleeding is to be expected, especially if the child has had a previous thoracotomy.
15. Manage postoperative pain.
16. Anticipate postoperative problems including damage to the phrenic, vagus, or recurrent laryngeal nerves.

Cardiologic Procedures

Cardiac Catheterization

This is usually an elective procedure, and older children will benefit from preoperative teaching, a visit to the catheterization laboratory, and familiarization with the procedures to be performed. Cardiac catheterization may be performed under general anesthesia or with a combination of sedation plus local or regional analgesia. The important prerequisites for gathering reliable catheterization data are as follows:

1. Hemodynamic parameters during sedation/anesthesia should be as close to awake values as possible.
2. Maintain a constant inspired O_2 throughout the procedure; room air is preferred if tolerated.
3. Spontaneous ventilation is preferred; controlled ventilation may change intracardiac shunts and modify intracardiac pressures.
4. The child should be maintained in an optimal physiologic state, i.e., normothermic and well hydrated.

Special Anesthesia Problems

1. The child may be seriously ill and in CHF.
2. The condition may further deteriorate during cardiac catheterization, especially if arrhythmias occur.
3. Contrast media may cause adverse effects.
4. Children with PAH are particularly prone to serious complications during cardiac catheterization and require special consideration.
5. Cardiac perforation with tamponade is always a possibility.

Anesthesia Management

When the procedure is to be performed under sedation, the following technique has proved satisfactory:

1. Establish an intravenous route using local analgesia.
2. Apply monitors (ECG, pulse oximeter, BP cuff, and temperature probe).
3. Maintain a thermoneutral environment, particularly in small infants, e.g., a forced air warming blanket, ± an overhead warmer.
4. Administer IV sedatives if hemodynamically tolerated. When combined with local or regional analgesia, only very small doses of drugs are required to ensure sleep, and very stable cardiovascular parameters are maintained.

5. Small infants may be offered a "sucrose soother" and often settle with this alone.
6. Caudal analgesia may be useful for some children, especially if bilateral femoral catheterization is necessary or if large catheters are to be inserted, e.g., for balloon dilation.
7. Angiography requires that the child remain absolutely still; adequate sedation that prevents movement is necessary. Contrast media can cause aggregation of erythrocytes and, rarely, anaphylaxis. The total dose administered should be recorded, especially in small infants and recommended limits observed.
8. The procedure is usually carried out in a darkened room.
9. When it is considered advisable to ventilate the lungs during the procedure, the same technique (propofol infusion) may be used with the addition of a suitable muscle relaxant, e.g., rocuronium, and tracheal intubation. Normocapnia should be maintained.
10. In some children, the response of the pulmonary circulation to hyperventilation, hyperoxia, or the inhalation of NO may be studied.
11. Post-catheterization the child should be monitored until the effects of sedation resolve and smooth awakening occurs. It is necessary that the child lie quietly to prevent bleeding and bruising at the catheter site; additional mild sedation may be necessary to achieve this state. The catheterization site should be examined for bleeding, and the pulses distal to arterial cannulation should be evaluated regularly. The child may be discharged from PACU when he/she is awake, with stable vital signs, and no evidence of vascular complications.

Interventional Cardiology

Sedation and/or general anesthesia are frequently required for complex interventional techniques. These include:

1. Balloon dilation of pulmonary, mitral, aortic valves, or re-coarctation of the aorta.

2. Occlusion of the ductus arteriosus.
3. Closure of septal defects or fistulas.
4. Balloon dilations and stent placements in conduits, pulmonary arteries, or veins.
5. Percutaneous placement of pulmonary valves.
6. Coiling of collateral vessels.

Special Problems

1. The child may be critically ill.
2. Absolute immobility is essential during the critical stages.
3. An urgent call for open operation if complications occur is a possibility. The heart may be perforated, vessels may be ruptured, or the occlusive device may become displaced. Complications are most likely during valve dilation procedures.
4. A steady hemodynamic state is required for measurements to be made.
5. Simultaneous TEE may be required to monitor results.

Anesthesia Management

1. Standard monitoring as per any open procedure. Two large-bore, reliable intravenous lines should be established. Inotropic medications and syringe pumps should be immediately available and defibrillator pads attached.
2. For some very simple procedures in older children, sedation with propofol with spontaneous ventilation and local analgesia may be suitable.
3. For more complex procedures, e.g., balloon dilation of a stenotic valve, "umbrella" closure of a septal defect, or those that require breath holding, tracheal intubation with neuromuscular block and controlled ventilation is preferred. Anesthesia may be maintained with a propofol infusion if hemodynamically tolerated. Be prepared for major life-threatening arrhythmias and hemodynamic instability during balloon dilations and stent placements.
4. Plans must be made for emergent transfer to the OR should a complication occur. Supplies of blood for rapid transfusion should be immediately available.

5. During the procedure, the anesthesiologist must be vigilant for signs of blood loss or cardiac tamponade.
   (a) Cardiac perforation manifests with hypotension and tachycardia with ectopic beats.
   (b) Cardiac tamponade manifests as hypotension with reduced cardiac motion on fluoroscopy that may be confirmed by ECHO. Emergent pericardiocentesis will be performed with continuous drainage; bleeding that does not resolve will require an emergent thoracotomy.
6. Children with PAH require special considerations:
   (a) During catheterization the response of the pulmonary vasculature to increased levels of oxygen and/or inhalation of NO may be assessed.
   (b) Anesthesia management should be conducted to prevent precipitating increases in PVR.
      - Excessive sedation leading to respiratory depression, increased $PaCO_2$, airway obstruction, and hypoxemia must be prevented. Hypoventilation should be prevented.
      - An adequate level of anesthesia should be ensured during potentially painful stimuli or instrumentation of the airway. Tracheal intubation should be avoided if possible in those with severe PAH.

Electrophysiologic Studies

Children may require anesthesia or sedation for electrophysiologic studies and radiofrequency catheter ablation of accessory conduction pathways for treatment of dysrhythmias, e.g., SVT. These procedures are not painful, except the initial vascular access and the actual ablation, but are generally prolonged and require immobility; consider inserting a urinary catheter and using a warming blanket. General endotracheal anesthesia with controlled ventilation is recommended.

Isoproterenol may be infused during the procedure to elicit dysrhythmias to find accessory conduction pathways. If ablation of such pathways is the goal, defibrillation pads should be in place before the procedure and antiarrhythmic drugs immediately at hand.

An important consideration is the possible effect of anesthesia or sedative drugs and anesthesia techniques on cardiac rhythm generation and conduction. Some anesthetics, e.g., dexmedetomidine and halothane, have much greater effects than others, e.g., propofol. Deep sedation or anesthesia with propofol or balanced anesthesia with nitrous oxide and low-dose isoflurane does not interfere with EP studies or the ability to trigger SVT or VT. Therefore these agents are acceptable during electrophysiologic studies.

Cardioversion

Cardioversion is usually an emergency procedure. The arrhythmia may be severe, markedly reducing cardiac output and producing shock.

Anesthesia Management

Preparation

1. Give 100% O_2 by mask until cardioversion can be performed.
2. Establish the fasting interval.
3. Prepare and check all equipment. Standard monitors are required no matter the location of the cardioversion.
4. Establish reliable intravenous access.

During the Conversion

1. Continue 100% O_2 by mask.
2. When ready to cardiovert, medicate with IV midazolam and induce anesthesia using a sleep dose of propofol (use etomidate or ketamine if cardiac function is poor).
   (a) If the child has a full stomach, perform an RSI as described above. Induce with propofol, ketamine, or etomidate (if a cardiomyopathy is present).

(b) As soon as anesthesia has been induced and good oxygenation achieved, countershock may be applied. Repeat propofol, ketamine, or etomidate doses as needed.

Post-procedure

1. The period of recovery is brief but the child should be closely monitored (including ECG) for several hours afterward.
2. If the trachea was intubated, remove the endotracheal tube after the child is fully conscious.

Anesthesia for Cardiac MRI

MRI studies provide a very important tool for mapping the anatomy of the heart. General anesthesia with intubation may be required if the child is unstable or if apneas are required for better imaging.

Special Anesthesia Problems

1. All considerations for sedation or anesthesia in the MRI unit must be observed (see Chap. 19).
2. The specific considerations of the child's cardiac disease must be addressed.
3. If tracheal intubation is required, children with potential difficult intubation should be intubated in the OR and then transferred to the MRI suite. All children should recover in a properly staffed and equipped PACU.

General Anesthetic Management

1. Apply the usual monitors.
2. The selected anesthetic technique depends on the physiologic status of the child and the needs of the radiologist; stable children may be induced by inhalation of sevoflurane or a titrated IV dose of propofol. Potentially unstable children may be

managed using an infusion of opioids and small doses of midazolam.
3. If breath holding will be required, a non-depolarizing agent should be used.
4. The lungs may be ventilated with an FIO_2 that is most appropriate for the specific cardiac defect and will maintain adequate oxygenation during the frequent apnea periods.

Anesthesia for Non-cardiac Surgery in Infants and Children with Congenital Heart Disease

CHD often occurs in association with other congenital defects, some of which may require surgery in the neonate or infant. Older children with CHD frequently require anesthesia for non-cardiac procedures, e.g., dental surgery. Some of these children have uncorrected cardiac lesions, others have undergone partial (palliation) procedures, and others have had complete repair of their defect. However, even after "complete repair" there may be important considerations, such as the need for prophylactic antibiotics (see Chap. 12) the presence of a pacemaker for heart block, or other residual defects. After repair of complex lesions, the post-repair physiology, e.g., post-Fontan repair, may require special perioperative considerations; the appearance of an intraoperative arrhythmia may be a very important observation indicating the potential for a more serious sudden cardiac event and should be reported to the child's cardiologist.

Identifying the Patient with Congenital Heart Disease

The first challenge may be to determine whether the child has CHD. Although some children with CHD may be diagnosed in utero, many still go unrecognized throughout the neonatal period. In neonates, the diagnosis of CHD can be quite difficult (see previous discussion). All neonates with defects that are commonly associated with CHD, e.g., midline defects including tracheoesophageal fistula, diaphragmatic hernia, and omphalocele, should be screened with an ECHO.

Older children may be found to have a previously undetected and undiagnosed murmur when examined before anesthesia. The problem is to determine whether significant heart disease is present and whether it is necessary to refer the child to a cardiologist. First, it is important to determine whether the child has normal exercise tolerance. It is very unlikely that a child with unlimited activity has a lesion that will cause problems during anesthesia. On physical examination, the characteristics of the murmur should be analyzed:

1. *Innocent murmurs* are soft, systolic, and not radiating; they may vary with position, may disappear on exercise, and are not characteristic of any lesion.
2. *Non-innocent murmurs* include all diastolic murmurs, all pansystolic and late systolic murmurs, all loud murmurs, all continuous murmurs (except venous hum), and all transmitted murmurs.

If a soft and presumably innocent murmur is heard in a healthy child, surgery usually is not delayed. If a murmur suggestive of a definite, previously undiagnosed cardiac lesion is heard, delay elective surgery and refer to a cardiologist. Emergency surgery must proceed, and the child should be managed with due regard for the cardiac disease; prophylactic antibiotics should be administered when indicated (see Chap. 12) and appropriate monitoring established.

Anesthesia Management

Preoperative

1. Many of the potential problems during non-cardiac surgery are similar to those associated with cardiac surgery, and the same considerations for each specific lesion apply. For major surgery, the child should be monitored as for cardiac surgery.

2. The anesthesiologist must clearly understand the pathophysiology of the child's heart disease and assess the current physical status (See heading above Diagnosis of Congenital Heart Disease, p446).
3. The child's current medications must be reviewed, particularly clarifying those which should be administered or withheld on the day of surgery.
4. Care must be taken to avoid excessive fluid restriction, especially in children with cyanotic CHD. The parents should be instructed to encourage clear fluids up until 2 h before the operation. If oral fluids cannot be taken, intravenous fluid therapy must be established.
5. Monitor SpO_2 if premedication is indicated. Apply a topical analgesic cream to the intravenous site.
6. Cardiopulmonary resuscitation equipment (including a defibrillator with paddles of suitable size) should be immediately available.
7. Check the coagulation status in children with cyanotic heart disease; coagulopathy is common in those with polycythemia.
8. Choose the anesthetic prescription:
   (a) Use extreme care with inhaled anesthetics or other cardiac depressants, especially in those at risk for or with a history of CHF or cardiomyopathy.
   (b) Avoid causing major changes in PVR or SVR, especially those with PAH.
      - Monitor and maintain ventilation and oxygenation.
      - Avoid vasodilating drugs
9. Administer antibiotic prophylaxis for children undergoing dental surgery with the cardiac defects listed (Table 12.1).
10. Routine prophylactic antibiotic therapy is not recommended for the prevention of infective endocarditis in children undergoing gastrointestinal or GU surgery. However, check with a cardiologist for their recommendations if in doubt.
11. Minimally invasive video assisted surgery is used for many procedures and provides the same advantages of decreased postoperative pain and more rapid recovery for the cardiac patient. However, the special considerations for these procedures (see Chap. 14) must be observed together with the

requirements dictated by the cardiac lesion. Provided intra-abdominal pressure is maintained at below 10 mmHg most children will tolerate these procedures.

12. For children with a Fontan who are scheduled for non-cardiac surgery, maintain the preload, prevent myocardial depression, and ensure that PVR remains optimal. While spontaneous ventilation is ideal, hypercapnia will attenuate pulmonary blood flow and reduce cardiac output; do not oversedate. If controlled ventilation is chosen, adjust settings to minimize the intrathoracic pressure (using brief inspiratory times, limited peak inspiratory pressure, and minimal PEEP). Euvolemia should be assured to maintain the preload.

Perioperative

1. After stable vital signs, establish a reliable intravenous route; remove all air bubbles from the intravenous lines, especially for children with right-to-left or bidirectional shunts.
2. Give 100% O_2 by mask unless the defect is an unrepaired single ventricle or large VSD with pulmonary over circulation.
3. Induce anesthesia with titrated doses of intravenous propofol, ketamine, or etomidate depending on the cardiac defect. Otherwise, induce anesthesia with sevoflurane, but beware of depressing the myocardium or triggering airway obstruction and hypoxemia-induced PAH.
4. Intubate the trachea for all but the most minor procedure. Give a suitable relaxant, but remember that if the circulation time is prolonged, there will be a longer delay before muscle paralysis is complete.
5. Children with less severe disease tolerate low concentrations of inhalational agents; for minor procedures, maintain anesthesia with N_2O and sevoflurane or isoflurane with spontaneous or assisted ventilation. Children with more severe disease and those with any history of CHF cannot tolerate potent inhalational anesthetics. These children should be managed with high-dose opioid, midazolam, and relaxant, with controlled ventilation.
6. Monitor the oxygen saturation recognizing that pulse oximeters yield less accurate readings at lower saturations.

7. For major non-cardiac surgery, insert an arterial and other lines and monitor the child as for cardiac surgery. Consider the effects of previous surgery, e.g., systemic-to-pulmonary shunts, in choosing the BP cuff location.
8. $PetCO_2$ may not correlate well and tends to underestimate $PaCO_2$ in those children with right-to-left shunts, but it does give valuable information as a trend indicator of cardiac output and pulmonary blood flow.
9. Replace blood and fluid deficits and losses as indicated.

Postoperative

1. Continue to monitor the child until the child has fully recovered from all effects of anesthesia. Transfer to the PICU or PACU as appropriate.
2. Give O_2 until recovery is complete. Those with cyanotic CHD have a reduced ventilatory response to hypoxemia.
3. Ensure adequate analgesia to limit oxygen demand.
4. Maintain IV fluids until oral intake is adequate, but avoid overhydration.

Suggested Reading

Agarwal HS, Wolfram KB, Saville BR, et al. Postoperative complications and association with outcomes in pediatric cardiac surgery. J Thorac Cardiovasc Surg. 2014;148:609–16.

Alkhatip AAAMM, Kamel MG, Farag EM, et al. Deep hypothermic circulatory arrest in the pediatric population undergoing cardiac surgery with electroencephalography monitoring: a systematic review and meta-analysis. J Cardiothorac Vasc Anesth. 2021;35:2875–88.

Andropoulos DB, Easly RB, Gottlieb EA, et al. Neurologic injury in neonates undergoing cardiac surgery. Clin Perinatol. 2019;46:657–71.

Black CS, Kushnood A, Holtby H, Hepburn L. Cardiac transplantation in children. BJA. Education. 2019;19:105–12.

Chen D, Du Y. Analysis of perioperative corticosteroid therapy in children undergoing cardiac surgery: systematic review and meta-analysis. Clin Cardiol. 2023;46:607–14.

Doshi RR, Qu JZ. Preoperative and postoperative anesthetic assessment for pediatric cardiac surgery patients. Int Anesthesiol Clin. 2004;42(4):1–13.

Elmitwalli I, Abdelhady E, Kalsotra S, et al. Use of high-flow nasal cannula versus other noninvasive ventilation techniques or conventional oxygen therapy for respiratory support following pediatric cardiac surgery: a systematic review and meta-analysis. Pediatr Anesth. 2024;34:519–31.

Garg RK, Thareen JK, Mehmood A, et al. Fast tracking after repair of congenital cardiac defects. Ind J Thorac Cardiovasc Surg. 2021;37:183–9.

Holtby HM. Anesthetic considerations for neonates undergoing modified Blalock-Taussig shunt and variations. Paediatr Anaesth. 2014;24:114–9.

Knott EM, Fraser JD, Alemayahu H, et al. Evaluation of cardiac function during laparoscopic gastrostomy in pediatric patients with hypoplastic left heart syndrome using intraoperative transesophageal echocardiography. J Laparoendosc Adv Surg Tech A. 2014;24:738–41.

Lam JE, Lin EP, Alexy R, Aronson LA. Anesthesia and the pediatric cardiac catheterization suite: a review. Paediatr Anaesth. 2015;25:127–34.

McNamara JR, McMahon A, Griffin M. Perioperative management of the Fontan patient for cardiac and noncardiac surgery. J Cardiothor Vasc Anaesth. 2022;36:275–85.

Murphy T. Anesthetist-delivered intraoperative transesophageal echocardiography in paediatric cardiac surgery. Pediatr Anesth. 2019;29:499–505.

Schlunt ML, Brauer SD. Anesthetic management for the pediatric patient undergoing deep hypothermic circulatory arrest. Semin Cardiothorac Vasc Anesth. 2007;11(1):16–22.

Sperotto F, Gearhart A, Hoskote A, et al. Cardiac arrest and cardiopulmonary resuscitation in pediatric patients with cardiac disease: a narrative review. Eur J Paediatr. 2023;182:4289–308.

Spiro J, Bauerle J, Njoku D. Anesthesia for children with congenital heart disease undergoing non-cardiac surgery. BJA Educ. 2024;24:458–67.

Twite MD, Ing RJ. Anaesthetic considerations in infants with hypoplastic left heart syndrome. Semin Cardiovasc Vasc Anesth. 2013;17:137–45.

Wacker J, Joye R, Genecand L, et al. Pulmonary vascular disease as a complication of pediatric congenital heart diseases. Transl Pediatr. 2023;12:1041–52.

Wadia RS, Bernier ML, Diaz-Rodriguez NM, et al. Update on perioperative pediatric pulmonary hypertension management. J Cardiovasc Vasc Anesth. 2022;36:667–76.

Orthopedics

16

Many children undergoing elective orthopedic surgery have multiple congenital anomalies and/or neuromuscular disease (see Appendix A). Underlying diseases, particularly those associated with muscle weakness, require special anesthesia care; even minor surgery may be fraught with major anesthesia complications.

General Principles

1. Children with orthopedic deformities may require repeated surgery and spend much time in the hospital; sympathetic management and the liberal use of preoperative sedation are particularly important.
2. Take a complete history. Neuromuscular diseases affect the doses of muscle relaxants; with myopathies, succinylcholine should be avoided (see Appendix A). Drug selection depends on the underlying disease and whether neuromonitoring will be needed. Children with cerebral palsy have contractures and must be positioned appropriately.
3. Scoliosis surgeries are extensive and may involve massive blood loss. To minimize blood transfusions, consider preoperative blood donation, autotransfusion, and acute normovolemic hemodilution. Amicar and tranexamic acid decrease blood loss.

J. Lerman, C. J. Coté, *Steward's Manual of Pediatric Anesthesia*,
https://doi.org/10.1007/978-3-032-24545-8_16

4. Malignant hyperthermia is more common in children with orthopedic diseases. (see Chap. 8).
5. Always establish a reliable IV route and confirm that blood is available.
   (a) A tourniquet effectively eliminates blood loss. When a tourniquet is inflated, heart rate and blood pressure increase progressively possibly the result of sympathetic stimulation. If inhaled agents are used to treat tourniquet-induced hypertension, the blood pressure may decrease precipitously when the tourniquet is released.
   (b) Hemodynamic and metabolic responses to tourniquet release in children are usually not clinically severe. A transient decrease in arterial pH associated with an increase in base deficit and carbon dioxide tension ($PaCO_2$) may occur, particularly after prolonged tourniquet times or bilateral tourniquets. General recommendations include:
      - Attempt to limit tourniquet times to <75 min.
      - Use controlled ventilation before and after tourniquet release to prevent respiratory acidosis.
      - Do not release bilateral tourniquets simultaneously.
      - In children in whom metabolic or respiratory acidosis is not easily compensated, i.e., those with renal disease or pulmonary disease, consider staged release of the tourniquet(s) and close monitoring of $PetCO_2$.
      - Serious complications of tourniquet use in children are very rare; however, pulmonary embolism on deflation has been reported in obese children. Consult the surgeon regarding prophylactic measures to prevent deep vein thromboses in such children.
      - Ensure that the tourniquet is removed from the limb as soon as it is deflated; residual pressure compromising perfusion of the limb has resulted in serious complications.
6. Postoperative pain may be substantive after orthopedic surgery. Begin pain management before emergence including regional analgesia when possible. Continuous peripheral nerve blocks using disposable pumps after limb or trunk surgery are effective.

7. Compartment syndrome may complicate orthopedic injuries, especially supracondylar fractures of the humerus and forearm, and tibial fractures. Effective analgesia may mask the presenting signs of this syndrome, i.e., increased pain, especially when the limb cannot be examined, e.g., in a cast. Compartment syndrome is sufficiently rare that withholding effective analgesia is unreasonable; there is no evidence to confirm that regional analgesic regimens delay the diagnosis of compartment syndrome. Effective postoperative pain relief should therefore be provided to every child. Increased analgesic requirements, breakthrough pain, or pain remote from the surgical site should prompt direct measurement of compartment pressure.
8. Urinary retention may occur in children who have lower limb surgery and are treated with a regional block that includes an opioid. This should be noted by post-anesthesia care unit (PACU) staff and treated as necessary.
9. Children with cerebral palsy frequently present for orthopedic surgery. They require special considerations (see Chap. 8).
10. Children with Duchenne muscular dystrophy who present for major scoliosis surgery require meticulous assessment of their cardiorespiratory status; anticipate bleeding (see later discussion and Appendix A).

Miscellaneous Orthopedic Procedures and Anesthesia Considerations

Hip Arthrogram

Hip arthrograms are performed in infants to assess the head of the femur and other aspects of the hip joint. As part of the procedure, a small amount of air may be injected into the joint to ensure that the tip of the needle is in the joint space before injecting contrast material; serious air embolism and cardiac arrest have occurred.

Recommendation: If a hip arthrogram is planned, determine whether air will be injected. Monitor the child very carefully during injection, eliminate nitrous oxide, and monitor for evidence of an air embolism.

Club Feet

Beware of the high incidence of myopathies in children with club feet; if the medical history or physical examination is suggestive of a myopathy, revise the anesthesia technique accordingly.

In some cases, regional analgesia combined with intravenous sedation may be optimal; caudal epidural analgesia may augment intraoperative management and provide postoperative analgesia.

Limb Fractures

Closed Limb Fractures

Injuries to upper limbs are common; regional analgesia may be appropriate in cooperative children and adolescents. If so:

1. Use an adequate dose of local anesthetic to produce a profound block.
2. Perform the block so it has time to become established before the surgery.
3. **Do not allow the surgeon to manipulate the limb until the block is satisfactorily established**.
4. If supplementary sedation is required, IV midazolam or a low-dose propofol infusion is usually satisfactory.

Fractures of the Forearm

1. A block of the brachial plexus via the axillary route or supraclavicular approach is appropriate (see Chap. 7); ultrasound guidance is preferred.
2. Intravenous blocks are usually not satisfactory for reduction of proximal fractures but may be effective for distal fractures.

Fractures of the Femur

1. A block of the femoral nerve with ropivacaine or bupivacaine is easy to perform and relieves pain and muscle spasms if traction is applied.
2. A catheter may be introduced to the femoral sheath and a continuous femoral nerve block maintained (see continuous femoral block Chap. 7).

General Anesthesia

Perioperative

Every child with a recent fracture must be considered to have a full stomach and an RSI should be performed. Vomiting frequently occurs during emergence from anesthesia; therefore, the child should be fully awake and in a lateral position before extubation.

Postoperative

1. Pain may be quite severe even after routine orthopedic surgery and should be controlled using systemic opioids, regional analgesia, and/or non-opioid analgesics, e.g., NSAIDs, dexmedetomidine, or ketamine, or a combination of these:
   (a) Regimens combining acetaminophen and a non-steroidal anti-inflammatory drugs (NSAIDs) are more effective than either drug alone. Acetaminophen, ibuprofen, or diclofenac augmented by incremental doses of opioids as required is a suitable basic regimen. Pain should be assessed using standard objective measures (see Chap. 20).
   (b) Patient-controlled analgesia (PCA) may be appropriate for many children over the age of 4 or 5 years (see Chap. 20).
   (c) Regional analgesia has shifted from neuraxial to peripheral nerve blocks. In children, regional blocks and catheters are inserted under general anesthesia. Ultrasonography should be used to place peripheral nerve blocks and catheters.
   (d) Peripheral nerve blocks are initiated in the operating room and continued through the PACU to the ward or even to

home using disposable elastomeric infusion pumps. The decision to continue an infusion at home will depend upon the social circumstances and the attitude and abilities of the parents. A postoperative infusion of ropivacaine is effective for most peripheral nerve blocks.

Scoliosis and Kyphoscoliosis

Scoliosis is more common than kyphoscoliosis in children, with adolescent idiopathic scoliosis occurring in ~3% of adolescents; more common in females (~80%) and is characterized by a thoracolumbar spinal curvature (left to right). This deformity is congenital (~15%), idiopathic (~65%), or secondary to neuromuscular disease (~20%) in origin. In contrast, kyphoscoliosis occurs in only ~0.1% of children, with Scheuermann's disease being the most common, although it also occurs in children with spina bifida, via genetics, and after trauma. The kyphotic deformity is an outward (dorsal, usually thoracic) curvature of the spine. Pulmonary function may be impaired, and some children with associated diseases (myopathies, cerebral palsy) may be severely disabled, wheelchair-bound, and physiologically debilitated.

Pulmonary Function

Changes in pulmonary function are related to the underlying cause, the speed of development of the scoliosis, and the severity of the curvature. The cardiorespiratory effects of scoliosis are summarized in Fig. 16.1.

The principal parental and patient concerns may include the cosmetic effect of the spinal, pelvic, and chest wall deformity, especially when the curvature increases during the years of rapid body growth. At this stage, respiratory symptoms are uncommon, although pulmonary function studies may be abnormal with normal lung volumes but reduced exercise tolerance. With progression, the mechanical effects of scoliosis on respiratory function become symptomatic even at rest.

Pulmonary function is relatively normal in most children who present for correction of idiopathic scoliosis with a curvature of

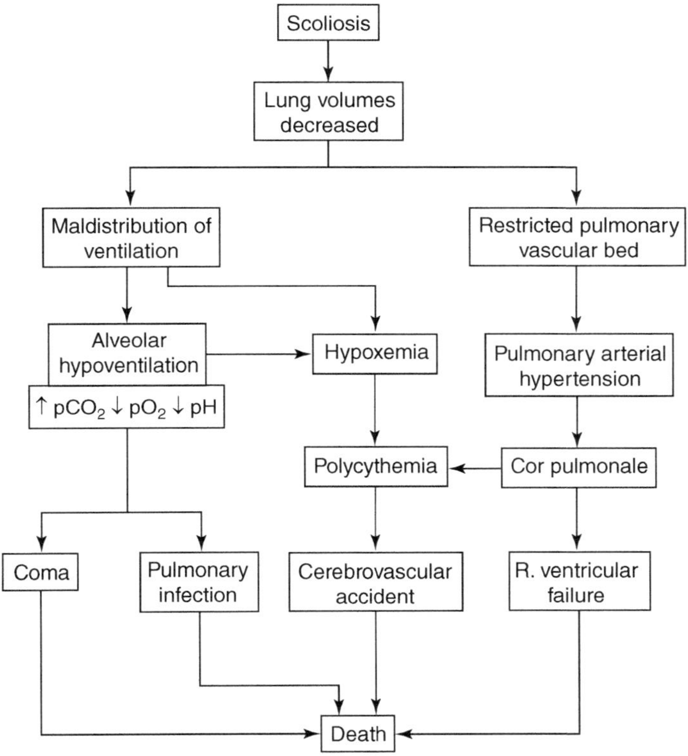

Fig. 16.1 Pathophysiology of the cardiorespiratory effects of kyphoscoliosis. Progressive alveolar hypoventilation, leading to hypoxia, may be accompanied by pulmonary hypertension and right ventricular failure. (Courtesy Henry Levison, MD, Former Director of Respiratory Physiology, The Hospital for Sick Children, Toronto)

less than 65%. Respiratory disability is more likely with congenital scoliosis and curvature of paralytic etiology.

The pulmonary abnormality follows a restrictive pattern, with reduced chest wall compliance. The vital capacity, FEV_1 (forced expiratory volume in 1 second), and the total lung capacity may be dramatically reduced and the functional residual capacity less so. The residual volume tends to be maintained. The elastic resistance of the chest wall may be high, increasing the work of breathing. If left untreated, severe and prolonged lung compression impairs gas exchange in later stages of the disease.

The High-Risk Scoliotic Child

Scoliosis surgery may be recommended for severely incapacitated children for the purpose of facilitating their ongoing care (such as sitting upright) and arresting the progression of cardiorespiratory compromise. There is a very high incidence of perioperative complications in this cohort and many require prolonged postoperative intensive care; however, the ultimate outcome is judged by many of these children and their caregivers to be worthwhile. It is very important that these children be optimally prepared for their surgery:

1. The nutritional status should be optimized.
2. The pulmonary system should be evaluated for reversible disease that might be improved by physiotherapy or antibiotic therapy. Those with neuromuscular disease and a preoperative $FEV_1 < 40\%$ of predicted are likely to need postoperative ventilation.
3. The cardiac status should be evaluated by echocardiogram, i.e., myocardial contractility, RV function, etc., and preoperative therapy initiated as indicated.

Surgical Procedures

1. Posterior spinal fusion may be performed using contoured metal rods to stabilize the spine until bony fusion occurs. In some children with a flexible spine, the deformity is corrected solely by a posterior fusion. Adjustable rods may be placed in young children to permit adjustments during growth.
2. In some, an anterior thoraco-abdominal approach may be used to remove the intervertebral discs or a hemivertebra to correct a lateral curve. This may be an open procedure or an endoscopic procedure in which case the special considerations for endoscopic surgery apply (see Chap. 14).
3. In others, the two procedures are combined: an anterior release followed by a posterior fusion. In this case, surgery is often prolonged and blood loss significant.

Special Anesthetic Problems

1. Anesthetic management should consider:
   (a) The severity and cause of the curvature. The more severe the curve, the more pulmonary function is impaired, and greater the likelihood of postoperative pulmonary failure.

   If the scoliosis is secondary to neuromuscular disease:
   - Pulmonary function impairment caused by the mechanical effects of the spinal curvature may be compounded by involvement of respiratory muscles in the disease process. Postoperative respiratory insufficiency is more likely.
   - Increased bleeding may be expected. This may results from altered vascular responses and platelet adhesion associated with myopathies, e.g., Duchenne muscular dystrophy.
   - Cardiomyopathy may occur in adolescents with Duchenne muscular dystrophy.
   - Selection of suitable drugs may be limited, e.g., avoid succinylcholine and inhalational anesthetics to prevent rhabdomyolysis if a myopathy is present. Titrate doses of non-depolarizing relaxants if required.

   (b) The degree of respiratory and cardiovascular impairment:
   - Surgery may be expected to stabilize the cardiorespiratory effects of the disease but may not result in improvement.
   - A further impairment of pulmonary function must be anticipated in the early postoperative phase and may require respiratory support.

   (c) The type of corrective procedure proposed.
   - Posterior fusion only.
   - Anterior and posterior fusion combined.
2. Preoperative assessment must include the following:
   (a) A detailed history and examination for disabilities, stamina, and the presence of related medical conditions.
   (b) Routine hematology, coagulation, biochemistry studies, and cross-match.

   (c) Pulmonary function studies, including blood gas analysis if feasible (these may not be possible in very young children due to lack of cooperation).
   (d) Echocardiogram to assess myocardial function, particularly adolescents, with very severe curves or an associated myopathy.
3. Be alert for signs of respiratory impairment, i.e., tachypnea at rest, severely reduced vital capacity, abnormal blood gas values, inability to cough effectively. Postoperative hypoventilation, secretion retention, and atelectasis are likely in response to pain, analgesic drugs, and immobilization that will further compound existing problems.
4. Severe impairment of respiratory function is not a contraindication to surgery provided appropriate resources are available for postoperative intensive respiratory care. Fixation of the spinal deformity is essential to prevent further deterioration of respiratory function but usually does not result in significant early improvement.
5. Children with a vital capacity less than 40% of normal or a Cobb angle of >69° may develop major postoperative respiratory complications and likely will require postoperative ventilation.

Corrective Surgery by the Posterior Approach

Special Anesthetic Problems

1. Pulmonary function may be severely impaired; ensure pulmonary function is optimal and an acute respiratory exacerbation is not present. If preoperative curvature correction has been achieved with an exoskeletal apparatus, intubation will likely be difficult; advanced airway adjuncts such as the GlideScope or a fiberoptic technique may be needed.
2. Preoperatively, the patient and family should be informed that once anesthesia has commenced, invasive lines will be inserted, that blood may be required during and after surgery, that sedation may be required postoperatively, and their breathing tube may remain in place postoperatively until it is safe to remove it. Also,

the patient should be warned that an intraoperative wake-up test may be needed, which means they will be asked to wiggle their toes, but will not feel pain, are unlikely to recall the wake-up, and will be re-anesthetized thereafter until surgery is complete.

3. Blood loss may be severe (in excess of 50% of the estimated blood volume [EBV]). Most bleeding originates from the vertebral veins, which become engorged if there is any pressure on the anterior abdomen. Blood loss is also related to the length of spine to be fused and to the surgeon's speed and expertise. Those with scoliosis secondary to a recognized neuromuscular disorder usually have a larger blood loss than those with idiopathic scoliosis. Alternatives to homologous transfusion should be considered:
   (a) Preoperative autologous blood donation.
   (b) Intraoperative moderate normovolemic hemodilution (hemoglobin not less than 8 Gm%) may be used. Hemoglobin may be increased preoperatively by administering oral ferrous sulfate and Vitamin C daily beginning 4 weeks before surgery, followed by twice-weekly intramuscular injections of erythropoietin commencing 2 weeks before surgery. The hematocrit (Hct) should not be allowed to exceed 55% preoperatively.
   (c) A cell saver may be used to salvage erythrocytes, however, transfusion of large volumes of washed cells may lead to dilutional coagulopathy. Fresh-frozen plasma should be available and administered if blood loss exceeds one blood volume.
   (d) Tranexamic acid or Amicar may be infused during surgery to attenuate blood loss.
4. Spinal cord function is usually monitored: the use of somatosensory-evoked potentials (SSEPs) has been augmented by the addition of motor-evoked potentials (MEPs), stimulating the cord above the level of the surgery and recording the electromyogram from the limbs.

   Anesthetic techniques to facilitate monitoring of evoked potentials limit inhalational agents to 0.5 MAC. A TIVA technique with <50% nitrous oxide is preferred. If MEPs are indicated, better results are obtained with minimal neuromuscular, i.e., two to four twitches on a train of four, or no blockade; this should be discussed with the neurophysiologist. A depth of anesthesia monitor is advised to facilitate a rapid recovery. For transcranial MEPs, a bite block should be inserted to prevent tongue and lip lacerations.

Despite the use of multimodal neurophysiologic monitoring, a wake-up test may still be required, i.e., a surgical misadventure or failure of the monitoring system. Fortunately, the anesthesia technique that provides for neurophysiologic monitoring also allows for a rapid wake-up test should this be required.

Every child should be awake at the end of the operation, so that both sensory and motor function can be tested.

5. Postoperative pain may be considerable; intraoperative intrathecal morphine administered by the surgeon has been effective for postoperative analgesia and may also facilitate intraoperative BP control and reduce blood loss. Otherwise, epidural analgesia or PCA should be planned and these options discussed with the child and family.
6. Visual loss is a rare (incidence <0.2%) but serious complication after spine surgery.
   (a) The most common ocular injury after surgery is a corneal abrasion. Far less common is visual loss because of posterior ischemic optic neuropathy (PION) (which occurs three times more frequently than anterior (AION)) or central retinal artery occlusion (CRAO)—especially when surgery is performed in the prone position.
   (b) Age: It rarely occurs in patients <18 years of age.
   (c) Factors associated with visual loss because of ION include preoperative anemia, prolonged surgery, intraoperative hypotension, low intraoperative hematocrit, and major blood loss. CRAO results from direct orbital compression.
   (d) A possible but unproven factor in the genesis of post-spinal visual loss is excessive intraoperative crystalloid administration, which increases intraocular pressure and causes periorbital edema.

   N.B. Visual loss recovers in 44% of those with ION but in none of those with CRAO.

Precautions that may reduce the risk of intraoperative visual loss include:

1. Staged procedures if the proposed operation is anticipated to be excessively prolonged (>6 h) or associated with large blood losses (>45% of the EBV).
2. Positioning:
   (a) Avoid pressure on the eyes—check frequently during surgery and document these assessments in the anesthesia record.
   (b) Position the head in a neutral forward position (no neck flexion, extension, or rotation) level with or above the heart.
3. Monitor the hematocrit and avoid markedly reduced values.
4. Administer balanced fluids to maintain euvolemia.
5. Induced hypotension is no longer recommended; a 15–20% reduction from baseline or a mean arterial pressure >65 mmHg or systolic pressure >80 mmHg is likely safe but unstudied.

Check the child's vision immediately upon awakening and seek consultation if there are any defects.

Anesthetic Management

Preoperative

1. Review the pertinent laboratory, echocardiographic, and pulmonary function studies.
2. Oral or IV midazolam premedication is usually preferred.
3. Avoid respiratory depressant drugs in those with impaired respiratory function.
4. Verify an adequate supply of blood and other fluid replacements is available.

Perioperative

1. If halo-gravity traction is in place, ensure that instruments to release the connecting rods are immediately available.
2. Tracheal intubation:

(a) In uncomplicated cases, induce anesthesia with propofol or thiopental followed by a low dose of an intermediate-acting relaxant, e.g., rocuronium 0.3–0.4 mg/kg, and intubate. If evoked potential monitoring is planned, allow the child to recover from the neuromuscular blockade, then confirm the function of the stimulating electrodes.

(b) If an exoskeletal apparatus is present, direct laryngoscopy may be difficult.
- Have difficult airway equipment immediately available.
- Select a suitable intubation technique, e.g., fiberoptic intubation or video laryngoscope.

3. Maintenance:

Generally, a balanced anesthetic with low-dose inhalation agent and opioid or propofol and opioid, i.e., total intravenous anesthesia [TIVA], depending on the neuromonitoring.

(a) Opioid infusions:
- Fentanyl-loading dose of 5 μg/kg; infusion rate of 3 μg/kg/h.
- Morphine-loading dose of 100 μg/kg; infusion rate of 10–30 μg/kg/h.
- Remifentanil infusion at 0.1 μg/kg/min and adjust to control the blood pressure.

(b) Low-dose isoflurane (0.5–1%), sevoflurane (1–1.5%), or desflurane (3–5%) to control the BP. Small doses of inhalation agent do not usually interfere with neurophysiologic monitoring. If MEPs are planned, neuromuscular blockade is generally permitted only for tracheal intubation.

(c) TIVA: This is a useful technique when multimodal neurophysiologic monitoring is to be performed. Low-dose propofol (100–150 μg/kg/min) administered with remifentanil (0.1–0.3 μg/kg/min) provides satisfactory anesthesia. The dose of propofol may be further modified based on anesthetic depth. The remifentanil infusion may be adjusted according to hemodynamic parameters. Other sedative drugs (dexmedetomidine and/or midazolam) may be administered to complement BP control, amnesia and prevent shivering postop.

   (d) Nitrous oxide >50% is avoided as it interferes with neurophysiologic monitoring.
   (e) Insert a nasogastric tube to treat possible postoperative ileus and a soft bite block to prevent dental damage and intraoral soft tissue lacerations from trans-cortical MEP stimulation.
4. Position the child to avoid pressure on the anterior abdominal wall. Periodically, assess the correct prone-suspended position to ensure that there is no abdominal pressure that would increase venous pressure and blood loss or external pressure on the eyes to obviate postoperative visual loss.
5. Monitor the following throughout:
   (a) Ventilation-esophageal stethoscope, airway pressure, $PetCO_2$.
   (b) Circulation—ECG, pulse oximeter, arterial line, and central venous pressure (CVP).
   (c) Temperature—rectal or esophageal probe.
   (d) Neuromuscular blockade—peripheral nerve stimulator.
   (e) Blood loss—gravimetric method and graduated suction bottles.
   (f) Urine output—indwelling catheter.
   (g) SSEPs and/or MEPs—before, during, and after correction.
   (h) Hematology and biochemistry—acid–base and blood gas status, Hct, and coagulation status as indicated by the duration and severity of the procedure.
   (i) Monitor the depth of anesthesia, although neurophysiological monitoring provides similar feedback.
6. Minimize blood loss by:
   (a) Proper positioning (see item 4 above).
   (b) Infiltration of the wound site (by the surgeon) with a dilute epinephrine/saline solution (up to 500 mL of 1:500,000 solution).
   (c) Controlled ventilation, maintaining $PaCO_2$ at 30–35 mmHg to avoid hypercarbia and vasodilation.
   (d) Moderate hypotensive techniques may be used, but the MAP should be maintained as described above. In the prone child, the spinal cord is above the heart and, if hypotension occurs, spinal cord ischemia may ensue, especially

while it is manipulated or stretched, leading to paraplegia. Do not combine a hypotensive technique with hemodilution.

(e) Acute normovolemic hemodilution, i.e., an alternative blood conservation method, requires:
  - A calculated volume of blood is withdrawn after induction to reduce the Hct to ~30%. Use the preoperative Hct and the EBV (in milliliters) to calculate the volume to be withdrawn:

$$\text{Volume withdrawn} = (\text{Hct} - 30) \times \text{EBV} / \text{Hct}$$

  - When the child is anesthetized and lines have been inserted, a weighed volume of blood is withdrawn via the arterial line into citrate-phosphate-dextrose bags for storage.
  - During blood withdrawal, a volume of warmed lactated Ringer's solution equal to three times the blood volume withdrawn is infused or 1:1 replacement with 5% albumen.
  - As surgery progresses, the blood that has been withdrawn is reinfused. This method results in loss of lower-Hct blood during surgery and conservation of the child's cells, clotting factors and platelets for reinfusion.
  - Monitor the oxygen tension (PaO_2) and pH to ensure an adequate tissue supply of oxygen.

(f) Both tranexamic acid and ε-aminocaproic acid decrease blood loss during spine surgery. The selected antifibrinolytic should be initiated after induction of anesthesia but before skin incision and continuously infused until the completion of surgery.

7. If the neurophysiologic recordings show any changes or cannot be obtained for technical reasons, or if the surgeon requires confirmation of spinal cord integrity after application of the distraction and compression apparatus or other manipulation, a wake-up test may be necessary:

(a) Discontinue inhaled anesthetics or TIVA infusions. Check the neuromuscular monitor for the extent of neuromuscular block (if present). Full antagonism is not advisable because it may lead to complications (see later discussion).
(b) Decrease ventilation to return the $PaCO_2$ to normal levels.
(c) Flood the wound with saline to reduce the potential for air embolization.
(d) Ask the child to move the toes (voluntary dorsiflexion and plantarflexion of the feet confirms spinal cord integrity). Beware of allowing the child to awaken too much; excessive movements may result in dangerous loss of position on the frame, and attempts to breathe spontaneously against the ventilator have been reported to result in air embolism.
(e) Have IV midazolam and propofol prepared to rapidly infuse as soon as the test has concluded.

Corrective Surgery by the Anterior Approach

For treatment of a curve in the lumbar region, the vertebral column is approached laterally on the convex side of the curvature. A thoracotomy is performed or using VATS; the diaphragm is divided at its peripheral attachments to provide access to the vertebrae.

N.B. This surgical trauma to the diaphragm and chest wall increases the risk of postoperative respiratory insufficiency.

Anesthesia management is the same as for the posterior approach with the following modifications:

1. Selective endobronchial intubation of the contralateral lung or placement of a bronchial blocker e.g., the Arndt endobronchial blocker, has proven useful for this procedure (see Chap. 14).
2. Serial blood gas measurements dictate the feasibility of continuing this technique throughout the procedure, but it is usually well-tolerated.

3. If bilateral ventilation is selected, ventilation of the exposed lung will be impeded by surgical packing and retractors. Periodically, expand the lung fully (to avoid prolonged atelectasis).

Spinal Osteotomy

Spinal osteotomy with wedge excision consists of local resection of deformed vertebrae. This procedure may result in excessive blood loss owing to the proximity of the vertebral and epidural venous plexuses.

Monitor blood loss by:

1. Gravimetric method by weighing the sponges and measuring suction losses.
2. Continuous CVP measurement and direct BP readings via an arterial line.
3. Clinical observation, e.g., urine output.

If massive transfusion (>1 blood volume) is required:

1. Use packed cells in recently thawed FFP.
2. Warm all blood and intravenous fluids.
3. Monitor coagulation indices, especially platelets.
4. Order platelet concentrates (1 unit/5 kg body weight) if the platelet count is less than 100,000/mm^3; administer platelets if <50,000/mm^3.
5. Monitor the acid–base status and correct acidosis.
6. If hypocalcemia is suspected (hypotension despite volume replacement, usually during rapid infusion of FFP), administer calcium chloride (10 mg/kg) or calcium gluconate (30 mg/kg) intravenously and repeat as indicated.
7. Activate a massive transfusion protocol (see Chap. 18) if massive uncontrolled hemorrhage continues.

Postoperative Care After Scoliosis Surgery

1. *Idiopathic*: For the child with idiopathic scoliosis and good preoperative pulmonary function:

(a) The child should be awake and the trachea extubated before leaving the operating room. Give supplemental oxygen and monitor SaO_2 and respirations during transport to PACU.
- Check for symmetric movement of the legs and feet.
- Check air bilateral breath sounds; pneumothorax is a possible complication.

(b) On arrival in the PACU:
- Continue O_2 by facemask.
- Provide a detailed handover of the intraoperative course to the PACU staff and document the vital signs.
- Supplement analgesia as necessary, e.g., morphine infusion, patient-controlled analgesia. Morphine requirements may be greater after a remifentanil infusion.
- Obtain radiographs of the chest and vertebral column, to rule out a pneumothorax.
- Obtain hemoglobin and coagulation values; administer additional blood products as indicated.

2. *Neuromuscular*: For the high-risk child with neuromuscular disease and impaired cardiopulmonary function.

(a) Transfer the child to the PICU intubated and ventilated if indicated; several days of IPPV may be required. Chest X-ray on arrival; check endotracheal tube and CVP catheter tip positions.

(b) Provide a detailed handover of the intraoperative course to the PICU staff.

(c) Postoperative pulmonary insufficiency may result from:
- Underlying neuromuscular disease and residual neuromuscular blockade.
- Acute conditions, e.g., pneumothorax, hemothorax, pleural effusion.
- Retention of secretions and atelectasis due to pain, analgesics, and/or immobilization.
- Perioperative aspiration of gastric contents.
- Postoperative alteration in thoracic mechanics.
- Fat embolism syndrome (rare, but may be fatal).

(d) Other medical complications may follow scoliosis surgery:
- Syndrome of inappropriate antidiuretic hormone secretion.
- Abdominal conditions; pancreatitis; cholelithiasis; superior mesenteric artery syndrome; ileus; pneumothorax; hemothorax; chylothorax.

Continuing Pulmonary Management

1. IPPV may be required for several days.
2. In some children, extubation may be possible with continuing assisted ventilation by means of non-invasive positive pressure ventilation.

Suggested Reading

Brigato P, De Salvatore S, Oggiano L, et al. Enhanced recovery after surgery for adolescent idiopathic scoliosis: a revised systematic review and meta-analysis. Spine Deform. 2025;13:647–65.

Choo S, Nuelle JAV. NSAID use and effects on pediatric bone healing: a review of the current literature. Children. 2021;8:821.

Chua ISY, Chong SL, Ong GYK. Intravenous regional anaesthesia (Bier's block) for pediatric forearm fractures in a pediatric emergency department-experience from 2003 to 2014. Injury. 2017;48:2784–7.

Fandino W. Strategies to prevent ischemic optic neuropathy following major spine surgery: a narrative review. J Clin Anesth. 2017;43:50–8.

McVey MJ, Lau W, Naraine N, et al. Perioperative blood conservation strategies for pediatric scoliosis surgery. Spine Deform. 2021;9:1289–302.

Muhly WT, Gurnaney HG, Ganesh A. Regional anesthesia for pediatric knee surgery: a review of the indications, procedures, outcomes, safety, and challenges. Local Regional Anesth. 2015;8:85–91.

Reysner M, Reysner T, Janusz P, et al. The influence of anesthesia on neuromonitoring during scoliosis surgery: a systematic review. NeuroSci. 2024;5:693–712.

Roddy E, Diab M. Rates and risk factors associated with unplanned hospital readmission after fusion for pediatric spinal deformity. Spine J. 2017;17:369–79.

Slattery C, Kark J, Wagner T, Verma K. The use of tranexamic acid to reduce surgical blood loss: a review basic science, subspecialty studies, and the

evolution of use in spine deformity surgery. Clin Spine Surg. 2019;32:46–50.
Sulton CD, Fletcher N, Murphy J, et al. Regional anesthesia as an alternative to procedural sedation for forearm fracture reductions in the pediatric emergency department. Pediatr Emerg. 2024;40:83–7.
Thirumala PD, Crammond DJ, Loke YK, et al. Diagnostic accuracy of motor evoked potentials to detect neurological deficit during idiopathic scoliosis correction: a systematic review. J Neurosurg Spine. 2017;26:374–83.
Yaszay B, Bartley CE, Sponseller PD, et al. Major complications following surgical correction of spine deformity in 257 patients with cerebral palsy. Spine Deform. 2020;8:1305–12.

Urology

17

General Principles

Anesthetic risk depends on the state of the child's renal function and any other disease process that may be present.

1. Most children who come for investigation or surgery of the lower urinary tract have normal renal function.
2. Surgery of the genitalia may have significant psychological effects on young children; effective postoperative analgesia may minimize these effects.
3. Many urologic procedures are now performed endoscopically, and the provisions for laparoscopy should be applied (see Chap. 14).
4. Many of those who require renal biopsy have mild renal dysfunction.
5. All children in renal failure are seriously ill and may present multiple problems.
6. Renal disease may be part of a syndrome and therefore requires consideration of all aspects of the condition (see Appendix A).

J. Lerman, C. J. Coté, *Steward's Manual of Pediatric Anesthesia*, https://doi.org/10.1007/978-3-032-24545-8_17

Infants and Children with Normal Renal Function

Minor Procedures

Children require general anesthesia for minor procedures such as cystoscopy, retrograde pyelography, circumcision, or hypospadias repair, and healthy children are almost all managed as outpatients.

Preoperative

1. Oral midazolam is a suitable premedication for anxious children, especially those who require repeat surgery.

Perioperative

1. Induce general anesthesia.
2. Maintain anesthesia with N_2O, O_2, and either sevoflurane or isoflurane by mask, laryngeal mask airway (LMA), or endotracheal tube.
3. Provide regional analgesia whenever possible (see Chap. 7). If the block is performed before surgery commences, fewer anesthetic drugs will be required during surgery, and awakening should be rapid and pain-free.
   (a) For circumcision: perform a penile (ring) or caudal block (see Chap. 7) using bupivacaine *without* epinephrine or ropivacaine. EMLA cream may be applied to the surgical site to augment the block.
   (b) For hypospadias repair, perform a caudal block (see Chap. 7). No clear relationship has been established between urethrocutaneous fistula, glans dehiscence, and the use of caudal block.

Postoperative

1. Children with a successful regional block are pain-free postoperatively. For those who did not receive a regional block or whose block was inadequate, supplementary analgesia will be required. Outpatients are usually discharged from the hospital 1 h after recovery. Most regional blocks wear off by 4 h after discharge, at which time additional analgesia (acetaminophen,

NSAIDs, or an opioid [e.g., oxycodone]) may be required. Instruct parents to administer a suitable analgesic *before* pain occurs.

Major Procedures

As for minor procedures with the following additions:

1. Use general endotracheal anesthesia, with either muscle relaxants and controlled ventilation or pressure support.
2. Establish reliable large-bore intravenous access, measure blood losses carefully, and replace fluids as indicated. Be prepared for a major hemorrhage.
3. Use regional analgesia to provide postoperative pain relief. For reimplantation of ureters, a single-shot caudal block provides analgesia for the first few hours, or an indwelling epidural catheter provides analgesia for up to 3 days. An intercostal nerve block or, preferably, a lumbar epidural block provides excellent analgesia after renal surgery and pyeloplasty. It is best to establish the block before surgery.
4. Children with dilated ureters may develop hypertension requiring treatment postoperatively.
5. For special considerations for Wilms tumor, see Chap. 14.

Children with Poor Renal Function or Renal Failure

These children may have many physiologic and emotional disturbances.

Special Anesthesia Problems

1. Anemia (usually normochromic, normocytic) may be present, but with standard care under the supervision of a renal unit, this should not be severe.

Anemia in renal failure is caused by:

(a) Decreased erythropoietin production. If erythropoietin is reduced, the hemoglobin concentration (Hb) will be 7–9 g/dL. Recombinant human erythropoietin therapy may not be effective if uremia is severe.
(b) Decreased erythrocyte survival and increased hemolysis.
(c) Increased bruising and bleeding from increased capillary fragility.
(d) Iron and/or folic acid deficiency.
(e) Bone marrow depression due to increased blood urea nitrogen (BUN).

The presence of anemia leads to a compensatory increase in cardiac output and increased red blood cell (RBC) 2,3-diphosphoglycerate (2,3-DPG), although the latter is minimal as the P_{50} values are similar to those in children with normal renal function.

Treatment with erythropoietin, supplemental iron, and vitamin C increases the Hb to approximately 10 g/dL, with possible further increases after a successful transplant. Blood transfusions may improve posttransplantation graft survival.

2. Coagulopathy may be caused by:
   (a) Increased capillary fragility.
   (b) Decreased adhesiveness of platelets.
   (c) Thrombocytopenia due to bone marrow depression.
   (d) Altered components of the coagulation cascade.
   (e) Drugs, e.g., heparin.

3. Acid-base imbalance:
   (a) Children produce more acid than adults; when urinary ammonia production decreases, a metabolic acidosis predominates and plasma bicarbonate decreases to 12–15 mEq/L. This is compensated to a variable degree by respiratory alkalosis.
   (b) In long-standing stable renal failure, H^+ displaces Ca^{2+} from bone and K^+ from intracellular fluid.
   (c) Lactated Ringer's solution is preferred to normal saline, as the latter causes a hyperchloremic metabolic acidosis, which increases the serum K^+ concentration.

4. Fluid and electrolyte changes. Children who have recently undergone dialysis (particularly hemodialysis) may be hypovolemic. The timing of the last dialysis and the volume of fluid removed are critical, as hypovolemia may cause precipitous hypotension at induction of anesthesia.
   (a) Children with polycystic kidneys or severe pyelonephritis (tubular damage is disproportionately greater than glomerular injury) are "sodium losers":
      - Normotension or slight hypotension is present.
      - Edema is infrequent.
      - Hypokalemia may be present.
      - Renal function is improved by an increased intake of sodium and water; sodium restriction may rapidly lead to severe hyponatremia.
   (b) Children with glomerulonephritis are often "sodium retainers"; salt retention, hypertension, and edema predispose them to cardiac failure.
   (c) Potassium shifts due to displacement of K+ from the cells by H+ lead to:
      - Increased serum K^+ concentrations.
      - Depressed excitability of muscles and nerves. This is particularly significant if the cardiac muscle is affected—further sudden increases in serum K^+, e.g., with succinylcholine (only if a peripheral neuropathy is present) or increased acidosis, may precipitate cardiac arrest.
   (d) Calcium shifts:
      - If displacement of Ca^{2+} by H^+ is prolonged, osteoporosis may develop.
   (e) Anion changes:
      - Plasma bicarbonate (HCO^{3-}) is decreased.
      - Plasma (SO_4^-), (HPO_4^-), and (Cl^-) are increased.
5. Cardiovascular problems:
   (a) Hypertension may result from abnormalities of extracellular fluid regulation, fluid overload, and derangement of the renin-angiotensin-aldosterone system:

- Hypertension in children secondary to sodium and water retention can be controlled by moderate salt restriction.
- In some children, the BP can be titrated against sodium and water content during dialysis.
- In others, diuretics and vasodilators are necessary.
- In a few, even large doses of antihypertensive agents fail to control the hypertension due to the overproduction of renin. Retinopathy and/or encephalopathy may develop, and bilateral nephrectomy may become necessary.
- A hypertensive crisis may occur in the perioperative period; an esmolol infusion is the treatment of choice.

(b) Congestive heart failure and associated pericardial effusion may occur with advanced renal failure as a result of hypertension, volume overload, anemia, electrolyte imbalance, and the effects of an arteriovenous (AV) fistula:
- Digitalis therapy is difficult to control.
- Pericardial effusion and tamponade may occur.

(c) Fatty degeneration of the myocardium may occur secondary to chronic renal failure.

6. Pulmonary:
   (a) The alveolar-arterial partial oxygen pressure difference (A-aDO_2) may be large.
   (b) Sodium and water retention, left ventricular failure, and hypoproteinemia contribute to the development of "uremic lung."
   (c) Pleural effusions may develop.
   (d) Recent evidence found that the severity of obstructive sleep apnea (OSA) increases with increasing chronic kidney disease; 50% had OSA with chronic kidney disease 2 (mild kidney disease).
7. Gastrointestinal disturbances:
   (a) Anorexia, nausea, and vomiting, due to bacterial breakdown of urea to ammonia in the gastrointestinal tract, may aggravate the water, electrolyte, and acid-base imbalance. Gastric emptying may be delayed.

8. Multiple medications:
   (a) Many of these children are receiving long-term steroid therapy with resultant osteodystrophy, Cushingoid state, and glycosuria; steroid supplementation is indicated perioperatively.
   (b) Antihypertensive polypharmacy: potential cardiovascular instability under anesthesia must be anticipated. Maintain beta-blockers preoperatively, but discontinue angiotension-converting enzyme (ACE) inhibitors 24 h before surgery to prevent hypotension and acute kidney injury (AKI).
   (c) Diuretic therapy may lead to K^+ depletion and thus to increased susceptibility to cardiac arrhythmias, especially if the child is receiving digitalis.
   (d) Antibiotics, e.g., gentamicin, may prolong the duration of non-depolarizing muscle relaxants.
   (e) Drugs that are highly protein-bound, e.g., azathioprine, may increase the bioavailability of other protein-bound drugs by displacing them from proteins.
   (f) Renal failure may affect the clearance of non-renal cleared drugs by altering hepatic cytochromes and transport mechanisms via the liver and intestines.
9. Strict asepsis should be maintained due to reduced immunity and an increased risk of infection.
10. Poor quality of life for family and child with potentially major emotional disturbances:
    (a) Resulting from chronic debilitating disease.
    (b) Heightened by the uremic state and knowledge of a life-threatening condition.

In summary, these children may have:

1. Reduced O_2 carrying capacity, which depends on a stressed cardiovascular system.
2. Incipient or apparent cardiac failure:
   (a) Left ventricular failure if hypertensive, hypervolemic, and anemic.
   (b) Right ventricular failure (late).
3. Greater risk of cardiac arrest, e.g., due to increased K^+ and acidosis.

4. Intolerance of excessive administration of blood and other fluids, as well as inaccurate replacement of electrolytes.
5. Cardiovascular instability due to long-term administration of antihypertensive drugs.
6. Coagulopathy.
7. Low resistance to infection.
8. Very low tolerance to further discomfort, however minor, e.g., finger prick, movement from one bed to another.

N.B. Many children with impaired renal function undergo hemodialysis regularly and therefore have an AV shunt or fistula, usually in the arm. Special care must be taken to ensure that this shunt is well-protected throughout the perioperative period. The shunt may be monitored using a gently applied Doppler flow meter; blood pressure should not be measured on that arm. The child must not be allowed to lie on that limb at any time.

Preoperative Assessment and Preparation

Pay careful attention to the following physical and psychological aspects:

1. Children in a dialysis program are usually dialyzed 12–18 h before surgery. Check the post-dialysis fluid and electrolyte status and body weight.
2. Plan ahead so that the child's discomfort is not increased and any necessary disturbances are minimized.
3. Psychological preparation and premedication are beneficial.
4. Check laboratory tests:
   (a) Blood transfusions may be given if deemed desirable and may help pretransplant. Packed RBCs are preferable.
   (b) Serum potassium: values less than 5 mEq/L are acceptable, even in an emergency; levels greater than 6 mEq/L are concerning.
      - If the serum K^+ level is increased, surgery is usually delayed until hemodialysis has been performed.
      - In an emergency in the absence of arrhythmias, the serum K^+ concentration can be reduced by giving 5 mL/kg glu-

cose as a 10% solution with 0.1 U/kg of regular insulin (maximum 10 U) followed by an infusion of insulin (0.1 U/kg/h) and $D_{10}W$ with 0.45 normal saline at maintenance rates (onset of effect ~15 min). Acute treatment of hyperkalemia with or without arrhythmias includes IV calcium (chloride or gluconate), bicarbonate, hyperventilation, and inhaled albuterol or salbutamol.

(c) Acid-base balance:
- A pH greater than 7.32 is acceptable; sodium bicarbonate ($NaHCO^{3}-$) may be indicated for correction of acidosis, even if sodium (Na^+) levels are increased.
- Correction must be cautious and gradual. Sudden correction may precipitate tetany or convulsions due to the resulting decrease in the serum calcium (Ca^{2+}) level.

Anesthesia Management

1. Meticulous attention to details of asepsis is essential.
2. For brief procedures, e.g., insertion of a peritoneal catheter, in a poor-risk child who is cooperative and emotionally stable, sedation and local anesthesia (1–2% lidocaine without epinephrine; maximum, 3 mg/kg) may be used.
3. For all other cases, and if in doubt, use general anesthesia.
4. Anesthesia drugs and renal failure:
   (a) Children with renal failure vary in their response to opioids. Morphine may exert a prolonged effect because of a failure to excrete/dialyze active metabolites (M6G); meperidine is no longer recommended for children due to the potential for metabolites to cause seizures. In contrast, fentanyl, alfentanil, and sufentanil are relatively safe because their metabolites are inactive. Remifentanil may be the ideal intraoperative opioid for children in renal failure.
   (b) Propofol and thiopental should be carefully titrated in reduced doses; less protein binding increases the free active fraction of drug. Ketamine and etomidate may cause less hypotension.
   (c) Inhalational anesthetics are eliminated via the lungs and hence are most useful but must be administered cautiously.

Fluoride nephrotoxicity does not occur with the current ether anesthetics.

(d) Succinylcholine may be used as a single dose, provided a peripheral neuropathy is not present. The serum potassium (K^+) concentration should be 5.5 mEq/L or less. Serum K^+ increases 0.5–1 mEq/L after succinylcholine in children with renal failure, but this produces no ECG changes because the hyperkalemia is chronic. If a peripheral neuropathy is present, or another factor that predisposes to hyperkalemia after succinylcholine, however, succinylcholine may cause greater increases in serum K^+ and arrhythmias. Succinylcholine should only be used if a rapid sequence induction is deemed necessary and should be preceded by a small dose (~10% of the intubating dose) of a non-depolarizing relaxant. Alternatively, high-dose rocuronium (1.2 mg/kg) may be used.

(e) Muscle relaxants, non-depolarizing: cisatracurium and rocuronium are drugs of choice in children with renal insufficiency. Rocuronium has a slower onset of action but a similar duration of action in children with and without renal failure. Pancuronium and gallamine are partially or completely excreted by the kidneys and should be avoided.

(f) Local anesthesia drugs have not been extensively studied in children with renal failure; they may be used in normal doses for "single-shot" techniques. Ropivacaine appears safe for long-term infusions, as impaired excretion of its metabolites is offset by non-renal metabolism.

Preoperative

1. Dose requirements for drugs in children with renal failure are more variable than in those with normal renal function, necessitating careful titration.
2. Continue antihypertensive medications, except ACE inhibitors, which should be discontinued 24 h before anesthesia.
3. Premedicate as indicated.
4. All medications and the timing of the last dose should be noted.

5. It is essential to avoid pressure on any shunt or fistula (*including blood pressure cuff*); continued monitoring with a Doppler flow meter is recommended.
6. Anticipate that vasoactive support may be needed. Appropriate dilutions and infusion pump setup are recommended.
7. Ensure that adequate supplies of blood and other fluids are available, including washed PRBCs.

Perioperative

1. Administer 100% O_2 by mask.
2. Apply monitors:
   (a) Precordial stethoscope.
   (b) ECG and pulse oximeter.
   (c) Automated blood pressure—*do not use a limb with a shunt or fistula.*
3. Ensure that the limb with the shunt or fistula is easily accessible and protected; monitor function with a Doppler or by palpation.
4. Anesthesia may be induced with IV propofol (2–4 mg/kg), thiopental (2–3 mg/kg), or, if dehydrated or recently dialyzed, with ketamine (1–2 mg/kg) or etomidate (0.3 mg/kg).
5. For tracheal intubation:
   (a) Avoid succinylcholine if a peripheral neuropathy is present. Consider pretreating with a low-dose non-depolarizing agent (~10% of the intubating dose) and limit succinylcholine to a single dose.
   (b) Alternatively, cisatracurium, rocuronium, or vecuronium may be used.
6. Maintain anesthesia with N_2O/O_2, an inhalation agent, and a non-depolarizing muscle relaxant.
7. Moderate controlled hyperventilation ($PaCO_2$ ~ 35 mmHg) helps offset the blood pH and encourages K^+ movement back into the cells.
8. Administer fluids as indicated to ensure an adequate blood volume for satisfactory BP, peripheral perfusion, and function of the AV fistula or shunt.
   (a) A balanced salt solution, e.g., plasmalyte or lactated Ringers, is recommended to replace preoperative deficits

and for perioperative maintenance. Normal saline may cause a non-anion gap acidosis, thereby increasing the serum K^+ greater than lactated Ringer's solution.

(b) Small blood losses can be replaced with a balanced salt solution.

(c) For significant blood losses, washed RBCs and salt-poor albumin are recommended.
- Check the Hb and hematocrit and maintain in the 6–7 g% range.
- Avoid over-transfusion.

9. At the end of surgery, antagonize muscle relaxants and extubate the trachea when full strength has returned and the child is awake.

Postoperative

1. Ensure adequate ventilation and oxygenation.
2. Carefully titrate opioids since repeated doses of morphine and its metabolites accumulate in renal failure; M6G cannot be removed by dialysis.
3. Ensure that the shunt or fistula is functioning and document this in the postoperative note.
4. Recheck Hb, electrolytes, and blood gases as indicated and return care to the child's nephrologist.

Renal Transplantation

Transplantation offers the chance of a relatively normal life for the child with chronic renal failure. Organs for transplantation are in very limited supply; meticulous anesthetic management is essential to maximize the chance for graft survival.

Anesthesia Management

Preoperative

1. General management is the same as for children in renal failure.
2. Discuss with the nephrologist and urologist to ascertain the child's exact present status regarding state of hydration, electrolyte and acid-base status, renal function, cardiopulmonary state, and coagulation issues.
3. If the child is not in optimal condition, e.g., volume overload, surgery may need to be postponed until after dialysis with the objective of implant within 24 h.
4. Review the immunosuppressive therapy plan, i.e., drug, dose, and timing. A typical plan includes administration of cyclosporine, methylprednisolone succinate (Solu-Medrol), azathioprine, and an antibiotic.

Perioperative

1. General management is the same as for children in renal failure.
2. After induction of anesthesia:
   (a) If indicated, insert a central venous line.
   (b) Check its position with a pressure tracing and/or radiograph.
   (c) Maintain the central venous pressure (CVP) at an acceptably high level to ensure diuresis (8–12 mmHg). Lactated Ringer's solution is the preferred initial maintenance fluid.
   (d) The objective is to adequately replace any existing deficits and ongoing losses.
3. An arterial line is not essential in uncomplicated cases. Leaving the radial artery untouched may be advantageous in case the child needs another shunt in the future.
   (a) If an external (Scribner) shunt is available, the arterial end may be used for monitoring and the venous end as an infusion route; careful aseptic technique is essential.
   (b) If an arterial line is indicated, insert the catheter in the radial artery (in the arm opposite to the fistula), use a

small-gauge cannula, and remove it as soon as possible to minimize damage to the artery.

4. Provided no significant coagulopathy is present, an epidural catheter may be placed to augment surgical anesthesia, improve hemodynamic stability, and ensure postoperative analgesia.
5. Transfuse with packed RBCs to obtain an Hct of ~35–40% at the end of surgery. Children with chronic renal failure tend to lose third-space fluid extensively; greater Hct and colloid administration may limit this effect and improve graft perfusion.
6. During vascular anastomosis and before the renal arterial clamp is released, 1 mg/kg of furosemide and 1 g/kg of mannitol IV is recommended. Anticipate a decline in blood pressure as the clamps are removed, and prepare for rapid fluid infusions. Some surgeons will request an RBC transfusion just before declamping.
7. Systolic blood pressure (100–120% of preoperative value) and a CVP >14 cm H_2O are preferred before the clamps are removed to initiate and maintain renal perfusion and function. Lighten the level of anesthesia and use a dopamine infusion of 5 μg/kg/min as necessary. A greater systolic pressure at this time increases graft perfusion, facilitates early function, and improves graft survival. Optimal results may be expected if the graft functions within 10 min.
8. The solution used to preserve the kidney has a high potassium concentration; hyperkalemia and acidosis should be anticipated after the arterial clamps are released, but this is rarely associated with a cardiac arrest. This may be a greater danger in small children.
9. Transplanting an adult kidney in a small infant can present problems. The kidney should be well-flushed by the surgeon before it is implanted to prevent hyperkalemia. Fluids must be rapidly infused as the clamps are released to fill the vascular space of the graft. The CVP should be increased to 15–20 mmHg in anticipation of unclamping. The danger of hyperkalemia (due to preservative fluid) and acidosis (due to clamping of the aorta or iliac artery) is increased. The acid-

base status should be frequently assessed; give calcium chloride or calcium gluconate and sodium bicarbonate as indicated. Dopamine infusions may need to be increased.

10. Maintain the CVP at an increased level, i.e., up to 15–20 mmHg, to produce good urine output. If the CVP is adequate but urine flow is still low:
    (a) Give furosemide (1–4 mg/kg IV).
    (b) If necessary, add mannitol (0.5–1 g/kg).
11. Anticipate the need to infuse large volumes of fluid, three to five times normal, i.e., 10–20 mL/kg/h, to compensate for third-space losses.
12. At the end of surgery, determine serum electrolyte concentrations:
    (a) If urine output is adequate, serum K^+ should be within the normal range.
    (b) If the serum K^+ is greater than 6 mEq/L and urine output is poor, continue moderate hyperventilation and plan dialysis or therapy with glucose and insulin.
13. With such an aggressive approach to fluid management, pulmonary edema may occur. In such cases, continue with controlled ventilation into the postoperative period and administer diuretics as indicated.

Postoperative

1. General management is the same as for children in renal failure. Ensure adequate postoperative analgesia; epidural analgesia is ideal.
2. The pulmonary status of all children should be monitored by pulse oximetry, blood gases, and chest radiography as indicated. Small infants with large implanted kidneys may be at risk for pulmonary complications, especially atelectasis. This may be a combined result of the abdominal surgery, the mass of the implanted kidney, and aggressive fluid therapy; the need to "push fluids" to ensure diuresis may result in pulmonary edema.
3. Extubation at the end of surgery in children with end-stage renal disease or after renal transplantation depends on several factors, including pulmonary, cardiovascular, and volume sta-

tus. In adults, sugammadex is more reliable than neostigmine to ensure extubation with fewer delayed reintubations, although the time to TOF >0.9 was greater than in those with normal renal function.

4. Renal function in the transplanted kidney is as follows:
   (a) Glomerular function is initially normal but wanes during the first 48 h as the kidney swells. Increased intravenous fluids are required to maintain diuresis at that time.
   (b) Some degree of tubular damage is always present, resulting in diuresis and loss of sodium; replacement of sodium and water is required. Other electrolytes must be infused as indicated.
   (c) Declining urine flow after 48 h despite fluid loading may be indicative of mechanical problems (vascular) or rejection of the transplant.
5. Hypoglycemia has been described as a late complication after renal transplantation in small children. This may be secondary to the use of β-blocking drugs.

Suggested Reading

Ahmed M, Fatima E, Shafiq A, et al. Continuation versus discontinuation of renin-angiotensin aldosterone system inhibitors before non-cardiac surgery: a systematic review and meta-analysis. J Clin Anesth. 2024;99:111679.

Jamil A, Gruner B, Jamil J, et al. Anemia management in pediatric chronic kidney disease: current challenges and treatment strategies. Ind J Hema Blood Transf. 2025;41:228–37.

Kim Y-S, Lim B-G, Won Y-J, et al. Efficacy and safety of sugammadex for the reversal of rocuronium-induced neuromuscular blockade in patients with end-stage renal disease: a systematic review and meta-analysis. Medicina. 2021;57:1259.

Kumar N, Joice RJ, Rajan RJ, et al. Prevalence of sleep disordered breathing in children with chronic kidney disease. Pediatr Neph. 2025;40(8):2661–8.

Liverman R, Chandran MM, Crowther B. Considerations and controversies of pharmacologic management of the pediatric kidney transplant recipient. Pharmacotherapy. 2021;41:77–102.

Mohidin B, Marks SD. Acute kidney injury in paediatric kidney transplant recipients. Pediatr Neph. 2025;40(7):2161–75.

Pere PJ, Ekstrand A, Salonen M, et al. Pharmacokinetics of ropivacaine in patients with chronic renal failure. Br J Anaesth. 2011;106:512–21.

Voet M, Cornelissen EAM, van der Jagt MFP, et al. Perioperative anesthesia care for the pediatric patient undergoing a kidney transplantation: an educational review. Pediatr Anesth. 2021;31:1150–60.

Xia Y, Yang Z, Li J, et al. Urethrocutaneous fistula and glans dehiscence formation of hypospadias surgery in patients receiving caudal block vs. non-caudal block: a meta-analysis. J Pediatr Urol. 2024;20:227–36.

Trauma and Burns 18

Children are commonly involved in accidents; trauma is the leading cause of death between 1 and 14 years of age. Even if the injury is relatively minor, some children require emergency anesthesia, the potential dangers of which may overshadow the injury.

Most children injured in accidents are previously healthy. Although considerations of past health are usually less important than in adults, a complete medical history should be solicited. From the time of arrival in the ED, the anesthesiologist should be present, contributing to the initial care while evaluating the child's condition for anesthesia and continuing care.

Basic trauma care involves three steps: primary survey, secondary survey, and definitive care. The primary survey involves initial resuscitation and stabilization: (a) airway, (b) breathing, (c) circulation, (d) disability (neurologic injury, modified Glasgow Coma Scale), and (e) exposure. Completely undress the child for full evaluation, but institute strategies to maintain thermoneutrality. The secondary survey focuses on additional, less life-threatening injuries (usually additional diagnostic testing). Definitive care involves transfer to the intensive care unit (ICU) or operating room (OR).

J. Lerman, C. J. Coté, *Steward's Manual of Pediatric Anesthesia*,
https://doi.org/10.1007/978-3-032-24545-8_18

Major Trauma

Diagnosis and treatment must proceed rapidly and simultaneously without interrupting resuscitative measures during anesthesia. The common major problems for the anesthesiologist include:

1. To secure and maintain a safe, reliable airway and to optimize ventilation and oxygenation.
2. To restore adequate organ perfusion and oxygen delivery with crystalloid, colloid, and blood replacement as needed.
3. To optimize cerebral perfusion pressure in children with a head injury.
4. To maintain body temperature.

N.B. Although injuries may appear limited to a single anatomic site or body system, consider the possibility that the injuries are widespread, e.g., a fractured femur may be obvious, but an undiagnosed ruptured liver could be life-threatening.

Initial Urgent Procedures

1. Ensure a safe and protected airway; optimize ventilation and oxygenation.
2. The cardiovascular status must be evaluated:
   (a) Correct hypovolemia.
   (b) Maintain or restore cardiac output.
3. Send blood for type and cross-match; immediately advise the blood bank if a massive transfusion protocol (>30 mL/kg blood loss and ongoing uncontrolled bleeding) must be activated (see Table 18.1).

Table 18.1 Massive transfusion protocol for immediate use

Number of units to be issued				
Protocol	Red cell units	Plasma	Platelets	Cryoprecipitate
Adult	6	4	One 5-pack	One 5-pack
Pediatric				
0–10 kg	1	1	1	1
11–20 kg	2	2	2	2
21–30 kg	3	3	3	3
41–50 kg	4	4	4	4
	5	5	One 5-pack	One 5-pack

Available from https://www.pathology.med.umich.edu/static/apps/cms/ckfinder/userfiles/238/files/Massive%20Transfusion%20Protocol%202014Nov20.pdf (Accessed June 12, 2025, Jerrold Lerman).

Establishing the Airway

Airway obstruction is common in head and facial injuries and can have a disastrous effect on the outcome:

1. Oxygen should be administered via a face mask to all children with head injuries as soon as possible, preferably at the trauma site.
2. For those with depressed consciousness, if simple positioning does not provide a clear airway or the gag reflex is absent, intubate the trachea without delay.
3. Do not insert oropharyngeal airways in unconscious children. Resistance to ventilation is greater than with a tracheal tube, and they do not prevent aspiration of gastric contents.
4. Injury of the cervical spine must be suspected in all trauma; immobilize the neck using sandbags, a plaster shell, or a bean-bag. The neck should not be moved. Note that a cervical spine injury may occur without radiologic evidence (known as SCIWORA, or *S*pinal *C*ord *I*njury *W*ith*o*ut *R*adiographic *A*bnormalities). Optimal airway management is the first priority; however, all airway manipulations should assume the presence of a cervical spine injury (see later discussion) and a full stomach. A supraglottic device, e.g., a laryngeal mask airway,

may be lifesaving for a difficult airway, but cervical spine stabilization is still critical during placement.

5. Consider foreign bodies (e.g., teeth, bone fragments, or food) in the mouth, pharynx, trachea, or bronchi, especially with facial injuries.
6. Assume that all trauma patients have a full stomach; perform a rapid-sequence intubation (RSI) to secure the airway. Succinylcholine does not increase intragastric pressure or the risk of regurgitation or increase intracranial pressure (ICP). The advantages of rapidly securing the airway and instituting controlled ventilation are the most important considerations. Be aware of potential neck injury; stabilize the spine, but do not exert traction on the neck. (Remember: a cervical spine injury is a relative contraindication to cricoid pressure.) Ensure that two functioning laryngoscope handles and size-appropriate blades are available, as well as two suction sources, should one become blocked with food or vomit, and an age-appropriate endotracheal tube and one size smaller fitted with a stylet.

   Awake laryngoscopy and intubation can increase ICP as much as coughing and crying, which may be detrimental in the head-injured child. In children with suspected increased ICP, deep sedation or general anesthesia is required for an RSI, using IV lidocaine 1–2 mg/kg, propofol 2–3 mg/kg (or thiopental 5 mg/kg), atropine 0.02 mg/kg, and succinylcholine 2 mg/kg are recommended. If succinylcholine is contraindicated, then use 1.2 mg/kg IV rocuronium. If the child is hypovolemic, ketamine, etomidate, or midazolam (with IV lidocaine and fentanyl) are acceptable alternative agents to induce anesthesia. Airway adjuncts such as a video laryngoscope, ProSeal-LMA, and fiberoptic bronchoscope should be immediately available for airway rescue.
7. Vomiting and aspiration may occur. If a history of the last food ingested is unavailable or ambiguous, point-of-care ultrasound (POCUS) may be used to assess the presence of foods in the gastric antrum. Immediately after intubation, check $PetCO_2$ and auscultate air entry to all lung regions; suction the bronchi via the tracheal tube if necessary. Examine chest radiographs

for tracheal tube position and evidence of lung pathology or aspirated foreign body.
8. Insert a gastric tube to decompress the stomach if POCUS is unavailable, especially in children with chest or abdominal injuries. Even children with relatively minor injuries often swallow large volumes of air, causing gastric distention that may interfere with ventilation and predispose them to regurgitation and aspiration. Do not pass a tube through the nose in children who may have a basal skull fracture.
9. Be alert to the possibility of pneumothorax/hemothorax.

Intravenous Therapy

Large-bore intravenous access must be established in the upper limbs or neck in children with injuries at or below the level of the thorax because flow through the inferior vena cava may be (or become) interrupted. If the source of hemodynamic instability is unknown, establish IV access in both upper and lower extremities. *Avoid central venous access in the neck in the presence of a head injury* to avoid obstructing cerebral venous return. *All intravenous fluids should be warmed since hypothermia rapidly develops in the injured child.*

Percutaneous cannulation of large veins, using rapid infusion catheters, is preferable. If successful venipuncture is taking more than 90 s, consider using a vein finder, ultrasound, or an intraosseous needle, e.g., Easy-IO. Internal jugular (IJ) or subclavian lines may be inserted if no other venous access is available; beware of further worsening the cardiorespiratory status if a pneumothorax or hemothorax occurs. A central venous catheter will be useful for ongoing management of the child, but it may be inserted after the initial acute fluid resuscitation.

Clues to blood volume status are as follows:

1. Cardiovascular indices:
   (a) Tachycardia, i.e., a heart rate in excess of 140 beats/min in infants or 100 beats/min in older children, suggests hypovolemia.

   (b) In infants, the systolic blood pressure (BP) varies directly with the intravascular volume and is a very good guide to volume status.
   (c) In adolescents, as in adults, hypovolemia stimulates early constriction of venous capacitance vessels. Therefore, the systolic BP may remain near normal despite a loss of up to 20% of the blood volume. The central venous pressure (CVP) may also be unchanged initially. When venoconstriction can no longer compensate and maintain the venous return to the heart, rapid decompensation may occur. At this point, the CVP decreases and becomes a more reliable guide to the adequacy of replacement of the blood volume. A 2–3 mmHg decrease in CVP may represent a loss of as much as 25% of the circulating blood volume in a healthy, supine child.
2. General appearance: Confusion, irrational behavior, pallor, mottling, sweating, and coolness of the skin, especially over the extremities, are signs of hypovolemia. Large differences between the skin and core body temperature indicate vasoconstriction and hypovolemia.
3. Urine output: Urine output should be assessed; a urine flow of ≥1 mL/kg/h indicates adequate renal perfusion and volume replacement.
4. Acid-base assessment: Metabolic acidosis (lactic acidosis) may result from impaired organ perfusion and is a confirmatory sign of a low circulating blood volume; this acidosis may be corrected with adequate volume replacement. Sodium bicarbonate administration is not recommended except in the presence of severe acidosis that may compromise cardiac contractility (i.e., pH <7.2) despite normocapnia or hypocapnia.

Selection of Fluids

The initial fluid resuscitation should consist of balanced salt solutions rather than blood products. If at all possible, do not transfuse uncross-matched universal donor blood; a rapid cross-match takes

~20 min. If blood loss is massive and it has accumulated in the chest cavity, consider autotransfusion.

A balanced salt solution, e.g., lactated Ringer's solution, expands the circulating blood volume, but if used in excess (> 100 mL/kg), pulmonary insufficiency and/or dilutional coagulopathy may result. An initial bolus of 20 mL/kg is appropriate for the hypotensive child and may be repeated. If the child has a head injury, use normal saline (isotonic) to reduce the potential for cerebral edema. *Dextrose-containing solutions should not be used* (except, very rarely, to treat documented hypoglycemia); hyperglycemia may occur and increase the severity of neurologic damage (blood glucose >200 mg/dL) with head injury.

Expansion of blood volume with 5% albumin may be effective in the immediate treatment of hypovolemia, but if large quantities are infused, "capillary leak" into the lungs may impair pulmonary function later.

Other plasma substitutes have been used, e.g., dextran 70 and hetastarch, but they have major side effects. Dextrans may impair coagulation, interfere with cross-matching, and cause transient temperature increases and rigors; we do not recommend their use in children. One systematic review and meta-analysis of hetastarch in adults reported a positive association with increased mortality and acute kidney injury; the authors recommended against using it for acute volume resuscitation. The starches also have long residence times in the reticuloendothelial system in humans; with limited pediatric safety data, we do not recommend their use.

Indications for Blood Transfusion It is seldom possible to measure blood loss associated with trauma, especially when large amounts may be lost from the intravascular volume but remain within hematomas, e.g., retroperitoneal or body cavities. Volume replacement must be judged on a case-by-case basis using patient-specific signs and symptoms. We recommend that sufficient fluid be replaced to restore euvolemia (with normal vital signs) and that blood be given in volumes sufficient to maintain the hematocrit (Hct) at ~21–25%.

The young child who is showing obvious signs of hypovolemia (pallor, sweating, tachycardia, and hypotension) has lost at least

25% of the blood volume. In the emergency situation, the weight of the average child may be predicted from the child's age using the following formulae (Table 18.2), and assume the blood volume to be 70 mL/kg; 25% of this total is the initial volume to be rapidly replaced, and then reassess the child's response. The need for additional fluid boluses or continuous infusion to maintain the BP, or deterioration after an apparently stable period, indicates persistent bleeding.

Children who have lost greater than one blood volume will require fresh-frozen plasma (FFP) to prevent dilutional coagulopathy. Packed cells resuspended in plasma (preferably recently thawed FFP) may be optimal.

Massive Blood Transfusion In children, a transfusion of >30 mL/kg packed red blood cells with ongoing blood losses warrants activation of a massive transfusion protocol. Transfusions of this order of magnitude may be required in severely injured children, e.g., after thoracoabdominal injury. One practical massive transfusion protocol (developed at the University of Michigan) for children alerts the blood bank to send set packs of blood products based on the child's weight (Table 18.1).

Serious problems begin to develop after the rapid infusion of 200% of the estimated blood volume, i.e., transfusion of ~140 mL/kg. These problems include:

1. Hypothermia and accompanying cardiac arrhythmias. Warm all blood and fluids to 40 °C.
2. Coagulation problems:
   (a) Dilutional thrombocytopenia and impaired platelet function:
      1. Check platelet count after each 50% blood volume replacement.

Table 18.2 Weight prediction from child's age

Age (years)	Predicted weight (kg)
<1	0.5 × age (months) + 4[a]
1–7	2 × age (year) + 9
8–12	3 × age (year)

[a]Graves et al. (2014)

   2. If the platelet count is less than 50,000/mm^3, administer platelet concentrates (0.1–0.3 units/kg). In general, ~40% of the initial platelet count is lost with the first blood volume, ~20% with the second blood, and ~10% with the third; e.g., after three blood volumes only ~30% of the initial platelet count remains.
 - (b) Deficiency of coagulation factors:
   1. Measure prothrombin time (PT) and partial thromboplastin time (PTT).
   2. If these are prolonged, give FFP (20 mL/kg). Generally this occurs after loss of 1–1.5 blood volumes; for blood loss, >1.5 blood volumes give one-third of the further volume replacement as FFP.
 - (c) Disseminated intravascular coagulation (DIC):
   1. Likely if bleeding increases at all sites, e.g., old venipuncture sites.
   2. Measure PT, PTT, clot lysis time, fibrinogen, and fibrin split product levels.
   3. Prolonged PT and PTT, low fibrinogen level, and the presence of fibrin split products suggest DIC.
   4. If DIC is suspected, enlist the aid of a hematologist if possible. Treatment must include removal of the cause, i.e., correction of hypovolemic shock and hypothermia, replacement of coagulation factors, and possibly heparinization.

3. Acidosis:
 - (a) Check acid-base status frequently.
 - (b) Correct severe metabolic acidosis with sodium bicarbonate (provided ventilation is not compromised).
4. Citrate toxicity (due to infusion of citrated blood or plasma):
 - (a) May cause more problems in infants and small children than in adults.
 - (b) Results in hypotension that persists despite adequate volume replacement. *N.B.* Remember that FFP and platelet suspensions contain more citrate per unit volume than whole blood. Significant hypocalcemia occurs when infusions exceed 1 mL/kg/min FFP.

   (c) May be diagnosed by measuring the ionized Ca^{++} concentration or by a prolonged rate-corrected QT interval on the ECG. If hypotension appears unresponsive to volume replacement, a therapeutic test of IV calcium chloride (10 mg/kg) or calcium gluconate (30 mg/kg) is justified.
   (d) Correct by slowly administering 10% calcium chloride 10–30 mg/kg while observing the ECG. Frequent small boluses (5–10 mg/kg calcium chloride or 15–30 mg/kg calcium gluconate) during rapid FFP infusions prevent serious hypocalcemia.
5. Serum potassium disturbances: Monitor serum K^+ levels periodically. Serious hyperkalemia is likely in the presence of a low cardiac output, after transfusing old cold blood through a central line, and with the use of a rapid infusion device. The cardiac manifestations of hyperkalemia (peaked T waves, ventricular irritability, and ventricular tachycardia) may be treated acutely by slow administration of intravenous calcium chloride 10–30 mg/kg, sodium bicarbonate 1–2 mmol/kg, hyperventilation, administration of a β-agonist, and, if more severe, with glucose, insulin, and Kayexalate. Repeat boluses of IV calcium may be required to convert and maintain normal sinus rhythm.
6. Posttraumatic pulmonary insufficiency. This is characterized by progressively decreasing pulmonary compliance, impaired gas exchange, and radiographic findings of diffuse infiltrates. The following factors may contribute:
   (a) Excess use of balanced salt solutions and/or albumin:
      1. Give diuretics (furosemide 1 mg/kg) if indicated.
   (b) Microembolization of the pulmonary vessels by infused particulate matter (platelet or leukocyte clumps):
      1. Filter all blood products prior to administration.
   (c) Damage to alveolar-capillary membrane:
      1. This results in low-pressure pulmonary edema.

Autotransfusion Autotransfusion can be lifesaving for some trauma patients. Advantages include the ready availability of warm compatible blood, although autotransfusion is contraindicated after abdominal trauma where there is a risk of bowel perforation and contamination.

Head Injury

Head injury is a major cause of pediatric mortality and morbidity, much of which might be reduced by effective, early medical intervention. Children with head injuries are less likely than adults to develop a mass lesion but are more likely to develop intracranial hypertension secondary to diffuse hyperemia and edema. This secondary brain injury, which occurs after the primary trauma, must be minimized if recovery is to be optimized. Early aggressive treatment is essential to ensure cerebral oxygenation, control ICP, and cerebral perfusion pressure (CPP = mean arterial blood pressure—ICP), and minimize cerebral edema. The Glasgow Coma Scale (GCS) and the Pediatric Modification (Table 18.3) are the most common metrics to assess the child's neurologic status. Most accept the "adult" GCS for use in children as young as 5 years and apply a modified "pediatric" GCS for those <5 years (although some limit its use to children <2 years).

Table 18.3 Glasgow Coma Scale with pediatric modification

Score	1	2	3	4	5	6
Eyes	No response	Open to pain only	Open to verbal stimuli	Open spontaneously		
Verbal	No response	Nonspecific Words or sounds / *Moans to pain*	Inappropriate words / *Cries to pain*	Confused / *Irritable cries*	Oriented, appropriate / *Alert, coos & babbles*	
Motor	No response	Responds to pain with decerebrate (extension) posturing	Responds to pain with decorticate (flexion) posturing	Withdraws in response to pain	Localizes painful stimulus / *Withdraws to touch*	Obeys commands / *Moves spont. & purposefully*

The GCS is the sum of the best scores in each of the three categories: *Eyes*, *Verbal*, and *Motor*, for a total score between 3 and 15. Split cells describe responses in two age groups: children >5 years and adults (left) and italicized text highlighted in amber for infants and children <2 years (right). For intubated children and those who are unconscious or preverbal, the *motor* response is considered the most important component of the scale.

Table 18.4 A GCS modifier: the pupil response and score

Pupil score	−2	−1	0
Pupil response	Neither pupil reacts to light	One pupil does not react to light	Both pupils react to light

To further qualify the brain injury, the pupil (P) response serves as an external metric of brain function that modifies the GCS score (Table 18.4).

The GCS-P score is the GCS score plus the pupil score; e.g., a GCS of 3 and a pupil score of −2 yield a combined GCS-P score of 1, indicating deep coma.

If consciousness is depressed (GCS < 8), airway obstruction may seriously compromise the prognosis. The first priority is to ensure a clear airway, excellent oxygenation, and optimal ventilation:

1. Oxygen should be administered, and the trachea should be intubated without delay; use a cuffed oral tube. Suitable drugs should be given to obtund the cardiovascular responses to intubation (see previous discussion). Nasal tubes (and nasogastric tubes) are contraindicated in children with basilar skull fractures; perforation of the cribriform plate may occur. Be aware of the possibility of SCIWORA; see later discussion.
2. Control ventilation to produce normocapnia pending further evaluation of the child's injuries. Extreme hyperventilation should be avoided ($PaCO_2$ < 30 mmHg) because it may compromise cerebral perfusion. $PaCO_2$ should preferably be checked by arterial blood gas analysis, as end-tidal CO_2 may be misleading, particularly in children with associated chest trauma.
3. Anesthesia should be continued as required, ideally with intravenous agents (e.g., titrated propofol, opioids, and muscle relaxants) to avoid hypotension. Inhalational agents should be limited to <1 MAC to prevent possible increases in ICP. MAP should be maintained to preserve CPP. Titrated opioids do not alter ICP, but if hypotension results, ICP may increase in head-injured patients.

4. Stabilize the hemodynamic state to ensure an optimal CPP. Glucose-free, isotonic fluids (normal saline) should be infused cautiously; excessive fluid therapy contributes to cerebral edema. If a vasopressor is required, neosynephrine is the drug of choice.
5. CT or MRI is generally recommended for any child with GCS <13 or with vomiting to accurately identify surgical lesions. The characteristic appearance of diffuse cerebral damage on the scan can obviate the need for craniotomy and permit early specific monitoring and therapeutic measures:
   (i) ICP monitoring—most commonly assessed with an extradural bolt connected to an external transducer. This is usually recommended for any child with a GCS < 8. Once ICP monitoring is established, the CPP is maintained at an optimal level (see below).
   (ii) Initiate treatment to control ICP and CPP:
      (a) Optimal positioning: 35°–45° head-up with the face positioned centrally. (Internal or external jugular lines should not be used in children with head injuries.)
      (b) Diuretics—mannitol and/or furosemide.
      (c) Consider hypertonic saline infusions.
      (d) Intermittent boluses of propofol may be effective in controlling ICP and seizures, but the use of infusions is controversial due to the risk of propofol infusion syndrome. Barbiturates may be more effective in controlling ICP and seizures in children than in adults, but thiopental is no longer available in the United States.
      (e) Controlled ventilation, preferably adjusted on the basis of measurements of ICP and CPP. Excessive hyperventilation ($PaCO_2$ < 30 mmHg) may be detrimental and is no longer recommended.
   (iii) Maintain optimal CPP (>40 mmHg in 0–5-year-olds, >50 mmHg in 6–17 years), hemoglobin values, and arterial oxygenation. Glucose-free isotonic or hypertonic fluids should be used for volume expansion. Vasoactive medications may be required to correct hypotension (see

later). Hyperglycemia should be avoided because it may exacerbate secondary brain injury. Fluid therapy must be guided by constant monitoring of physiologic and biochemical variables. Endocrine functions (especially pituitary/hypothalamic) may be disturbed after head injury, which may lead to:
   (a) Diabetes insipidus, with a large urine volume and hypernatremia.
   (b) Inappropriate secretion of antidiuretic hormone (SIADH) with oliguria and hyponatremia.
   (c) Hyperglycemia is common after head injury, secondary to catecholamine release, but should not exceed >200 mg/dL. Hypoglycemia may develop later and should be corrected.
(iv) Control of seizure activity, as evident clinically or by EEG monitoring.
(v) Control body temperature:
   (a) To maintain normothermia and prevent hyperthermia, which commonly follow brain injury.
   (b) Prophylactic moderate hypothermia (32–33 °C) is not recommended.
(vi) When all else fails to control ICP, a decompressive craniectomy may be required. If this is performed, be alert to the possibility of sudden severe hypotension as the dura is opened—especially in cases with a major midline shift.

Caution: Head injuries do not normally cause shock. When anesthetizing or caring for a child with a head injury, be alert for evidence of other injuries. Do not ascribe signs of hypovolemic shock—i.e., tachycardia, hypotension—to the head injury. If such signs are present, search for other sources of bleeding (intra-abdominal, intrathoracic, or in the limbs).

Cervical Spine Injury

Spinal Cord Injury Without Radiologic Abnormality (SCIWORA) is most common in children <8 years of age, especially those involved in motor vehicle accidents. High cervical spinal cord injury may result in apnea and cardiac arrest and should be considered in children with absent vital signs. This contrasts with the lower cervical and upper thoracic spine injuries that occur in older patients.

The anesthesiologist must ensure a rapid, safe tracheal intubation of the injured child while minimizing additional injury to the spinal cord. Early relief of an obstructed airway and controlled ventilation are essential for optimal recovery.

Techniques of intubation other than by direct vision are more difficult (and often more prolonged) in children. Hence, direct laryngoscopy and intubation are recommended, complemented by manual inline stabilization (avoiding traction on the neck). Airway adjuncts such as a video laryngoscope may be particularly valuable to minimize neck movement during laryngoscopy but may prolong the time to tracheal intubation.

Thoracoabdominal Injury

Blunt abdominal trauma is most commonly managed conservatively in children; bleeding from the spleen or liver can be assessed by scanning techniques and usually resolves spontaneously. Surgery is necessary for penetrating wounds, and if continued bleeding causes hemodynamic instability, laparoscopy may be employed to assess intra-abdominal injuries.

The initial assessment must evaluate possible physiologic consequences and the additional effect of anesthesia on the child's condition. In those with intrathoracic injuries, the anesthesiologist's prime concerns are the pulmonary contusion/trauma, possible hemothorax/pneumothorax, the amount of blood lost, and the problem of securing a safe airway (possible tracheal disruption).

Special Anesthesia Problems

1. Major hemorrhage requiring massive blood transfusion (see Chap. 6 and Table 18.1).
2. The possibility of a full stomach (food or blood); always use a cuffed tube.

3. Impaired cardiorespiratory function (in children with diaphragmatic or thoracic trauma); significant pulmonary contusion and serious arrhythmias may follow blunt thoracic trauma.

Immediate Management

1. Prepare for transfusion:
   (a) Insert a wide-bore (a rapid infusion catheter is preferable) cannula into an upper limb or neck vein.
   (b) Send blood for type and cross-match; immediately advise the blood bank if massive transfusion is likely.
   (c) Insert a central venous cannula via a second upper limb or neck vein (use the femoral vein if a head injury is present) for measurement of CVP and to provide an alternative route for transfusion and vasopressors if necessary.
   (d) Place a urine catheter to assess ongoing renal perfusion and function (blood in the urine may indicate renal fracture or disruption).
2. Assess the extent of hypovolemic shock.
3. Infuse appropriate solutions with the use of a blood warmer (boluses of 20 mL/kg balanced salt solution initially).
4. Never infuse large volumes of cold fluids (or blood) via a central vein.

Anesthesia Management

Preoperative

1. Before induction of anesthesia, begin to restore euvolemia, time-permitting. This may require rapid infusions of balanced salt solutions, albumin, and/or blood products, depending on the severity of the trauma and blood loss.
2. Assure adequate supplies of blood in the operating room (OR).
3. Premedication is usually unnecessary, although low-dose opioids may be used.

4. In hypovolemic children, titrate all IV drug doses to avoid hypotension.
5. Ensure availability of a rapid infusion device to provide rapid administration of warmed blood and fluid.
6. Prepare appropriate vasopressors and set up administration pumps through a separate IV with multiple stopcocks and a continuous carrier solution.
7. Prepare transducers for arterial and central venous access lines.

Perioperative

Induction

1. Prepare and check all necessary equipment (two blades, two handles, two suctions) and drugs for RSI and tracheal intubation (see above).
2. Before induction of anesthesia, reassess the child's physiologic status.
3. Preoxygenate as tolerated.
4. Check patency of intravenous lines.
5. Connect monitoring equipment.
6. Consider the possibility of persistent hypovolemia:
   (a) If hypovolemia has been corrected, induce anesthesia with propofol or thiopental, atropine, and succinylcholine, or high-dose rocuronium.
   (b) For emergent surgery in hypovolemic children, induce with ketamine (2 mg/kg) or etomidate (0.3 mg/kg).
7. Position the child supine for intubation.
8. Do not inflate the lungs before laryngoscopy (ventilation may precipitate vomiting). Cricoid pressure may be considered, although it is contraindicated if cervical spine injury may be present. Release cricoid pressure after the tracheal tube is placed and the cuff inflated.
9. Do not give any drugs (except atropine and possibly low-dose fentanyl and midazolam) to moribund patients before intubating the trachea.

Maintenance

1. Give O_2, fentanyl, and a non-depolarizing neuromuscular relaxant (rocuronium, vecuronium, or pancuronium). N_2O may cause distention of air-containing spaces, e.g., bowel and pneumothorax, and should be avoided. Only low concentrations of inhalational agents should be used initially; midazolam may be indicated to reduce the risk of awareness.
2. Control ventilation to produce a near-normal $PetCO_2$, but confirm $PaCO_2$ with arterial blood gases because of possible large $\dot{V}/\dot{Q}$ mismatch. If the hypovolemia is uncorrected, avoid positive end-expiratory pressure and adjust the inspiratory-expiratory ratio to give a low mean intrathoracic pressure. Use a passive or heated humidifier.
3. Monitor ventilation, heart rate and rhythm, temperature, BP, CVP, SaO_2, $PetCO_2$, and urine output. A processed EEG monitor may provide useful trend information in older children.
4. Insert an arterial cannula for direct BP monitoring and for repeated blood sampling for serial determination of the acid-base status, blood gases, Hct, and coagulation studies.
5. Insert a multi-lumen CVP line to provide for monitoring and drug infusions.
6. Maintain body temperature with a forced air warming mattress.
7. Be prepared to treat sudden hypotension as the abdomen is opened in the child who has massive intra-abdominal bleeding.

Postoperative

1. In the absence of chest injury, significantly impaired pulmonary function, or a need for damage control abdominal packing, remove the tracheal tube after antagonizing the muscle relaxant with the child awake and responding and in a lateral position.
2. In the child with thoracic injuries or impaired pulmonary function who remains unconscious—or whose condition is otherwise labile—continue ventilatory support and re-evaluate later in the intensive care unit.
3. Plan postoperative pain relief.

Special Considerations

1. Overt or suspected hepatic injury: the elimination half-lives of drugs that are metabolized by the liver may be increased. Hence, repeat doses of such drugs, e.g., barbiturates and opioids, should be delayed to prevent excessive blood concentrations. Drugs that avoid hepatic elimination, e.g., cisatracurium and remifentanil, are preferred.
2. Overt or suspected renal injury is usually treated conservatively unless the child is hemodynamically unstable. Trauma patients with acute renal failure as a complication of prolonged hypovolemia and hypotension require special attention: Maintain an adequate mean arterial pressure, administer mannitol (0.25 mg/kg), and avoid drugs that are excreted predominantly via the kidneys.
3. Ruptured diaphragm: Rupture of the diaphragm is more common in children than adults and may be overlooked because respiratory distress is usually not severe. This condition requires thoracoabdominal repair:
   (a) Insert a gastric tube to decompress the upper gastrointestinal tract.
   (b) N_2O is contraindicated as in most cases of chest injury.
4. Injury to chest wall and lungs:
   (a) In young children, the ribs are relatively soft and less likely to fracture; however, the injury may separate the costochondral junctions, and this, in association with fractures of posterior ribs, may lead to "flail chest." If this results in hypoventilation, intubate the trachea and control the ventilation.
   (b) Trauma to the chest wall is usually accompanied by contusion of the underlying lung, even when there are no rib fractures. This results in shunting of blood through damaged lung tissue and the need for O_2 therapy and possibly for positive pressure ventilation.
   (c) Pneumothorax, hemothorax, or both may be present. If these are suspected, insert appropriate chest drains before induction. These injuries are suspected in the child with grunting respirations and may occur without rib fracture.

5. Overt or suspected tracheal or bronchial injury:
   (a) If there is evidence to suggest such injury, or if subcutaneous emphysema of the face, neck, or chest is present, bronchoscopy is required to define the extent of the damage.
   (b) Induce anesthesia with sevoflurane in O_2 or IV propofol (deep anesthesia/sedation is needed to avoid coughing and straining). Maintain spontaneous ventilation and avoid positive pressure, which may increase any air leak. Avoid N_2O.
   (c) Give lidocaine (1.5 mg/kg IV), wait for 3 min, and then perform laryngoscopy and topicalize the larynx with lidocaine. The bronchoscope may then be inserted.
   (d) During bronchoscopy, sevoflurane in 100% O_2 may be continued via the bronchoscope; alternatively, anesthesia may be continued with a propofol infusion or a combination of sevoflurane and propofol.
   (e) If thoracotomy is required and damage is limited to one bronchus, intubate the uninjured main bronchus using a fiberoptic scope to guide correct placement (see Chap. 4).
   (f) If a tracheal injury is present as a temporizing measure, pass the tracheal tube past the site of injury, almost to the carina. Check bilateral ventilation and allow spontaneous respirations. In some cases a tracheostomy may be required.
6. Injury to the heart and pericardium is rare in children but may occur in association with severe thoracic trauma. Cardiac contusion may result in changes in ventricular function assessed by echocardiography; the ECG may show nonspecific ST changes but most often is unchanged.
7. Injuries to the great vessels are less common than in adults, owing to the greater elasticity and mobility of the mediastinal structures; however, a widened mediastinum indicates the need for immediate exploration.
   (a) If cardiac tamponade develops secondary to hemopericardium (Beck's triad: hypotension, raised jugular venous pressure, muffled heart sounds), induction of anesthesia is very hazardous because the fixed low cardiac output cannot compensate for any drug-induced alterations in systemic vascular resistance.

(b) If the hemopericardium is small and the child is hemodynamically stable and can lie flat, general anesthesia may be induced with ketamine anesthesia, and the airway secured with an endotracheal tube. The cardiologist or surgeon may then drain the pericardium, leaving a pigtail catheter to prevent further fluid accumulation. If, however, the child is short of breath and cannot lie flat or is hypotensive, the child is positioned recumbent with oxygen administered by facemask, while the surgeon drains the pericardium under local anesthesia alone or in combination with sedation (e.g., ketamine).

Acute Burns and Scalds

Children are often the victims of burns and scalds. Extensive burns have widespread systemic effects: massive fluid shifts occur, plasma protein is lost, and all the major organ systems are affected. The physiologic response to acute burns may be divided into early (first 72 h after injury) and late (4 days to weeks after injury) (Table 18.5):

Table 18.5 Systemic effects of burn injury

System	Early	Late
Cardiovascular	↓ CO due to decreased circulating blood volume, myocardial depressant factor	↑ CO due to sepsis ↑ CO 2–3 times > baseline for months (hypermetabolism) Hypertension
Pulmonary	Upper airway obstruction due to edema Lower airway obstruction due to edema, bronchospasm, particulate matter ↓ FRC ↓ Pulmonary compliance ↓ Chest wall compliance	Bronchopneumonia Tracheal stenosis ↓ Chest wall compliance

(continued)

Table 18.5 (continued)

System	Early	Late
Renal	↓ GFR (a) Secondary to ↓ circulating blood volume (b) Myoglobinuria (c) Hemoglobinuria Tubular dysfunction	↑ GFR 2° to ↑ CO Tubular dysfunction
Hepatic	↓ Function 2° to ↓ circulating blood volume, hypoxia, hepatotoxins	Hepatitis ↑ Function due to hypermetabolism, enzyme induction, ↑ CO ↓ Function due to sepsis, drug interactions
Hematopoietic	↓ Platelets ↑ Fibrin split products, consumptive coagulopathy, anemia	↑ Platelets ↑ Clotting factors Anemia of burns due to ↓ erythropoietin
Neurologic	Encephalopathy Seizures ↑ ICP	Encephalopathy Seizures ICU psychosis
Skin	↑ Heat, fluid, electrolyte loss	Contractures, scar formation, difficult intubation
Metabolic	↓ Ionized calcium	↑ Oxygen consumption ↑ Carbon dioxide production ↓ Ionized calcium
Pharmacokinetics	Altered volume of distribution Altered protein binding Altered pharmacokinetics Altered pharmacodynamics	Tolerance to opioids, sedatives Enzyme induction, altered receptors Drug interactions

Adapted with permission (Table 34-2 in "Burn Injuries"). Nichols et al. (2024)

Early refers to the first 24–72 h after injury; *late* refers to days to weeks after injury

CO cardiac output, *FRC* functional residual capacity, *GFR* glomerular filtration rate, *ICP* intracranial pressure, *ICU* intensive care unit

1. Direct injury to the upper airway and lungs may cause obstruction secondary to edema, bronchospasm, or sloughed tissue early after a burn (see further). Later, pulmonary function may be affected by infection (pneumonia), acute respiratory distress syndrome (ARDS), or pulmonary vascular changes.
2. Hypovolemia and a circulating myocardial depressant factor may lead to early cardiac dysfunction. After day 3, a hypermetabolic state occurs with a marked increase in cardiac output (2–3 times baseline) to maintain oxygen delivery; this will persist until the child is fully grafted (see Table 18.5).
3. Circulating myoglobin and hemoglobin can directly damage the kidneys. Hypovolemia may cause acute tubular damage, especially if compounded by hypoxia. After day 3, the marked increase in cardiac output increases GFR, which in turn dramatically reduces the half-life of many drugs excreted by the kidneys. In addition, hypertension occurs in approximately 50% of children with extensive burn injury. This is mediated by increased renin, endogenous catecholamines, atrial natriuretic factor, and aldosterone production. Some children require a β-blocker or calcium channel blockers to control the hypertension.
4. The liver may be damaged as a result of hypotension, hypoxemia, inhaled toxins, or sepsis. After day 3, marked increases in hepatic blood flow will increase excretion of medications metabolized by the liver.
5. Anemia of burns (decreased erythropoietin production), thrombocytopenia, and a consumptive coagulopathy may occur. Later, a notable thrombocytosis and increased fibrinogen may occur; a sudden decrease in platelet count often heralds developing sepsis.
6. Gastric distention, intestinal ileus, and bleeding secondary to stress ulcers may develop; abdominal compartment syndrome may occur. Appropriate antacid therapy is indicated.

The anesthesiologist will be involved in the early treatment, which consists of the following:

1. Airway management and fluid resuscitation
2. Fasciotomy (electrical burns on day 1 improve blood flow to extremities and digits) and/or escharotomy (flame or scald burns on day 2–3 improve adequacy of chest wall excursion)
3. Debridement and grafting (day 3–5 and beyond)

Special Anesthesia Problems

1. Airway and pulmonary involvement may lead to airway obstruction, severe intrapulmonary shunting, and respiratory failure; edema of the tissues surrounding the upper airway may occur very rapidly and make intubation extremely difficult (intubate the trachea as soon as possible). Airway burns should be suspected in all children involved in enclosed-space fires (house/automobile), where inhaled temperatures may reach 1000 °F. Carbonaceous material in the mouth and nose or burned facial hair and/or eyebrows is a common warning sign. These children may have macroglossia, macrouvula, epiglottitis, and glottic edema (croup) simultaneously.

   Early tracheal intubation with a cuffed tube is advised; any delay in intubation may render the airway impossible to secure due to swelling. Thermal injury is limited to the upper airway, but inhalation of products of plastic combustion, such as NO_2 or SO_2, carry these gases far down the tracheobronchial tree, and they combine with water to form sulfuric and nitric acid, causing a distal chemical airway burn. Loss of ciliated epithelium and other respiratory protective mechanisms predisposes to early infection and airway obstruction. Bronchospasm is common. Acid aldehydes may cause pulmonary edema, and inhaled cyanide may poison the cytochrome oxidase system. Carbon monoxide (CO) poisoning is the most common cause of impaired oxygen delivery after burns and necessitates therapy with 100% oxygen to reduce the CO elimination half-life (from ~4 h to ~30 min).
2. Maintenance of fluid balance and renal function: several formulas may be used to calculate fluid regimens for the burned patient; these are based on the burn area (excluding erythema).

The Parkland formula prescribes 4 mL/kg of lactated Ringer's solution for each 1% of burn area, whereas the Brook formula prescribes 0.45 mL/kg crystalloid and 1.5 mL/kg colloid for each 1% of burn area. One-half of these amounts is given in the first 8 h, and the other half over the next 16 h. Note that these formulas underestimate fluid requirements in children who weigh less than 10 kg, who should receive their normal maintenance requirements as well. It should be further noted that the "rule of 9s" does not apply to toddlers and that burns of the head may account for 20% of the body surface area (it is easy to underestimate the severity of a burn). Many other resuscitation fluid regimens have been used, and all are effective; see Romanowski et al. for more discussion and additional resuscitation formulae. In practice, fluid therapy should be adjusted.

3. Preventing hypothermia: Loss of normal skin severely impairs the patient's ability to conserve heat. Warming the operating room to maximal values (32 °C), a forced air warming device, and a radiant lamp are essential; do not unwrap all of the dressings at one time.
4. In children with extensive burns: as dictated by the child's clinical and biochemical status, urine output is the primary metric for hydration. Do not use glucose-containing solutions for fluid resuscitation, as life-threatening hyperglycemia may occur. Hyperosmolar, hyperglycemic non-ketotic coma may occur in association with burns; glucose-containing fluid administration should be guided by measured blood values.
5. Acute gastric dilation: This commonly occurs and increases the risk of regurgitation. The stomach should be decompressed, and special care should be taken during induction and emergence from anesthesia. For subsequent surgery, jejunal feeding tubes should not be removed.
6. In children with extensive burns:
   (a) Monitoring may be difficult.
   (b) Sites for intravenous infusions may be limited; subclavian and femoral lines are common.
7. Circumferential thoracic burns: These may lead to severely compromised ventilation requiring multiple escharotomies to restore chest wall compliance.

8. Danger of infection: Extreme care must be taken to observe strict asepsis with invasive procedures.
9. Electrical burns: electrical current travels along neurovascular bundles; such an injury can produce a compartment syndrome, which will require immediate operative fasciotomies to preserve extremity function. Look for evidence of both entrance and exit wounds, and assume everything in between may have been damaged.

Anesthesia Management

Preoperative

1. If the fire occurred in a closed space or involved burning hydrocarbons, suspect respiratory tract burns:
   (a) Look for evidence of burns around the face, e.g., singed eyebrows.
   (b) Carefully assess the airway, as children with airway burns may have considerable swelling of the pharyngeal and laryngeal tissues, rendering intubation difficult.
   (c) Early tracheal intubation with a cuffed tube is essential before massive upper airway edema forms. This tube should be meticulously secured with cloth tracheostomy tape, as adhesive tape cannot be used on burned tissue. Mark the appropriate distance of insertion at the level of the nares or dentition with indelible ink so that misplacement with later dressing changes is less likely. Accidental extubation must be prevented, as reintubation may be impossible if upper airway edema ensues.
   (d) If the airway is already intubated, ensure that the tracheal tube is properly placed and secured.
2. Check the adequacy of fluid and blood replacement:
   (a) The Hct should be maintained at 25–30%. Ensure adequate blood products are in the OR.
   (b) The bladder should be catheterized, and urine output maintained at least 1 mL/kg/h.
   (c) FFP or platelets may be required to correct documented deficiencies.

If the child is receiving intravenous alimentation, reduce the rate to two-thirds during anesthesia to avoid hyperglycemia.

3. Establish a thermoneutral environment (see above), including warmers for blood and intravenous fluids.
4. Analgesics and hypnotics should be given to prevent pain during transportation to the OR.

Perioperative

General endotracheal anesthesia may be required, but remember:

1. In acute burns, use conservative dosing of propofol or thiopental if the child's volume status is uncertain; ketamine may be useful in such circumstances. Generally, the child is induced in the hospital bed to prevent pain upon movement to the OR table.
2. Succinylcholine is contraindicated (after the first 24 h) because it may cause cardiac arrest secondary to massive potassium release from muscle.
3. Resistance to non-depolarizing muscle relaxants is increased in proportion to the burn area. Larger doses of rocuronium, 1.8–2.0 mg/kg, may be required for rapid sequence intubation. Muscle relaxants must be titrated to achieve their desired effects. Monitor the neuromuscular blockade. Antagonism of very large doses of relaxants is not a problem.
4. Potent inhalational agents may cause hypotension in those with extensive burns in the acute phase but may be useful in controlling blood pressure during the hypertensive phase. Generally, a high-dose opioid technique with a background inhalation agent is most useful. Alternatively, TIVA with a propofol infusion and an opioid or ketamine greatly simplifies the anesthetic management of burned or scalded children.
5. Infusions of vasopressors should be immediately available at the time of first excision and grafting, as bacterial sepsis may lead to severe hypotension after induction of anesthesia.

For burn dressing changes:

(a) Give atropine (0.02 mg/kg) and midazolam (50–100 mcg/kg) IV, followed by ketamine (1–2 mg/kg) IV and supplemented doses as needed.
(b) Alternatively, if IV access is not available, induce anesthesia with ketamine (4–6 mg/kg) IM combined with atropine (0.02 mg/kg) and midazolam (50–100 μg/kg) IM. After an IV is placed, further incremental doses of ketamine (1–2 mg/kg) may be titrated.
(c) A combination of propofol (1 mg/kg) and ketamine (1–2 mg/kg) IV, followed by a propofol infusion, is another alternative.

For all children:

1. Carefully monitor the following:
   (a) Cardiac rate via an esophageal stethoscope and the ECG plus pulse oximeter. The oximeter probe may be placed on the tongue or at the corner of the mouth if no other site is available.
   (b) BP—place a sterile BP cuff at any available site; for severe burns, insert an arterial line.
   (c) Temperature—core temperature measured either esophageally and/or rectally.
   (d) Blood loss—it is often difficult to estimate loss. Replacement must then be dictated by cardiovascular parameters and urine output. Blood loss is far greater with tangential excision of eschar until bleeding is observed from viable tissue, compared with full-thickness eschar excision. Blood loss can be greatly reduced if the surgeon administers subcutaneous saline with dilute epinephrine (1:2,000,000 = 0.5 μg/mL) into both the donor and excised areas. Beware of fluid overload when large quantities of tumescent solution are injected; this must be considered in overall fluid management, as late pulmonary edema may occur as this fluid is absorbed.
   (e) CVP—consider utility versus danger of introducing infection. A CVP may be the only venous access available with

large burns. Large-caliber access should be sought to rapidly deliver a large volume of blood if required. Avoid rapidly transfusing cold, old blood products via the central line to prevent cardiac dysfunction due to hyperkalemia in packed red blood cells and hypocalcemia from the citrate in FFP. Short-term cannulation of a femoral vessel with a single-lumen catheter may be indicated just for the procedure and may be removed afterward.

2. Significant blood loss necessitates the administration of large volumes of replacement fluids. Anticipate coagulation problems with massive transfusions.
3. Beware of hypocalcemia. Chronic low levels of ionized calcium have been described in burn patients. Plasma and platelet suspensions contain more citrate per unit volume than whole blood; give calcium chloride (5–10 mg/kg) or calcium gluconate (15–30 mg/kg) if unexpected hypotension occurs. If transfusion exceeds 1 mL/kg/min, anticipate hypocalcemia and administer calcium during these rapid infusions.

Postoperative

1. Order maintenance fluids:
   (a) Crystalloid fluids to maintain urine output at more than 1 mL/kg/h.
   (b) PRBCs to maintain the Hct at 25–30%.
   (c) Albumin may be indicated to maintain total serum protein at 2–3 g/dL.
   (d) Electrolyte supplements as indicated by serial determinations.
2. Order analgesics by continuous infusion as required. Burn patients require constant nursing supervision so that a generous dosage of analgesics can be safely administered. Long-term infusions of ketamine and/or dexmedetomidine have been found to reduce total opioid requirements in children with extensive burns. Children with extensive burn injuries may become tolerant to opioids and sedatives, requiring up to 1–3 mg/kg/h of morphine and 1–3 mg/kg/h of midazolam to

maintain adequate analgesia and sedation. Additional bolus doses may be required.

3. Respiratory insufficiency may occur in the first 24 h after a burn, even if the chest appears clear initially. Rhonchi and a decreasing level of arterial oxygenation are often the first signs of deteriorating pulmonary function. Inhaled β_2-adrenergic agents may be useful, as may nebulized acetyl cysteine and heparin. In severe airway burns, beware of the possibility of sudden airway obstruction because of sloughed mucosa. Bronchoscopy may be required.
4. Proton pump inhibitors and antacids should be administered to protect against stress ulcers. Burn patients may require larger than usual doses to reduce acid secretion.
5. Children who have been intubated for a period in the intensive care unit are at increased risk for development of postextubation stridor. The ETT should not be removed until there is a detectable leak around the tube. After extubation, they require careful monitoring for 24–48 h, and treatment with racemic epinephrine, helium, and O_2 or even reintubation may be required.
6. Long-term administration of opioids and benzodiazepines may be associated with late withdrawal symptoms. Transition to oral methadone and gradual withdrawal of benzodiazepines reduce this risk.

Gunshot Wounds

Deaths from gunshot wounds in children in the United States now exceed those from motor vehicle trauma. The free access to weapons and guns in the home contributes to this toll. The epidemiology varies by age and geographic location.

Anesthesiologists should be particularly aware of the tissue damage caused by modern high-velocity bullets. Tissue over an extensive area surrounding the path of the bullet is damaged or destroyed by the energy of the projectile. This is of particular importance when such wounds occur in the upper chest or neck region, with the damage at the exit wound being far greater than the entrance wound. Tissue swelling can be expected to spread to involve a wide surrounding area, possibly jeopardizing the airway. The airway should be secured as early as possible, before distortion of the anatomy progresses further. If the child is relatively stable, ensure that adequate blood products are in the room and checked; otherwise, O-negative blood is necessary. Adequate venous access must be established in the upper extremities before incision, as tamponade of the intra-abdominal or intrathoracic wound will be relieved upon surgical incision, and rapid hypotension may ensue. Be prepared for rapid transfusion and the need for vasopressors.

Minor Trauma

Children with minor trauma must be provided with anesthesia that is safe, pleasant, and suitable for a young patient to facilitate rapid discharge from the hospital. Usually there is no extreme urgency in these cases, permitting a considered approach to the selection of both the anesthetic and the optimal time for surgery. However, fractures with vascular compression may require immediate intervention.

Gastric emptying may be substantively delayed after even minor injury, resulting in a full stomach. There is no safe interval between the last food ingested and the injury that guarantees an empty stomach. Currently, POCUS is being used increasingly to detect the presence and quantity of gastric contents. Hence, we recommend using a regional technique or inducing general anesthesia and a rapid-sequence induction followed by extubating the trachea while awake. The use of a laryngeal mask airway in children with minor injuries has been complicated by aspiration.

Although metoclopramide may help to speed gastric emptying, neither regional analgesia nor general anesthesia should be administered without fasting unless surgery is needed urgently. The need to convert an unsatisfactory regional anesthesia to general anesthesia arises more frequently in children than in adults.

Suggested Reading

Borgialli DA, Mahajan P, Hoyle JD Jr, et al. Performance of the pediatric Glasgow Coma Scale score in the evaluation of children with blunt head trauma. Acad Emerg Med. 2016;23:878–84.

Brennan PM, Murray GD, Teasdale GM. Simplifying the use of prognostic information in traumatic brain injury. Part 1: the GCS-Pupils score: an extended index of clinical severity. J Neurosurg. 2018;128(6):1612–20.

Cercueil E, Henriet A, Barbe C, et al. Diagnostic accuracy of qualitative gastric ultrasound assessment for detecting high gastric fluid volume in children: a prospective randomised study. Anaesthesia. 2025;80:636–44.

Cochran ED, Machchhar A, Qiao J, Chung DH. Caught in the crossfire: 10-year experience with pediatric firearm injury at a single institution. J Am Coll Surg. 2025;240:588–95.

Demirel A, Özgünay ŞE, Eminoğlu Ş, et al. Ultrasonographic evaluation of gastric content and volume in pediatric patients undergoing elective surgery: a prospective observational study. Children (Basel). 2023;10(9): 1432.

Figaji A. An update on pediatric traumatic brain injury. Childs Nerv Syst. 2023;39(11):3071–81.

Fraser Doh K, Chaudhary S, Ruest SM, et al. Variability in firearm injury among major pediatric trauma centers a cross the USA. Trauma Surg Acute Care Open. 2023;8(1):e001014.

Graves L, et al. A comparison of actual to estimated weights in Australian children attending a tertiary children's hospital, using the original and updated APLS, Luscombe and Owens, Best Guess formulae and the Broselow tape. Resuscitation. 2014;85:392–6.

Kochanek PM, Tasker RC, Carney N, et al. Guidelines for the management of pediatric severe traumatic brain injury, Third Edition: update of the Brain Trauma Foundation Guidelines. Pediatr Crit Care Med. 2019;20(3S Suppl 1):S1–s82.

Lannon MM, Duda T, Martyniuk A, et al. Pediatric craniocerebral gunshot injuries: a national trauma database study. J Trauma Acute Care Surg. 2022;92:428–35.

Lui A, Kumar KK, Grant GA. Management of severe traumatic brain injury in pediatric patients. Front Toxicol. 2022;4:910972.

Madhivathanan PR, Corredor C, Smith A. Perioperative implications of pericardial effusions and cardiac tamponade. BJA Educ. 2020;20(7):226–34.

Nassar JY, Al Qurashi AA, Albalawi IA, et al. Pediatric burns: a systematic review and meta-analysis on epidemio logy, gender distribution, risk factors, management, and outcomes in emergency departments. Cureus. 2023;15(11):e49012.

Nichols JH, Coté CJ, Martyn JAJ. In: Coté CJ, Lerman J, Anderson BJ, editors. A practice of anesthesia for infants and children. 7th ed. Philadelphia: Elsevier; 2024. Chapter 34.

Pelizzo G, Calcaterra V, Marinaro M, et al. Metabolic and hormonal changes in pediatric burn patients: mechanisms, evidence, and care strategies. Eur Burn J. 2025;6:17..

Romanowski KS, Palmieri TL. Pediatric burn resuscitation: past, present, and future. Burns Trauma. 2017;5(1):26.

Strobel AM, Fey R. Emergency care of pediatric burns. Emerg Med Clin N Am. 2018;36:441–58.

Zhang JK, Hongsermeier-Graves N, Savic B, et al. Pediatric cervical spine trauma: a narrative review. Clin Spine Surg. 2024;37:416–24.

Anesthesia Outside the Operating Room

19

Remote Anesthesia

Almost one-third of all anesthetics are provided in non-operating room locations for a variety of medical investigations or procedures in infants and children of all ages. However, anesthesia services in remote locations may be associated with serious complications, similar to those in the operating room.

Equipment for the Remote Location

Each area should be fully equipped to provide safe anesthetic care and for any resuscitation that might be required. Each area should be provided with:

1. Primary and backup oxygen supplies (checked O_2 tank), and means to provide intermittent positive-pressure ventilation (IPPV).
2. Facilities for gas scavenging if any inhalation anesthetics are used.
3. Functioning suction apparatus.
4. Good lighting.
5. Electrical outlets (operating room standards).

J. Lerman, C. J. Coté, *Steward's Manual of Pediatric Anesthesia*, https://doi.org/10.1007/978-3-032-24545-8_19

6. Means of immediate communication to the operating room personnel.
7. Equipment to transport the child while anesthetized.
8. Facilities and staff for the preparation and recovery of children according to published guidelines.[1]
9. Fully equipped, provisioned, and regularly checked resuscitation cart and defibrillator in the immediate vicinity.

In addition, all drugs and equipment that are needed to manage the child during the anesthetic must be provided:

1. Standard ASA monitors, including pulse oximetry, electrocardiography (ECG), $PetCO_2$, blood pressure, and body temperature.
2. Airway supplies: age and size-appropriate facemasks, laryngoscope blades, tracheal tubes, oropharyngeal airways, laryngeal mask airways, suction catheters, and breathing circuits.
3. Appropriate, regularly serviced anesthesia equipment and infusion pumps.
4. All necessary drugs for anesthesia and sedation, syringes, a variety of IV catheters, intravenous fluids, and fluid administration sets.
5. Emergency resuscitation drugs and equipment (pediatric-size pads for the defibrillator).
6. Forced air warmer in specific situations (cardiac cath lab).

Administrative Procedure for Remote Anesthesia

A pre-procedure evaluation should be performed as for OR patients. Children who require anesthesia in remote locations may be scheduled for urgent or semi-urgent cases; this should not exclude a full assessment.

[1]Guidelines for monitoring and management of pediatric patients before, during, and after sedation for diagnostic and therapeutic procedures: Coté CJ, Wilson S, American Academy of Pediatrics, American Academy of Pediatric Dentistry. Pediatrics 2019:143(1);e20191000.

1. A complete evaluation should be performed and reviewed just before sedation/anesthesia.
2. Informed consent should be obtained or confirmed to be on file, e.g., a serial consent for children undergoing multiple radiation treatments.
3. A detailed anesthesia record should be completed.
4. The child should be recovered in an appropriately staffed and equipped area for children or be safely transported to the pediatric postanesthesia care unit (PACU).
5. A recovery record should be completed.
6. The child should be evaluated by an anesthesiologist when the child has recovered and is ready for discharge; where appropriate, this might be delegated using standard written criteria.

General Principles

1. The technique chosen should result in minimal (if any) postanesthesia sequelae.
   (a) Use short-acting drugs that will not delay recovery and are not associated with postoperative nausea and vomiting; when possible, avoid opioids, barbiturates, and ketamine. Propofol and/or dexmedetomidine are ideal.
   (b) Most children can be managed with an oxygen mask or nasal prongs and a support to extend the neck. Occasionally, an oral or nasopharyngeal airway may be required. The laryngeal mask airway (LMA) is a useful alternative; in some, tracheal intubation may be required. In general, tracheal intubation is avoided in remote locations to abbreviate the recovery time.
   (c) When repeated anesthetics are needed, access to a venous port is advantageous for both the anesthesiologist and the child.

Diagnostic and Therapeutic Medical Procedures

Computed Tomography (CT)

1. CT scans require absolute immobility of the child. Since current scan times are exceedingly brief, even when contrast is given, they are completed within 10 min. Hence, many children for CT scanning can be managed without anesthesia, and, for the others, the anesthetic plan must be tailored accordingly. Small infants can be fed, bundled, and restrained during the procedure without sedation. Older cooperative children may not require any form of sedation or anesthetic, as they can be distracted and entertained for the short time necessary to complete a scan. It is sometimes necessary to sedate or anesthetize infants and children less than 3 years old, cognitively challenged children, and those with significant comorbid disease or injury.
2. Intravenous sedation alone is suitable for many children:
   (a) A propofol infusion is preferred.
   (b) The child should be monitored with standard ASA monitors. All equipment required to establish an airway and ventilate the lungs should be immediately available.
3. If general anesthesia with airway instrumentation is required, use only plastic materials in the breathing circuit; metal components distort the image. Be aware that the metal spring in some LMA cuffs and tracheotomy tubes may cause an artifact; the spring should be taped away from the field.
4. Intravenous contrast media may be needed to enhance images. Very rarely, reactions may occur; be aware to limit the dose in children with renal dysfunction.

Magnetic Resonance Imaging

Magnetic resonance imaging (MRI) scans are used increasingly to avoid radiation exposure that is associated with CT scans. They are used to define anatomic or physiologic anomalies and increasingly to define vascular anatomy [magnetic resonance angiography (MRA)], e.g., in children with congenital heart disease. The basic component of the MRI system is a powerful superconducting magnet, which presents important safety issues for the patient and the anesthesiologist, particularly the need for MRI-compatible equipment:

1. The space is very confined, which limits access to the child should an emergency occur; this limited space may frighten children with claustrophobia. It is helpful if the walls in the MRI room are covered in bright, colorful murals to reduce children's fears. Additionally, loud sudden noises (approximately 95 dB) and vibrations may scare the awake child; hence, the need for deep sedation or general anesthesia. Noise-canceling MRI-safe headphones carrying music will help distract older children.
2. Ferromagnetic materials (containing iron, cobalt, or nickel) are MRI unsafe, as they are highly attracted to the magnet and become dangerous, life-threatening projectiles (Zone IV scanner). All equipment, including oxygen tanks, IV poles, laryngoscope blades and handles, etc., which are taken into the unit must be MRI-compatible (non-ferromagnetic). Any "doubtful" items must be tested with a magnet in Zone II before being brought into the scanner room.
3. It is essential that the child and accompanying parent are screened for implanted devices that might incorporate ferromagnetic material (see list at www.radiologyinfo.org/en/info/safety-mr). These could be dangerously attracted to the magnet; their function could be affected by the magnetic field, e.g., cardiac pacemaker, implanted defibrillator, transthoracic or transvenous pacing wires, or vagal nerve stimulator; or they could seriously damage adjacent tissues, e.g., implanted prostheses, wires or vascular clips, cochlear implants, and metal foreign bodies. Cell phones, watches, credit cards, parking receipts, some pens, etc. may be damaged or attracted to the magnet and must not enter the scanning room (Zone IV). Firearms may spontaneously discharge, causing death or injury, so police in particular must be carefully screened. Programmable VP shunts or vagal nerve stimulators must be

adjusted before and, if necessary, reprogrammed after the MRI. All implanted devices and pumps must be checked for MRI compatibility (see website above) and reprogrammed as needed after the MRI. This situation may require a call to the manufacturer. MRI is contraindicated in children with non-removable ferromagnetic implanted material.

4. The magnetic field may cause burns by inducing currents and heat in circinate wire leads (ECG or pulse oximeter cables) or temperature probes. Prevent direct contact between the cables and the child's skin, avoid loops in the cables, and ensure that the cables are directed out of the center of the bore (not the sides) to minimize current induction. MRI-compatible ECG and pulse oximetry equipment must be used to reduce the risk of burns. Tattoos pigmented with dyes that contain ferromagnetic metals may produce a burning sensation at the tattoo site.
5. The magnetic field may affect the performance of anesthesia delivery systems; syringe pumps may be unreliable or attracted to the magnet. Alternatively, the infusion pump may be placed outside of the scanner room to avoid interference from the magnet by using extra-long infusion lines threaded through a conduit in the wall of the scanner room. Note that the distance may require up to 5 lengths of pressure tubing; multiple extension IV tubings are generally avoided because the high resistance sensed by the pump when several lengths are combined may cause the pump to alarm or the infusion rate to decrease.
6. MRI scanning is motion-sensitive; if the child moves, an entire scan sequence may need to be repeated.
7. The child may have a major life-threatening illness with the need for vasopressor support or invasive monitoring. This necessitates using long infusion lines to keep the pumps outside of the scanner room, which may interrupt infusions, resulting in cardiovascular instability. Arterial line transducers may need extended lines to keep the transducer out of the scanner room.
8. The child may have a difficult airway. In such a case, tracheal intubation should be performed outside of the scan-

ner room to allow use of special airway adjuncts such as the GlideScope® or a fiberoptic bronchoscope, or alternately, the airway should be secured in the operating room and then the anesthetized child should be transported to the MRI unit.

9. Resuscitation equipment *cannot* be brought into the MRI scan room should it be required. If resuscitation is required, the child must be rapidly extracted from the scanner room and transferred to an adjacent room where resuscitation equipment resides.
10. Higher power magnets (3 T) may reveal that equipment previously found to be safe and reliable in the environment of a 1.5 T unit may be unsafe and/or unreliable in a 3 T unit. Implanted devices are graded according to their susceptibility to the magnetic fields in an MRI scanner: MR safe, MR unsafe, and MR conditional (see website above). The shielding installed and the distance a piece of equipment is sited from the magnet are also vital safety concerns. Even some MRI-compatible anesthesia machines will trigger an alarm should the machine be placed too close to the magnet. The anesthesiologist should be very familiar with the safety concerns of the local unit.
11. Gadolinium-based contrast agents are commonly used to enhance blood vessels in MRI imaging; they very rarely cause anaphylaxis. Of greater concern is that it is poorly cleared and may result in nephrogenic systemic fibrosis (NSF) with multiorgan involvement. Hence, the FDA has published a warning about the unknown long-term effects, in particular comparing the two types of contrast material (linear and macrocyclic), with the retention longer in the latter formulations. The FDA advises that the drug can be used in children <2 years but recommends against use in those with renal impairment (GFR <30 mL/min/1.73 m^2). **N.B**. Radiology departments now have guidelines for gadolinium dose based on weight, creatinine, and BUN values, and these charts should be consulted.

Monitoring During MRI Scans

Monitoring during the scan is essential; a plastic precordial or esophageal stethoscope (without a thermistor probe) may be used, and MRI-compatible equipment is essential:

1. MRI-compatible pulse oximetry must be used continuously; it is essential to avoid loops in the cable leads to the child—otherwise currents may be induced and the child may be burned.
2. Continuous monitoring of expired carbon dioxide tension ($PetCO_2$) is standard of care.
3. Blood pressure may be measured with automated NIBP machines fitted with nylon connections.
4. The ECG may be monitored using non-ferromagnetic fasteners, cables, and electrodes.
5. Temperature may be monitored using probes that have radiofrequency filters. Insulating the infant from the cool ambient magnet temperature is important; however, children may increase their body temperature slightly during long MRI scans, but hypothermia is a greater concern.
6. MRI-compatible monitoring devices are available with a remote slave monitor outside the MRI scanner room, allowing the anesthesiologist to remain outside and be able to view the patient via a window. However, for scans that require breath-holding, the anesthesiologist will remain in the scanner room to start and stop the ventilator. Each multichannel monitoring device must be tested for compatibility with the local MRI magnet.

Management for Magnetic Resonance Imaging

Satisfactory immobilization of the child during the scanning process may be achieved by intravenous deep sedation/anesthesia or general anesthesia with an LMA or tracheal tube.

Intravenous Deep Sedation/Anesthesia

An intravenous propofol infusion is the most reliable and efficient method, although some providers use combinations of dexmedetomidine, midazolam, and propofol.

1. The child should fast as per ASA fasting guidelines.
2. The vast majority of scans are performed on outpatients. Anesthesia is induced by inhalation, and IV access is established. The propofol infusion is started at 250 μg/kg/min in toddlers and at 350–400 μg/kg/min in neonates, infants, and those cognitively impaired. Alternately, if IV access has been established, the propofol infusion is supplemented with several small IV boluses of propofol to rapidly establish a steady-state brain concentration to prevent movement.
3. The cervical spine is extended using a shoulder roll to maintain a patent upper airway because the head fixation device slightly flexes the neck. Oxygen may be delivered by baffled nasal prongs, which delivers oxygen through one ala and aspirates gas for carbon dioxide analysis through the second. Alternatively, an oxygen facemask with a 16-ga IV catheter placed near a naris, to which the CO_2 sampling line is connected, may be used. If airway obstruction is a concern or the head moves excessively during a brain scan, then an LMA may be required. The adequacy of ventilation is monitored via the $PetCO_2$.
4. If the child moves, an IV bolus of propofol is administered, and the infusion rate is increased until movement ceases.
5. After 15–20 min, the infusion rate may be reduced to 200 μg/kg/min, and after a further 15–20 min (in older children), the rate may be further reduced to 150 μg/kg/min. Hypotension and/or apnea are rare events at these infusion rates, and recovery is rapid even if the infusion rate is unchanged.
6. The airway is usually well-maintained during propofol sedation; however:
   (a) If airway obstruction occurs, reposition the head.

(b) If obstruction persists, consider inserting an oral or nasopharyngeal airway or a laryngeal mask airway, in order of escalating importance.
(c) If obstruction persists or ventilation/oxygenation is poor, the trachea may require intubation.

7. At the end of the scan, the infusion is discontinued; recovery in an appropriately staffed and equipped pediatric recovery area is usually complete within 20–30 min.

General Anesthesia

1. General anesthesia with an LMA or tracheal intubation and controlled ventilation may be required for seriously ill children, especially those with central nervous system disease, neonates, children with multiple injuries, and those who require abdominal MRI scans, as these often require periodic breath-holding. There is no pain and/or stimulation during MRI scans, so neither opioids nor an excessive depth of anesthesia is required to complete the scans.

   A common anesthetic prescription is to induce with sevoflurane, nitrous oxide, and oxygen; establish venous access; and administer 1 mg/kg IV propofol to facilitate inserting the LMA; and then reduce the inspired sevoflurane concentration to 1.5–2.0% in 50% nitrous oxide while maintaining spontaneous respirations or pressure support with 5 cm PEEP. At the end of the scan, administer an additional 0.5–1 mg/kg propofol and remove the LMA; this reduces the risk of laryngospasm and emergence delirium.
2. Children with known difficult airways should have their airway secured outside of the scanner with all the usual difficult airway adjuncts or intubated in the operating room and transported to the scanner.

Special Considerations for Cardiac MRI Imaging

Cardiac imaging in the MRI unit successfully demonstrates the exact anatomy of congenital heart diseases and is a valuable diagnostic tool. To obtain consistent images, the scan must be successfully ECG "gated" to the cardiac cycle and obtained at a standard phase of ventilation, which can similarly be achieved by respiratory gating ("free breathing"). Anesthesia or sedation for these children must recognize all the implications of their heart disease. Comprehensive monitoring should be provided appropriate for their pathology. In many cases, tracheal intubation with paralysis and a low-dose inhalation agent is required to facilitate scanning with breath holding; other patients can be managed using deep sedation with propofol. The technique chosen must balance the severity and type of cardiac anomaly and the needs of the cardiologist.

Other Radiologic Procedures

General anesthesia is often necessary for cerebral angiography because the procedure may be prolonged and uncomfortable, and the child must remain immobile throughout.

Special Anesthesia Problems

1. Intracranial pressure (ICP) may be increased.
2. The radiologic examination may require special positioning and tilting of the child.
3. It may be difficult to maintain body temperature in infants.
4. Special attention must be paid to the total load of contrast material (mg/kg) particularly in infants with compromised renal function; low ionic contrast solutions are preferred. Reactions to contrast media may occur; though this is now quite rare with the use of nonionic agents.
5. It is desirable for children to recover rapidly so that their neurologic status can be assessed.

Anesthesia Management

Preoperative

1. Review the child's neurologic status and other underlying medical conditions.
2. Check for a history of allergy, asthma, prior anesthetic experiences, or previous reactions to radiologic contrast media.
3. Avoid premedication if ICP is increased.

Perioperative

1. An intravenous induction with propofol or thiopental followed by a non-depolarizing muscle relaxant.
2. For children with increased ICP, give lidocaine 1.5 mg/kg IV and a short-acting opioid, e.g., fentanyl 2 µg/kg, to attenuate the hypertensive response to laryngoscopy and intubation.
3. Insert an endotracheal tube. A nasal or armored tube should be used if the tube may become kinked during the procedure.
4. Maintain anesthesia with sevoflurane or a propofol infusion.

Cerebral Arteriography

1. If a tumor or an arteriovenous malformation (AVM) is suspected, maintain anesthesia with N_2O, a low concentration of an inhalational agent, and a muscle relaxant. It is recommended to maintain mild hyperventilation ($PetCO_2$ of 30-35 mmHg), confirmed using arterial blood gases obtained by the radiologist, since this degree of hypocapnia improves radiographic definition by constricting the normal vessels while abnormal vessels remain dilated.

   N.B. If an AVM is suspected, preoperative management and induction of anesthesia should be as outlined in Chap. 9.
2. Monitor the total volume of contrast medium and flush fluid to avoid fluid overload, especially in small infants with AVMs.
3. A transient bradycardia with hypotension may occur at the time of injection into the carotid artery owing to baroreceptor activity; atropine prevents this response.

Postprocedure Management

1. The child must be awake or sedated with a patent airway before transfer to PACU. After angiography, apply pressure over the catheterization site to prevent hematoma formation or dislodging of a clot at the puncture site; this is achieved if the child is sedated and/or immobile with a dose of dexmedetomidine or a combination of a low dose of opioid and midazolam.
2. Check arterial puncture sites frequently for vessel patency and/or hematoma formation.

Additional Possible Complications

In addition to the complications that may develop during administration of any anesthetic, some special problems may occur during neuroradiologic procedures.

1. Hypothermia is common because of the difficulty keeping warming blankets and heating lamps in place because the child's position changes frequently and the angiography suite is usually cold.
2. An acute increase in ICP, leading to brain stem herniation, is commonly associated with bradycardia. In this event:
   (a) Hyperventilate the lungs.
   (b) Request that a ventricular tap be performed as soon as possible.
   (c) Give an osmotic diuretic (mannitol 0.5–1 g/kg or furosemide 0.5–1 mg/kg IV) and atropine to counter the bradycardia.
3. Allergic reactions to contrast media (hives, bronchospasm, and hypotension) may occur, but these reactions are less frequent with nonionic contrast media.
4. Stroke may occur if the embolizing glue or coil plugs a blood vessel inadvertently.

Reactions to Contrast Media

1. Although very rare in children, the anesthesiologist must be prepared for this complication.
2. Minor allergic reactions, e.g., skin rashes, are treated with diphenhydramine (1 mg/kg IM or IV).
3. Major anaphylactic shock or bronchospasm must be treated aggressively as follows:
   (a) Ventilate with 100% oxygen; cardiopulmonary resuscitation as required.
   (b) Epinephrine 1–10 μg/kg IV (depending upon the severity of the reaction), followed by an epinephrine infusion of 0.05–0.2 μg/kg/min as needed.
   (c) Hydrocortisone 2–5 mg/kg IV.
   (d) Intravenous fluids as necessary to maintain the blood pressure.
   (e) H1 blocker (diphenhydramine 1–2 mg/kg IV) and H2 blocker (ranitidine 1.5 mg/kg IV).
   (f) Transfer to an ICU environment for continued treatment and observation.

Radiation Therapy

Infants and small children usually require general anesthesia or deep sedation to render them immobile for the period of radiotherapy. Treatments may have to be repeated daily or twice daily for many days. Therefore, a technique should be used that minimally interferes with the child's lifestyle and nutrition and causes the least emotional upset; sedation with propofol is very effective.

These children usually have central venous access to facilitate their care; this can be used to administer anesthetic drugs, but:

1. Be meticulous with aseptic precautions to prevent catheter infection.
2. Carefully flush the catheter clear of propofol after the treatment. Residual propofol in the catheter might predispose to

infection or to unexpected apnea when flushed later in PACU, on the ward, or at home.

3. Flush the system with an appropriate heparin solution so as to preserve device function and avoid clotting.

Alternatively, an intravenous catheter should be painlessly introduced (using a topical anesthetic cream) at the first treatment and maintained by the use of a splint and "Hep-lock" connection for use during subsequent sessions. For radiotherapy to the head region, a fiberglass mask, molded to the child's face during pre-radiation therapy planning CT scan sessions, that locks into position is used.

Expired CO_2 is monitored by inserting an IV catheter into the oxygen mask and locating the tip near the nose or mouth for optimal sampling. SaO_2 and NIBP monitoring are routine. All parameters can be monitored by closed-circuit television when the patient care team leaves the radiation suite during treatment. Recovery is very rapid after even repeated propofol sedations. The child must be recovered in an appropriately staffed and equipped pediatric recovery facility.

Invasive Medical Procedures (Oncology)

Children who need lumbar puncture, bone marrow aspiration, or other painful procedures should be provided with optimal sedation and analgesia. This is particularly important for the child with a malignant disease who requires repeated sessions; an optimal management plan should be instituted at the outset of treatment. Apart from the use of well-selected sedative and analgesic drugs, there are some other important considerations:

1. The child and the parents must be well-prepared and know what to expect. Psychological preparation and behavioral training may be of value.
2. The procedure should be performed with parents present in an area equipped with oxygen, suction, and emergency

equipment to deal with potential complications; this equipment can be discreetly covered but should be immediately available.

3. A suitably equipped and staffed recovery area must be provided, and the parents should be allowed to remain with the child during awakening.

Suggested Routine

1. Fasting as for elective general anesthesia.
2. The child's current health status should be reassessed, and informed consent for the procedure obtained or on file for serial treatments.
3. If the child does not have an established intravenous route (e.g., Hickman line or venous port), place topical local anesthetic cream over a suitable vein as soon as the child arrives at the clinic to establish pain-free access. If the Hickman line is to be accessed, meticulous asepsis is mandated.
4. If the child is anxious, premedicate with oral or intravenous midazolam.
5. Further sedation is provided with propofol, supplemented if necessary by small doses of fentanyl. It is preferable to avoid opioids as they increase the risk of postprocedure nausea and vomiting. Small doses of ketamine (0.25–1 mg/kg) may be added to provide additional analgesia. This will not usually increase vomiting but may delay recovery.
6. During the procedure, standard ASA monitoring should be used.
7. Age- and size-appropriate equipment to establish an airway and ventilate the lungs should be immediately available.
8. Monitor ventilation continuously as the child may be positioned in the lateral decubitus position or even prone. Usually a clear airway is maintained without the need for tracheal intubation. Minor degrees of airway compromise usually can be corrected by repositioning the head or by insertion of an oropharyngeal airway.

Gastrointestinal Endoscopy

Infants and children may require anesthesia during diagnostic upper or lower endoscopy and for therapeutic procedures such as injection of esophageal varices and percutaneous endoscopic gastrostomy.

Esophagogastroduodenoscopy (EGD)

There are several methods to maintain the airway for upper endoscopy and therapeutic procedures: an unprotected airway or a tracheal tube. Most procedures are performed with an unprotected airway in the lateral decubitus position, which facilitates drainage of oropharyngeal fluids from the mouth and emptying of stomach contents via a gastroscope. In such cases, anesthesia is induced with sevoflurane, an IV is placed, and anesthesia is maintained with either intermittent boluses of propofol or a continuous infusion of propofol (with or without remifentanil). There is little need for opioids as these are non-painful procedures. Care should be taken to prevent nerve compression in the lateral decubitus position. A second approach is to topicalize the larynx with local anesthetic and intubate the trachea. Anesthesia may be maintained with either a propofol infusion, titrated to the child's requirements or sevoflurane ± nitrous oxide. This approach is indicated for infants <10 kg, for obese children, or those with abnormal airway anatomy, since the gastroscope may cause upper airway obstruction. Tracheal intubation is also indicated for injection of varices in children of any age, along with placement of a large-bore intravenous access in case an urgent transfusion is required. Another approach is to place an LMA. After the larynx is topicalized, an LMA one size smaller than that estimated by weight is inserted and the scope is passed. Alternatively, the LMA may be placed with a deflated cuff and, after the endoscopist passes the scope, the LMA cuff is reinflated. The esophagus and stomach should be emptied of all air at the end of the procedure before the endoscope is removed and the child is allowed to wake up. If a child is to undergo insertion of a gastrointestinal camera (PillCam), then intubation may be the safest method to manage the airway since this device is quite large and could accidentally be deployed, obstructing the airway.

Colonoscopy

Colonoscopy usually follows the EGD in a combined procedure or is a separate procedure. Anesthesia may be continued as per the EGD (e.g., a propofol infusion) or with 70% N_2O administered by an anesthesia facemask and headstrap or an LMA with supplemental doses of propofol as needed. Tracheal intubation is usually unnecessary. In young children, anesthesia is maintained using either a propofol infusion with oxygen delivered by nasal prongs or facemask or with sevoflurane through an LMA or tracheal tube after induction of anesthesia. The child will be positioned either in the left lateral decubitus position or supine and care must be directed at preventing nerve compression. The extent of abdominal distention caused by insufflation of air into the bowel should be monitored. The endoscopist should be encouraged to remove all air possible before terminating the procedure.

Percutaneous Endoscopic Gastrostomy (PEG)

Insertion of a PEG requires tracheal intubation, with the addition that the skin area at the proposed gastrostomy site should be infiltrated with a long-acting local anesthetic.

Suggested Reading

Ageel M. Review of pediatric sedation and anesthesia for radiological diagnostic and therapeutic procedures. J Radiat Res Appl Sci. 2024;17(1):100833.

Banka P, Geva T. Advances in pediatric cardiac MRI. Curr Opin Pediatr. 2016;28(5):575–83.

Coté CJ, Wilson S. Guidelines for monitoring and management of pediatric patients before, during, and after sedation for diagnostic and therapeutic procedures. Pediatrics. 2019;143(6):e20191000.

Cronin JA, Shen C, Rana S, et al. Association between magnetic resonance imaging in anesthetized children and hypothermia. Pediatr Qual Saf. 2019;4(4):e181.

Guimarães Ferreira Fonseca L, Garbin M, Bertolizio G. Anesthesia for pediatric magnetic resonance imaging: a review of practices and current pathways. Curr Opin Anaesthesiol. 2023;36(4):428–34.

Hartjes KT, Dafonte TM, Lee AF, et al. Variation in pediatric anesthesiologist sedation practices for pediatric gastrointestinal endoscopy. Front Pediatr. 2021;9:709433.

Landrigan-Ossar M, Setiawan CT. Pediatric anesthesia outside the operating room: safety and systems. Anesthesiol Clin. 2020;38(3):577–86.

McFarlan CS, Anderson BJ, Short TG. The use of propofol infusions in paediatric anaesthesia: a practical guide. Pediatr Anesth. 1999;9(3):209–16.

Saretta F, Caimmi S, Mori F, et al. Radiocontrast media hypersensitivity reactions in children. Medicina (Kaunas). 2022;58(4):517.

Shah A, Aran S. A review of magnetic resonance (MR) safety: the essentials to patient safety. Cureus. 2023;15(10):e47345.

Shah R, D'Arco F, Soares B, et al. Use of gadolinium contrast agents in paediatric population: Donald Rumsfeld meets Hippocrates! Br J Radiol. 2019;92(1094):20180746.

Postoperative Care and Pain Management

20

The Post-anesthesia Care Unit

General Management

All children should be transported to the post-anesthesia care unit (PACU) in the lateral decubitus position with the head extended to provide an unobstructed airway. We recommend that the transport bed be equipped with an oxygen tank with adequate supply of oxygen and equipment for bag-mask ventilation. All children should receive oxygen and/or be monitored with SpO_2 during transport to PACU. Evidence suggests that decreases in SpO_2 during transport are most likely due to airway obstruction. *However, administering oxygen while monitoring SpO_2 renders the oximeter an insensitive metric of hypopnea; respirations should be monitored by observing chest movements, mist in the facemask, by feeling exhaled breathing, and/or portable capnography.* A member of the anesthesia team should be positioned at the head of the bed facing forward to allow continuous observation and monitoring of the child. If the airway is in doubt, do not leave the OR until respirations are adequate and unobstructed. If airway obstruction occurs while on route to the PACU, digital pressure to the condyle of the mandible behind the pinna will open the upper airway and stimulate breathing.

J. Lerman, C. J. Coté, *Steward's Manual of Pediatric Anesthesia*,
https://doi.org/10.1007/978-3-032-24545-8_20

In the PACU, the anesthesiologist:

1. During the transfer of the child to the care of the PACU nurses (see later discussion), the team should summarize the child's underlying medical and surgical conditions, the operative procedure, and any associated issues, e.g., bleeding, vascular compromise; describe the size of the tracheal tube used, distance of insertion, and ease of intubation; provide the timing and doses of antibiotics, analgesics, antiemetics, intravenous fluid therapy, and blood loss and replacement; and describe the anesthesia technique including any complications and their management. Specific orders should be given for any continuing anesthesia care, e.g., continuous epidural or patient-controlled analgesia.
2. After care has been transferred, the record should be completed by recording the initial vital signs obtained in the PACU and documenting the patients condition at the time of transfer.
3. Postoperative (PACU) orders, including pain and anti-emesis orders, intravenous fluids, and respiratory therapy, are then completed.
4. Every child should receive oxygen via facemask or nasal prongs as tolerated. The anesthesiologist should remain with the child in PACU until airway patency is confirmed, the vital signs are stable, and the PACU nurses are ready to accept care of the child. *A child who still requires an oropharyngeal airway or tracheal tube may still need an anesthesiologist at the bedside.*

Small infants (younger than 3 months of age) may not rapidly convert to mouth breathing if the nasal passages are blocked, e.g., after cleft lip or palate repair. If such obstruction occurs, an oropharyngeal or nasopharyngeal airway should remain in situ until the child is fully awake.

The progress of recovery is documented with a post-anesthesia scoring system along with regular recording of vital signs. Supplemental oxygen should be administered until the child can maintain an SpO_2 >90% in room air; SpO_2 should be monitored until the child is fully awake and ready for discharge.

Once the child awakens, has stable vital signs, and is free from pain, the parents may rejoin their child in PACU. This decreases the child's anxiety and reduces crying and/or the need for additional sedation. It also clarifies whether the child is crying because of emergence delirium, pain, or the absence of a parent.

After ketamine anesthesia, it is recommended that the child recovers in a quiet, dimly lit area with minimal tactile and auditory stimulation to minimize the risk of nightmares. If delirium and/or hallucinations develop, IV midazolam or remimazolam may be considered.

Complications in PACU

To successfully extubate the airway without complications, it is incumbent on everyone to recognize the stages of emergence from anesthesia.

Emergence from inhalational anesthesia follows three stages as depicted in Fig. 20.1. Notably, the success rate of emergence from anesthesia without complications increases with time. During the early (first) phase of arousal, the child begins to swal-

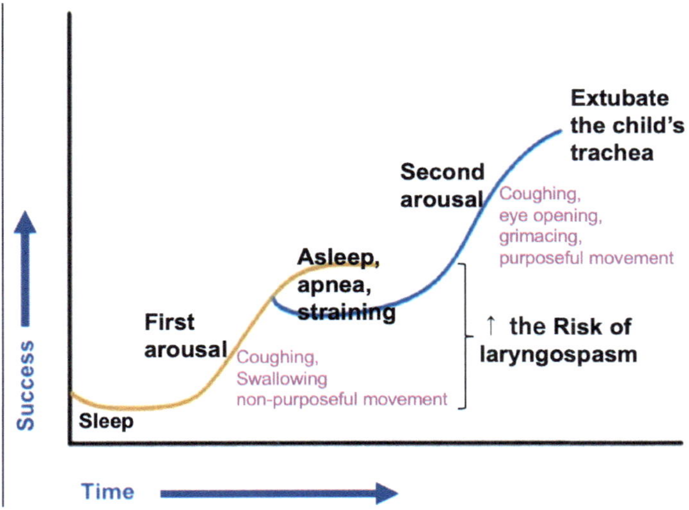

Fig. 20.1 Stages of arousal after inhalational anesthesia in children. (By J. Lerman)

low, cough, and move non-purposefully. Extubation of the airway at this time presents a very high risk of laryngospasm and desaturation. Once this period passes (lasting up to several minutes), the child will become apneic (or breathholding), unresponsive, and/or strains with tense rectus abdominis musculature. Once this stage passes and the child enters the late (second) phase of arousal, the risk of airway complications diminishes and the likelihood of an uneventful emergence increases. As arousal proceeds, the child coughs more vigorously on the tracheal tube, begins to grimace, show purposeful movement, and opens their eyes spontaneously. At this stage, the respiratory rate becomes regular, SaO2 is >95%, and the pupils are convergent. The oropharynx should then be suctioned. Laryngeal reflexes may be tested by gently tapping the endotracheal tube connector to elicit a gag reflex that is not followed by breathholding. Once these signs are present, the cuff of the endotracheal tube should be deflated, which will also stimulate a gag reflex, indicating that it is safe to proceed with extubation with a minimal risk of laryngospasm. As soon as the tracheal tube has been removed, apply a facemask with oxygen and positive airway pressure.

Laryngospasm

Laryngospasm may occur during emergence and is more likely in children with blood or secretions in the pharynx, those with a history of URTI, or those with a history of second-hand smoking (see Chap. 8). Laryngospasm should be managed by bag-mask ventilation with 100% oxygen, maintaining positive airway pressure, and subluxing the temporomandibular joint (TMJ). Propofol or a short-acting muscle relaxant may be required; tracheal reintubation should not be delayed if desaturation progresses and/or bradycardia occurs. If laryngospasm persists, a very small dose of succinylcholine (0.2 mg/kg) will be salutary. Non-cardiogenic pulmonary edema may follow immediately upon relief of severe laryngospasm. If this occurs, treat with continued positive-pressure ventilation, furosemide, fluid restriction, and supplemental oxygen as indicated.

Postoperative Stridor

Postoperative stridor may develop due to subglottic edema (especially after endoscopy), in children with a history of croup or Down syndrome, those who were intubated as neonates, and after the use of an over-sized endotracheal tube. Stridor usually appears within 30–60 min after extubation. Infants with laryngomalacia preoperatively may manifest a similar degree of airway obstruction postoperatively. The use of humidified oxygen and intravenous dexamethasone may reduce subglottic edema. If stridor persists, racemic epinephrine by spontaneous respirations or preferably intermittent positive-pressure breathing may be salutory. If racemic epinephrine is used, the child should be observed for an extended period of time for possible rebound edema. It is rarely necessary to reintubate the airway in the PACU for persistent severe stridor; in such cases, a smaller diameter tube that is accompanied by an audible leak should be used.

Emergence Delirium

Delirium occurs most commonly but not exclusively in children 2–6 years of age after sevoflurane or desflurane anesthesia, with a reported incidence of ~10%. It is characterized by the presence of restless, thrashing, and inconsolable behaviors; disorientation; failure to establish eye contact; and a lack of purposeful movement and awareness of their surroundings. The delirium dissipates spontaneously within 10–20 min, without intervention or sequelae. The incidence may be attenuated by pretreatment with propofol, opioids, dexmedetomidine, clonidine, or NSAIDs (ketorolac). The Pediatric Anesthesia Emergence Delirium scale has been validated as a metric to confirm the diagnosis of emergence delirium in children (threshold >12) although differentiating delirium from perioperative pain remains a challenge. Small doses of propofol or fentanyl generally treat delirium in the PACU.

Shivering and Rigidity

Shivering and rigidity may occur during recovery after anesthesia in both hypothermic and normothermic children. The use of a forced air warmer during surgery pre-empts the decrease in core temperature perioperatively. Shivering increases the metabolic rate and oxygen consumption; it may be treated with a single dose of meperidine (0.25 mg/kg IV) or dexmedetomidine (0.5 μg/kg IV slowly).

Nausea and Vomiting

Postoperative nausea and vomiting (PONV) is troublesome and a leading cause of delayed discharge from the hospital or, more rarely, of unplanned admission. The incidence of PONV can be greatly reduced by invoking several general measures:

1. Avoid the indiscriminate use of opioids; a single dose dramatically increases PONV. Use alternative analgesic drugs, e.g., nonsteroidal anti-inflammatory drugs (NSAIDs) or regional analgesia when possible.
2. Administer large volumes (up to 30 mL/kg) of balanced salt solution intraoperatively.
3. Delay administering oral fluids postoperatively until the child asks for them or expresses thirst.
4. Do not rush to mobilize the child, especially after eye surgery.

Nausea and vomiting are more common in children after specific surgeries, e.g., strabismus correction, adenotonsillectomy, and hernia repair, after opioids, and after nitrous oxide for >2 h especially in teenagers. The frequency of vomiting is reduced by administering prophylactic multimodal antiemetic therapy (dexamethasone and a serotonin-receptor antagonist, such as ondansetron) and large volumes of intravenous fluids (20–30 mL/kg). The addition of the NK-1 antiemetic, aprepitant, given orally (40 mg)

Table 20.1 Antiemetic IV drug doses for children

Dimenhydrinate	0.5 mg/kg (maximum 25 mg)
Dexamethasone[a]	75–150 μg/kg (maximum 8 mg)
Ondansetron	50–100 μg/kg (maximum 4 mg)
Droperidol	10–15 μg/kg (maximum 1.25 mg)
Metoclopramide	0.15 mg/kg (maximum 10 mg)

[a]Not a rescue antiemetic

preoperatively in adolescents is a powerful adjunct complementing dual antiemetic therapy. In the presence of at least 2 prophylactic antiemetics, substituting TIVA for inhalational anesthesia for maintenance, only marginally reduces postoperative vomiting. In children with unexpected nausea and vomiting or when the above therapies fail, rescue antiemetic medication is indicated (Table 20.1).

Ondansetron is the most effective antiemetic for PONV. If dexamethasone was not given intraoperatively, it may be given postoperatively but should be given slowly to reduce the risk of perineal irritation. Dimenhydrinate and metoclopramide are both moderately effective antiemetics and cause little sedation; they may be used for protracted vomiting in PACU. Droperidol in doses adequate to combat nausea and vomiting may cause sedation, with delayed recovery and discharge.

Duration of Stay in PACU

The duration of stay in PACU depends on the nature of the surgery (airway or major cavity surgery), duration of surgery, and age of the child. Children remain in the PACU until they are fully awake and recovered from anesthesia, generally between 30 min and 2 h. Postoperative complications, e.g., stridor after airway surgery or instrumentation of the airway, or bleeding after a biopsy or tonsillectomy, will prolong the PACU stay. Older children with lower respiratory tract wheezing and persistent desaturation may require deep-breathing and coughing exercises and chest physiotherapy.

Each child should be discharged from the PACU by an anesthesiologist. If however the discharge order from the PACU is delegated to the nurse, specific written clinical criteria should be documented. If an anesthetic complication occurs, the child must be re-evaluated by the anesthesia team before PACU discharge. If the child receives IV opioids in the PACU, they should be monitored for an additional 30–60 min to ensure they remain pain-free, and breathe adequately. They should be reassessed by an anesthesiologist before discharge.

Management of Pain

The biochemical and nervous components of the pain perception pathways begin to develop at ~7–8 weeks of gestational age, and the capacity to feel pain is likely present by ~20–22 weeks of gestation. Studies suggest that inadequate treatment of pain in infants may lead to increased sensitivity to pain later in life.

There are many reasons why pain in children is undertreated:

1. Infants cannot tell us when they feel pain, and it is sometimes difficult to determine whether they are crying because they are in pain or for another reason.
2. The older child's response to pain differs from that of the adult; often children in pain are quiet and withdrawn, failing to announce their discomfort.
3. Physicians are at times uncertain of the safety of the analgesic drugs given to infants; this has led to an ultraconservative approach in prescribing opioids.
4. Many physicians are also unsure of the correct dosage of analgesics for infants and children.
5. Healthcare providers have overestimated the danger of children becoming addicted to opioids.

All infants and children can experience pain. Postoperative pain management should be planned during the preoperative evaluation and discussed with the child and parents; consent for additional procedures, e.g., a continuous catheter for a regional block,

Table 20.2 A pain scale for preverbal and nonverbal infants (**FLACC** Scale)

Score			
Category	0	1	2
Face	No particular expression or smile	Occasional grimace or frown, withdrawn, disinterested	Frequent to constant quivering chin, clenched jaw
Legs	Normal position or relaxed	Uneasy, restless, tense	Kicking or legs drawn up
Activity	Lying quietly, normal position, moves easily	Squirming, shifting back and forth, tense	Arched, rigid, or jerking
Cry	No cry (awake or asleep)	Moans or whimpers, occasional complaint	Crying steadily, screams or sobs, frequent complaints
Consolability	Content, relaxed	Reassured by occasional touching, hugging, or being talked to; distractable	Difficult to console or comfort

Reproduced with permission of Merkel SI et al.: The FLACC: A behavioral scale for scoring postoperative pain in young children. Pediatr Nurs 23:392, 1997

should be obtained if indicated. Tools are available to assess the severity of the pain (pain scoring systems) even in developmentally delayed children and neonates, e.g., FLACC scale, Table 20.2. Nurse and parent-controlled pain delivery systems are available for children who are unable to communicate due to age or cognitive impairment. Multiple analgesic strategies are available including patient-controlled analgesia (PCA), NSAIDs, non-opioid analgesics, e.g., dexmedetomidine or ketamine, nerve blocks, and continuous catheter techniques. For outpatients, it is most important that the parents have written instructions to manage pain after discharge:

(a) Analgesic drugs must be administered before pain becomes excessive and additional doses repeated by schedule rather than waiting until the pain is severe. The only exception being the child with OSA in whom opioids could pose a threat to their safety. Approaches such as alternating acetaminophen/ibuprofen at fixed intervals are recommended.

(b) The "analgesic gap" as regional analgesia wears off must be anticipated (most often manifest by the child becoming irritable or quiet) and suitable analgesics administered in advance.

(c) Parents should be provided with and instructed on using pain assessment tools, e.g., visual analog scales (VAS), to guide analgesic dosing.

Assessment of Pain

For optimal pain management, it is essential to establish regular, objective pain level assessments recorded on the medical record. For infants, the level of pain is assessed by physiologic or behavioral indices. Indices of pain include tachycardia, tachypnea, increased blood pressure, sweating, facial expressions, posture, and crying. Of the behavioral indices, facial expression may be most reliable, but crying characteristics and body movement (especially flexion of the limbs) are also useful. The opinions of the parent and of the child's nurse in interpreting these behavioral signs are very useful. These indices are incorporated into a numeric scale that can be scored and recorded (Table 20.2).

Older children may be asked to self-report their pain using one of a variety of pain scales such as the Wong-Baker FACES Pain Rating Scale (Fig. 20.2). They may also be asked to rate their pain

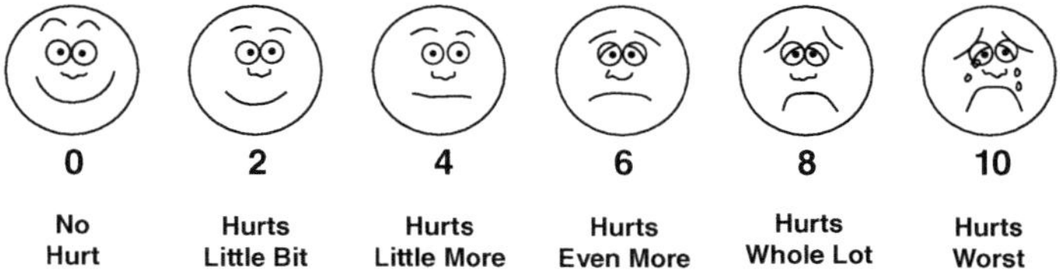

Fig. 20.2 Wong-Baker FACES pain rating scale. (©Reproduced with permission of Dr. Donna L. Wong and Mosby Inc. Wong DL, et al. (eds): Nursing Care of Infants and Children, 6th ed. St. Louis, Mosby-Year Book, 1999)

on a color scale or to report it by coloring their pain on a body outline. Adolescents can be assessed with the use of standard adult self-report scales. Note, however, that at this age psychological and emotional factors may influence the response to a greater extent than younger children.

When treating pain at any age, it is essential to monitor the response to therapy with an objective scoring system. Pain scores should be regularly recorded on the patient's chart.

Postoperative Pain

Postoperative pain has adverse physiologic and psychological effects. Optimal postoperative pain relief reduces oxygen consumption and cardiorespiratory demands, promotes early ambulation, and speeds recovery. In addition, postoperative emotional disturbance is reduced if pain is well controlled.

Systemic Analgesic Drugs

After minor procedures without a regional block or local anesthetic infiltration, systemic analgesic is indicated in PACU. Doses for analgesics in common use are listed in Table 20.3. Meperidine is no longer recommended for perioperative analgesia in children because of the risk of seizures associated with its metabolite, normeperidine, after repeat doses; a single dose of meperidine is indicated to treat shivering.

The appropriate drug should be chosen for the magnitude of the pain, and a satisfactory effect should be confirmed. It is preferable to administer the first analgesic dose before the child emerges from general anesthesia—for example, for tonsillectomy give 0.05–0.2 mg/kg IV morphine during surgery (if no OSA is present), and for minor superficial surgery give acetaminophen, 15 mg/kg PO or ~40 mg/kg PR preoperatively, or 15 mg/kg IV, after induction of anesthesia. *Do not* cut suppositories of acetaminophen (or any other drug) as the acetaminophen may not be evenly distributed throughout the suppository. Remember that peak blood levels after rectal acetaminophen are achieved

Table 20.3 Common dosages for systemic analgesics in PACU

For minor procedures:
Acetaminophen, 10–20 mg/kg PO, or 30–40 mg/kg PR loading dose followed by 20 mg/kg q6h, maximum 75–90 mg/kg/24 h; 15 mg/kg IV for children & 7.5 mg/kg IV for infants <10 kg, maximum 75 mg/kg/24h children, 60 mg/kg/24h infants & 50 mg/kg/24h neonates
Ibuprofen, 5–10 mg/kg PO
Ketorolac, 0.5 mg/kg IM or IV to a max of 15 mg
Tramadol[a], 1–2 mg/kg q6h (contraindicated in children after tonsillectomy)
For major procedures:
Morphine, 0.05–0.2 mg/kg IV q5-10 min and repeated until pain is controlled
Hydromorphone, 5–15 μg/kg IV q10 min. Repeat as needed.
Oxycodone[a], 0.05–0.2 mg/kg po q4–6 h in second stage recovery
Hydrocodone[a], 0.05–0.1 mg/kg po q4–6 h in second stage recovery

[a]These opioids are subject to CYP2D6 polymorphisms that may result in a drug overdose (in ultrarapid metabolizers) or inadequate analgesia (in poor metabolizers)—see text

60–180 min after rectal administration, so the suppository must be administered immediately after induction; this route is not appropriate for brief procedures. Multiple suppositories with several strengths may be simultaneously administered to achieve the desired ~40 mg/kg PR dose. Avoid intramuscular injections in awake children; give analgesics by the intravenous, rectal, or oral route.

Mild Analgesics and NSAIDS

Acetaminophen. Acetaminophen is a mild analgesic and antipyretic drug, but it provides good analgesia and antipyresis after minor procedures. It is safe for use in neonates, but metabolism and elimination are delayed compared with adults, so repeat doses should be given at 6–8 h rather than 4-h intervals. Excessive doses can cause hepatic failure; the total daily dose should not exceed 90 mg/kg (maximum daily dose for IV acetaminophen in children is <75 mg/kg, see Table 20.3). *Make sure that clear instructions are given to parents about dosage after the child is discharged.*

After major surgery, acetaminophen combined with opioids reduces the dose of the latter, thereby reducing the risk of respiratory depression. Acetaminophen does not affect surgical bleeding. Postoperatively, oral acetaminophen dosing is 10–15 mg/kg q4 to 6 h; IV acetaminophen is given q6 to 8 h to infants <10 kg as 7.5 mg/kg and to children 11–50 kg as 15 mg/kg IV (see Table 20.3 for maximum daily doses). Children >50 kg may receive 1 g IV q6h. IV acetaminophen should be infused over 15–20 min; the dosing in infants should be carefully checked as a number of cases of several-fold overdoses have been reported.

Diclofenac

Diclofenac has been widely used in children and may be administered orally, intravenously, or rectally. It is effective for arthritic pain and pain after minor surgical procedures. Suggested pediatric dosing is 0.3 mg/kg IV, 0.5 mg/kg rectal, and 1 mg/kg oral every 8 h. After tonsillectomy, it reduces the need for opioids and hence reduces PONV. It does not significantly affect bleeding or clot strength in children after tonsillectomy.

Ibuprofen

Ibuprofen, an NSAID, may be given by either the oral or rectal route, 5–10 mg/kg every 6 h. It reduces the child's postoperative opioid requirements; however, it can cause gastrointestinal upset (nausea, vomiting, and diarrhea) and decrease platelet aggregation, which could increase bleeding.

Ketorolac

Ketorolac is a potent analgesic. The recommended single IV dose is 0.5 mg/kg to a maximum of 15 mg. In common with other NSAIDs, ketorolac inhibits platelet aggregation and is not recommended when bleeding may be a problem. Impaired bone healing after ketorolac remains controversial. Other serious but uncommon potential side effects include gastrointestinal hemorrhage, interstitial nephritis, and acute renal failure. Once hemostasis has been achieved, it is our practice to ask the surgeon if ketorolac can be administered given its potential negative effects on platelet function and bone healing.

Celecoxib

Celecoxib reduces morphine requirements in children undergoing tonsillectomy after 6 mg/kg PO preoperatively followed by 3 mg/kg q12h PO for 3 postoperative days. There was no effect on postoperative bleeding.

Parecoxib

Paracoxib is prodrug that is converted to the active metabolite valdecoxib with a peak analgesic effect at ~0.5 h; it has no effect on platelet function. Dosing in children is 0.75 mg/kg IV (max. 40 mg) q 6-12 h for opioid sparing.

Opioids

Morphine is the most widely used analgesic for infants and children. It produces effective analgesia together with sedation and a useful degree of euphoria. In children, an IV dose of 0.05-0.1 mg/kg is administered every 7–10 min until the child is comfortable by continuous infusion/PCA (see later discussion).

Codeine is a prodrug that is converted via CYP450 2D6 to the active analgesic, morphine. Most children convert codeine to morphine efficiently (intermediate isoforms of 2D6) although some populations carry polymorphisms of CYP2D6 that either severely limit the conversion of codeine to morphine resulting in almost no analgesia (slow metabolizers) or very rapidly convert codeine to morphine (ultrarapid metabolizers) resulting in excessive plasma concentrations of morphine that could depress respiration. As a result, codeine has become proscribed and is no longer available in most children's hospitals since the FDA issued a black box warning in response to deaths after tonsillectomy in children with OSA (see Chap. 3). This drug is no longer recommended for routine use or postoperative analgesia in children.

Hydromorphone (*Dilaudid*) is a long-acting opioid that is 5–7 times more potent than morphine in the IV form. Thus, the IV analgesic dose in children is 5–15 μg/kg. Its elimination half-life is ~2.5 h. Hydromorphone may be given as an alternative postoperative analgesic to morphine.

Hydrocodone (0.05–0.1 mg/kg) is also a long-acting oral opioid commonly used for postoperative analgesia. This drug is metabolized by CYP2D6 to the active metabolite hydromorphone and subject to the same polymorphism issues as codeine, which may result in either minimal analgesia in slow metabolizers or a morphine overdose in ultrarapid metabolizers. Therefore, we recommend caution with its use.

Oxycodone (*Oxycontin*) (also containing acetaminophen in some formulations) is most commonly prescribed as an oral analgesic but is also approved for IV, IM, and sublingual routes in some countries. Single doses of oxycodone via all routes are 0.05–0.2 mg/kg every 6 h. It is also used in older children to assist transition from PCA to oral analgesics. Its side effect profile is similar to that of morphine. However, it too is subject to the problems associated with polymorphisms of 2D6 (slow or ultrarapid metabolizers), as the active form of oxycodone is its metabolite, oxymorphone.

Tramadol is a synthetic opioid; a dose of 1–2 mg/kg IV provided good pain relief in children after tonsillectomy. However, tramadol is also subject to variable metabolism due to the CYP2D6 polymorphisms that can lead to accumulation of active metabolites. The FDA has now contraindicated its use in children <12 years for pain management and under 18 years of age after tonsillectomy.

Continuous Morphine Infusions

A continuous infusion of morphine, using a dilute solution administered by a designated patient-controlled analgesia (PCA) pump, provides for a constant level of analgesia with good sedation and is appropriate for many children after major surgery. The child must have close nursing supervision and be monitored by pulse oximetry. The dose administered should be frequently titrated against the observed and recorded pain level.
Recommended doses for continuous infusions of morphine:

1. Children >1 year: Loading dose, 0.1 mg/kg IV; infusion, 10–20 μg/kg/h with PCA bolus doses of 10–30 μg/kg and lockout of 8–15 min. The loading dose may have to be repeated to establish an initial satisfactory level of analgesia. PCA is indicated for those who are old enough to understand how the system functions to provide analgesia. Younger children may benefit from a similar system for pain management that may use either nurse or parent-controlled analgesia. All children receiving continuous infusions with intermittent PCA boluses must be closely observed for sedation and slowing of respirations; rescue naloxone should be immediately available.
2. Infants <1 year: Loading dose, 0.05 mg/kg IV; infusion, 5–15 μg/kg/h. These infants should be carefully monitored during the infusion, usually in an ICU setting, and for 24 h after the infusion is discontinued to detect respiratory depression.
3. Reduced morphine infusion rates may be indicated after cardiac surgery in children of all ages, especially those receiving vasopressors, which commonly reduce clearance rates.

Patient-Controlled Analgesia

PCA for children older than 5 or 6 years of age offers the advantage of excellent pain relief while avoiding requesting pain relief and delaying in receiving it; it also provides some degree of autonomy since they can be "in control." Most children are familiar with computer games and have no problem mastering the principles of PCA. It is important that a safe regimen be established and that both child and parents be reassured that the system has an appropriate lockout time and total dosage safeguards. The parents (and other adults) should be warned not to trigger the PCA for the child. Evidence suggests that parents or nurses can effectively and safely manage PCA for a child who is unable to do so for age, cognitive, or physical reasons. If such an approach is used, an educational program for the surrogate user must be delivered successfully before they are allowed to participate. *Always be aware that overdose is a potential complication when well-meaning parents are allowed to push the PCA button.*

All children treated with opioids should have a loading dose. Whether a background infusion is used to supplement boluses is controversial, but in children a continuous infusion of a small dose of opioid complemented with PCA supplements may give the best results in terms of both pain control and sleep pattern.

The regimen used should be tailored to the child's age, underlying medical/surgical conditions, and the type of surgery, e.g., morphine requirements vary with the type of surgery: orthopedic surgery > general surgery > spinal surgery. It is convenient to adjust the background infusion rate to suit the type of surgery (Table 20.4). On occasion the background infusion is not initiated until the second postoperative day due to residual analgesic effects from intraoperative opioids and residual anesthesia.

Table 20.4 Common dosages for patient-controlled analgesia

	Morphine	Hydromorphone	Fentanyl
Loading dose	0.05–0.2 mg/kg	0.1–0.15 μg/kg	0.5–1 μg/kg
Infusion	10–20 μg/kg/h	2–4 μg/kg/h	0.1–0.5 μg/kg/h
PCA bolus	10–30 μg/kg	2–6 μg/kg	0.2–0.5 μg/kg/h
Lockout time	8–15 min	8–15 min	5–10 min
4-h limit	250–400 μg/kg	50–80 μg/kg	7–10 μg/kg

Note: Smaller doses should be administered to infants; track sedation scores and respiratory rate over time. Write orders that describe the lower limit of SpO_2 and respiratory rates to trigger deep breathing, supplemental O_2, stopping infusions, and when to notify the Pain Service

Side effects of PCA include the following:

1. *Nausea and vomiting*: These may be troublesome and require a reduction in the opioid dose. Management will include either an antiemetic or an infusion of low-dose naloxone (0.25 μg/kg/h), the latter is also effective for pruritus.
2. *Excessive sedation*: Monitor children carefully and have naloxone ready to treat excessive narcosis and respiratory depression. It may be prudent to keep naloxone and a bag-mask oxygen source at the bedside. Anticipate that another healthcare provider who is unaware that the child is receiving a PCA, may order a "stat dose" of an analgesic or sedative drug, that leads to respiratory depression. Orders for children with PCA pumps should specifically state that no additional sedative or analgesic drugs are allowed without notifying the PCA team.

Regional Analgesia for Postoperative Pain

Pain after many procedures can be effectively treated using regional analgesia and should be used whenever possible. Frequently blocks do not require supplemental analgesics, or at the most, only mild analgesics or NSAIDs, e.g., acetaminophen. Regional analgesic techniques avoid the side effects of opioids and allow the child to rapidly return to full wakefulness and activity after major surgery. These blocks are performed using surface landmarks, e.g., caudal epidural block, nerve stimulation, or most preferably with ultrasound guidance. The use of ultrasound increases success rates, decreases drug doses, and reduces the number of needle passes for a successful block. Provision must be made for transition to systemic analgesics as the block dissipates. Parents should be instructed to administer an analgesic, e.g., acetaminophen or another analgesic, in anticipation of this need. After major surgery, appropriate nerve blocks, e.g., TAP block, adductor canal block, or intercostal block, may reduce the need for opioids and facilitate earlier mobilization.

The possibility that a regional block established before the surgical incision (preemptive analgesia) may modulate total postoperative pain by preventing biochemical changes ("windup") within the central nervous system is appealing, but well-designed studies have been disappointing. Regional blocks performed before the surgical incision do provide intraoperative analgesia, reducing the dose of general anesthetic drugs required, indicating that the block is well established before emergence.

The maximum doses of local anesthetics are listed in Table 7.2. The common doses of local anesthetics and opioids for continuous caudal epidural analgesia are listed in Table 7.3. Note that many concentrations of opioids have been used, but the minimally effective dose with the minimal risk of complications should be sought, especially in infants <6 months of age.

Studies of complications after pediatric regional analgesia procedures strongly suggest that peripheral nerve blocks are associated with fewer complications than neuraxial blocks. Hence, whenever there is a choice, a peripheral nerve block is advised. Peripheral nerve and neuraxial blocks as well as their complications and treatments are detailed in Chap. 7.

Postoperative Care for the Outpatient

Many children require no analgesics immediately after surgery, especially if a regional block has been performed (e.g., for hernia, see Chaps. 7 and 14), but beware of the "analgesic window," which may occur later at home as the block wears off. Analgesics should be initiated before the block wears off rather than waiting for pain to occur. Parents should be instructed on the dose of analgesics and reinforced with written instructions. Acetaminophen alternating with ibuprofen every 3 h around the clock may obviate the need for opioids, depending on the severity of the postoperative pain. More potent analgesics are seldom required for outpatients, but hydrocodone (lortab elixir), oxycodone, and tramadol may be indicated. Although few complications have been reported, these opioids are subject to the same metabolic pathways as codeine; thus they should be used with caution and the dosing carefully prescribed particularly in obese children (see Chap. 3). Parents should be instructed regarding the treatment of postoperative pain as more complex procedures are being performed in the day surgery unit. Educating parents regarding the use of visual analog scores or other means to assess their child's pain and instructing them to record the scores over time is helpful.

Many children will ingest oral fluids before discharge; however, it is unwise to "push" oral fluids before the child is ready to drink since doing so increases the incidence of PONV. A useful method of fluid administration is to offer Popsicles ad lib or apple juice, especially to children who have undergone tonsillectomy or adenoidectomy (see Chap. 11).

Every child should be discharged from the post-anesthesia care unit (PACU) by the anesthesiologist or his/her designee; in many cases standard discharge criteria may be used. Infants may be taken home when they have fully recovered. Children should be assessed for street fitness and able to walk out; if dizzy or nauseated, discharge should be delayed. If the anesthesiologist determines that a child is unfit for discharge, overnight admission is recommended.

Children must be accompanied home by an adult, who preferably should not also be the driver of the vehicle. This is especially important for infants placed in a car seat, as they may fall asleep and obstruct their airway. Children should not ride a bicycle or engage in dangerous activities for 24 h after discharge. A brochure containing basic information and a follow-up phone call is recommended. Parents must be encouraged to seek advice if postoperative problems develop.

Complications After Pediatric Outpatient Surgery

Complications are rare after pediatric ambulatory surgery, with 0.19–3.5% of children requiring readmission. The most common reasons for admission are PONV or a surgical complication, although prophylactic antiemetics and other strategies outlined above have dramatically reduced the incidence. Airway surgery may result in croup or stridor, necessitating an overnight admission.

Complications that may occur at home include vomiting, cough, sleepiness, sore throat, and hoarseness. Postdischarge vomiting after tonsillectomy (14%) correlated only with perioperative opioid administration. Bleeding after adenotonsillectomy at home may occur in the first 24 h postoperatively known as primary or surgical bleeding or within the first 7–10 days known as secondary or late bleeding. Primary bleeding often requires a return to the operating room to cauterize the bleeding spot, whereas secondary bleeding is managed in the ED with conservative management, i.e., hydration and either tranexamic acid or Amicar, and only if bleeding persists is a return to the operating room warranted.

Suggested Reading

Archer V, Cloutier Z, Park L, Briatico D, Walton JM. Intravenous acetaminophen for postoperative pain control after open abdominal and thoracic surgery in pediatric patients: a systematic review and meta-analysis. Pediatr Surg Int. 2022;39(1):7.

Efune PN, Minhajuddin A, Szmuk P. Incidence and factors contributing to postdischarge nausea and vomiting in pediatric ambulatory surgical cases. Pediatr Anesth. 2018;28:257–63.

Kim MS, Coté CJ, Cristoloveanu C, et al. There is no dose-escalation response to dexamethasone (0.0625-1.0 mg/kg) in pediatric tonsillectomy or adenotonsillectomy patients for preventing vomiting, reducing pain, shortening time to first liquid intake, or the incidence of voice change. Anesth Analg. 2007;104(5):1052–8.

Lerman J, Ingelmo P. Emergence delirium in children: do the studies reflect reality? Pediatr Anesth. 2024;34:493–4.

Murto K, Lamontagne C, McFaul C, et al. Celecoxib pharmacogenetics and pediatric adenotonsillectomy: a double-blinded randomized controlled study. Can J Anaesth. 2015;62(7):785–97.

Packiasabapathy S, Rangasamy V, Horn ND, Hendrickson M, Renschler JS, Sadhasivam S. Personalized pediatric anesthesia and pain management: problem-based review. Pharmacogenomics. 2020;21(1):55–73.

Pessano S, Gloeck NR, Tancredi L, et al. Ibuprofen for acute postoperative pain in children (review). Cochrane Database Stemat Rev. 2024:CD015432.

Ringblom J, Wahlin I, Proczkowska M, et al. Measurement properties of the pediatric anesthesia emergence delirium scale: a confirmatory factor analysis-based study. Pediatr Anesth. 2025;35:155–62.

Sueda A, Kagawa T, Kojima T. Day surgery in children: 15-year analysis of unplanned admissions at a Japanese tertiary children's hospital. J Anesth. 2025;39:215–22.

Tan L, Taylor E, Hannam JA, Salkeld L, Salman S, Anderson BJ. Pharmacokinetics and analgesic effectiveness of intravenous parecoxib for tonsillectomy ± adenoidectomy. Paediatr Anaesth. 2016;26(12):1126–35.

Vittinghoff M, Lonnqvist PA, Mossetti V, et al. Postoperative pain management in children: guidance from the Pain Committee of the European Society for Paediatric Anaesthesiology (ESPA Pain Management Ladder Initiative) Part II. Anaesth Crit Care Med. 2024;43:101427.

Appendix A: Anesthesia Implications of Syndromes and Unusual Disorders[1]

This Appendix summarizes the descriptions of common and rare pediatric syndromes and their anesthetic implications. Space limits a complete literature review for each condition, but we have included those features that hold the most significant anesthetic implications. *When possible, the referenced literature should be consulted before anesthesia* is undertaken. A list of several excellent resources for syndromes in pediatric anesthesia follows below.

There are now more than 10,000 medical syndromes recorded, so it is inevitable that this list is incomplete. Although the number of syndromes has increased and existing syndromes have become better understood in part because of genetic studies, anesthesiologists may still encounter unreported difficulties and complications. When in doubt as to the identity and implications of a particular syndrome, the anesthesiologist should prepare to take into account all possible associated disorders.

Recurring challenges are common in many of these syndromes. In particular, the choices of anesthetic drugs and technique, airway management, and the congenital heart defects will determine the optimal anesthetic prescription. The reader is encouraged to consult the chapters within the manual when planning the anesthetic prescription, review literature sources, combine that infor-

[1] Originally adapted from Jones EP, Pelton DA: Can Anaesth Soc J 23:207, 1976 and extensively augmented and revised.

J. Lerman, C. J. Coté, *Steward's Manual of Pediatric Anesthesia*,
https://doi.org/10.1007/978-3-032-24545-8

mation with the particular syndrome, and then devise the optimal strategy within their practice and experience.

Suggested Reading

Baum VC, O'Flaherty JE, editors. Anesthesia for genetic, metabolic, & dysmorphic syndromes of childhood, 3rd ed. Lippincott, Philadelphia; 2015.

Jones KL, Jones MC, Del Campo M, editors. Smith's recognizable patterns of human malformation, 8th ed. Elsevier, Philadelphia; 2021.

Kliegman RM, St. Geme III JW, editors. Nelson textbook of pediatrics, 22nd ed. Elsevier, Philadelphia; 2024.

Open Reference Sites

Rare diseases at OrphanAnesthesia. https://www.orphananesthesia.eu/en/rare-diseases/published-guidelines.html.

Syndromes and rare disease in pediatrics: anesthesia. https://sites.uclouvain.be/anesthweekly/MRP_ENG/index.html?Achondroplasie.html.

Syndrome	Issues	Anesthesia concerns
Achondroplasia	Dwarfism due to fibroblastic growth factor (FGFR3) on chromosome 4 Maxillary hypoplasia Possible OSA Odontoid hypoplasia Atlantoaxial instability Foramen magnum stenosis	***Intubation may be difficult*** Consider in-line cervical spine stabilization Possible hydrocephalus IV may be difficult
Acrocephalopolysyndactyly	See Carpenter syndrome, Saethre-Chotzen syndrome	
Acrocephalosyndactyly	See Apert syndrome	
Adrenogenital syndrome	Inability to synthesize hydrocortisone Virilization of females	Assess electrolytes Supplemental corticosteroids are needed for anesthesia
Adrenoleukodystrophy	See Leukodystrophy	
Aicardi syndrome	Absent corpus callosum Infantile spasms, marked myotonia & drowsiness Repeated aspiration pneumonia	Sensitive to muscle relaxants; observe for residual weakness
Alagille syndrome	Bile duct disorder with cholestasis Hepatosplenomegaly May have cardiac (97%), vertebral, ocular, facial, and neurologic abnormalities Autosomal dominant, variable presentation	Assess cardiac & hepato-biliary status Caution with liver metabolized drugs RSI if regurgitation risk Caution with positioning, possible osteoporosis from vitamin D deficiency,

(continued)

Syndrome	Issues	Anesthesia concerns
Albers-Schönberg disease	Disorder of osteoclasts and bone overgrowth (marble bone disease, osteopetrosis) Macrocephaly with frontal bossing Obligate mouth breathing (overgrowth of nasopharyngeal bones) Hydrocephalus and pneumocephalus possible Brittle bones, pathologic fractures Anemia from marrow sclerosis Hepatosplenomegaly	***Possible difficult airway*** Check hemoglobin and Ca^{++} Maintain anti-seizure medications Care in moving, positioning, restraints; brittle bones Avoid nitrous oxide (pneumocephalus)
Albright hereditary Osteodystrophy	Ectopic bone formation Hypocalcemia (pseudohypoparathyroidism) Possible cardiac conduction defects Seizures Cataracts	Monitor ECG for conduction defects Check electrolytes Avoid hyperventilation if hypocalcemic Titrate muscle relaxants; possible residual weakness
Albright-Butler syndrome	Renal tubular acidosis Hypokalemia Osteomalacia with rickets Renal calculi	Assess renal status Check and correct electrolytes Caution with renally excreted drugs
Aldrich syndrome	See Wiskott-Aldrich syndrome	
Alexander disease	See leukodystrophy	
Alpha-mannosidosis	Developmental delay Short, stiff, unstable cervical spine Skeletal and muscle abnormalities Impaired pulmonary function & infections	***Assess for difficult airway*** Preop anxiolysis & antiemetics ***May require in-line cervical spine stabilization***

Alport syndrome	Associated cardiac anomalies including dissection of coronary arteries and aortic dilation Nephritis & other renal pathology Renal failure in second to third decade Nerve deafness	Assess ECG for A-V conduction defects Assess renal status Caution with renally excreted drugs
Alström syndrome	Obesity; diabetes after puberty Glomerulosclerosis Hepatic dysfunction Blindness by 7 years; hearing loss Dilated cardiomyopathy	Assess cardiac status, renal & hepatic functions Diabetic and obesity considerations Adjust drug dosing accordingly
Amaurotic familial idiocy	See Gangliosidosis GM2 (Tay-Sachs disease)	
Amyotonia congenita (infantile muscular atrophy)	Anterior horn cell degeneration Progressive muscle weakness & respiratory failure Risk of aspiration pneumonia	Unpredictable response to muscle relaxants Monitor respiratory status
Amyotrophic lateral sclerosis	Degeneration of motor neurons Progressive muscular weakness and respiratory failure Prone to aspiration pneumonia	Check baseline ventilatory status (spirometry) ***Avoid succinylcholine:*** hyperkalemic cardiac arrest possible Sensitive to sedatives, respiratory depressants & muscle relaxants
Analbuminemia	Extremely low level of serum albumin (4–100 mg/dL) Hyperlipidemia with early artherosclerosis	***Decreased protein binding resulting in greater unbound drug concentrations (e.g., propofol)*** ***Manage as for coronary artery disease***
Analphalipoproteinemia	See Tangier disease	

(continued)

Syndrome	Issues	Anesthesia concerns
Andersen disease (GSD Type IV)	Deficiency of glucosyl transferase (glycogen branching enzyme deficiency) Ranges in severity from perinatal death to slow progressive death by third decade Hypotonia, respiratory distress, cardiomyopathy, cirrhosis, and liver failure	Preop liver function tests, platelet count, glucose Possible liver transplant candidate Preop cardiac consult
Andersen syndrome	Dysmorphic features Severe midfacial hypoplasia with mandibular prognathism; abnormal structure and angle of mandible (triangular facies) Potassium channelopathy; associated periodic paralysis and long Q-T interval Kyphoscoliosis	***Possible airway difficulties*** Monitor ECG for long Q-T syndrome ***Avoid succinylcholine***
Angelman syndrome	Genetic defect in maternal 15q chromosome in 75%, affecting $GABA_{A\beta}$ subunit receptors response to anesthetic drugs Vagal hypertonia Mental retardation Craniofacial anomalies Drooling, ataxia, seizures, paroxysmal laughter, muscle atrophy	***Possible difficult airway*** Usually uncooperative Continue anticonvulsants Caution with IV hypnotics and muscle relaxants Propofol, inhaled agents, and opioids safe Prophylactic anticholinergic to limit vagal overactivity

Angioedema (hereditary angioneurotic edema)	Episodic brawny edema extremities, face, trunk, airway & abdominal viscera Lasts 4 h to 1 week Etiology: (1) Deficiency of C1 esterase inhibitor (20% of normal) levels or (2) normal levels of dysfunctional type of C1 esterase inhibitor Accumulation of vasoactive substances → increased Vascular permeability → edema usually painless; often induced by trauma or vibration Recurrent abdominal pain, diarrhea hemoconcentration leading to hypotension, shock, pharyngeal edema (usually develops slowly) Most deaths from laryngeal edema (mortality 33%)	Check complement assay Assess hematocrit, fluid status, treatment history, drug reactions Note voice change or dysphasia Prophylaxis: C1 esterase inhibitor (C1INH) replacement therapy or fresh frozen plasma for 1–3 days, preoperatively Extreme care when instrumenting the airway Danazol (androgen) may be indicated Acute attack: epinephrine, steroids, antihistamine (in case diagnosis is a true anaphylaxis), fresh frozen plasma or purified C1 inhibitor If pharyngeal edema develops: tracheal intubation for 24–72 h Treatment with antifibrinolytic and hormonal agents ***Emergent tracheotomy may be required***
Angio-osteohypertrophy	See Klippel-Trénaunay-Weber syndrome	
Anhidrotic ectodermal Dysplasia	See Christ-Siemens-Touraine syndrome	
Antley-Bixler syndrome	Craniosynostosis with midface hypoplasia, choanal atresia Cardiac, gastrointestinal, and renal anomalies	± ***Difficult airway, early tracheostomy may be required*** Possible respiratory problems Assess cardiac & renal status

(continued)

Syndrome	Issues	Anesthesia concerns
Apert syndrome	Craniosynostosis with flat facies, hypertelorism, exophthalmos Maxillary hypoplasia, narrow ± cleft palate Fused tracheal rings (Bamboo trachea) Possible increased ICP Congenital heart disease ± Hydronephrosis, polycystic kidney Syndactyly (*unique feature*)	***Difficult mask airway;*** oral intubation easy Assess renal and cardiac status
Arachnodactyly	See Marfan syndrome	
Arima syndrome	Brain stem malformation Congenital amaurosis and psychomotor retardation Polycystic kidneys with associated renal dysfunction or failure Possible hepatic failure	Assess renal and hepatic functions, electrolytes Possible hyperkalemia on ECG Caution with renally or hepatic excreted drugs
Arthrogryposis multiplex congenita (multiple congenital contractures)	Retrognathia, possible cleft palate ± Klippel-Feil syndrome with fusion of cervical vertebrae ± torticollis CHD in 10% Thoracolumbar scoliosis Non-MH hypermetabolism & hyperthermia	***Difficult airway due to TM joint dysfunction*** Assess cardiac status Tachycardia & hyperthermia unrelated to MH Regional anesthesia with ultrasound is effective
Arthroosteoonychodysplasia	See Nail-patella syndrome	

Asphyxiating thoracic dystrophy	See Jeune syndrome	
Asplenia syndrome	Absent spleen Malposition of abdominal organs Complex cardiac anomalies Cyanosis and heart failure Prone to overwhelming infection	Assess cardiac status; adjust drug dosing Use sterile techniques, possible reverse isolation
Ataxia telangiectasia	Cerebellar ataxia Skin and conjunctival telangiectasia Decreased serum IgA or IgE → defective immunity → recurrent pulmonary and sinus infections Bronchiectasis Severe anemia possible RES malignancy in 10%	Check hemoglobin & treat anemia Assess pulmonary status Use sterile technique (reverse isolation) Oxygen postop
Bardet-Biedl syndrome	Developmental delay Possible bifid epiglottis Obesity; diabetes; renal and cardiac defects Hypertension Pigmentary retinopathy Polydactyly	Assess cardiac and renal status Assess endocrine status (glucose) Use contrast with caution

(continued)

Syndrome	Issues	Anesthesia concerns
Bartter's syndrome	Hypokalemic, hypochloremic metabolic alkalosis Normotensive but hypovolemic Chloride reabsorption defect with urinary potassium loss Juxtaglomerular cell hyperplasia Hyperaldosteronism Prostaglandin overproduction and activation of the renin-angiotensin-aldosterone system	Check acid-base status Electrolyte abnormalities difficult to correct ***Anticipate hemodynamic instability*** Invasive monitoring may be required Consider regional anesthesia
Beare-Stevenson syndrome	Cervical spine & foramen magnum abnormalities Craniosynostosis with cloverleaf skull, proptosis, choanal atresia, cleft palate Hydrocephalus	***± Difficult airway including intubation*** ***Use in-line cervical spine stabilization*** Eye care may be important Assess postop ventilation
Becker syndrome	See Duchenne muscular dystrophy	
Beckwith-Wiedemann syndrome (visceromegaly; infantile gigantism)	Genetic defect, chromosome 11 Birth weight >4000 gm, macroglossia regresses with age; may require partial glossectomy Omphalocele; visceromegaly; hyperviscosity syndrome (polycythemia) Hypoglycemia up to 4 months Congenital heart defect	***± Difficult airway***, cleft palate Assess glucose status & hematocrit Nasopharyngeal airway may be required postop

Behçet syndrome	Ulcerations of mouth (may extend to esophagus) and genital area Uveitis, iritis, conjunctivitis, skin lesions Possible associated vasculitis, & myocardial, and CNS involvement Risk for sepsis	Assess cardiac status preop ± ***Difficult airway if pharynx scarred*** Use sterile techniques May require supplemental steroids
Berardinelli-Seip syndrome	See Lipodystrophy	
Binder syndrome	Maxillonasal dysplasia	May require maxillary advancement with postoperative wiring Airway precautions postoperatively
Blackfan-diamond syndrome	Craniofacial and cardiac defects Congenital idiopathic RBC aplasia Hepatosplenomegaly; possible hypersplenism, thrombocytopenia Treatment with steroids and repeated transfusions Hemochromatosis & leukemia may develop	Assess cardiac, coagulation and liver function status Treat anemia; have platelets available Administer steroids as needed
Bland-White-Garland syndrome	Left coronary artery arising from the pulmonary trunk Myocardial ischemia leading to acute heart failure and sudden death	Assess cardiac status preop (echocardiogram) ***Anesthesia as for coronary artery disease*** May be difficult to wean from bypass due to left ventricular dysfunction
Bowen syndrome	See cerebrohepatorenal syndrome	

(continued)

Syndrome	Issues	Anesthesia concerns
Brachmann-de Lange syndrome	Craniofacial malformation Associated cardiac and GI malformations Hirsutism and strabismus Gastroesophageal reflux; aspiration with frequent pulmonary infections	Assess cardiac and respiratory status ***± Difficult airway***
Branchio-Oto-Renal (BOR) syndrome (Melnick-Fraser syndrome)	Branchial cysts or fistulae Hearing loss, external ear malformations & pre-auricular pits Renal abnormalities	***Anticipate bradycardia associated with sevoflurane anesthesia: treat with atropine or epinephrine*** Assess renal status
Brugada syndrome	Na^+ channel defect leading to right bundle branch block, ST segment elevation Fatal arrhythmias (ventricular tachycardia and fibrillation) with anatomically normal heart	Monitor ECG perioperatively ***Apply defibrillator pads preoperatively*** Caution with drugs that affect Na^+ channels (local anesthetics), avoid parasympathetics ***Anticipate the need to treat arrhythmias***
Camurati–Engelmann disease (progressive diaphyseal dysplasia)	Cortical thickening of long bones Pathologic skull and bone fractures with skeletal pain, muscle weakness Cranial nerve compression	***± Difficult airway*** Careful positioning due to brittle bones Sensitivity to muscle relaxants
Canavan disease	See leukodystrophy	

Cantrell pentalogy	Recti abdominal wall defects above the umbilicus Agenesis of sternum (ectopia cordis) and diaphragm Pericardial defect and cardiac septal and valvular defects (Tetralogy of Fallot, TGA)	Assess cardiac status Anesthesia as appropriate for the cardiac defect
Capillary angioma with thrombocytopenic purpura syndrome	See Kasabach-Merritt syndrome	
Carcinoid tumors	Carcinoid tumors secrete vasoactive peptides, causing flushing, hypotension Carcinoid syndrome rare in children but occurs with malignant carcinoid tumors (in appendix) Cardiac fibrosis (carcinoid heart disease) may be present	Assess cardiac status for valvular disease Avoid drugs that stimulate the sympathetic system (i.e., ketamine) or release histamine Octreotide may be indicated for control of carcinoid manifestations
Cardioauditory syndrome	See Jervell-Lange-Nielsen syndrome	
Carpenter syndrome (acrocephalopolysyndactyly)	Obesity; developmental delay Craniosynostosis (oxycephaly), peculiar facies, proptosis, hypoplastic mandible Associate cardiac defects (pulmonary artery stenosis) Syndactyly	Assess cardiac status ± ***Difficult airway*** Eye protection for proptosis
Catch 22 syndrome	See DiGeorge syndrome	

(continued)

Syndrome	Issues	Anesthesia concerns
Central core disease	Muscular dystrophy Hypotonia without muscle wasting MH risk/precautions	Assess respiratory status ***Full MH precautions*** Sensitive to respiratory depressants; avoid muscle relaxants when possible
Cerebral gigantism	See Sotos syndrome	
Cerebrohepatorenal syndrome (Bowen syndrome, Zellweger syndrome)	Neonatal jaundice, hepatomegaly, polycystic kidneys, hypotonia, coagulopathy Dysmorphic facies, developmental delay Congenital heart disease may be present GERD leading to recurrent pneumonia	Assess cardiac, pulmonary status, hepatic and coagulation status ± ***Difficult intubation*** Adjust drugs and doses based on organ dysfunction
Charcot-Marie-Tooth syndrome (peroneal muscular atrophy)	Hereditary polyneuropathy; muscle weakness in legs and arms Cardiac involvement: arrhythmias, conduction defects, cardiomyopathy Not an MH risk	Assess cardiac status Monitor for ECG conduction defects Expect usual responses to nondepolarizing muscle relaxants
CHARGE association	**C**oloboma Congenital **H**eart disease Choanal **A**tresia **R**enal abnormalities **G**enital hypoplasia **E**ar defects Possible laryngomalacia	***Difficult airway & intubation; worsens with age*** Assess cardiac status Possible impaired renal function Treat hypoprothrombinemia with FFP

Chédiak-Higashi syndrome or Beguez Cesar syndrome	Disorder of neutrophil function, histiocyte infiltration of organs Partial albinism; immunodeficiency, pancytopenia; hepatosplenomegaly, recurrent bacterial infections Developmental delay, neurologic disorders Steroid and cytotoxic therapy	Use sterile technique (reverse isolation) Supplemental steroids, Thrombocytopenia; may require platelet transfusions
Cherubism (fibrous dysplasia of jaw)	Fibrous painless dysplasia of mandible and maxilla Intraoral masses may obstruct airway	Mask ventilation and tracheal intubation may be very difficult Profuse bleeding during resection of the mass
Chotzen syndrome	see Saethre-Chozten syndrome	
Christ-Siemens-Touraine syndrome (anhidrotic ectodermal dysplasia)	Absence of sweating and tearing leads to unexplained hyperthermia Poor mucus formation → persistent respiratory infections	Monitor temperature; be prepared to cool
Chronic granulomatous disease	Inherited disorder of leukocyte function Recurrent infections; poor pulmonary function Multiple organ system involvement; 95% with hepatomegaly, risk of portal hypertension Thrombocytopenia may be present GI lesions may predispose to regurgitation and aspiration	Assess respiratory and coagulation status, check platelet count Use sterile technique (reverse isolation) Rapid sequence induction Caution with drugs metabolized in the liver

(continued)

Syndrome	Issues	Anesthesia concerns
CINCA syndrome	Chronic infantile neurologic cutaneous articular syndrome Genetic autoinflammatory syndrome; repeated fever, skin and joint inflammation Progressive developmental delay, muscle wasting & facial dysmorphia	***Possible difficult airway due to facial dysmorphia*** TIVA recommended to reduce stress/inflammation Caution with muscle relaxants
Cockayne syndrome (Neill-Dingwall syndrome)	Dysmorphic dwarfism, developmental delay with premature senescence with hypertension, atherosclerosis, and renal disease Ataxia, peripheral neuropathy, and flexion contractures Microstomia, micrognathia Survival beyond second decade unusual	Assess ECG for evidence of myocardial ischemia Difficult airway; smaller size tracheal tube ***Manage as an adult with coronary artery disease***
Collagen diseases (dermatomyositis; polyarteritis nodosa; rheumatoid arthritis; systemic lupus erythematosus)	Systemic connective tissue diseases with variable systemic involvement Pulmonary infiltration with fibrosis Osteoporosis, fatty infiltration of muscle Anemia Renal involvement common Steroid therapy Risk of fat embolism	Assess renal and pulmonary status Temporomandibular or cricoarytenoid arthritis with ***limited mouth opening: ± difficult airway*** Supplemental steroid therapy may be indicated

Congenital heart block	1% of CHD, associated with other lesions Defect in conduction between AV node and bundle of His, or within bundle of His Supraventricular arrhythmias Up to 20% develop CHF and Stokes-Adams attacks Heart rates <55 poorly tolerated by infants; muted response to chronotropic drugs	Preoperative cardiology consultation ***Consider preoperative insertion of a temporary transvenous pacemaker or transcutaneous pacing via pads*** Transesophageal pacing may or may not be effective
Congenital hypothyroidism	Glossomegaly; goiter Decreased thyroid hormone synthesis Low cardiac output, hypotension Sensitive respiratory center Hypothermia; hyponatremia Umbilical hernia	Ensure euthyroid preop ± ***Difficult airway*** Use warming blanket Monitor glucose Cautious use of cardiac and respiratory depressants Decreased drug metabolism
Congenital Insensitivity to Pain and Anhidrosis (CIPA)	Auto recessive deficient nerve growth factor Insensitive to pain, temperature Inability to sweat Delayed gastric emptying	Anesthesia to block tactile hyperesthesia and unpleasant sensations; use BIS Monitor temperature RSI may be indicated
Congenital long QT syndrome	See Jervell and Lange-Nielsen syndrome	
Congenital oculofacial paralysis	See Moebius syndrome	

(continued)

Syndrome	Issues	Anesthesia concerns
Conradi Hünermann syndrome (chondrodysplasia epiphysealis punctata; chondrodysplasia calcificans congenita; koala bear syndrome)	Dwarfing; microcephaly; micrognathia Developmental delay Congenital heart disease and renal anomalies Congenital cataracts X-linked dominant from mutations in the emopamil-binding protein gene: lethal in males	Assess cardiac and renal status ± ***Difficult airway***
Cooley anemia	See Thalassemia major	
Cori disease	See von Gierke disease	
Cornelia de Lange syndrome	Short stature, microcephaly, developmental delay Micrognathia, high-arched palate Macroglossia, cleft palate, short neck Congenital heart disease in 30% Pulmonary aspiration common	Assess cardiac status ***Possible difficult intubation*** One report of respiratory depression after midazolam
Costello syndrome	Developmental delay & growth Short neck, choanal atresia, macroglossia Papillomata orally, nasally & anally CHD in 30%, hypertrophic cardiomyopathy in 20% Hypopituitarism, hypothyroid, hypoadrenal, and hypoglycemia	Assess cardiac status ± ***Difficult airway*** Check endocrine status May need stress dose steroids Monitor blood glucose
Cretinism	See congenital hypothyroidism	

Cri du chat syndrome	Chromosome 5p deletion causing developmental delay, catlike cry, microcephaly, hypertelorism Micrognathia, laryngomalacia, small larynx; abnormal ears CHD may be present	Assess cardiac status ± ***Difficult intubation; small size tube may be needed*** Possible post-extubation croup
Crouzon syndrome, Craniofacial dysostosis of Crouzon	Craniosynostosis, hypertelorism Maxillary hypoplasia ± large tongue Ocular proptosis due to shallow orbits	***Difficult mask ventilation***; intubation usually easy Potential for eye injury; strict eye precautions
Cutis laxa	Elastic fiber degeneration: pendulous skin, frequent hernias Recurrent pulmonary infections, emphysema and cor pulmonale Arterial fragility	Assess pulmonary status Upper airway obstruction due to soft tissue laxity Difficulty maintaining IV lines due to tissue fragility
Dandy-Walker syndrome	See hydrocephalus (Chap. 9)	
Deletion 9p syndrome	Chromosome 9 partial deletion causing developmental delay, trigonocephaly, dysmorphic facies, microstomia, cleft palate, choanal stenosis Associated cardiac and renal diseases Gastroesophageal reflux with repeat pulmonary aspirations	Assess cardiac, pulmonary and renal status ± ***Difficult airway*** Expect to use a smaller diameter tracheal tube
Dermatomyositis	See collagen disease	

(continued)

Syndrome	Issues	Anesthesia concerns
DiGeorge syndrome (Catch 22 syndrome, deletion 22q syndrome, Velocardiofacial syndrome, third and fourth brachial arch/pharyngeal pouch syndrome)	Chromosome 22 defect; immune deficiency susceptible to fungal and viral infections Aortic arch and cardiac abnormalities Thymus and parathyroids absent; expect low serum Ca^{2+} causing tetany and stridor Often associated with recurrent pulmonary infections	Assess cardiac status ***Difficult airway (short trachea)*** Use sterile technique (reverse isolation) ***Irradiate donor blood to prevent GVHD*** Check calcium levels; an infusion may be required
Donohue syndrome	See leprechaunism	
Down syndrome	See trisomy 21, Chap. 6	
Duchenne muscular dystrophy	X-linked recessive mutation in dystrophin gene on chromosome 21 Presents with progressive pseudohypertrophy of muscles, male dominance Subclinical until 6 years of age! Cardiomyopathy in adolescents Becker syndrome, milder variant, later onset but occurs in both sexes	Assess cardiac status in adolescents TIVA is preferred ***Succinylcholine contraindicated (hyperkalemic cardiac arrest)*** Monitor muscle relaxation prone to respiratory depression, regional analgesia preferred
Dutch-Kentucky syndrome	See Trismus pseudocamptodactyly	

EEC syndrome (ectrodactyly, ectodermal dysplasia, and cleft lip and palate)	Congenital anomaly complex: limbs, CNS, anemia, and GU Developmental delay in 8% Disordered temperature control Cleft lip/plate, conjunctivitis; respiratory tract infections	Preop pulmonary assessment Care with skin, positioning Protect eyes ***Tracheal intubation may be difficult*** Warming blanket
Edwards syndrome (trisomy 18)	Developmental delay and dysmorphia Micrognathia in 80%, hypotonia Congenital heart disease in 95% Renal malformations in 5%–80% Infant death common	Assess cardiac and renal status ± ***Difficult airway*** Caution with renally excreted drugs
Ehlers-Danlos syndrome (cutis hyperelastica)	Collagen abnormality with hyperelasticity Dissecting aortic aneurysm Fragile blood vessels ECG conduction abnormalities Defective platelet function Associated cardiac, pulmonary, and gastrointestinal malformations	Preoperative cardiac status Spontaneous pneumothorax ***May need in-line cervical spine stabilization*** May need platelet transfusions Monitor ECG for conduction abnormalities Difficult to maintain IV access

(continued)

Syndrome	Issues	Anesthesia concerns
Eisenmenger syndrome	Increased pulmonary vascular resistance (pulmonary hypertension) with R-to-L shunt Polycythemia increases viscosity Profound cyanosis, fatigue, dyspnea, clubbing and cardiac failure Often associated with Down syndrome	Assess cardiac status and consult cardiologist R-to-L cardiac shunt may increase with hypoxia, hypercarbia, or acidosis Caution hemodiluting as oxygen-carrying capacity decreases Hypovolemia not well-tolerated Avoid increases in PVR (e.g., hypercarbia, hypoxemia, & acidosis) Avoid drugs that decrease SVR (vasodilators) Caution with ventilation to maintain lung volume but minimize increased intrathoracic pressure
Elfin facies syndrome	See Williams syndrome	
Ellis-van Creveld syndrome (chondroectodermal/ mesoectodermal dysplasia)	Tetrad of dwarfism, polydactyly, ectodermal dysplasia and CHD (50%) Abnormal maxillae, cleft palate, cleft lip, peg teeth Chest wall defects with poor lung function May have hepatorenal disease Death in infancy	Assess cardiac and renal status ± ***Difficult airway*** Anticipate poor respiratory function postoperatively Caution with hepatically metabolized drugs
Eosinophilic granuloma	See Histiocytosis X	

Epidermolysis bullosa (Herlitz syndrome)	Skin cleavage at dermal-epidermal injunction leading to blisters/scars Simplex form (chromosome 17) mild, 70% cases affect hands and feet, little scarring Dystrophic form (chromosome 12)-severe Junctional: rare, either mild or severe, begins in infancy Kindler syndrome: rare skin blisters then poikiloderma Pressure lesions to mouth, airway, and skin Laryngeal, digital scarring, esophageal strictures Dilated cardiomyopathy <4% by 8 years of age	Assess airway for scarring; gentle laryngoscopy if required Lubricate soft face mask, small tracheal tube Possible postoperative laryngeal obstruction due to bulla formation *Avoid ALL tape*; wrap rather than use tape Place well lubricated ECG pads under the patient Lubricate conjunctiva, avoid eyelid tape
Erythema multiforme	See Stevens-Johnson syndrome	
Escobar syndrome (multiple pterygium syndrome)	Facial anomalies Progressive disease Severe kyphoscoliosis Multiple joint contractures	***Difficult airway; worsens with age*** IV access may be limited Caution with padding and positioning
Eulenburg periodic paralysis	See paramyotonia congenita	

(continued)

Syndrome	Issues	Anesthesia concerns
Fabry disease (angiokeratomas corporis diffusum)	X-linked lipid storage disorder Cervical spine fusion Hypertension and myocardial ischemia possible Renal failure Lipid deposition in blood vessels causes pain and fever crises; corneal opacities	Assess cardiac function and renal status Monitor for cardiac ischemia Adjust drug doses if renally impaired
Familial cerebellar vermis agenesis syndrome	See Joubert syndrome	
Familial dysautonomia	See Riley-Day syndrome	
Familial osteodysplasia	See Andersen syndrome	
Familial periodic paralysis	Periodic muscle weakness secondary to hypokalemia or hyperkalemia Muscle weakness in the hypokalemic variety is caused by massive uptake of K^+ into muscles decreasing the serum K^+	Monitor serum K^+, glucose, and the ECG Maintain normal K^+, glucose and temperature ***Avoid succinylcholine***
Familial xanthomatosis	See Wolman disease	
Fanconi syndrome (anemia with renal tubular acidosis)	Usually secondary to cystinosis Proximal tubular defect; impaired renal function, acidosis, potassium wasting, dehydration Older children may have thyroid and pancreatic dysfunction secondary to cysteine deposition	Assess and correct electrolyte and acid-base abnormalities Caution with renally excreted drugs Possible metabolic or endocrine defects

Farber disease (lipogranulomatosis)	Sphingomyelin deposition; visceral lipogranulomas especially in CNS Oral deposits can distort the anatomy Systemic involvement can lead to cardiac and renal failure	Preop cardiac and renal status ± ***Difficult airway*** in the presence of oral deposits
Favism (glucose-6-phosphate dehydrogenase [G6PD] deficiency)	Risk of spontaneous/induced hemolytic anemia from drugs, fava beans, or infection	Avoid drugs that cause hemolysis (e.g., acetylsalicylic acid, phenacetin, sulfonamides, quinidine, methylene blue) Correct anemia if necessary (rare)
Fetal alcohol syndrome	Neonatal abnormalities due to excessive maternal alcohol consumption Developmental delay Craniofacial anomalies: microcephaly, microphthalmia, hypoplastic upper lip, flat maxilla Associated cardiac defects (especially VSD), & renal abnormalities	Assess cardiac & renal status ± ***Difficult airway***
Fetal face syndrome	See Robinow syndrome	
Fibrodysplasia ossificans progressiva	See Myositis ossificans	
Focal dermal hypoplasia (Goltz syndrome)	Papillomas of mucous membranes (airway) and skin Ontogenic cysts Giant cell tumors of bone	Papillomas in the airway may impair ventilation and tracheal intubation

(continued)

Syndrome	Issues	Anesthesia concerns
Forbes-Cori disease (GSD type III)	Physical findings similar to von Gierke disease GSD Type I) Deficient glycogen debranching enzyme Variable cardiac and skeletal muscles and liver involvement	Preop cardiac and liver function Titrate muscle relaxants
Fragilitas ossium syndrome	See Osteogenesis imperfecta	
Freeman-Sheldon syndrome (whistling face syndrome)	Autosomal or X-linked recessive inheritance Progressive congenital myopathy and dysplasia; limb contractures Micrognathia, microstomia, hypertelorism Kyphoscoliosis	***Very difficult airway due to microstomia, micrognathia*** ***Associated "jaws of steel" response to succinylcholine*** Possible MH susceptibility
Friedreich ataxia	Progressive degeneration of cerebellum, lateral and posterior column of spinal cord Myocardial degeneration and fibrosis leading to heart failure and arrhythmias Scoliosis Diabetes in 10%	Assess cardiac function and metabolic state including diabetes TIVA with propofol and remifentanil is recommended Avoid muscle relaxants if possible
Gangliosidoses GM1, type 1 GM1, type 2 GM2 (Tay-Sachs disease: Sandhoff disease)	Invariably fatal <10 years of age Acute onset in infancy or childhood, rapid neurologic decline with blindness, seizures, death by 2 years Pulmonary infiltrates Cardiomyopathy Tay-Sachs predominantly in Ashkenazi Jewish heritage	Assess cardiac status and pulmonary status preop Preop anti-seizure medications Monitor for perioperative cardiorespiratory complications

GAPO syndrome (Growth retardation, Alopecia, Pseudo-anodontia, and Optic atrophy)	Growth retardation, optic atrophy Facial anomalies, short neck, macroglossia, unerupted teeth Associated with dilated cardiomyopathy Possible pulmonary hypertension Glaucoma	Assess cardiac status ± ***Difficult airway***; sitting position improves airway Avoid increases in pulmonary vascular resistance Glaucoma precautions
Gardner syndrome	Familial polyposis of colon Bone tumors, sebaceous cysts, fibromas Associated with bowel adenocarcinoma and intussusception	No specific anesthesia problems
Gaucher disease	Cerebroside accumulation in CNS, liver, spleen due to enzyme deficiency Calcified cardiac valves Pulmonary disease from aspiration (pseudobulbar palsy) Hepatosplenomegaly; hypersplenism may cause thrombocytopenia	Assess cardiac & pulmonary status preop Check platelet count Surgical bleeding; treat coagulopathy and anemia
Glanzmann disease (thrombasthenia)	Abnormal platelet function Bleeding risk with any surgical procedure	No specific therapy for bleeding; platelet transfusions may be ineffective Consider recombinant activated factor VII plus antithrombolytic agents May have history of steroid therapy
Glucose-6-phosphate dehydrogenase (G6PD) deficiency	See favism	

(continued)

Syndrome	Issues	Anesthesia concerns
Glycogen storage diseases (GSD):		
Type 0	See Lewis disease	
Type I	See von Gierke disease	
Type II	See Pompe disease	
Type III	See Forbes-Cori disease	
Type IV	See Andersen disease	
Type V	See McArdle disease	
Type VI	See Hers disease	
Type VII	See Tarui disease	
Type VIII	See hepatic phosphorylase kinase deficiency	
Goldenhar syndrome (oculoauriculovertebral syndrome, hemifacial microsomia)	Hypoplasia of zygomatic arch and mandible (85% unilateral) Possible cleft tongue, palate Occipitalization of atlas, cervical vertebral defects CHD in 35% Tracheoesophageal fistula	50:50 chance it is a ***very difficult airway***, particularly if right sided Airway becomes increasingly difficult with age ***Prepare for a surgical airway*** ***In-line neck stabilization***
Goltz syndrome	See focal dermal hypoplasia and Gorlin-Golt syndrome	
Gonadal dysgenesis	See Turner syndrome	

Gonosomal aneuploidy with tubular dysgenesis	See Klinefelter syndrome	
Gorham syndrome (disappearing bone disease)	Massive osteolysis and lymphangiomatosis Pathologic fractures with neurologic and respiratory complications Cervical spine subluxation Severe kyphoscoliosis Thoracic deformity leads to respiratory failure Pleural effusions or chylothorax may occur	***± Difficult airway*** ***In-line cervical spine precautions*** ***Avoid succinylcholine as fasciculations could fracture bones*** Caution with protein bound drugs if chylothorax has caused hypoproteinemia Caution with transport and positioning
Gorlin-Chaudhry-Moss syndrome	Craniofacial dysostosis Patent ductus arteriosus Dental and eye anomalies	***± Difficult airway***
Gorlin-Goltz syndrome (basal cell nevus syndrome)	Multiple nevoid basal cell carcinomas Mandibular prognathism Multiple jaw cysts and fibrosarcomas Incomplete segmentation of cervical and thoracic vertebrae Kyphoscoliosis, hypertelorism Congenital hydrocephalus	***± Difficult airway*** Extension of the cervical spine may be limited Increased ICP may be unrecognized

(continued)

Syndrome	Issues	Anesthesia concerns
Grönblad-Strandberg syndrome (pseudoxanthoma elasticum)	Degeneration of elastic tissue in cardiovascular system, skin & eyes Rupture of arteries, especially in the gastrointestinal tract Arterial calcification with occlusion of cerebral and coronary arteries	Assess cardiac status ***Manage as for adult with severe coronary artery disease*** Prevent tachycardia and hypertension (rupture of aneurysms) IV access difficult to maintain Avoid arterial access & NG tube (bleeding)
Guillain-Barré syndrome (acute [idiopathic] polyneuritis)	Acute progressive polyneuropathy, progressive peripheral neuritis, often involving cranial nerves with bulbar palsy, hypoventilation, and hypotension Some require tracheotomy and ventilatory support Early plasma exchange and immunotherapy limits the progression	***Do not use succinylcholine for at least 3 months after the onset of polyneuritis and until lower motor neuron deficit resolves*** May have serious hemodynamic instability
Hallervorden-Spatz disease (pantothenate-kinase-associated neurodegeneration PKAN)	Progressive neurologic deterioration due to iron accumulation in basal ganglia Onset is at 7–15 years or earlier Possible dementia Dystonia, rigidity or cheoreoathetosis, dysarthria, dysphonia, dysphagia Trismus, scoliosis Airway obstruction and desaturation during posturing	Assess pulmonary status ***± Difficult airway*** Inhalation induction relaxes posturing and trismus ***Avoid succinylcholine (⇑ K^+ release may intensify rigidity)*** Responses to other anesthetics are normal

Hallermann-Streiff syndrome (oculomandibulofacial syndrome)	Congenital disorder affecting growth, cranial and dental development Malar hypoplasia with micrognathia and hypoplasia of rami and anterior displacement of TMJ; narrow high-arched palate	***± Difficult intubation***
Hand-Schüller-Christian syndrome	See Histiocytosis X	
Harlequin syndrome	Skin color changes with demarcation line bisecting the body Hemifacial sweating and flushing due to unilateral sympathectomy	No contraindications to routine anesthesia Hemifacial flushing may develop
Hecht-Beals syndrome	Developmental delay Mandibular contractures Kyphoscoliosis, arachnodactyly Multiple congenital joint contractures	***Possible difficult airway due to limited mouth opening***
Hemangioma with thrombocytopenia	See Kasabach-Merritt syndrome	

(continued)

Syndrome	Issues	Anesthesia concerns
Hemolytic uremic syndrome	Occurs in children 1–2 years old after gut infection followed by renal failure, hemolytic anemia and thrombocytopenia Cardiac, pulmonary, CNS (seizures), and coagulopathy Hepatosplenomegaly with secondary thrombocytopenia and prolonged prothrombin time	Assess respiratory, cardiac, and coagulation status Give anti-seizure medications preop Correct electrolyte, acid-base, and coagulation abnormalities May have full stomach: RSI Short-acting medications, avoid hepatic and renal drug excretion paths
Hemorrhagic telangiectasia	See Osler-Rendu-Weber syndrome	
Hepatic phosphorylase kinase deficiency (GSD type VIII)	Genetics: Xp222-p221 Mild form of GSD Growth retardation Hepatomegaly; increased liver glycogen concentration; hypoglycemia and fasting hyperketosis, hypertriglyceridemia	Assess liver status Avoid prolonged fasting Monitor glucose levels and consider infusing glucose-containing solution
Hepatolenticular degeneration	See Wilson disease	
Herlitz syndrome	See epidermolysis bullosa	
Hermansky-Pudlak syndrome	Albinism Bleeding diathesis due to platelet abnormality Life-threatening pulmonary fibrosis	Assess pulmonary status Thrombocytopenia may require platelet transfusions

Hers disease (GSD Type VI)	Chromosome 14q21-q22 mutation Liver phosphorylase deficiency Short stature, hepatomegaly, cirrhosis, hypoglycemia, ketosis	Preop liver assessment Avoid prolonged fasting Preop glucose concentration
Histiocytosis X (eosinophilic granuloma: Hand-SchüllerChristian disease, Letterer-Siwe disease)	Osteolytic lesions in bones and lesions in viscera (larynx, lungs, liver, and spleen) Laryngeal fibrosis and loose teeth Hypersplenism, pancytopenia, anemia, purpura, hemorrhage Hepatic involvement Pulmonary infiltration, cor pulmonale Diabetes insipidus if sella turcica is involved May be treated with chemotherapy and/or radiotherapy	Assess cardiorespiratory status Correct anemia, coagulation defects and electrolytes ± ***Difficult airway*** Beware of loose teeth May require stress dose steroids
Holt-Oram syndrome (heart-hand syndrome)	Upper limb abnormalities CHD in 80% (usually ASD) but arrhythmias may occur with normal cardiac anatomy Possible sudden death from arrhythmia, pulmonary embolus or coronary occlusion	Assess cardiac status Upper limb venous system may be abnormal causing difficult venous cannulation ± ***Difficult airway*** Difficulty positioning BP cuff

(continued)

Syndrome	Issues	Anesthesia concerns
Homocystinuria	Kyphoscoliosis Thromboembolic phenomena due to intimal thickening Osteoporosis Possible hypoglycemia	Consult hematologist to reduce the risk of thromboembolism IV fluids to maintain urine output Pneumatic stockings may be indicated Infuse dextrose and monitor glucose levels ***Avoid nitrous oxide (impairs conversion of homocysteine to methionine and increases levels of homocysteine)***
Hunter syndrome (mucopolysaccharidosis type II)	Similar, but less severe than Hurler syndrome (see below)	Assess cardiac status Manage as per Hurler syndrome ***Difficult airway from macroglossia, limited neck extension***; LMA not always effective ***Possible need for in-line cervical spine stabilization*** Delayed emergence Post-obstructive pulmonary edema reported

Hurler syndrome (mucopolysaccharidosis type I H)	Developmental delay; dwarfing Coarse (gargoyle) facies; macroglossia, short neck, abnormal tracheobronchial cartilages, odontoid hypoplasia and atlanto-axial instability Coronary artery disease at young age with valvar and myocardial involvement OSA Sudden death beyond age 7 years Hepatosplenomegaly ± Increased intracranial pressure Kyphosis, limb contractures	Assess cardiac status *Manage as an adult with severe coronary artery disease* Upper airway obstruction, nasal/oral airways and LMA may not relieve upper airway obstruction due to lymphoid hyperplasia ***Very difficult intubation; have fiberoptic and video laryngoscope available*** ***In-line cervical spine stabilization for unstable C-spine*** Reduce opioids for OSA
Hurler-Scheie compound syndrome (type I HS)	See Scheie syndrome	
Hutchinson-Gilford syndrome	See Progeria	
Hyalinosis, cutaneous-Mucosal syndrome	See Urbach-Wiethe disease	
Hyperekplexia "startle disease"	See stiff baby syndrome	
Hypospadias, dysphagia syndrome	See Opitz-Frias syndrome	

(continued)

Syndrome	Issues	Anesthesia concerns
I-cell disease (mucolipidoses)	Chronic pulmonary disease Stiff neck, atlantoaxial subluxation Cardiac involvement; valvar insufficiency Hurler-type bone changes, severe joint limitation Death in childhood, but may live 1 or 2 decades	Assess cardiac status (echocardiogram and ECG) Assess pulmonary status ***Difficult airway*** ***Use In-line cervical spine stabilization*** Caution with cardiac depressant drugs
Idiopathic thrombocytopenic purpura	Autoimmune disease resulting in destruction of platelets in the spleen High-dose steroids and γ-globulin is effective to increase the platelet count Splenectomy is rarely recommended in children	May have a history of steroid use Platelet transfusions may be ineffective ***Avoid NSAIDs and intramuscular injections***
Infantile muscular atrophy, SMA type 1	See Werdnig-Hoffmann disease	
Ivemark syndrome	See asplenia syndrome	
Jervell and Lange-Nielsen syndrome	Congenital deafness and cardiac conduction defects: arrhythmias and syncope Drug-induced long QT syndrome Diagnosed by peaked T waves, prolonged Q-T interval on ECG Ventricular fibrillation during anesthesia Sudden death may occur	Assess cardiac status (ECG) Consult with cardiologist Anticipate arrhythmias; pretreat with β-blockers to decrease risk Avoid atropine TIVA with propofol and opioids may be the optimal technique Possible hypoglycemia with β-blockade

Jeune syndrome (asphyxiating thoracic dystrophy)	Ciliopathy Severe thoracic malformation leading to neonatal asphyxia, associated with pulmonary hypoplasia Associated high rate of cervical spine instability Cystic renal changes, may progress to renal insufficiency and failure	***Consider in-line cervical spine stabilization*** Assess pulmonary and renal status Avoid high pressure ventilation (hypoplastic lungs)
Joubert syndrome (Mohr syndrome variant or Oral-facial-digital syndrome)	Developmental delay Cerebellar vermis dysplasia or agenesis and brain stem cysts Hypotonia, ataxia, jerky eye movements, and tongue protrusion Abnormal respirations with alternating tachypnea and apneic spells	Life-threatening perioperative respiratory problems Very sensitive to anesthetic agents and opioids Postoperative apnea monitoring; consider caffeine
Juvenile hyaline fibromatosis	Multiple subcutaneous nodules with flexion contractures large and small joints and radiolucent bone destruction Limited neck and temporomandibular joint mobility Gingival hyperplasia Systemic manifestations may involve pleura, lung, renal, & digestive system Nerve and vessel entrapments	***± Difficult airway due to neck and jaw immobility*** Assess for evidence of other organ involvement Careful positioning and padding required

(continued)

Syndrome	Issues	Anesthesia concerns
Kabuki syndrome	Developmental delay & craniofacial anomalies CHD in 50% Hypotonia; many develop scoliosis	Assess cardiac status preop ± ***Difficult airway***
Kartagener syndrome	Dextrocardia Situs inversus Immotile abnormal cilia; deficient mucus clearance Sinusitis, bronchiectasis	Assess pulmonary status preop Involve respiratory physiotherapy Use aseptic technique (reverse isolation)
Kasabach-Merritt syndrome	Hemangioma that suddenly increases in size Thrombocytopenia, hypofibrinogenemia → purpura, bleeding, anemia, increased fibrinolytic activity Therapies include radiotherapy, embolization, steroids, and chemotherapy	Correct anemia, hypovolemia, and coagulation defects preop Anticipate major blood loss Consider invasive monitoring FFP and platelet transfusions may be required Stress dose steroids

Kawasaki disease (mucocutaneous lymph node syndrome)	Acute febrile exanthematous disease Vasculitis with cardiac involvement (20%) (pancarditis, valvular dysfunction, arrhythmias, & coronary artery vasculitis with aneurysms) Cardiac effects range from asymptomatic ECG changes to congestive failure and myocardial infarction Salicylates used to reduce coronary lesions Biliary tract or bowel symptoms may require laparotomy; 10% have hepatic involvement CNS vasculitis manifested as headaches to seizures and death	Assess cardiac status and consult with cardiologist preop Continue anti-seizure medications ***Anesthetize as for an adult with coronary artery disease*** Monitor for cardiac ischemic changes (leads V_5 and II) Prepare with vasoactive and antiarrhythmic drugs
Kenny-Caffey syndrome	Dwarfism with normal intellect Macrocephaly, mandibular hypoplasia and thoracic skeletal abnormalities Anemia, hypocalcemia Recurrent aspiration	± ***difficult airway***; have videolaryngoscope and LMAs prepared Monitor ionized calcium
Ketouria, branched-chain	See Maple syrup urine disease	
Kinky hair disease	See Menkes syndrome	

(continued)

Syndrome	Issues	Anesthesia concerns
Klinefelter syndrome	Confined to males Sex chromosome defect (47 XY XXY) Ambiguous genitalia at birth Reduced intelligence, behavior issues Vertebral collapse due to osteoporosis May have diabetes mellitus	No anesthesia specific issues Standard diabetes management Careful positioning due to osteoporosis
Klippel-Feil syndrome	Congenital fusion of two or more cervical vertebrae leading to neck rigidity Occipital encephalomyelocele Arnold-Chiari malformation and/or scoliosis Associated rib defects, cardiac and renal disease	Assess cardiac and renal status ***Airway may be very difficult; prepare for a surgical airway*** Extubate until fully awake
Klippel-Trénaunay-Weber syndrome (angio-osteohypertrophy)	Hemangiomas with bone hypertrophy Macrocephaly, scoliosis, & pectus excavatum Severe bleeding may occur from hemangiomas Thrombocytopenia AV fistulas and anemia led to high cardiac output & possible heart failure	Assess cardiac status Correct coagulopathy Usually not a difficult airway Be prepared for massive blood loss
Krabbe disease	See leukodystrophy	

Laing distal myopathy	Autosomal dominant variant, MYH7 Begins in distal muscles of hands and feet before 5 years of age Mild proximal weakness after 10 years	No relation to MH Several myosin heavy chain variants; cardiomyopathy in some
Lamellar ichthyosis	Disorder of keratinization with widespread severe scaling Severe dental disease Microstomia	± ***Difficult airway*** LMA may be useful Prone to thermal instability Difficult IV access and fixation
Larsen syndrome	Multiple congenital dislocations: knees, elbows, hips Characteristic facies with abnormal laryngeal anatomy (epiglottis, arytenoids) & tracheomalacia Abnormal and unstable cervical spine Kyphoscoliosis Associated CHD and respiratory problems	Assess cardiac and respiratory status ***Difficult airway with subglottic stenosis*** ***In-line stabilization during laryngoscopy***
Laurence-Moon-Biedl syndrome	Developmental delay, pigmentary retinopathy Spastic paraplegia Associated CHD and renal anomalies	A assess cardiac and renal status

(continued)

Syndrome	Issues	Anesthesia concerns
Leigh disease	Mitochondrial myopathy, infancy or child Hypotonia, somnolence, deafness, optic atrophy, pyramidal tract signs Altered respiratory patterns that may cause sudden infant death syndrome Impaired intracellular metabolism 2° to deficiencies in the respiratory chain and pyruvate dehydrogenase Older children have neurologic deterioration and respiratory failure General anesthesia may be followed by respiratory failure and death	Assess pulmonary status Treat acute infections Ensure adequate hydration with normal saline; ***avoid lactated Ringer's solution*** Administer glucose and monitor levels Treat acidosis Consider TIVA
LEOPARD syndrome (Noonan syndrome with multiple lentigines-NSML)	**L** for lentigines **E** for ECG conduction defects **O** for ocular hypertelorism **P** for pulmonary stenosis **A** for abnormal genitalia **R** for growth retardation **D** for deafness/hearing loss	Assess cardiac status Avoid tachycardia Prepare vasoactive and antiarrhythmic drugs ± ***Difficult airway*** See Noonan syndrome

Leprechaunism	Severe insulin resistance (hyperplastic islets of Langerhans) due to a mutant insulin receptor gene; hypothyroidism Severe developmental delay Hypoglycemia, renal tubular dysfunction Elfin face with mandibular hypoplasia Lungs may be dysmorphic Death before 1 year of age	Assess pulmonary and renal status ***± Difficult airway*** ***Administer glucose-containing solutions and monitor glucose***
Lesch-Nyhan syndrome	Disorder of purine metabolism in males Developmental delay, growth retardation, & choreoathetosis Aggressive self-destructive behavior Hypertension and coronary artery disease Hyperuricemia leading to renal calculi and renal failure by 20 years of age Tracheal diverticulum reported	Assess cardiac and renal status ***Manage as adult with coronary artery disease as appropriate*** Caution with drugs excreted by the kidney Preop sedation for behavior
Letterer-Siwe disease	See Histiocytosis X	

(continued)

Syndrome	Issues	Anesthesia concerns
Leukodystrophy (Alexander disease, Canavan disease, Krabbe disease, Pelizaeus-Merzbacher disease, adrenoleukodystrophy, metachromatic leukodystrophy)	Inherited lysosomal storage disorder of myelin formation Progressive degenerative disease with spasticity, gait disturbance, poor motor development, seizures, extrapyramidal movements, and choreoathetosis Disordered swallowing and gastroesophageal reflux lead to aspiration pneumonia Acid-base abnormalities may occur	Assess pulmonary status preop Give anti-seizure medications preop For copious secretions give antisialogogue ***Avoid succinylcholine due to risk of hyperkalemia*** Use glucose-containing solutions; avoid lactated Ringer's solution Adrenal dysfunction may require steroid supplement
Lewis disease (GSD Type 0)	Autosomal recessive deficiency in hepatic glycogen synthase production of glycogen on chromosome 12p122 Ketotic hypoglycemia; fatty liver Short stature, liver normal size, weakness	Assess liver function Avoid prolonged fasting Consider perioperative glucose infusions Hyperthermia reported after sevoflurane; consider TIVA
Lipodystrophy with diabetes (Seip syndrome, Berardinelli-Seip syndrome)	Loss of all body fat May develop dilated cardiomyopathy Fibrotic liver failure leading to portal hypertension Hypersplenism with thrombocytopenia Nephropathy with renal failure Diabetes	Assess cardiac and renal status Assess coagulation status and platelet count Considerations for diabetes; monitor blood glucose Caution with drugs metabolized by liver and those excreted by the kidneys
Lipogranulomatosis	See Farber disease	

Loeys-Dietz syndrome	Defect in growth factor-beta receptors that leads to a dilated aortic root, hypertension, tortuous vessels, joint laxity & bruising Cervical spine instability Kyphosis	Assess cardiac status and aortic root preop ***Assess cervical spine preop*** ***± Difficult airway*** Review antihypertensive medications Maintain normal heart rate and blood pressure Prepare to treat hyper/hypotension
Long QT syndrome	See Jervell and Lange-Nielsen syndrome (Romano-Ward syndrome)	
Lowe syndrome (oculocerebrorenal syndrome)	Affects males Developmental delay Glomerulosclerosis leads to renal failure Hypotonia Renal tubular acidosis, proteinuria, sodium and potassium wasting, osteoporosis, and rickets Cataract, glaucoma	Assess renal status Correct electrolyte and acid-base balance Avoid hyperventilation or excess glucose infusion Caution with drugs excreted by kidneys
Lupus erythematosus disseminatus	See collagen diseases	
Maffucci syndrome	Enchondromatosis and hemangiomas with malignant changes Gastrointestinal bleeding from hemangiomas Orthostatic hypotension Pathologic fractures	Anticipate possible airway hemangioma Anticipate orthostatic changes Sensitive to vasodilating medications Position carefully to protect hemangiomata and avoid pathologic fractures
Mandibulofacial dysostosis	See Treacher Collins syndrome	

(continued)

Syndrome	Issues	Anesthesia concerns
Mannosidosis Type I	Primary metabolic deficiency of α-mannosidases A and B → lysosomal accumulation of mannose-rich substrates Abnormal neutrophil immunologic function Hurler-like skeletal changes Gargoyle-like facies, developmental delay Hepatosplenomegaly & recurrent infections and early death,	Assess for hepatic dysfunction and hypoventilation ± ***Difficult airway***
Maple syrup urine disease (MSUD, branched-chain ketonuria)	Inability to metabolize leucine, isoleucine, and valine leading to the cumulation of branched-chain amino acids and ketoacids Episodes of hypoglycemia	Consult with child's endocrinologist Check acid-base balance Check serum glucose before, during, and after anesthesia Administer 10–15 mg/kg/min glucose infusion until oral intake is reestablished
Marfan syndrome (arachnodactyly)	Chromosome 15 defect for fibrillin Tall, thin, mostly males with narrow facies and high-arched palate Cervical spine instability, scoliosis, kyphosis, pectus excavatum Dissecting aortic aneurysm Aortic & mitral valve insufficiency Spontaneous pneumothorax in 4%	Assess cardiac and pulmonary status ***Assess stability of the cervical spine preop*** ***Avoid hypertension*** Caution with cardiac depressant drugs

Maroteaux-Lamy syndrome (mucopolysaccharidosis type VI)	Normal intellect; short stature Kyphoscoliosis with poor lung reserve; chronic respiratory infections Myocardial involvement with heart valve thickening, cardiomyopathy, fibroelastosis and conduction defects Heart failure by 20 years of age Hypersplenism with thrombocytopenia and anemia	Assess cardiac and pulmonary status preop Check hemoglobin and platelet count **± *Difficult airway*** ***Possible odontoid hypoplasia-cervical spine stabilization*** May require postoperative ventilation
Marshall-Smith syndrome	Skeletal dysplasia; prone to non-traumatic fractures with dysmorphic facies and micrognathia Possible atlantoaxial instability Laryngomalacia and tracheomalacia Respiratory tract anomalies Hypotonia	Assess ***lateral neck films for atlantoaxial instability and treat accordingly*** **± *Difficult airway***; may require an oral or nasal airway Reconsider muscle relaxants if hypotonia is present Caution with positioning due to fragile bones

(continued)

Syndrome	Issues	Anesthesia concerns
Mastocytosis syndrome (urticaria pigmentosa)	Abnormal aggregates of histamine- and heparin-containing mast cells Skin lesions with brownish-red maculopapular rash on trunk Mast cell degranulation with systemic histamine and heparin release occurs with trauma, temperature changes, alcohol, and drugs (including salicylates, morphine, papaverine, polymyxin, vancomycin and atropine) Gastroesophageal reflux often present Even minor surgical procedures have led to generalized anaphylaxis and death	Avoid stimuli and drugs known to degranulate mast cells Prophylactic treatment with antihistamines and steroids recommended Inhalation and propofol/rocuroniums are safe ***Avoid amphotericin B, anticholinergics, dextran, dextromethorphan, vancomycin; ketorolac, atracurium, succinylcholine, benzocaine, chloroprocaine, tetracaine, procaine; caution with NSAIDs*** Bleeding secondary to heparin release may require a dose of protamine
McArdle myopathy (GSD Type V)	Muscle phosphorylase deficiency Myocardium may be involved Possible ECG abnormalities Possible rhabdomyolysis with succinylcholine Myoglobinuria may led to renal failure May have false positive MH contracture test; MH never reported	Assess cardiac status ***Avoid succinylcholine*** Monitor ECG for arrhythmias Avoid tourniquets that might damage muscle tissue Infuse dextrose-containing solution throughout surgery

Meckel syndrome (dysencephalia splanchnocystica)	Occipital encephalocele, microcephaly, micrognathia, cleft epiglottis Associated CHD Cystic renal dysplasia Hepatic duct proliferation and fibrosis Polydactyly Most die during infancy	Assess cardiac and renal status ± ***difficult airway*** Care with drugs excreted by liver or kidneys
Median cleft face syndrome (Burian's syndrome or frontonasal dysplasia FND)	Various degrees of cleft face: cleft nose, lip, forehead and palate Lipomas and dermoids over frontal bone Possible encephalocoele Possible choanal atresia	Assess for associated defects ± ***Difficult airway*** Be wary of nasal encephalocele
Medium chain acyl-CoA dehydrogenase deficiency (MCAD)	Disorder of fatty acid metabolism secondary to a deficient mitochondrial enzyme Hypoglycemia, seizures & coma Tachyarrhythmias with carnitine	Assess ECG preop Avoid prolonged fasting and Lactated Ringer's solution: infuse Normal saline Give anti-seizure medications preop Administer glucose and check blood glucose perioperatively ***Avoid propofol infusions due to its high fat content***
Melnick-Fraser syndrome	See Branchio-Oto-Renal (BOR) syndrome	

(continued)

Syndrome	Issues	Anesthesia concerns
Menkes syndrome (kinky hair disease)	X-linked disorder of copper metabolism Onset in infancy: developmental delay and growth retarded Seizures and progressive cerebral degeneration Gastroesophageal reflux leads to aspiration pneumonia Death from seizures or pneumonia	Give anti-seizure medications preop Succinylcholine is relatively contraindicated Risk of aspiration Prone to hypothermia and postoperative ventilation
Metaphyseal dysplasia	See Pyle disease	
Methylmalonyl-coenzyme A mutase deficiency	Autosomal recessive defect of protein metabolism leads to high plasma methylmalonic acid levels leading to vomiting, acidosis, dehydration and hyperammonemia Anesthesia and surgery may increase protein metabolism and acidemia	Avoid excessive fasting Maintain intravascular volume Monitor blood gases, electrolytes, and ammonia level ***Avoid nitrous oxide*** (may exacerbate the metabolic defect)
Moebius syndrome	Congenital paralyzes of sixth and seventh cranial nerves; unable to smile Micrognathia, limb deformities Feeding difficulties and aspiration; may cause chronic pulmonary problems	Assess respiratory status ± ***Difficult airway*** May be sensitive to opioids Central apnea may occur; monitor respiration postop
Mohr syndrome	See Joubert syndrome	

Morquio syndrome (mucopolysaccharidosis type IV)	Normal intellect but severe dwarfing Mildly coarse facies, short neck Odontoid hypoplasia, unstable atlantoaxial spine may lead to spinal cord compression Aortic incompetence late-onset Kyphoscoliosis with poor lung function Pulmonary hypertension by second decade	Assess cardiac and pulmonary status ± ***Difficult intubation*** ***Assess C-spine preop; may require in-line cervical spine stabilization***
Moschcowitz disease (thrombotic thrombocytopenic purpura)	Hemolytic anemia and thrombocytopenia Arteriolar and capillary disease Neurologic damage Renal damage Treatment with plasmapheresis and steroids; possibly splenectomy for resistant cases	Assess platelet count & hemoglobin: Consult hematologist for platelet transfusions Assess renal function Possible steroid supplement Caution with drugs excreted by kidneys Avoid IM injections
Moyamoya disease	Severe carotid artery stenosis Fine network of vessels around the basal ganglia appears as a "puff of smoke" Initially have transient ischemic attacks then paroxysmal hemiplegia Treatment is low dose aspirin or calcium channel blockers and by surgical revascularization using a scalp artery to the pial surface of the brain	Avoid hypocapnia, which may cause cerebral ischemia Maintain cerebral perfusion pressure (surgeon may request inotropic intervention) Isoflurane may be useful as a cerebral vasodilator Propofol may provide cerebral protection Maintain hydration (1.5 x maintenance) Scalp blocks may be useful during neurosurgery
Mucocutaneous lymph node syndrome	See Kawasaki disease	

(continued)

Syndrome	Issues	Anesthesia concerns
Mucopolysaccharidoses Type I H, I HS, II, VII Type III Type I S, IV, VI	Affects bones and intellect Affects intellect only Affects bones only See previous classifications: I H: Hurler syndrome I S: Scheie syndrome; formerly classified as type V HS: Hurler-Scheie compound (see Scheie syndrome) II: Hunter syndrome III: Sanfilippo syndrome IV: Morquio syndrome V: Formerly Scheie syndrome VI: Maroteaux-Lamy syndrome VII: Sly syndrome, β-Glucuronidase deficiency	***May be difficult to intubate*** LMA may not relieve obstruction Assess cardiac status preop Thickened dura and odontoid hypoplasia may compress spinal cord; consider preoperative MRI At risk for post-obstructive pulmonary edema Early stem cell therapy may reduce the difficulty of airway management later
Multiple endocrine adenomatosis: MEN1 (type 1) MEN2 (type 2)	See Wermer syndrome See Sipple syndrome	

Muscle, eye, brain disease (MEB)	A form of muscular dystrophy Eye disease: glaucoma, strabismus, nystagmus Severe muscle weakness, bedridden Secretion retention	***Avoid succinylcholine (possible rhabdomyolysis and hyperkalemia)*** Caution with all muscle relaxants
Muscle phosphofructokinase deficiency (GSD Type VII)	See Tarui disease	
Myasthenia congenita	Similar to myasthenia gravis in older children See myasthenia gravis (Chap. 14)	Avoid respiratory depressants & muscle relaxants Possibility of cholinergic crisis with anticholinesterase therapy
Myofibrillar myopathy	Skeletal, cardiac, and smooth muscle involved in progressive disease Risk of respiratory failure, cardiomyopathy, conduction defects, & sudden death Contractures and rigidity	Assess cardiac status ***± Difficult airway*** ***Do not use succinylcholine (rhabdomyolysis, hyperkalemic cardiac arrest)*** Caution with muscle relaxants Risk of MH is unknown

(continued)

Syndrome	Issues	Anesthesia concerns
Myositis ossificans (fibrodysplasia ossificans progressiva)	Bony infiltration of tendons, fascia, aponeuroses, and muscle Neck and mouth may become ossified Thoracic compliance greatly reduced if thorax is involved leading to respiratory failure Minor trauma can lead to tissue ossification	Assess respiratory function ± ***Difficult airway*** Forced manipulation of jaw may cause local progression of disease; fiberoptic intubation May need steroids Avoid IM injections Carefully pad and prevent trauma to joints and tissues
Myotonia congenita (Thomsen disease)	Decreased ability to relax muscles after contraction Diffuse muscle hypertrophy of muscle (similar to myotonia dystrophica) Paradoxical response to nondepolarizing muscle relaxants possible (generalized muscle spasms)	***Avoid succinylcholine (causes profound muscle spasms, masseter spasm possible hyperkalemia)*** Use short-intermediate acting nondepolarizing muscle relaxants with caution TIVA recommended
Myotonia dystrophica (myotonic dystrophy, Steinert disease)	Weakness and myotonia in neonate Possible cardiomyopathy with cardiac conduction defects and arrhythmias Endocrine abnormalities (hypothyroidism, diabetes) Reduced pulmonary function Esophageal motility disorder; dysphagia, GERD, aspiration Ptosis, cataracts, frontal baldness	Assess cardiac and respiratory status ***Do not use succinylcholine (causes myotonia in 50%)*** Cautious use of myocardial depressants drugs Monitor ECG Nondepolarizing relaxants may produce incomplete relaxation Use sugammadex to antagonize muscle relaxants

Nager syndrome	Micrognathia, fishlike face, cleft palate (similar to Treacher Collins) Cervical spine anomalies Associated CHD (tetralogy of Fallot) Limb deformities	Assess cardiac function ***Possible very difficult airway; prepare for a surgical airway*** Upper airway obstruction may necessitate tracheostomy in the neonate
Nail-patella syndrome (arthroosteoonychodysplasia)	Dysplasia of nails and absent or hypoplastic patella Fragile teeth May have "lilac horns" abnormality of elbows Possible nephropathy Vasomotor instability Distal sensory changes	Caution during laryngoscopy (fragile teeth) Assess renal status Anticipate vasomotor instability Decrease the dose of drugs excreted by the kidneys
Nemaline rod myopathy	Congenital myopathy may be related to central core disease and therefore MH, but no cases of MH have yet to be reported myopathy Associated CHD Dysmorphic features, micrognathia, slender face, high-arched palate Pharyngeal incompetence leads to aspiration pneumonia Respiratory failure	Assess cardiac and pulmonary status ***± Difficult airway*** ***Avoid succinylcholine and inhalation agents*** Brisk vagal responses noted; atropine or glycopyrrolate may be indicated Possible central sensitivity to depressant drugs Possible MH precautions

(continued)

Syndrome	Issues	Anesthesia concerns
Neonatal hypoglycemia, symptomatic	Symptomatic hypoglycemia in infants: small for gestational age, of diabetic mothers, and premature infants See also Beckwith syndrome	Start IV glucose infusion preop and monitor blood glucose Avoid glucose boluses to preclude rebound hyperglycemia
Neurofibromatosis	See von Recklinghausen disease	
Nevoid basal cell carcinoma syndrome	See Gorlin-Goltz syndrome	
Niemann-Pick disease (see also Wolman disease)	Hepatosplenomegaly and accumulation of sphingomyelin and other lipids throughout the body Developmental delay, epilepsy, ataxia May have coronary or valvular heart disease Diffuse foam cell infiltration of lungs leads to pulmonary insufficiency and pneumonia Bone marrow infiltration leading to anemia and thrombocytopenia Death by 3rd to 15th year	Assess cardiac, pulmonary, and coagulation status Anesthesia as for adults with coronary artery disease and myocardial ischemia Caution with drugs metabolized by the liver Anticipate ventilation difficulties due to pulmonary restrictive disease and ascites
Noack syndrome	See Pfeiffer syndrome	

Noonan syndrome	Short stature, web neck, hypertelorism, and mild developmental delay; similar to Turner syndrome Cardiac anomalies in 50–80%: pulmonary stenosis most common, hypertrophic cardiomyopathy, also ASD, VSD Micrognathia, hydronephrosis, platelet dysfunction	Assess cardiac, renal and coagulation status ± ***Difficult airway*** Caution with renally excreted drugs
Oculoauriculovertebral syndrome	See Goldenhar syndrome	
Oculocerebrorenal syndrome	See Lowe syndrome	
Oculodento-osseous dysplasia (ODOD)	Mandibular dysplasia, cleft palate Small nose with anteverted nostrils Generalized defect of bony modeling; thick ribs, abnormal long bones Microphthalmia	± ***Difficult airway*** Care with laryngoscopy, brittle teeth
Oculofacial paralysis, congenital	See Moebius syndrome	
Ollier syndrome (see Maffucci syndrome)	Dwarfism Multiple chondromas within bones Pathologic fractures 25% risk for skeletal, brain or visceral malignancy	± ***Difficult airway*** ***Possible airway hemangioma*** Position carefully

(continued)

Syndrome	Issues	Anesthesia concerns
Opitz-Frias syndrome (Opitz G syndrome, hypospadias, dysphagia syndrome)	X-linked or autosomal dominant; males >females Craniofacial anomalies: micrognathia, laryngeal and/or tracheal cleft, subglottic stenosis Pulmonary hypoplasia Dysphagia, achalasia, recurrent aspiration	***Difficult airway; require smaller tracheal tube*** Assess pulmonary status GERD, aspiration risk, possible RSI
Oral-facial-digital syndrome (Mohr syndrome)	Hypoplastic mandible and maxilla; cleft lip and palate; lobed tongue Possible tracheomalacia and laryngomalacia Hydrocephalus, corpus callosum anomaly Polycystic kidneys	Assess respiratory and renal status ± ***Difficult airway*** Caution with drugs excreted by the kidneys if renal function impaired
Osler-Rendu-Weber syndrome (hemorrhagic telangiectasia)	Massive capillary and venous dilation High incidence of pulmonary and hepatic AV fistulae Massive hemoptysis possible	Assess pulmonary and hemoglobin status; preoperative internal hemorrhage Anticipate massive hemorrhage Ensure adequate venous access

Osteogenesis imperfecta (fragilitas ossium)	Congenita—stillbirth or rapidly fatal Tarda-Pathologic fractures, blue sclera, deafness Osteoporosis → kyphoscoliosis → lung pathology Fragility of vessels results in subcutaneous hemorrhage Dentine deficiency causes carious, fragile teeth	Extreme care in positioning to prevent breaking bones ***Care with intubation; teeth are easily broken*** Difficulty in maintaining IV due to fragile vessels Intraoperative hyperthermia (not MH) during inhaled anesthesia
Osteopetrosis	See Albers-Schonberg disease	
Papillomatosis larynx and trachea	Difficult laryngoscopy Pulmonary hypertension	***Potentially difficult intubation*** Avoid seeding papilloma into trachea Laser precautions May require special airway technique such as apneic oxygenation with intermittent intubation
Paramyotonia congenita (Eulenburg periodic paralysis)	Cold-induced myotonia Paroxysmal weakness Serum K^+ may be high or low	Assess serum K^+ concentration ***Avoid succinylcholine*** Unpredictable response to nondepolarizing muscle relaxants (See also myotonic dystrophy)

(continued)

Syndrome	Issues	Anesthesia concerns
Patau syndrome (trisomy 13 syndrome)	Developmental delay Microcephaly, micrognathia, cleft lip or palate Associated cardiac anomalies (usually VSD and/or dextrocardia) Possible spinal malformations	Assess cardiac status ± ***Difficult airway***
Pelizaeus-Merzbacher disease	See leukodystrophy	
Pendred syndrome	Sensorineural deafness Goiter; incomplete block of thyroxine production May be euthyroid or hypothyroid	Ensure that patient is euthyroid preoperatively otherwise as for cretinism
Periodic paralysis	See familial periodic paralysis and paramyotonia congenita	
Pfeiffer syndrome	Cloverleaf skull (bicoronal craniosynostosis) with proptosis, hypertelorism, small mandible, OSA, and hydrocephalus Normal intelligence, high mortality	***Prepare for a difficult airway*** If hypoxic at night, reduce opioid dose

PHACE syndrome	**P**osterior fossa brain malformations **H**emangiomas **A**rterial anomalies; **C**oarctation of the aorta **C**erebral perfusion via the vertebral arteries **E**ye defects (PHACE) May be associated with bilateral carotid artery agenesis Airway hemangioma may be present Renal artery stenosis may cause hypertension	Assess cardiac status Risk of cerebral ischemia Potential airway hemangiomas Consider monitoring cerebral oxygenation Have antihypertensive medications at hand
Phenylketonuria	Phenylalanine hydroxylase deficiency Risk for B12 deficiency Possible megaloblastic anemia Vomiting, CNS irritability, developmental delay, hypertonia, seizures	Ensure megaloblastic anemia is resolved preoperatively Maintain anti-seizure medications Glucose infusion and monitor levels perioperatively (tendency to hypoglycemia) ***Nitrous oxide is contraindicated as it irreversibly oxidizes the cobalt in vitamin B12 and has led to subacute spinal cord degeneration*** Sensitive to opioids and other CNS depressants
Pierre Robin sequence	Triad: micrognathia, glossoptosis and respiratory distress in the first 24 h after birth High-arched, cleft palate, nurse prone Associated CHD May require tongue suture, intubation, or tracheostomy	Assess cardiac status ***May be a very difficult airway: prepare a video laryngoscope, LMA, fiberoptic bronchoscope and prepare for a surgical airway*** Extubate fully awake

(continued)

Syndrome	Issues	Anesthesia concerns
Plott syndrome	Vocal cord paralysis, psychomotor retardation and sixth nerve palsy Stridor at rest, respiratory distress Cyanotic or choking spells	***Anticipate airway obstruction*** Possible perioperative aspiration risk
Poland syndrome	Absent or hypoplastic pectoral muscles with chest wall deformity Ipsilateral syndactyly or microdactyly Associated CHD, renal and gastrointestinal anomalies Extreme form: Mobius syndrome	Assess cardiac and renal status Controlled ventilation is recommended for the chest deformity
Polyarteritis nodosa	See collagen disease	
Polycystic kidneys	Associated cysts in liver, pancreas, spleen, lungs, bladder, and thyroid (one-third) Cerebral aneurysms in 15%	Assess pulmonary and renal status Lung cysts may lead to pneumothorax; avoid high peak inflation pressures Prevent hypertension (possible associated cerebral aneurysm)
Polyneuritis, acute	See Guillain-Barré syndrome	

Pompe disease (GSD Type II; acid maltase deficiency gene)	Lysosomal enzyme deficiency causes pathologic accumulation of glycogen in lysozymes of most tissues e.g., cardiac, skeletal muscles Cardiomyopathy, conduction defects, muscle hypotonia Macroglossia Death from cardiorespiratory failure before 2 years Lifespan has been extended using recombinant human α-glucosidase enzyme (rhGAA)	Assess cardiac function and rhythm ***± Difficult airway from macroglossia*** Use muscle relaxants with caution TIVA is recommended
Porphyrias	Paralysis Autonomic imbalance—hypertension, tachycardia Abdominal pain precipitated by drugs, stress, infection High incidence of diabetes	Avoid prolonged fasting and dehydration ***Avoid barbiturates and other precipitating IV agents (i.e., etomidate, ketamine, hydantoin, derivatives, sulfonamides, antipyretics, or hypoglycemic agents)*** Safe drugs: atropine, glycopyrrolate, propofol, succinylcholine, N_2O, inhaled agents, all nondepolarizing agents, opioids (except diclofenac), epinephrine, neostigmine, chloral hydrate, diphenhydramine, chlorpromazine, and local anesthetics Diabetic precautions if indicated

(continued)

Syndrome	Issues	Anesthesia concerns
Prader-Labhart-Willi syndrome	May have a small mouth or mandible Hypothalamic type "Pickwickian syndrome" Two phases: Neonate: hypotonia, poor feeding, reflexes absent Second phase: hyperactive, uncontrollable polyphagia, thermoregulation disturbed, developmental delay Extreme obesity leading to cardiorespiratory failure	***± Difficult airway*** Possible hypoglycemia so infuse IV glucose solution perioperatively and measure glucose Difficult IV cannulation Low-grade pyrexia reported during scoliosis, strabismus, or hernia surgery; no MH risk OSA common; reduce opioid dosing if chronic nocturnal saturation <85%
Progeria (Hutchinson-Gilford syndrome)	Premature aging starts at 6 months to 3 years Small mouth Coronary artery disease (CAD), cardiomegaly, hypertension Diabetes may be present Death from CAD before 10 years Thin fragile skin and blood vessels	Assess cardiac status preoperatively, particularly for evidence of CAD and myocardial ischemia ***± Difficult airway*** ***Anesthesia as for adults with CAD and myocardial ischemia*** ***Avoid tachycardia and hypertension*** Administer glucose-containing solutions and check glucose values perioperatively

Proteus syndrome	Cervical vertebral deformity Cystic lung lesions; scoliosis is common Variable disease with overgrowth of connective tissues, bone, skin lesions (nevi), and abnormal distribution of fat Vascular malformations may be present Pulmonary emboli without venous thrombosis have been reported	Assess pulmonary status for cystic lesions If cysts present, avoid N_2O and high peak inflation pressures; possible pneumothorax ± ***Difficult airway***
Prune-belly syndrome	Agenesis of abdominal musculature Renal anomalies Poor cough Risk of postoperative atelectasis, respiratory infections, and respiratory failure	Assess renal function ± ***Difficult airway*** ***Secure the airway with an RSI:*** intubate and control ventilation Caution with renally excreted drugs
Pseudohemophilia	See von Willebrand disease	
Pseudohypoparathyroidism	See Albright osteodystrophy	
Pseudoxanthoma elasticum	See Grönblad-Strandberg syndrome	
Pyle disease (metaphyseal dysplasia)	Craniofacial abnormalities Enlarged mandible Cranial nerve paralyzes	± ***Difficult airway***

(continued)

Syndrome	Issues	Anesthesia concerns
Rett syndrome	Disabling neurologic disorder affecting females Cardiac arrhythmias (long QT syndrome) Vasomotor instability Irregular respirations: hyperventilation alternating with apneic spells Developmental delay, autism, seizures, scoliosis, abnormal pain sensation	Assess cardiac and pulmonary status Maintain anti-seizure medications Precautions for long QT syndrome; prevent tachycardia MEP should not be monitored if seizure history High risk for respiratory complications including postoperative apnea Insensitive or hypersensitive to pain
Reye syndrome	Severe metabolic encephalopathy Fatty degeneration of viscera (especially liver) Hyperaminoacidemia Increased intracranial pressure → death Abnormal coagulation Suspected cofactor is ingestion of ASA (aspirin) during prodromal illness Rare in the past 25 years	Anesthetize for investigation of and decompression of increased ICP Patients may be receiving steroids and controlled hypothermia Caution with drugs metabolized by the liver
Rheumatoid arthritis (see collagen diseases)	TMJ mobility limited; hypoplastic mandible Cricoarytenoid arthritis; narrow larynx Cervical spine subluxation rigid cervical spine Associated myocarditis, valvular disease, especially aortic insufficiency Steroid therapy Anemia	***± Difficult airway*** ***Cervical spine in-line stabilization may be needed*** Supplemental steroid coverage Care with positioning, contractures, and padding Assess cardiac status

Rieger syndrome	Hypodontia Maxillary hypoplasia Malformations of anterior chamber of eye	± ***Difficult airway***
Riley-Day syndrome (familial dysautonomia)	Recessive disorder of autonomic ganglia and sensory neurons in Ashkenazi Jews Deficiency of dopamine-β-hydroxylase; autonomic dysfunction and decreased sensation, paroxysmal hypertension, and orthostatic hypotension Emotional lability, absent lacrimation, abnormal sweating, poor sucking and swallowing Recurrent aspiration pneumonia and chronic lung disease Dysautonomic crisis (vomiting, profuse sweating, heart rate and hemodynamic instability) can occur in response to stress	Avoid prolonged fasting Premedication with midazolam and H_2-receptor antagonist Parental presence may help Atropine can be given Maintain euvolemia Sensitive to anesthetic agents ***Respiratory center unresponsive to*** CO_2***: use opioids with caution*** Aspiration risk, take precautions
Robinow syndrome (fetal face syndrome)	Limb-shortening, midface hypoplasia and spinal deformities, CHD, renal disease, and hypoplastic genitalia May be associated with Crigler-Najjar liver disease	Assess cardiac, hepatic, and renal status Assess coagulation factors if Crigler-Najjar suspected ± ***Difficult airway***
Romano-Ward syndrome	See Jervell and Lange-Nielsen syndrome	

(continued)

Syndrome	Issues	Anesthesia concerns
Rubinstein-Taybi syndrome	Developmental delay, microcephaly, broad thumb and great toes Maxillary hypoplasia, narrow palate Associated cervical vertebral anomalies Associated CHD (pulmonary stenosis) Repeated aspiration → chronic lung disease	Assess cardiac and pulmonary status ***± Difficult intubation*** ***Use in-line cervical spine stabilization*** Possible postoperative respiratory depression or apnea
Russell-Silver syndrome	See Silver-Russell dwarfism	
Saethre-Chotzen syndrome	Acrocephalosyndactyly III, premature closure of cranial sutures with syndactyly Hypoplastic maxilla, hypertelorism Malformed ears Mutation in TWIST1 gene, usually intelligent	***± Difficult airway***
Sandhoff disease	See gangliosidosis GM2	
Sanfilippo syndrome (mucopolysaccharidosis type III)	CNS malfunction progresses to developmental delay and dementia Emotional disturbance and agitation Mildly coarse facial features No hepatosplenomegaly, cardiac problems, or major bone problems	***± Difficult intubation*** See mucopolysaccharidoses No specific anesthesia problems

Sanjad-Sakati syndrome	Dysmorphic features Congenital hypoparathyroidism, hypocalcemia, hyperphosphatemia, seizures, dwarfism, developmental delay, and dysmorphic features Recurrent pulmonary infections Confined to Arabic children	Assess respiratory status, ionized calcium, and electrolytes ± ***Difficult airway*** Preop anti-seizure medications
Scheie syndrome (mucopolysaccharidosis type I, formerly classified as type V)	Macrocephaly, micrognathia, coarse facies, OSA May have aortic insufficiency ± Hepatosplenomegaly Mild joint stiffness	Assess cardiac and hepatic status See mucopolysaccharidoses Monitor for OSA; reduce the dose of opioids if nocturnal desaturation nadir is <85%
Schwartz-Jampel syndrome (see myotonia and paramyotonia)	Dwarfism, microstomia, micrognathia, cleft palate Myotonia limiting joint movement Thermoregulatory disorder Normal intellect but developmental delay in 25%	***Difficult intubation*** ***Succinylcholine contraindicated; possible abnormal response to nondepolarizing relaxants, avoid inhalation agents***

(continued)

Syndrome	Issues	Anesthesia concerns
Scleroderma	Diffuse cutaneous stiffening; scarring May have hemifacial atrophy May have cardiac fibrosis or cor pulmonale May have pulmonary fibrosis Esophageal dilation leads to GERD Raynaud phenomena rarely present Therapy may include steroids, methotrexate, Ca^{++} channel blockers	Assess cardiac and pulmonary status ± ***Difficult airway*** Decreased pulmonary compliance Supplemental steroids may be indicated Difficult IV access Risk of hypothermia
Sebaceous nevi syndrome, linear	Linear nevi from forehead to nose May have coarctation and/or hypoplasia of aorta Hydrocephalus Developmental delay	Assess cardiac status May have increased ICP
Seckel syndrome	Autosomal recessive disorder, developmental delay Dwarfism Microcephaly ("Birdlike" facies) prominent maxilla, micrognathia	***Difficult mask ventilation and intubation*** Difficult venous access
Seip syndrome	See lipoatrophy with diabetes	

Shy-Drager syndrome	Orthostatic hypotension, lability of pulse and blood pressure Diffuse degeneration of central and autonomic nervous systems Decreased sweating Hypersensitivity to catecholamines and angiotensin	Caution with potent inhalation anesthetics Restore euvolemia Treat hypotension with IV fluids and phenylephrine Vasopressin may be the best agent to treat refractory hypotension Use muscle relaxants with caution
Silver-Russell dwarfism	Short stature, skeletal asymmetry, micrognathia Low birth weight Endocrine abnormalities Café au lait spots	± ***Difficult mask ventilation and intubation*** Assess endocrine status Monitor blood glucose level Prone to hypothermia Titrate muscle relaxants
Sipple syndrome (multiple endocrine adenomatosis type 2 (MEN 2))	Autosomal dominant Three forms: MEN 2A, familial medullary thyroid cancer, and MEN 2B Triad of medullary carcinoma of thyroid (100%), pheochromocytoma (in 40–50%), and parathyroid disease MEN 2A differs from 2B with the former including primary hyperparathyroidism (20–30%) MEN 2B less common than 2A, presents with mucosal neuromas as earliest sign	See pheochromocytoma Assess for multiple endocrine disorders For MEN 2B, assess for muscular hypotonia before using muscle relaxants

(continued)

Syndrome	Issues	Anesthesia concerns
Sleep apnea syndromes	Three types: Central sleep apnea due to CNS immaturity, trauma, infections or neoplasms and primary central alveolar hypoventilation Apnea occurs without evidence of respiratory muscle activity Obstructive sleep apnea due to obesity, adenotonsillar hypertrophy, Pierre Robin sequence, and congenital airway obstruction; accompanied by increased respiratory muscle activity. CO_2 response blunted Opioid sensitivity may be increased Mixed forms include daytime somnolence, loud snoring, night terrors, nocturnal enuresis, restless sleep, restless sleep, insomnia, fatigue and hyperactive behavior	Review polysomnogram with attention to the nocturnal desaturation: ***if nadir is <85% decrease the opioid dose by 30–50%*** Assess opioid sensitivity by titrating opioids for apnea during spontaneous respiration after intubation Use opioid sparing approach: acetaminophen, ibuprofen, dexmedetomidine and ketamine Awake extubation, monitor postoperatively for apnea
Sly syndrome (Mucopolysaccharidosis type VII or β-glucuronidase deficiency)	Genetics 7q11.21 Mild to moderate developmental delay Dwarfism, stiffness, short stature Repeated pneumonia in first year of life Thrombocytopenia, anemia, and hepatosplenomegaly	No specific anesthesia considerations beyond those listed for mucopolysaccharidoses in general

Smith-Lemli-Opitz syndrome	Inborn error of cholesterol synthesis Microcephaly, micrognathia, cleft palate Developmental delay, skeletal anomalies Hypotonia, thymic hypoplasia; susceptibility to infections	Use sterile technique ± ***Difficult airway*** Use muscle relaxants with caution Muscle rigidity with inhalational agents described, but not MH or rhabdomyolysis Consider TIVA
Sotos syndrome (cerebral gigantism)	Macrocephaly Dilated cerebral ventricles but normal ICP, developmental delay Cardiac and GU anomalies in minority Hypotonia Reduced immune response Accelerated growth in childhood	Assess cardiac status Use aseptic technique, extra padding and positioning head Hyperthermia, not MH, has been reported
Spinal muscle atrophy	Degeneration of anterior spinal neurons Progressive muscle weakness Possible bulbar dysfunction Intellect and sensation normal	± ***Difficult airway*** ***Avoid succinylcholine*** Caution with relaxants; may have prolonged effect Monitor blood glucose
Steinert disease	See Myotonia dystrophica	

(continued)

Syndrome	Issues	Anesthesia concerns
Stevens-Johnson syndrome (erythema multiforme)	Urticarial lesions, erosions in the mouth, eyes, genitalia Possible hypersensitivity reaction to exogenous agents Possible myocarditis, pericarditis hypovolemia or pleural blebs. Care similar to burn injury Some on high-dose steroids	Assess cardiac and fluid status, need for supplemental steroids ***Use sterile technique (reverse isolation)*** Oral lesions: Avoid intubation and insertion of esophageal stethoscope Gentle pharyngeal suctioning Use soft face mask with vaseline gauze on skin If intubation is required, ***secure tracheal tube with tracheostomy tape; do not use adhesive tape*** Cover ECG pads with lubricant; place beneath the patient Prewarm the operating room to 35–37 °C Monitor for arrhythmias and ventricular fibrillation Ketamine should be considered
Stickler syndrome	Autosomal dominant with midface hypoplasia, micrognathia, cleft palate “Moon-face” appearance Spinal abnormalities and mitral valve prolapse are common	Assess cardiac status ± ***Difficult airway (as in Pierre Robin sequence)***
Stiff baby syndrome (hyperekplexia, “startle disease”)	Severe muscle rigidity at birth persisting several years Exaggerated startle response Life-threatening spasms terminated by flexing the head and legs toward the trunk	Use muscle relaxants with caution Resistance to succinylcholine but normal responses to nondepolarizing muscle relaxants

Still disease (juvenile rheumatoid arthritis)	See collagen diseases	
Sturge-Weber syndrome	Cavernous angioma over trigeminal nerve distribution, usually unilateral Possible laryngeal and tracheal involvement Glaucoma Intracranial calcification, seizures and developmental delay	Port wine stains Care with airway instrumentation; possible undiagnosed laryngeal or tracheal angioma Preop seizure medications Glaucoma precautions
Subacute necrotizing encephalomyelopathy	See Leigh disease	
Supravalvar aortic stenosis with idiopathic infantile hypercalcemia	See Williams syndrome	
Tangier disease (analphalipoproteinemia)	Accumulation of cholesterol in large orange tonsils, spleen and lymph nodes Premature CAD Thrombocytopenia, anemia Low plasma high density lipoproteins Peripheral neuropathy	Assess cardiac/coronary status, platelet counts, and hemoglobin ***Manage as an adult with CAD*** Monitor for cardiac ischemia Avoid tachycardia and hypertension
TAR syndrome	See Thrombocytopenia with absent radius	

(continued)

Syndrome	Issues	Anesthesia concerns
Tarui disease (GSD Type VII)	Muscle phosphofructokinase deficiency Affects skeletal muscle and erythrocytes Neither glycogen nor glucose can be used as metabolic fuels May have myoglobinuria, rhabdomyolysis, muscle cramps, exercise intolerance, hemolytic anemia and hyperuricemia Reduced RBC life span (13–16 days) Features similar to McArdle disease	Assess renal status and Hb level Monitor glucose levels; infuse dextrose No specific anesthesia complications reported
Tay-Sachs disease	See gangliosidosis GM2	
Telangiectasis, hemorrhagic	See Osler-Rendu-Weber syndrome	
Thalassemia major (Cooley anemia)	Hb synthesis slow: persistent Hb F Hemosiderosis after multiple transfusions Splenectomy to reduce transfusions	Assess cardiac and liver function, and Hb ***Prominent maxilla: difficult airway*** ***Asceptic technique post-splenectomy***
Thomsen disease	See myotonia congenita	
Thrombasthenia	See Glanzmann disease	
Thrombocytopenia with absent radius (TAR syndrome)	Chromosome 1q21.1 deletion Episodic thrombocytopenia precipitated by stress, infection, surgery Associated CHD (30%) e.g., ASD, TOF At risk for cerebral hemorrhage Associated tracheoesophageal fistula and renal anomalies	Assess cardiac function (if CHD present), platelet count, and renal function Consult with hematologist Avoid elective surgery in first year (35%–40% mortality from intracranial hemorrhage)

Thrombocytopenia with eczema and repeated infections	See Wiskott-Aldrich syndrome	
Thrombotic thrombocytopenic purpura	See Moschcowitz disease	
Tourette syndrome	Complex neuropsychiatric disorder Attention deficit disorder progresses to spasmodic repetitious movements May exhibit coprolalia (profane speech) and echolalia (repetitions) Migraine headaches	Establish rapport with patient and family; preop sedation Continue medications Pimozide may prolong QT interval
Treacher Collins syndrome (mandibulofacial dysostosis)	Micrognathia with slanting jawbone, microstomia, aplastic zygoma, choanal atresia, microtia, coloboma, cleft palate Airway becomes more difficult with age CHD Normal intelligence, hearing impaired Associated cervical spine deformity	Assess cardiac status ***Increasingly difficult intubation as ages*** ***Use in-line cervical spine precautions*** ***A surgical airway may be required***
Trismus pseudocamptodactyly (Dutch-Kentucky syndrome)	Microstomia due to enlarged coronoid process Short stature, foot deformities	***Extremely difficult intubation; prepare for a surgical airway***
Trisomy 13 syndrome	See Patau syndrome	
Trisomy 18	See Edwards syndrome	

(continued)

Syndrome	Issues	Anesthesia concerns
Trisomy 21 Down syndrome	Macroglossia Cervical spine subluxation Congenital subglottic stenosis Associated CHD (atrioventricular communis, ventricular septal defect) Duodenal atresia Congenital leukemia Hypotonia	Assess cardiac status ***Subglottic narrowing*** ***May require in-line cervical spine stabilization*** Risk of postintubation stridor
Tuberous sclerosis (TSC)	Neurocutaneous condition with hamartoma growth in body Cardiac rhabdomyomas, benign, occur up 90% of neonates, resolve spontaneously Tumors may be found in brain, lungs, and kidneys; also in the upper airway and atria Possible pyelonephritis and renal failure Seizures	Assess cardiac and renal status Cardiac tumors may cause outflow tract obstruction, particularly in infants Continue anti-seizure medications Caution with radiocontrast material during repeat MRI assessments Possible cardiac arrhythmias
Turner syndrome (gonadal dysgenesis)	XO females; infantile genitalia, webbed neck, short stature Narrow maxilla, micrognathia Coarctation of aorta, dissecting aortic aneurysm (adolescents) or pulmonary stenosis Renal anomalies in 50% Hypothyroidism	Assess cardiac and renal status ***± Difficult airway*** Hypertension may require treatment Ensure euthyroid

Urbach-Wiethe disease (cutaneous mucosal hyalinosis)	Hoarseness or aphonia (eosinophilic hyaline-like deposits in larynx and pharynx) and skin eruption Thick tongue Thick mucus membranes, dry, and friable Possible seizure disorder	Avoid anticholinergics ± ***Difficult airway*** Gentle laryngoscopy and intubation to prevent mucosal trauma Vocal cords may be thickened Continue anti-seizure medications preop
Urticaria pigmentosa	See Mastocytosis syndrome	
VACTERL association	Random association of defects: **V**ertebral anomalies **A**nal atresia **C**ardiac anomalies **T**racheoesophageal fistula **E**sophageal atresia **R**enal anomalies **L**imb defects	Assess cardiac and renal status ± ***Difficult airway*** Anesthesia management dictated by considerations of individual lesions
VATER association	Random association of defects: **V**ertebral **A**nal atresia **T**racheoesophageal fistula **E**sophageal atresia **R**enal anomalies	Assess cardiac and renal status ± ***Difficult airway*** Anesthesia management dictated by considerations of individual lesions

(continued)

Syndrome	Issues	Anesthesia concerns
Velocardiofacial syndrome	A phenotypic variant of the 22q deletion syndrome, distinct from DiGeorge syndrome Associated CHD, OSA Facial anomalies, speech difficulties, learning disability Long-term risk of psychiatric disorders	Assess cardiac status ± ***Difficult airway*** ***Possible OSA;*** if the nocturnal saturation nadir is <85% reduce opioid dose
Very long-chain acyl coenzyme A dehydrogenase deficiency	Disorder of fatty acid metabolism Associated cardiomyopathy, liver failure, rhabdomyolysis, and hypoglycemia	Assess cardiac liver status Minimal fasting Administer glucose infusions perioperatively ***Propofol infusion contraindicated due to emulsion vehicle*** ***Avoid succinylcholine***
von Gierke disease (Type I GSD)	Most common GSD, 90% cases Developmental delay, short stature Early onset, marked hepatomegaly, renal hyperplasia, hypoglycemia, lactic acidosis, hyperlipidemia, hyperuricemia Impaired neutrophil function, stomatitis Bleeding diathesis secondary to impaired platelet aggregation and deficient von Willebrand factor Severe hypoglycemia is unresponsive to glucagon and epinephrine Possible seizures, malignancies, hypertension	Preop assess renal and hepatic statuses, glucose, electrolytes, and platelet count Brief preop fast; consider perioperative IV glucose infusion; avoid lactated Ringer's solution ± ***Difficult intubation*** ***Caution with propofol infusions; possible postoperative pancreatitis***

von Hippel-Lindau syndrome	Retinal angiomas and cerebellar hemangioblastomas Associated pheochromocytoma May have pulmonary, pancreatic, hepatic, adrenal, and renal cysts Paroxysmal hypertension due to cerebellar tumor or pheochromocytoma	Assess renal and hepatic statuses, Rule out pheochromocytoma; if present institute preoperative management Hypertensive crises may occur
von Recklinghausen disease (neurofibromatosis)	>5 café au lait spots are diagnostic Tumors may occur within the CNS and peripheral nerve trunks; larynx, trachea, and right ventricular outflow tract Kyphoscoliosis in 50%; neck may be unstable Pulmonary problems due to fibrosing alveolitis "honeycomb (cystic) lung" Renal artery dysplasia common; systemic hypertension may occur Pheochromocytoma in 1%	Assess cardiac, pulmonary, and renal status for tumors Assess upper airway for tumors ***May need in-line cervical spine stabilization*** Care with renally excreted drugs

(continued)

Syndrome	Issues	Anesthesia concerns
von Willebrand disease (pseudohemophilia)	Prolonged bleeding time (↓von Willebrand factor & ↓ factor VIII activity; defective platelet adhesiveness) Several variants determine treatment: Use DDAVP for type 1 and some type 2 patients, but may exacerbate others Use factor VIII concentrates for types 2 and 3 Bleeding controlled using fresh frozen plasma, cryoprecipitate, or product concentrates (e.g., Humate P®, Alphanate®, Wilate®, or Koate HP) Consult a hematologist	Consult with surgeon and hematologist to develop optimal management strategy Monitor factor VIII levels and bleeding time Product concentrates and antifibrinolytics may be effective
Weaver syndrome	Skeletal overgrowth leads to craniofacial abnormalities and digital abnormalities Relative micrognathia, midfacial hypoplasia, short neck, anterior larynx	***± Difficult airway*** ***Airway may become easier with age***
Weber-Christian disease (chronic nonsuppurative panniculitis)	Necrosis of fat in retroperitoneal tissue leading to adrenal insufficiency In pericardium, restrictive pericarditis In meninges, seizures	Assess cardiac and renal status, assess seizure risk Maintain blood volume Caution with renally excreted drugs

Werdnig-Hoffmann disease (infantile muscular atrophy, SMA type 1)	Onset in infancy, hypotonia Severe scoliosis in <1 year of age Chronic feeding problems, >95% have gastrostomy tube by 2 years of age Chronic respiratory problems Most die before puberty	Assess severity of pulmonary status and hypotonia ***Succinylcholine is contraindicated*** Cautious use of muscle relaxants and respiratory depressant drugs
Wermer syndrome (multiple endocrine adenomatosis type 1 (MEN1))	Autosomal dominant mutation on chromosome 11 Hyperparathyroidism (90%), anterior tumors of pituitary (40%), insulinomas of the pancreas (60%) Carcinoid tumors occur in 3% Asymptomatic adrenal tumors in 20–73% Renal failure from kidney stones	Preop assess for renal and pituitary functions, carcinoid tumor and glucose levels Consider monitoring and/or perioperative glucose infusion Caution with renally excreted drugs
Werner syndrome	Premature aging starts at 13 years Short stature, diabetes (in 50%) Possible coronary artery disease and CHF	Assess cardiac and diabetes preop ***Manage as for adults with CAD, avoid tachycardia and hypertension***
West syndrome	Developmental delay, infantile spasms Hypsarrhythmia seizures on EEG Possible ketogenic diet	Preop anti-seizure medications Avoid glucose-containing solutions with a ketogenic diet Infuse lactated Ringer's solution
Whistling face syndrome	See Freeman-Sheldon syndrome	

(continued)

Syndrome	Issues	Anesthesia concerns
Williams syndrome (elfin facies syndrome)	Elfin facies Micrognathia Cardiac defects; supravalvular aortic stenosis, pulmonary artery obstruction, critical coronary artery stenosis-prone to sudden death Associated hypercalcemia "Party personality" Very high anesthetic risk and difficult to resuscitate Renal abnormalities may be present	Assess cardiac and renal status preop and calcium ***Potentially difficult airway*** ***High risk of cardiac arrest without provocation!*** ***Intravenous induction with an opioid based anesthetic is recommended; also inhaled induction possible*** Establish euvolemia Stress dose steroids as indicated
Wilson disease (hepatolenticular degeneration)	Decreased ceruloplasmin Copper deposits in liver and CNS motor nuclei Renal tubular acidosis Hepatic failure due to fibrosis	Assess renal, hepatic and coagulation statuses Avoid muscle relaxants that depend on hepatic or renal paths for excretion (e.g., cisatracurium)
Wilson-Mikity syndrome	Prematurity (<1500 g birth weight) Severe chronic lung disease leading to generalized fibrosis with cystic interstitial emphysema, repeated chest infection, and aspiration Right ventricular failure Steroids to prevent pulmonary fibrosis	Assess cardiac & pulmonary statuses May require stress dose steroids

Wiskott-Aldrich syndrome	Decreased production of microplatelets (thrombocytopenia) Autoimmune coronary vasculitis Hypersusceptible to eczema, asthma, severe herpes simplex infections, and lymphoid malignancy due to T and B-cell function defects Death before 10 years despite stem cell transplant	Assess cardiac status ***If coronary vasculitis is present, manage as adult with CAD*** ***Irradiate blood products prevent graft-versus-host reaction*** ***Use sterile technique (e.g., reverse isolation)***
Wolff-Parkinson-White syndrome (WPW)	Anomalous conduction path between atria and ventricles resulting in short P-R interval (delta wave) Prolonged QRS with phasic variation (40%) Prone to paroxysmal supraventricular tachycardia (SVT), other cardiac defects	Review cardiac status with cardiologist preop Avoid atropine TIVA may be preferred technique
Wolman disease (familial xanthomatosis, also Hemophagocytic lymphohistiocytosis)	Failure to thrive, adrenal calcification resembles Niemann-Pick disease with hepatosplenomegaly, hypersplenism Thrombocytopenia Foam cell infiltration (of all tissues, including myocardium-death by 6 months	Assess cardiac, pulmonary, and hepatic statuses Assess platelet count
Worster-Drought syndrome	A form of cerebral palsy with childhood onset epilepsy	Preop seizure medications postoperative apnea possible
β-glucuronidase deficiency	See Sly syndrome	
Zellweger syndrome	See cerebrohepatorenal syndrome	

Appendix B: Cardiopulmonary Resuscitation, Including Neonatal Resuscitation

The purpose of cardiopulmonary resuscitation (CPR) is to restore pulmonary and cardiovascular function and prevent neurologic damage. It begins with *basic life support,* which consists of artificial ventilation and circulation by whatever means are available, for the purpose of preventing clinical death from progressing to biologic death before other remedial measures (i.e., *advanced life support*) can be instituted. In children, the most common cause of cardiac arrest is respiratory failure with a variable period of progression/deterioration.

The overall success rates for pediatric CPR and long-term survival without neurologic deficit in children are greater than in adults with 40% of children surviving to hospital discharge. Those who do survive may have poor long-term outcomes because most arrests in children result from hypoxia, and by the time the heart stops, the brain has already sustained hypoxic damage. Every effort must be directed at rapidly diagnosing and treating depressed ventilation and hypoxemia. Outcomes after "within hospital cardiac arrest" exceed those after "outside hospital cardiac arrest" possibly because children are generally healthy; outside hospital arrest outcomes are also improving because bystander CPR skills and AEDs are more widely available.

J. Lerman, C. J. Coté, *Steward's Manual of Pediatric Anesthesia*,
https://doi.org/10.1007/978-3-032-24545-8

Prevention of Cardiac Arrest

Precipitating factors in cardiac arrest in children include:

1. Respiratory failure:
   (a) Due to airway obstruction, central respiratory depression, or primary pulmonary disorders.
   (b) Secondary to pulmonary aspiration.
   (c) Secondary to neurologic and neuromuscular disorders (e.g., seizure, residual neuromuscular weakness).
2. Hypovolemia.
3. Toxicity (drugs, poisons, toxins).
4. Primary cardiac disorders, particularly severe aortic stenosis and Fontan physiology.

Prevention requires:

1. Recognition of the potential causes (respiratory failure)
2. Constant surveillance

Special Hazards for Children Undergoing Anesthesia

Factors that rapidly lead to life-threatening events in infants and children:

1. During anesthesia or sedation, the upper airway may become partially or totally obstructed by:
   (a) Laryngospasm (common); due to small amounts of mucus or blood or light anesthesia (see Chap. 4).
   (b) Hypertrophic adenoids and/or tonsils.
   (c) Relative macroglossia, especially in infants and toddlers associated with:
      (i) Flaccid muscles in the upper airway during anesthesia.
      (ii) Iatrogenic displacement or compression of submental soft tissue and tongue.

(iii) Failure to extend the neck.
(iv) Failure to sublux the temporomandibular joint (at the coronoid process).
(v) Premature removal of an artificial airway.

(d) Regurgitated gastric contents.

Remember: Neonates are obligate nose breathers, but if their nasal passages are not patent, an oral airway is needed.

2. Ventilation may be compromised if the stomach becomes inflated from:
   (a) Excessive peak inspiratory pressures during facemask ventilation
   (b) Partial airway obstruction
   (c) Crying and swallowing air

   After securing the airway with a tracheal tube, decompress the stomach.
3. Blood volumes are small—a small blood loss may cause hypovolemia.

Routine Precautions

Preoperative

1. Atropine should be immediately available for neonates/infants who are scheduled for laryngoscopy/tracheal intubation, those at risk for reflex bradycardia (succinylcholine), or having surgery that may elicit vagal reflexes, e.g., strabismus repair. In infants and children, vagal reflexes are brisk and may lead to severe bradycardia and/or cardiac arrest. The greater the delay in giving atropine, the greater the time until it increases the heart rate. NB. The most common cause of bradycardia is hypoxemia; atropine does not correct hypoxemia. Ventilation with oxygen corrects hypoxemia!
2. Always give 100% O_2 before intubation since the speed and severity of the desaturation are inversely related to age: neonates >> infants > children > adolescents.
3. Select the tracheal tube size based on the child's age, check for a leak at 20–30 cmH_2O peak inflation pressure, confirm the presence of $EtCO_2$, secure it firmly, and check for proper

tracheal depth and bilateral breath sounds after positioning (see Chap. 4). Position and support the tracheal tube to avoid kinking.

Perioperative

1. Maintain a patent airway and adequate ventilation.
2. Monitor the following continuously (Do not disable the alarms):
   (a) Heart and lung functions using the ECG, NIBP, SaO_2 and $EtCO_2$
   (b) Body temperature
   (c) Blood loss
3. Read all drug labels; accurately calculate diluted drugs or use small volume syringes, but ensure correct doses are administered.
4. Accurately assess fluid and blood losses and replace as indicated, even a small loss may be significant in an infant. Establish a reliable and adequately sized IV access before incision.
5. Rapid infusion of blood products may cause hyperkalemia (old whole blood or irradiated blood) or hypocalcemia (FFP), especially when administered into a central vein in small infants.
6. Prevent unintentional pressure on the chest and abdominal walls from dressings, hands, and surgical staff leaning on the drapes.
7. If problems become apparent, advise all members of the team (especially the surgeon) immediately.

Postoperative

Note: Cardiac arrest may occur in the post-anesthesia care unit (PACU).

1. For all infants and all ill children: do not extubate the trachea until the child has recovered from anesthesia, is breathing reg-

ularly, and is reacting vigorously. Monitor SaO_2 during transport and have oxygen and a means to bag/mask ventilate during transport. Delivering oxygen may mask hypoventilation!

2. If possible, transport all children to the PACU in the lateral (recovery) position, with the upper leg flexed at the hip and knee and overlying the lower leg and the neck moderately extended (the "tonsil" or "recovery" position) by placing the upper hand under the jaw.
3. In the PACU:
   (a) Immediately assess SaO_2, ECG, and NIBP.
   (b) Provide a full report to the PACU nursing staff regarding medical conditions, surgical issues, medication doses and time of administration, blood loss and replacement, and anticipated possible PACU problems.
   (c) Ensure that the child remains positioned with a clear airway.
      (i) Administer humidified O_2 by mask until the child can maintain their SaO_2 on room air.
      (ii) Ensure that vital signs are recorded and reported to you if changes occur.
   (d) Do not leave until the vital signs are stable and all nursing questions have been addressed.
   (e) Before discharge from the PACU, ensure that the danger of drug-induced respiratory depression has passed and the child has returned to their baseline condition.
   (f) Some neonates and infants need to be stimulated to maintain ventilation.
   (g) All former preterm infants less than 65 weeks post-menstrual age and those with a history of chronic respiratory disease should be monitored with an apnea alarm for at least 24 h or until they are 12 h apnea-free (see Chap. 2).
   (h) Children with obstructive sleep apnea (OSA) may require extended observation and monitoring. Those with severe OSA should be treated with either opioid-free analgesics or reduced opioid doses, as they may have chronic hypoxia-induced opioid sensitivity (see Chap. 11).

Treatment of Arrhythmias

Arrhythmias that cause hemodynamic compromise or those that might progress to cardiac arrest must be promptly treated. The advice of a pediatric cardiologist should be obtained.

Supraventricular Tachycardia (SVT)

(a) Heart rates >220 bpm in infants or >180 bpm in children suggest SVT. SVT may be difficult to differentiate from sinus tachycardia, but the history and the heart rate usually clarify the diagnosis.

(b) Vagal maneuvers (Valsalva maneuver, breath holding, or placing ice on the face) constitute initial therapy. If vagal maneuvers fail, then administer adenosine, as a rapid IV bolus and if this fails, try amiodarone (Appendix C for dosing). If circulatory instability is present, synchronized electrical cardioversion (0.5–1 joule/kg) is recommended (See further).

Ventricular Tachycardia (VT) and Fibrillation (VF)

(a) For VT (QRS >0.12 s) with hypotension but with a palpable pulse, immediate synchronized cardioversion is recommended. Children with less hemodynamic compromise should be assessed for the cause of the VT and may be sedated before cardioversion.

(b) For pulseless VT (pVT) and VF, immediate defibrillation is indicated. If this is unsuccessful or VT recurs, amiodarone 5 mg/kg IV may be considered (See below).

Shockable Rhythms (VF and pVT)

1. After starting CPR assess if the rhythm is shockable.
2. If the rhythm is shockable (0.5–1 J/kg) and continue CPR for 2 min while establishing IV or intraosseous access (IO).

3. If the rhythm has not converted, then shock again doubling the power to 4 J/kg. Administer epinephrine 10 μg/kg (0.1 ml/kg of a 1:10,000 solution up to a max of 1 mg). Reassess after 2 min.
4. If the shockable rhythm persists, repeat with 4 joules/kg up to a max of 10 joules/kg in incremental steps. Administer epinephrine 0.01 mg/kg at 3–5-min intervals. Treat reversible causes of cardiac arrest: 7 "H's" [**h**ypoxia, **h**ypovolemia, **h**ydrogen ion (acidosis) [Note that bicarbonate is associated with worse outcomes and is no longer recommended unless to assist with treatment of **h**yperkalemia, sodium channel blocker/tricyclic antidepressant toxicity], **h**ypoglycemia, **h**yperkalemia or **h**ypokalemia, and **h**ypothermia] and 5 "T's" [**t**ension pneumothorax, cardiac **t**amponade, **t**oxins, **t**hromboembolic event, and **t**rauma]. Administer amiodarone (IV/IO) 5 mg/kg. Repeat x3 doses for refractory VF or pVT. Consider lidocaine 1 mg/kg loading dose. [Note that calcium is no longer recommended as it is associated with worse outcomes unless used to treat hyperkalemia, hypocalcemia, calcium channel blocker overdose, or hypermagnesemia.]

Non-shockable Rhythm (Asystole & Pulseless Electrical Activity [PEA])

Asystole and PEA are the most common ECG findings in infants and children with cardiac arrest. In the presence of PEA (QRS complexes in the absence of palpable pulses), CPR should be continued for 2 min and followed by epinephrine (0.01 mg/kg IV or IO). If venous access has not been established, give 0.1 mg/kg epinephrine intratracheally (diluted to a larger volume for better mucosal absorption).

CPR should continue for 2 min after which the airway should be intubated. Underlying causes of the asystole and PEA should be sought: the 7 "H's" and 5 "T's" (See above). Repeat as needed.

Cardiopulmonary Resuscitation

The guidelines for cardiopulmonary resuscitation and neonatal resuscitation outlined here are based on the most recent American Heart Association 2020 recommendations for infants and children.

Basic Life Support

N.B. For basic life support in hospitals, use a bag and mask as soon as possible to prevent the risk of infection from using mouth-to-mouth resuscitation to hospital personnel. Ensure that such equipment is immediately available and functioning in all patient-care areas.

Do not leave the child. Call for help and equipment, including an automated external defibrillator AED.

When called to resuscitate a child, assess the situation immediately according to the following priorities:

A. Check Ventilation
   1. *If there are respiratory efforts with a patent upper airway:*
      (a) Position the child in the lateral position (recovery position) to maintain a clear airway and decrease the risk of aspiration.
      (b) Give O_2 by mask as soon as it becomes available.
   2. *If respiratory efforts are present, but there is evidence of airway obstruction* (breath sounds absent, intercostal retraction, flaring of lateral chest margins, cyanosis):
      (a) Pull the tongue or mandible forward (by pressing behind the mandibular condyles) and remove any foreign matter from the pharynx, keeping the mouth slightly open.
      (b) Extend the neck if necessary (Caution if neck injury—but remember that ventilation is the priority).
      (c) Give O_2 by mask.
      (d) Check for improved chest movement and breath sounds.

B. If there are no respiratory efforts or ventilation appears inadequate:
   1. Begin positive-pressure ventilation.
   2. Ventilate directly, mouth to mouth if necessary; the small infant face necessitates application of your mouth to the infant's mouth and nose. Once airway equipment is available remember that an infant's tidal volume is small (8–10 mL/kg); therefore, only puffs are necessary. Ensure that the chest expands adequately with each breath (20–30 breaths/min).

C. *If a pulse is not palpable within 10 s (brachial, femoral, or carotid artery) or the heart rate is <100 bpm in an infant or <80 bpm in a toddler begin chest compressions.* One rescuer performs 30 compressions, then 2 breaths and this sequence is repeated until a second rescuer arrives. Two rescuers perform 15 compressions and two breaths. *Check for a pulse every 2 min.* ("Push Hard, Push Fast"):
   (a) The site of compression in an infant is one finger-breadth below the intermammary line; in a child, it is over the lower sternum, one finger-breadth above the xiphisternum. In an infant, two thumb-encircling hand chest compressions may be used; in a child, the heel of the hand should be used See Figure.
   (b) Depth of compression: one-third to one-half of the anteroposterior diameter of the chest; between compressions, release completely to allow the chest wall to recoil fully.
   (c) The rate of chest compressions is 100/min for infants, children, and adolescents.
   (d) Do not interrupt the compressions for ventilation.

   If the pulse is 60 or greater, continue with ventilation only.

D. Check for a shockable rhythm every 2 min (a pediatric programmable automated external defibrillator (AED) is preferred for children <8 years of age). *If a shockable rhythm is present, give one shock and resume CPR for 2 min. If a shockable rhythm is absent, resume CPR for 2 min until prompted by an AED; repeat this sequence until initiating Advanced Life Support.*

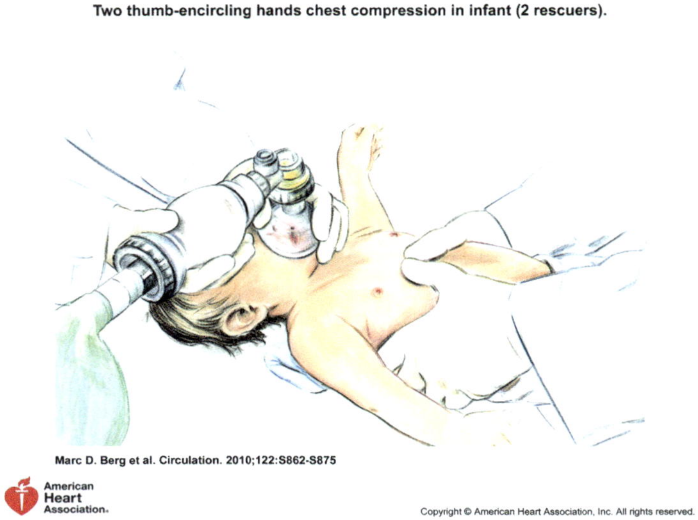

Fig. Infant external cardiac compressions. In 2025, the American Heart Association (AHA) adopted two thumb chest compressions (encircling the chest with two-hands) in infants to ensure adequate cardiac output during CPR. For a single rescuer who cannot apply two-thumb compressions, the heel-of-one-hand technique may be used. The AHA no longer recommends two-finger chest compressions in infants. (From Todres D, Rogers MC: Method of external cardiac massage in the newborn infant. J Pediatr 86:781, 1975, with permission)

Defibrillation

Use the AED as soon as possible. Early defibrillation is recommended for children who have VF and pVT. These are more likely in the scenario of a sudden, unexpected arrest, especially in children with congenital heart disease.

1. For infants and children weighing less than 20 kg, use pediatric defibrillator plates (diameter of 4.5 cm for infants and 8 cm for children). However, a pediatric programmable AED is preferred even if the pads seem oversized provided the pads do not touch each other.

2. Set the AED to deliver shocks appropriate to the child's size (to maximize the chance of success and minimize the danger of electrically induced myocardial damage); the initial setting should be 0.5–1 joules (watt-seconds)/kg increasing to 2 J/kg if ineffective.
3. Give one shock and immediately resume CPR for 2 min. If this is unsuccessful, the power should be doubled to 4 joules. This allows the AED to reassess the rhythm.
4. Many AED's have the potential to detect pediatric "shockable" rhythms in children <8 years of age and can be adjusted to deliver the appropriate energy to each shock. Ensure that AEDs installed for children conform to these requirements. Even without a pediatric dose attenuator, an AED is preferred over a standard manual defibrillator.
5. Initially, children who are digitalized should be treated with a reduced power since normal doses of countershock may cause ventricular fibrillation, which may be difficult to convert to sinus rhythm. Subsequently, the power setting is gradually increased.

Advanced Life Support

Most children in cardiac arrest require:

1. Continued ventilation and oxygenation as the first line of therapy.
2. Secure the airway by rapidly intubating the trachea; a cuffed tracheal tube is preferred. A laryngeal mask airway may be useful in some instances. Exhaled CO_2 detection is recommended to quickly confirm a successful intubation and to ensure adequate pulmonary circulation with chest compressions. Do not delay ventilation during lengthy attempts at intubation: ventilation is essential and intubation is optional.
3. Assess definitive ECG diagnosis of cardiac activity and defibrillation if indicated.
4. Establish an intravenous (IV) or intraosseous (IO) route for drug administration; intratracheal drug administration may

be considered for some drugs. After IV or IO access is established, blood or fluid losses should be replaced initially with crystalloids and later with colloids (plasma or blood). Dextrose-containing solutions are best avoided, as hyperglycemia may compromise cerebral survival. If hypoglycemia is suspected, it should be confirmed by blood glucose determination and treated accordingly.
5. Supportive drugs, primarily epinephrine (see below).
6. Waveform capnography or capnometry should be used to confirm correct ETT placement and the adequacy of chest compressions. An expired CO_2 of 10–20 suggests adequate pulmonary circulation with chest compressions.

Drug Therapy

Although subsequent drug therapy is necessarily individualized, a standard initial protocol is advantageous.

1. Epinephrine: To be maximally effective, it must be given intravenously (preferably into a central vein) or, if this is not possible, by the IO route.
   (a) Initial and subsequent doses: 10 μg/kg (0.1 ml/kg of a 1:10,000 solution).
   (b) High-dose (100 μg/kg) epinephrine is no longer recommended (except possibly in the treatment of β-blocker overdose).
2. Vasopressin has been successful in some cases of prolonged cardiac arrest but has not resulted in increased survival to a neurologically intact hospital discharge.
3. Dopamine infusion may be required for continued hypotension and poor tissue perfusion; 5–20 μg/kg/min may be titrated to achieve the desired effect.
4. Sodium bicarbonate administration is no longer recommended as a routine, but it might be considered in prolonged cardiac arrest for documented continuing severe metabolic acidosis despite adequate ventilation, oxygenation, and chest compressions. It may also be useful in the treatment of hyperkalemia, hypermagnesemia, or tricyclic antidepressant overdose.

N.B. Administration of excessive doses of sodium bicarbonate produces hyperosmolarity, hypernatremia, hypokalemia, decreased ionized calcium, impaired cardiac action, and possibly severe alkalosis after recovery.

5. Calcium is no longer recommended except as the definitive treatment for hyperkalemic-induced arrhythmias or arrest and citrate-induced hypocalcemia.
6. Glucose: Documented hypoglycemia should be treated by glucose infusions. Otherwise, avoid any glucose administration because hyperglycemia (glucose >200 mg/dl) may compromise neurologic outcome after a hypoxic event. Preterm infants may require exogenous glucose to prevent hypoglycemia.

Route of Administration of Drugs

Inject epinephrine into a central line, if one is available; otherwise, use a peripheral IV or IO line. The tracheal route is only used as a last resort.

Intracardiac injections should not be made. Damage to the heart and coronary arteries and/or a pneumothorax may result.

Post-resuscitation Care

Emphasis is placed on this as being critical to a favorable outcome.

1. Maintain normocarbia and oxygen saturation between 94% and 99%: hyperventilation may be harmful and should be avoided.
2. Hypothermia (32–34 °C) may be considered for 12–24 h in children who remain comatose after CPR.
3. Prevent hyperthermia.
4. Support hemodynamics using vasoactive drugs (e.g., dopamine) to improve the circulatory status.
5. Target blood glucose levels to achieve normal levels.

6. Restrict fluid replacement: avoid large infusions of crystalloid solutions once cardiovascular stability is ensured.
7. Monitor for post-arrest seizure activity and treat with phenobarbital and/or phenytoin (Dilantin) as indicated.
8. Obtain an early neurologic consultation.
9. Maintain cerebral perfusion pressure

Neonatal Resuscitation

The anesthesiologist is frequently called upon to assist at or manage the care of the neonate immediately after birth. Neonatal resuscitation is based on detailed knowledge of the normal physiologic changes that occur during transition to extrauterine life (see Chap. 2) plus knowledge regarding health issues of the mother or the fetus that may affect the infant at or after delivery.

Most infants require little help. Those born at term, with clear amniotic fluid, who are crying or breathing and have good tone are dried, kept warm, and require no further interventions. Others require rapid intervention to prevent serious sequelae. Most often infants at risk are recognized before birth, and preparations are made for their immediate resuscitation on delivery, although infants with no antenatal signs of distress may also require urgent intervention after birth.

Immediate Assessment of the Neonate

A rapid assessment must be made to determine the extent of stepwise treatment that is required. This determination is made based on respirations, heart rate, and color during the first minute after delivery.

Procedures for Neonatal Resuscitation

These recommendations are based on the American Heart Association and the American Academy of Pediatrics 2023 recommendations.

1. Assess Respirations—term gestation, good tone, good cry → routine care, position airway, clear secretions as needed.
2. If respirations or breathing are inadequate, then dry the baby, position the airway, clear secretions, and stimulate the baby.
3. If apneic or gasping, clear the airway. If breathing is labored or cyanosis persists, reposition and clear the airway, apply a pulse oximeter, and consider assisted or controlled ventilation. In preterm infants, positive end-expiratory pressure of 5 cm H_2O maintains lung volumes and may avoid intubation. An initial inspired oxygen of 21% is preferred but may be increased gradually if hypoxemia persists.
4. If apnea persists or gasping respirations are present with a heart rate < 100 bpm, initiate positive-pressure ventilation and apply a pulse oximeter and an ECG monitor. Each 30 s of delayed positive-pressure ventilation increases prolonged hospitalization or death by ~16%! Respirations should be assisted at a rate of 40–60 per minute with peak inflation pressures up to 30 cm H_2O in term infants and 20–25 cm H_2O in preterm infants. A T-piece system with pressure manometer is preferred over a self-inflating bag, although the latter should be available as a backup. Avoid hypocapnia.
5. If the heart rate remains <100 bpm, confirm chest movement and breath sounds and place a tracheal tube if needed. A laryngeal mask airway is a less secure airway.
6. If the heart rate remains <60 bpm despite adequate assisted ventilation for 30 s, then intubate if the airway has not been secured, initiate chest compressions (two-thumb chest encircling technique, ratio 3:1 compression/ventilation ratio), ventilate with 100% oxygen, and consider placing an umbilical venous catheter for rescue access. The intraosseous route is a reasonable alternative.
7. If heart rate remains below 60 bpm, administer intravenous epinephrine (0.01–0.03 mg/kg IV or 0.05–0.1 mg via tracheal tube) every 3–5 min, and consider hypovolemia and a pneumothorax as possible causes.

Meconium

Intrapartum suctioning has not been demonstrated to reduce the incidence of meconium aspiration syndrome and is no longer recommended. Tracheal suctioning should be performed on meconium-stained depressed infants before stimulation. Meconium-stained vigorous infants do not require suctioning.

Post-resuscitation Care

1. Temperature control; hyperthermia is bad and increases the risk of mortality and morbidity. Hypothermia with defined protocols is recommended for infants at risk for hypoxic ischemic encephalopathy older than 35 weeks gestational age; the efficacy of such therapy in younger infants is unclear.
2. Check blood glucose levels; treat hypoglycemia and avoid hyperglycemia.

The Preterm Infant

Some special considerations are necessary for the very small infant:

1. Special care must be taken to prevent heat losses; immediately dry and place the infant on a warm mattress under a heating lamp. Use humidified oxygen.
2. Infants weighing greater than 1000 g should be given O_2, suctioned, and stimulated as needed.
3. Infants weighing less than 1000 g will likely require early tracheal intubation and ventilation. Be prepared to intervene rapidly unless the infant is in satisfactory condition.
4. Any preterm infant who displays respiratory difficulty should have their trachea intubated to provide optimal ventilation and oxygenation.

Suggested Reading

Duff JP, Topjian AA, Berg MD, et al. 2019 American Heart Association focused update on pediatric advanced life support: an update to the American Heart Association guidelines for cardiopulmonary resuscitation and emergency cardiovascular care. *Circulation*. 2019;140(24):e904–14.

Holmberg MJ, Ross CE, Fitzmaurice GM, et al. Annual incidence of adult and pediatric in-hospital cardiac arrest in the United States. Cir Cardiovasc Qual Outcomes. 2019;12(7):e005580.

Kaczmarski P, Karuga FF, Szmyd B, et al. The role of inflammation, hypoxia, and opioid receptor expression in pain modulation in patients suffering from obstructive sleep apnea. Int J Mol Sci. 2022;23(16).

Pruitt CM. Pediatric out-of-hospital cardiac arrest: more common than we thought? Resuscitation. 2020;153:260–1.

Topjian AA, Raymond TT, Atkins D, et al. Part 4: pediatric basic and advanced life support: 2020 American Heart Association guidelines for cardiopulmonary resuscitation and emergency cardiovascular care. Circulation. 2020;142(16):S469–523.

Trevisanuto D, Roehr CC, Davis PG, et al. Devices for administering ventilation at birth: a systematic review. Pediatrics. 2021;148(1).

Yamada NK, Szyld E, Strand ML, et al. 2023 American Heart Association and American Academy of Pediatrics focused update on neonatal resuscitation: an update to the American Heart Association guidelines for cardiopulmonary resuscitation and emergency cardiovascular care. Circulation. 2024;149(1):e157–66.

Appendix C: Drug Doses

Preoperative Period

N.B. Avoid intramuscular drugs (IM) as they are painful and may cause sterile abscesses. If multiple IM drugs are necessary, combine them into a single syringe whenever possible.

Premedications

Sedatives

Midazolam (Versed): 0.5–0.75 mg/kg PO (20 mg maximum dose), 0.2 mg/kg intranasally (IN) (up to 10 mg), 1.0 mg/kg per rectum (PR) (up to 20 mg), or 0.1 mg/kg IM (up to 10 mg), or 0.05–0.1 mg/kg IV (2 mg/dose maximum).
Clonidine: 4 µg/kg PO, or 1–2 µg/kg IN.
Dexmedetomidine: 2.5 µg/kg PO or 1 µg/kg IN.
Ketamine: 5–10 mg/kg PO, 2–8 mg/kg IM ± glycopyrrolate 0.2 mg IM.
Lorazepam (Ativan): for adolescents, 1–2 mg PO.
Midazolam/ketamine mixture: 0.3–0.5 mg/kg midazolam combined with 2–3 mg/kg ketamine ±0.02 mg/kg atropine PO (may cause considerable sedation—monitor).

J. Lerman, C. J. Coté, *Steward's Manual of Pediatric Anesthesia*,
https://doi.org/10.1007/978-3-032-24545-8

Antacids

Ranitidine: 2–5 mg/kg PO or 1.5 mg/kg IV or IM.

Famotidine: 0.25–0.5 mg/kg IV or 0.5 mg/kg PO; max. IV dose is 20 mg > 3mo; max PO dose: 1 mg/kg term to 1 year & 20 mg > 1 year.

Sodium citrate: 0.4 mL/kg PO.

Antiemetics

Aprepitant: 40 mg PO for adolescents >12 years.

NSAIDS

Acetaminophen: 15 mg/kg PO (maximum dose 650 mg).

Tramadol: 10 mg/kg PO syrup or 50 mg tablet for children >12 years. 1–2 mg/kg IV.

Gastric Motility Agents

Metoclopramide: 0.15 mg/kg IV.

Topical Local Anesthetics (Cover all Topicals with an Occlusive Dressing)

EMLA (eutectic mixture of local anesthetics): Prilocaine (2.5%) and *Lidocaine* (2.5%). Apply to skin for 60 min <3 months; up to 90 min >3 months before IV cannulation. Caution: limit the dose to manufacturer recommendations for EMLA cream in neonates as prilocaine may cause methemoglobinemia.

Amethocaine gel (Ametop®): Tetracaine (4%). Apply to skin 45 min before IV cannulation Caution: not recommended for neonates.

Ela-Max (4% Lidocaine): Apply to skin 30 min before IV cannulation.

S-Caine Patch: Eutectic mixture of 70 mg *lidocaine* and 70 mg *tetracaine*. Apply 20 min before IV cannulation.

Intraoperative Period

Induction Agents

Propofol (Diprivan): infants 1.5–2 mg/kg, children 2.5–3.5 mg/kg IV.

Etomidate: 0.25–0.3 mg/kg IV (avoid in septic shock).

Ketamine: 2 mg/kg IV or 4–8 mg/kg IM (plus atropine 0.02 mg/kg IM/IV).

Methohexital: up to 2 mg/kg IV, or 15–25 mg/kg of a 1% or 20–30 mg/kg of a 10% solution PR.

Thiopental sodium (Pentothal): neonates, up to 3–4 mg/kg; infants (1 month–1 year); children, up to 5–6 mg/kg IV.

Neuromuscular Blocking drugs (Monitor Train of Four Twitch Response)

Succinylcholine: infants, 2 mg/kg IV; children >1 year, 1 mg/kg IV or 4–5 mg/kg IM.

Rocuronium: 0.3–1.2 mg/kg IV, repeat doses 0.15 mg/kg. Also, infants 1 mg/kg IM and children 1.8 mg/kg IM for intubation. Infusion rate for maintenance: 10–12 µg/kg/min.

Cisatracurium: 0.1–0.2 mg/kg IV. Repeat doses 0.03 mg/kg IV. IV infusion for maintenance: 2–3 µg/kg/min.

Vecuronium: 0.1 mg/kg IV, repeat doses 0.05 mg/kg/h IV (duration greater in neonates/infants).

Pancuronium: infants and children 0.1 mg/kg.

Antagonism of Neuromuscular Blockade

Atropine 0.02 mg/kg or *glycopyrrolate* 0.01 mg/kg followed by *neostigmine* 0.05 mg/kg-administer IV slowly *OR*.

Sugammadex 2–4 mg/kg IV slowly (up to 16 mg/kg for profound blockades).

Analgesics: Opioids and NSAIDs

Fentanyl: Bolus doses 1–2 μg/kg IV prn.
IV infusion: loading dose 5 μg/kg IV, then 2–4 μg/kg/h IV.

Hydromorphone (Dilaudid): 0.01–0.02 mg/kg IV.

Morphine: 10–100 μg/kg IV prn.
IV infusion: loading dose 100 μg/kg IV, then 40–60 μg/kg/h IV.

Remifentanil: Loading dose—0.5–2 μg/kg IV.
IV Infusion: 0.05–0.3 μg/kg/min.

Acetaminophen: 10–15 mg/kg PO q4-6h (maximum 90–100 mg/kg daily) (650 mg maximum single dose); 10 mg/kg q6h IV (maximum 75 mg/kg daily) or 30–40 mg/kg single dose PR followed by 20 mg/kg q6h (maximum 4 doses).

Ketorolac: 0.2–0.5 mg/kg IV (maximum dose in a 70 kg adult is 15 mg).

Celecoxib: 10 mg/kg IV.

Parecoxib: 0.9 mg/kg in 2-year-olds; 0.75 mg/kg in 2–7 year-olds; 0.65 mg/kg 7–12 year-olds.

Antiemetics

Dexamethasone: 0.0625–0.15 mg/kg IV (maximum 8 mg).

Ondansetron: 0.05–0.15 mg/kg IV.

Metoclopramide: 0.15 mg/kg IV.

Fosaprepitant: 4 mg/kg IV for 6 mos to <12 year (max. 150 mg in adults mg)(FDA approved for oncologic patients only); ≥12 years 150 mg IV.

Local Anesthetics: Recommended safe maximum doses (see Table 7.2, Chap. 7), have intralipid immediately available

Local Anesthetic Systemic Toxicity (LAST): See Chap. 7 Regional Analgesia Techniques.

Ancillary Drugs

Antibiotics

The doses below are for a single IV administration. The smaller dose should be given to neonates <1 week of age (limited liver and renal functions). Antibiotics should be infused over several minutes only (i.e., *never* give antibiotics as IV boluses!) to minimize adverse reactions. Some antibiotics must be infused over a prolonged period (e.g., vancomycin). Regimens for antibiotic prophylaxis against subacute bacterial endocarditis are listed in Chap. 12. Note that both dose (mg/kg) and intervals between dosing for some medications vary considerably with gestational age, e.g., gentamicin loading dose in a 25-week gestation infant *5 mg/kg/48 h*; in a 32-week gestation infant *5 mg/kg/36 h* in a full term infant *4 mg/kg/12 h*, and in infant >44 weeks gestation *2–2.5 mg/kg/8 h*. Check with pharmacy.

Ampicillin[1]*:* 25–100 mg/kg.
Cefazolin: 20–40 mg/kg.
Cefoxitin: 20–40 mg/kg.
Cefotetan: 40 mg/kg.
Cefuroxime: 20–50 mg/kg.
Clindamycin: 5–10 mg/kg.
Gentamicin: 2.0 mg/kg (see above for age adjustments).
Benzyl penicillin[1]*:* 30,000–50,000 IU/kg.
Vancomycin[1]*:* 10–15 mg/kg infused over at least 1 h.

Corticosteroids

Dexamethasone (Decadron): 0.2–0.5 mg/kg IV (maximum 10 mg).
Methylprednisolone (Solu-Medrol): 5–25 mg/kg IV slowly over 10 min.
Hydrocortisone sodium succinate (Solu-Cortef): 1–5 mg/kg IV over 8–10 min.

[1]Use caution in children with renal failure.

Cardiovascular Drugs (Titrate Infusions to Effect)

Adenosine: 100 µg/kg as a *rapid IV bolus*. Repeat up to maximum dose 0.3 mg/kg or 12 mg.

Amiodarone: loading dose 5 mg/kg infused over 30–60 min IV.

Amrinone: loading dose 0.75 mg/kg IV; infusion 3–5 mg/kg/min in neonates, 5–10 mg/kg/min in children.

Calcium chloride: 5–15 mg/kg IV or *Calcium gluconate:* 10–30 mg/kg IV.

Dopamine/dobutamine: 5–20 µg/kg/min infusion.

Epinephrine: 0.1–1 µg/kg/min infusion.

Esmolol: 100–500 µg/kg IV, 50–100 µg/kg/min infusion.

Hydralazine: 0.1–0.2 mg/kg IM or IV.

Isoproterenol: 0.025–0.1 µg/kg/min infusion.

Lidocaine: 1–2 mg/kg IV.

Milrinone: 50–100 µg/kg loading dose over 15–30 min (reduce loading dose if hypotension occurs) followed by 0.5–1.0 µg/kg/min infusion.

Norepinephrine: 0.1–1 µg/kg/min infusion.

Nitroglycerin: 1–10 µg/kg/min infusion.

Phenoxybenzamine: loading dose 0.25 mg/kg × 4 over 2–4 h; maintenance, 0.25 mg/kg q6h.

Phentolamine: 0.2 mg/kg IV.

Phenylephrine: 0.1–1 µg/kg/min infusion.

Procainamide: 5–15 mg/kg IV.

Propranolol: 0.01–0.1 mg/kg IV over 10 min.

Prostaglandin E_1*:* 0.05–0.1 µg/kg/min (starting dose). (Maintenance infusion rate, e.g., after PDA open, may be between 0.005 and 0.4 µg/kg/min).

Sodium nitroprusside: 0.5–10 µg/kg/min infusion.

Verapamil: 0.1–0.3 mg/kg IV. (Do not give to infants younger than 1 year of age.)

Diuretics

Furosemide (Lasix): 1–2 mg/kg IV.

Mannitol: 0.5–1.0 g/kg IV (administer over several minutes to prevent hypotension).

Anticonvulsants

Diphenylhydantoin (Dilantin): loading dose 15–20 mg/kg IV slowly; maintenance, 2.5–5 mg/kg bid IV or PO.

Phenobarbital: loading dose 10 mg/kg IV; maintenance, 1.5–2.5 mg/kg bid IV.

Bronchodilators

Salbutamol (Albuterol): loading dose 5–6 μg/kg IV; infusion 0.1–1.0 μg/kg/min; inhaled aerosol 100 μg dose q6h. (See Chap. 8).

Aminophylline: loading dose 5 mg/kg over 30 min IV; infusion 1 mg/kg/h (if no recent doses). Monitor blood levels (therapeutic range is 10–12 μg/mL).

Postoperative Period

Analgesics

Acetaminophen (Tylenol): 10–20 mg/kg q4-6h PO, max single dose 650 mg, or 30–40 mg/kg dose PR loading dose followed by 20 mg/kg q6h (maximum daily dose 90–100 mg/kg); 10 mg/kg q6h IV (max. daily dose <75 mg/kg).

Diclofenac: 1 mg /kg PO or PR.

Hydromorphone: Bolus dose: 0.01–0.02 mg/kg IV q3–4 h. Infusion rate: 3–5 μg/kg/h.

Ibuprofen: 10 mg/kg PO.

Ketorolac: 0.25–0.5 mg/kg IV (max. 15 mg in adults, ceiling effect).

Morphine: 0.05–0.1 mg/kg IM or IV.

Morphine infusion: For children, 10–30 μg/kg/h IV. For infants, infuse half the rate as in children.

Caudal or epidural morphine: 30 μg/kg single dose.

Spinal morphine (preservative free): 10 μg/kg single dose.

Nalbuphine: 0.1–0.2 mg/kg IV (maximum 5 mg/kg). IV Infusion 0.1–0.2 mg/kg/h.

Oxycodone: 0.1–0.2 mg/kg PO q4h.
Tramadol: 1.0–2.0 mg/kg q6h PO for children >4 years of age.

Opioid Antagonist

Naloxone (Narcan): 0.5–2 μg/kg IV or IM. This drug should be titrated IV slowly until respirations have been restored. The same dose should be given IM to prevent recrudescence

Antiemetics

Dimenhydrinate (Gravol, Dramamine): 0.5–1 mg/kg IV slowly or IM or 2 mg/kg PR.
Diphenhydramine (Benadryl): 0.5–1 mg/kg IV slowly (may cause phlebitis and sedation).

Drugs Infusions

These formulas are designed to permit medications to be infused with limited fluid volumes (*N.B.* Weight = the child's weight in kilograms).

Dopamine or dobutamine:
(Weight × 6) mg of drug in 100 mL; then 1 mL/h = 1 μg/kg/min.
In the case of neonates and infants <10 kg use:
(Weight × 30) mg of drug in 100 mL; then 1 mL/h = 5 μg/kg/min.

Epinephrine:
(Weight × 0.6) mg of drug in 100 mL; then 1 mL/h = 0.1 μg/kg/min.

Sodium nitroprusside or nitroglycerin:
(Weight × 6) mg of drug in 100 mL; then 1 mL/h = 1 μg/kg/min.

Isoproterenol:
(Weight × 0.15) mg of drug in 100 mL; then 1 mL/h = 0.025 μg/kg/min.

Phenylephrine (1 mL [10 mg] in 100 mL normal saline = 100 μg/mL) 2–10 μg/kg bolus dose.

Vasopressin (0.5 mL [20 units/mL solution] in 50 mL normal saline = 200 milliunits (mU)/mL); administer at 0.3–2 mU/kg/min. *Note that it is very easy to miscalculate the infusion rate.*

Prostaglandin:

(Weight × 60) μg of drug in 20 mL; then 1 mL/h = 0.05 μg/kg/min.

Hemostatic Medications

Desmopressin: 0.3 μg/kg by slow infusion over 20 min.

ε-Aminocaproic acid (Amicar): Loading dose: 100–200 mg/kg (maximum 5 g) IV diluted and infused slowly over 20–60 min followed by a continuous infusion during surgery at 10–15 mg/kg/h.

Tranexamic acid: Loading dose 10–100 mg/kg IV followed by an infusion during surgery at 1–10 mg/kg/h.

Index

J. Lerman, C. J. Coté, *Steward's Manual of Pediatric Anesthesia*,
https://doi.org/10.1007/978-3-032-24545-8

D

N

GPSR Compliance

The European Union's (EU) General Product Safety Regulation (GPSR) is a set of rules that requires consumer products to be safe and our obligations to ensure this.

If you have any concerns about our products, you can contact us on ProductSafety@springernature.com

In case Publisher is established outside the EU, the EU authorized representative is:

Springer Nature Customer Service Center GmbH
Europaplatz 3
69115 Heidelberg, Germany

Batch number: 10755079

Printed by Printforce, the Netherlands